Transcatheter Therapy in Pediatric Cardiology

Transcatheter Therapy in Pediatric Cardiology

Editor

P. SYAMASUNDAR RAO

Department of Pediatrics
University of Wisconsin Medical School
Madison, Wisconsin

WILEY-LISS

A JOHN WILEY & SONS, INC., PUBLICATION

NEW YORK • CHICHESTER • BRISBANE • TORONTO • SINGAPORE

Address All Inquiries to the Publisher
Wiley-Liss, Inc., 605 Third Avenue, New York, NY 10158-0012

Library of Congress Cataloging-in-Publication Data
Transcatheter therapy in pediatric cardiology / editor, P. Syamasundar
  Rao.
      p.   cm.
    Includes bibliographical references and index.
    ISBN 0-471-58827-X
    1.   Congenital heart disease in children—Treatment.   2.   Cardiac
catheterization in children.   3.   Arterial catherterization in
children.   I. Rao, P. Syamasundar, 1941–
    [DNLM: 1. Balloon Dialatation—in infancy & childhood.   2.   Balloon
Dilatation—methods.   3.   Heart Catheterization—in infancy &
childhood.   4.   Heart Catheterization—methods.   5.   Heart Diseases—
in infancy & childhood.   6.   Heart Diseases—surgery.   WS 290 T772]
RJ426.C64T73   1993
617.4'1059—dc20
DNLM/DLC   92-48794
for Library of Congress   CIP

The text of this book is printed on acid-free paper.

To my parents,
P.V.B. Krishna Rao and Savithramma

To my wife and children,
Hymavathi, Vijay, Madhavi, and Radhika

P.S.R.

Contents

Contributors xi

Foreword
William B. Strong xiii

Preface
P. Syamasundar Rao xv

Acknowledgments xvii

1. **Historical Aspects of Therapeutic Catheterization**
   P. Syamasundar Rao 1

2. **Balloon Atrial Septostomy: Current Perspective**
   Langford Kidd 7

3. **Blade Atrial Septostomy**
   Sang C. Park and William H. Neches 17

4. **Technique of Balloon Valvuloplasty/Angioplasty**
   P. Syamasundar Rao 29

5. **Mechanism of Balloon Valvuloplasty/Angioplasty**
   Mohinder K. Thapar and P. Syamasundar Rao 45

6. **Balloon Pulmonary Valvuloplasty for Isolated Pulmonic Stenosis**
   P. Syamasundar Rao 59

7. **Balloon Valvuloplasty for Aortic Stenosis**
   P. Syamasundar Rao 105

8. **Balloon Valvotomy in Atrioventricular Valve Stenoses**
   Muayed Al-Zaibag and Mutrada Halim 129

 9. **Balloon Dilatation of Fixed Subaortic Stenosis**
    Zuhdi Lababidi. 143

10. **Balloon Angioplasty of Native Aortic Coarctation**
    P. Syamasundar Rao. 153

11. **Balloon Angioplasty for Aortic Recoarctation Following
    Previous Surgery**
    P. Syamasundar Rao. 197

12. **Balloon Angioplasty for Peripheral Pulmonary Artery Stenosis**
    Albert P. Rocchini 213

13. **Role of Balloon Dilatation and Other Transcatheter Methods in the Treatment
    of Cyanotic Congenital Heart Defects**
    P. Syamasundar Rao 229

14. **Balloon Dilatation of Stenotic Bioprosthetic Valves**
    P. Syamasundar Rao 255

15. **Balloon Dilatation of Other Congenital and Acquired Stenotic Lesions of the
    Cardiovascular System**
    P. Syamasundar Rao and Mohinder K. Thapar 275

16. **Catheter Closure of the Ductus Arteriosus**
    Lee Benson 321

17. **Transcatheter Closure of Atrial Septal Defects**
    Larry A. Latson 335

18. **Transcatheter Closure of Heart Defects: Role of "Buttoned" Devices**
    P. Syamasundar Rao and E.B. Sideris 349

19. **Role of Embolization Therapy in the Treatment of Infants and Children**
    Jean S. Kan 371

20. **Transcatheter Retrieval of Intravascular/Intracardiac Foreign Bodies**
    P. Syamasundar Rao 377

21. **Transcatheter Ablation in the Treatment of Childhood Dysrhythmia**
    Paul C. Gillette, Christopher L. Case, and Vicki L. Zeigler 393

22. **Balloon Valvuloplasty/Angioplasty: International Experience**
    P. Syamasundar Rao 401

22a. **Balloon Valvuloplasty/Angioplasty: The Brazilian Experience**
    Valmir F. Fontes 403

22b. Balloon Valvuloplasty/Angioplasty: The British Experience
Christopher Wren   421

22c. Balloon Valvuloplasty/Angioplasty: The Hong Kong Experience
Roxy N.S. Lo, Maurice P. Leung, and K.C. Lau   433

22d. Balloon Valvuloplasty/Angioplasty: The Indian Experience
Savitri Shrivastava and Vishva Dev   445

22e. Balloon Valvuloplasty of Pulmonic Stenosis: The Saudi Arabian Experience
M.A. Ali Khan   457

22f. Balloon Valvuloplasty/Angioplasty: The Spanish Experience
José Suárez de Lezo, Alfonso Medina, Manuel Pan, Miguel Romero,
Enrique Hernández, Djordje Pavlovic, and Francisco Melián   471

23. Conclusions and Future Directions
P. Syamasundar Rao   493

Index   503

Contributors

Muayed Al-Zaibag, M.D., Adult Cardiology Division, Riyadh Armed Forces Hospital, Riyadh 11159, Saudi Arabia **[129]**

M.A. Ali Khan, M.D., F.R.C.P.(E.), Division of Pediatric Cardiology, Riyadh Armed Forces Hospital, and Department of Pediatrics, King Saud University, Riyadh 11159, Saudi Arabia **[457]**

Lee Benson, M.D., F.R.C.P.(C.), Department of Pediatrics, The Variety Club Cardiac Catheterization Laboratories, The Hospital for Sick Children, Toronto, Ontario M5G 1X8, Canada **[321]**

Christopher L. Case, M.D., South Carolina Children's Heart Center, Medical University of South Carolina, Charleston, SC 29425 **[393]**

Vishva Dev, M.D., D.M., Department of Cardiology, Cardio-Thoracic Centre, All India Institute of Medical Sciences, New Delhi 110 029, India; present address: 8585 Burton Way, Los Angeles CA 90068 **[445]**

Valmir F. Fontes, M.D., Division of Pediatric Cardiology and Hemodynamic Laboratory, Institute Dante Pazzanese of Cardiology, São Paulo, SP 4012 Brazil **[403]**

Paul C. Gillette, M.D., South Carolina Children's Heart Center, Medical University of South Carolina, Charleston, SC 29425 **[393]**

Mutrada Halim, M.D., Adult Cardiology Division, Riyadh Armed Forces Hospital, Riyadh 11159, Saudi Arabia **[129]**

Enrique Hernández, M.D., Unidad de Cardiologia, Hospital del Pino, University of Las Palmas, Las Palmas de Gran Canaria, Spain **[471]**

Jean S. Kan, M.D., Division of Pediatric Cardiology, The Helen B. Taussig Children's Cardiac Center, The Johns Hopkins University School of Medicine, Baltimore, MD 21205 **[371]**

Langford Kidd, M.D., F.R.C.P., Division of Pediatric Cardiology, The Helen B. Taussig Children's Cardiac Center, The Johns Hopkins University School of Medicine, Baltimore, MD 21205 **[7]**

Zuhdi Lababidi, M.D., Department of Pediatrics, Division of Pediatric Cardiology, University of Missouri School of Medicine, Columbia, MO 65212 **[143]**

The numbers in brackets are the opening page numbers of the contributors' articles.

Larry A. Latson, M.D., Division of Pediatric Cardiology, University of Nebraska Medical Center, Omaha, NE 68198-2166 **[335]**

K.C. Lau, M.B.B.S., F.R.C.P., D.C.H., Department of Paediatrics, University of Hong Kong, The Grantham Hospital, Hong Kong **[433]**

Maurice P. Leung, M.B.B.S., M.R.C.P., D.C.H., Department of Paediatrics, University of Hong Kong, The Grantham Hospital, Hong Kong **[433]**

Roxy N.S. Lo, M.B.B.S., F.R.C.P., D.C.H., Department of Paediatrics, University of Hong Kong, The Grantham Hospital, Hong Kong **[433]**

Alfonso Medina, M.D., Unidad de Cardiologia, Hospital del Pino, University of Las Palmas, Las Palmas de Gran Canaria, Spain **[471]**

Francisco Melián, M.D., Unidad de Cardiologia, Hospital del Pino, University of Las Palmas, Las Palmas de Gran Canaria, Spain **[471]**

William H. Neches, M.D., Cardiology Division, Children's Hospital of Pittsburgh, Pittsburgh, PA 15213 **[17]**

Manuel Pan, M.D., Servicio de Cardiologia, Hospital Reina Sofía, University of Córdoba, 14004 Córdoba, Spain **[471]**

Sang C. Park, M.D., Cardiology Division, Children's Hospital of Pittsburgh, Pittsburgh, PA 15213 **[17]**

Djordje Pavlovic, M.D., Servicio de Cardiologia, Hospital Reina Sofía, University of Córdoba, 14004 Córdoba, Spain **[471]**

P. Syamasundar Rao, M.D., Department of Pediatrics, Division of Pediatric Cardiology, University of Wisconsin Medical School, University of Wisconsin Children's Hospital, Madison, WI 53792-4108 **[1,29,45,59,105,153, 197,229,255,275,349,377,401,493]**

Albert P. Rocchini, M.D., Division of Pediatric Cardiology, University of Minnesota, Minneapolis, MN 55455, and Division of Pediatric Cardiology, University of Michigan, Ann Arbor, MI **[213]**

Miguel Romero, M.D., Servicio de Cardiologia, Hospital Reina Sofía, University of Córdoba, 14004 Córdoba, Spain **[471]**

Savitri Shrivastava M.D., D.M., Department of Cardiology, Cardio-Thoracic Centre, All India Institute of Medical Sciences, New Delhi 110 029, India; present address: Department of Cardiology, Sanjay Gandhi Postgraduate Institute of Medical Sciences, Lucknow 226 011, India **[445]**

E.B. Sideris, M.D., Pediatric Cardiology, Amarillo TX **[349]**

José Suárez de Lezo, M.D., Servicio de Cardiologia, Hospital Reina Sofía, University of Córdoba, 14004 Córdoba, Spain **[471]**

Mohinder K. Thapar, M.D., Department of Pediatrics, Division of Pediatric Cardiology, University of Texas Medical School, Houston TX 77030 **[45,275]**

Christopher Wren, M.D., Department of Pediatric Cardiology, Freeman Hospital, Newcastle upon Tyne NE7 7DN, England **[421]**

Vicki L. Zeigler, R.N., M.S.N., South Carolina Children's Heart Center, Medical University of South Carolina, Charleston, SC 29425 **[393]**

Foreword

The late Bill Rashkind and his colleague Bill Miller initiated the era of therapeutic intervention when they introduced the atrial balloon septostomy to palliate the infant with transposition of the great arteries. Can the young cardiologist even imagine the foresight and courage that is required? Today catheter intervention is commonplace both in pediatrics and in internal medicine. The advances are rapid as both technology and skills improve. In 1990 in my orientation address to incoming freshman, I stated that laser catheterization was in the future. In 1991 I had to say, "This is the future." The progress from the experimental-developmental laboratory to clinical use is so rapid that a book such as P. Syamasundar Rao's *Transcatheter Therapy in Pediatric Cardiology* is essential to provide a perspective at a moment in time.

From 1972 to 1982, Dr. Rao and I were associates at the Medical College of Georgia. I had the wonderful opportunity to observe and learn firsthand from my colleague. Before he left the MCG he was cooperating with Dr. Rashkind in his initial studies of umbrella closure of atrial septal defects. He has progressed a long way since those initial endeavors. I can only say that I am proud to have been associated with this pediatric cardiologist, who, I believe, embodies all of the attributes of one of the best-of-the-best. He is a physiologist, a superb clinician who interacts beautifully with children and their families, and an educator.

All three of these characteristics are demonstrated in this monograph. It is his awareness of "where we are" and "where we need to go" that is so relevant. As an international expert, he has been able to bring together many of the leaders in this emerging discipline. This book should provide the necessary details to form a relatively common framework from which developments can systematically progress. The broad spectrum of contributors provides a breadth of diversity that will answer questions and provide challenges.

I believe that this comprehensive text will facilitate the development of our exciting discipline—pediatric cardiology. As we progress, it is crucial that we also stop to reflect to be sure that what we are doing is in the best interests of "our children."

William B. Strong, M.D.
Augusta, Georgia

Preface

Over the past five and a half decades, the techniques for correction of heart defects have advanced to such a degree that almost every cardiac defect can be corrected. The few that cannot be corrected can be effectively palliated, or cardiac transplantation can be performed. The 1940s and 1950s witnessed surgical correction of simpler lesions, introduction of palliative surgical procedures for more complex defects, and the beginnings of open heart surgery. In the 1960s and 1970s, further refinement of these techniques evolved, employing these surgical procedures in infants and neonates, and applying concepts and procedures to a variety of complex cyanotic heart defects. The continued progress of these and other innovative procedures was observed in the 1980s. Concurrent with these developments, advances occurred in prosthetic valves (mechanical and biological) and in cardiac transplantation. While these surgical procedures have salvaged many a patient who would have died but for the availability of the surgery, there is some mortality, and by necessity, significant morbidity.

There were attempts as early as the mid-'50s to accomplish the objective of improving hemodynamics by less invasive transcatheter means. Rashkind's balloon atrial septostomy, described in the mid-'60s, was another such attempt, and was for many years the only major transcatheter therapeutic measure available, effectively replacing surgical atrial septostomy in the neonate. In those children in whom Rashkind's balloon septostomy was not successful because of a thick lower margin of the foramen ovale, Park's blade atrial septostomy was used. With the advent of balloon angioplasty for coronary artery stenotic lesions following Grüntzig's work, similar balloon dilatation techniques were extended by Kan to children with pulmonic stenosis. Several workers followed the lead and applied this technique to relieve other obstructive lesions in the heart and great vessels. Concurrently, transcatheter closure of cardiac septal defects evolved in the 1980s following the early pioneering work of Porstmann, King, and Rashkind. Thus the 1980s witnessed enormous growth of interventional pediatric cardiology. The balloons, blades, coils, and umbrellas should now be added to the therapeutic armamentarium available to the pediatric cardiologist. With the advances in both surgical and transcatheter methods, there has been a gradual change in the treatment approach to children with cardiac defects: catheter intervention instead of surgery, and surgical intervention instead of allowing the pathologist to examine the heart.

The purpose of this book is to unify and review the decade of advances in interventional pediatric cardiology and to present the state-of-the-art of this exciting new discipline. Although a substantial portion of the volume deals with balloon angioplasty/valvuloplasty, the book includes chapters dealing with balloon and blade atrial septostomy, transcatheter closure of cardiac septal defects, selective embolization of abnormal blood vessels, transcatheter removal of foreign bodies, transcatheter ablation of conduction bundles, and other transcatheter measures. While a number of chapters have been authored by my associates and myself, I have taken the liberty to tap the resources and expertise of other workers in the field. A section on international experience is also included. Although the presentations focus on the pediatric age group, the same principles, by and large, can be applied to adult patients with congenital or acquired stenotic lesions. Attempts to avoid repetition have been made, but some degree of duplication is unavoidable to preserve the continuity of discussion.

It is hoped that this book will provide useful information to pediatric cardiologists and to internist cardiologists caring for adults with congenital heart disease in their day-to-day management of patients with congenital cardiac defects. It should serve as a reference work to many physicians in pediatrics, cardiovascular surgery, neonatology, and pediatric intensive care. The volume should also serve as source material for other health care professionals, including nurses, social workers, catheterization laboratory technologists, and echocardiography technicians. It is hoped that this book will answer many questions in interventional pediatric cardiology, stimulate further interest in transcatheter therapy, and promote research to resolve unsettled issues in this new and exciting field.

P. Syamasundar Rao, M.D.
Madison, Wisconsin

Acknowledgments

I have made liberal use of case material that I encountered at King Faisal Specialist Hospital and Research Center, Riyadh, Saudi Arabia, and at the University of Wisconsin Medical School/Children's Hospital, Madison, Wisconsin, in several chapters of this book. I acknowledge the contributions to these data made by past and present colleagues at these institutions in the areas of pediatric cardiology, cardiovascular surgery, and adult cardiology. These colleagues include Drs. J. Al-Halees, M. Brais, P.S. Chopra, D. Ende, M.E. Fawzy, O. Galal, V.K. Gupta, J.M. Levy, F. Kutayli, M.K. Mardini, H.N. Najjar, L. Solymar, M.K. Thapar, and A.D. Wilson. In addition, there were many trainees who also contributed to the clinical material.

I express my sincere gratitude to all those who helped me in the book's preparation. First, I thank Dr. Philip M. Farrell, Chairman, Department of Pediatrics, University of Wisconsin Medical School, for providing a mileu to foster academic activities such as the writing of this book. I make special mention of Drs. Allen D. Wilson and Paramjeet S. Chopra for their unreserved support of my catheter intervention vagaries and for their help in gathering data on many children the results of whose therapies are included in several chapters of this volume. Ms. Pat Smith, our clinical nurse specialist, has been of immense help in effective communication with parents, and I thank her for this and for keeping clinicians and parents sane during the evolution of the pediatric cardiology interventional procedures. I also thank Ms. Jan Ewenko for her diligent work in the performance of the echocardiographic studies reported here.

I appreciate the efforts of each of the contributors in preparing high-quality chapters. Patrick Carey and Rebecca Langhough of the Department of Biostatistics, University of Wisconsin-Madison, contributed to the statistical analyses reported in several chapters of this book, and I thank them. The staff of the cardiac catheterization laboratory, University of Wisconsin Hospital and Clinics, were very helpful in allowing collection of data related to interventional procedures. I make special mention of Daniel Kolk and Joyce Tackle for their help in this regard.

The photographs and illustrations were prepared with the help of Mr. E.A. Joseph and his staff in the Department of Medical Photography and with the help of Ms. L.A. Henson and her staff in the Department of Medical Illustrations at the Clinical Sciences Center of the University of Wisconsin-Madison; many thanks to them for their fine work. I make special mention of several of these dedicated workers: Mark Anderson, Geoff Bosner, Patricia Dvorak, Christopher Jakel, Joan Kozel, Jon Powell, Grant Sanders, and Betsy True. Several figures and tables are reproduced from several publications of ours, and I thank the publishers and the journals, namely, the *American Heart Journal*, the *American Journal of Cardiology*, *Annals of Saudi Medicine*, the *British Heart Journal*, *Catheterization and Cardiovascular Diagnosis*, *Clinical Cardiology*,

Current Problems in Cardiology, the *International Journal of Cardiology*, the *Journal of the American College of Cardiology*, the *Journal of Cardiovascular Ultrasonography* (*Journal of Technical Methods*), and the *Journal of Interventional Cardiology*. I also acknowledge that the preparation of some of the illustrations used in this volume was supported in part by a grant from the Oscar Rennobohm Foundation, Inc., Madison, Wisconsin.

Nanette Kelsey spent long hours in preparing multiple revisions of the chapters and was of immense help, and I appreciate her efforts and thank her for uncompromised cooperation. Finally, I thank Mr. Thomas E. Mackey, Jr., Ms. Louise C. Page, Mr. John Hanley, and the staff of the Wiley-Liss Division, John Wiley & Sons, Inc., for their patience in waiting for long-overdue manuscripts and for their help and advice in the preparation of the manuscripts and photographs.

P.S.R.

1

Historical Aspects of Therapeutic Catheterization

P. Syamasundar Rao, M.D.

Department of Pediatrics, Division of Pediatric Cardiology,
University of Wisconsin Medical School, University of Wisconsin
Children's Hospital, Madison, Wisconsin 53792-4108

The conventional treatment of choice for structural abnormalities of the heart and blood vessels, whether congenital or acquired, is surgical correction. During the last decade there has been an enormous increase in the use of transcatheter techniques to improve or correct structural defects in the cardiovascular system. Although the major advances and their application to treat cardiovascular defects in children have occurred during the last decade, the concepts and innovations can be traced back to the 1950s. This chapter will review historical aspects of the origin of transcatheter methods. I have made all efforts to present the information accurately, mostly based on priority of publication. However, oversight of some literature is possible, especially since earlier publications are not completely indexed.

In 1953, Rubio-Alvarez et al. [1] reported their experience in performing pulmonary valvotomy by a transcatheter technique. To the best of my knowledge, this was the first attempt to treat congenital heart defects via a catheter. These authors used a ureteral catheter with a modified tip and a wire passed through it. The tip of the catheter could be bent and the wire kept straight; the latter was used to cut the fused pulmonary valve commisures. They attempted to emulate Brock's closed pulmonary valvulotomy [2]. They used this procedure in a 10-month-old child and reduced the pulmonary valve gradient from 72 to 59 mmHg, a modest improvement. They also noted clinical and phonocardiographic improvements. They suggested that this method is comparable to Brock's operation, but has the advantage of not requiring anesthesia and thoracotomy. The following year (1954), they reported their results at the second World Congress of Cardiology [3]. The published abstract indicates that they had performed valvulotomy in at least one other patient in whom they observed disappearance of cyanosis and improvement in arterial oxygen saturation, presumably related to decreased or abolished interatrial right-to-left shunting following relief of pulmonary valve obstruction. It also appears [3] that the authors used the same technique to relieve tricuspid valve stenosis in several patients. The catheter tricuspid valvotomy resulted in clinical improvement, decreased mean right auricular (atrial) pressure, and increased right ventricular pressure. Thus began transcatheter therapy to relieve obstructive lesions of the heart. Unfortunately, they published no subsequent reports, and there is no other published information by other investigators about adopting this technique.

A decade later, Dotter and Judkins [4] described a gradual dilation technique for recanalization of narrowed and occluded peripheral arteritis. They developed this technique following both inadvertent passage of a catheter retrograde into the aorta through an "occluded" iliac artery for performing abdominal aortogram and experiments in cadavers [5].

Their technique involved passage of 0.05 inch guidewire across the stenotic lesion followed by passage of a Teflon catheter of 0.1 inch diameter over the guidewire. Larger dilating catheters (e.g., 0.2 inch) are passed over the first catheter, as necessary [4]. This type of progressive dilation of arterial stenotic lesions was accomplished in nine patients; 15 such procedures on 11 lower extremities were performed. Clinical and angiographic improvement was noted in most patients. Scheduled amputations were averted in some patients. Short-term patency was good. Failures (of the procedure) were not associated with harmful side effects. Long-term follow-up of some patients of the initial cohort [5] showed continued patency of these vessels 9–14 years later. The authors concluded [4] that transluminal recanalization is an effective alternative to surgical reconstruction and that it is a safer and more attractive alternative to amputation.

In 1966, Rashkind and Miller [6], in a 2 page article, reported one of the most significant advances of that time; they positioned a double-lumen, balloon-tipped catheter in the left atrium (from the femoral vein to right atrium and from there into the left atrium via the patent foramen ovale), inflated the balloon with diluted radiopaque liquid, and rapidly withdrew the catheter into the right atrium, tearing the lower margin of the patent foramen ovale and producing an atrial septal defect. They performed this procedure in six puppies, and on follow-up 1 hour to 2 months after the procedure the sacrificed animals showed good-sized atrial septal defects. A similar procedure was successfully performed in three infants, aged 15 hours to 6 weeks, with transposition of the great arteries. Follow up 4–9 months following transcatheter atrial septostomy revealed that these infants are clinically well. The authors suggested that balloon atrial septostomy is useful in palliating patients with transposition of the great arteries with inadequate intracardiac mixing and that it serves as an alternative to surgical atrial septostomy so that a "corrective" Mustard procedure could be performed beyond age 6 months. They cited avoidance of anesthesia, thoracotomy, pericardiotomy, and chest wall scarring as an advantage over the surgical atrial septostomy. The authors also suggested that the balloon septostomy may be effective in temporizing patients with Ebstein's anomaly of the tricuspid valve, tricuspid atresia, and total anomalous pulmonary venous connection with inadequate interatrial communication [6]. Rashkind's balloon atrial septostomy was the major interventional pediatric cardiology procedure for two to three decades, and only now has it been surpassed by other balloon dilation procedures because of the advent of the arterial switch procedure for correction of transposition of the great arteries in the first few days of life.

Porstmann and associates [7] have developed a technique for transcatheter closure of patent ductus arteriosus. The technique involves cannulation of both a femoral artery and a femoral vein. A catheter is inserted into the femoral artery, either percutaneously or via cut-down, advanced into the aorta and then into the patent ductus arteriosus, and from there into the right heart and inferior vena cava. A long guidewire (300 cm) is advanced from the arterial catheter into the right heart and retrieved by a catheter retrieval system via the femoral vein, and the wire is exteriorized. This wire serves as a track over which a ductal closure Ivalon foam plug will be guided into the ductus from the aortic side. An Ivalon plug, appropriate to the size and shape of the patent ductus arteriosus, is prepared/chosen based on the ductal anatomy determined by aortic cineangiography prior to the procedure. The plug is then inserted over the guidewire into the femoral artery with the help of a tubular applicator. Once in the femoral artery, the plug is advanced over the guidewire with the help of a pushing catheter until the plug is positioned into the ductus, the ductal closure is confirmed by aortic angiography, and the guidewire is removed from the venous side, taking care not to dislodge the plug. A more detailed report was published in 1971 [8], in which the authors described successfully closing the patent ductus arteriosus in 56 of the 62 patients in whom the procedure was attempted. There was no mortality, and the morbidity was minimal. All successfully closed ductuses remained closed over a 4.5 year follow-up period. They concluded [7,8] that transfemoral catheter closure of ductus arteriosus constitutes a sound alternative to surgery in adults and older children with patent ductuses that are not larger than their femoral arteries.

While the above described techniques are useful and had varying influences on the clinical practice of cardiovascular medicine, a major impact was observed after Grüntzig and coworkers [9–14] modified the original technique of Dotter and Judkins. A double-lumen catheter with a nonelastic balloon was developed by Grüntzig [9] that he and his colleagues used in dilating stenotic lesions of the iliac and femoropopliteal arteries [10], renal arteries [11], and coronary arteries [12–14]. In one report describing their 18 month experience, they used percutaneous transluminal coronary angioplasty (PTCA) in 50 patients [14]; the technique was successful in 32 patients, reducing the stenosis from 84% (mean) to 34% and the transstenotic peak gradient from a mean of 58 mmHg to 19 mmHg. The cardiac function improved in 29 patients, and acute deterioration requiring emergency bypass surgery was observed in 5 patients. Grüntzig and associates concluded that patients with single vessel disease appear suitable for PTCA and that patients with short history of pain indicating the presence of a soft, distensible atheroma are likely to respond to PTCA. They suggested that 10%–15% of patients scheduled for bypass surgery are likely candidates for PTCA and that a prospective randomized trial will be necessary to evaluate the usefulness of PTCA in comparison with surgical management.

In 1976, King, Mills, and their associates reported transcatheter closure of atrial septal defects in human subjects [15,16] following their initial experimentation in dogs [17]. A 17-year-old girl with clinical and cardiac catheterization data confirming ostium secundum atrial septal defects had her defect sized with a balloon catheter. The defect measured 25 mm [15]. A delivery catheter, loaded with a 35 mm umbrella device, was inserted into the right saphenous vein (at its junction with the femoral vein) by cut-down and advanced into the left atrium across the atrial defect. The left atrial umbrella was opened in the body of the left atrium. The umbrella was gently withdrawn and positioned against the atrial septum. By slowly withdrawing the capsule, the right atrial umbrella was opened. Then both umbrellas were locked across the atrial defect by an internal locking mechanism built into the catheter–umbrella delivery system. After having made sure that the umbrellas are locked and that the device is in place, the catheter delivery system is disconnected from the device by complex but well-described maneuvers [15]. With this method they were able to close the 25 mm atrial defect in the 17-year-old patient successfully [15]. They subsequently reported closure of atrial septal defects in four additional patients, aged 17 to 75 years [16]. They concluded that nonoperative closure of atrial septal defect may offer an attractive alternative to open heart surgery in certain patients.

Despite the success with Raskind's balloon atrial septostomy [6] in neonates and young infants, inadequate results were observed in older infants and children, presumably related to thick interatrial septum. To circumvent this problem, Park et al. [18] developed a catheter with an extendable blade. The clinical applications began after animal experiments [19]. The blade atrial septostomy catheter is introduced into the saphenous vein by cut-down or into the femoral vein percutaneously, and the catheter tip passed across the interatrial communication into the left atrium. After having made sure that the catheter tip is in the left atrium, the blade control wire is advanced so as to extend the blade. The catheter is then rotated so that the blade faces inferiorly, anteriorly, and to the left. The entire catheter–blade system is slowly withdrawn into the right atrium with the blade open. Some resistance is usually felt as the blade cuts the atrial septum. The blade is then folded back into the catheter by withdrawing the wire. This is followed by conventional balloon atrial septostomy to enlarge the atrial defect further [18]. Measurement of hemodynamic data and balloon sizing of the atrial defect are performed prior to and following the procedure. Park and associates performed this procedure in seven patients, two with transposition of the great arteries and five with mitral atresia complex. They were aged 1 month to 9.5 years (median 4 months). Improvement in oxygen saturation (in transposition patients) and decreases in the left atrial pressure and the pressure difference between atria (in mitral atresia cases) occurred in each child. The size of the atrial septal defect, as measured by balloon pullback, increased in each case. The authors concluded that blade atrial septostomy is a safe and effective procedure for enlarging interatrial defects even in patients with thick interatrial septum, and that it avoids thoracotomy.

Semb and associates [20] introduced a 5 Fr Berman angiographic catheter into the pulmonary artery, inflated the balloon, and withdrew it forcefully into the right ventricle in a 2-day-old infant with pulmonary stenosis, severe tricuspid insufficiency, and severe systemic arterial desaturation (50%), presumably secondary to interatrial right-to-left shunting. This resulted in a decreased transpulmonary valvar gradient and rapid improvement in the patient's condition. The infant was taken off the respirator 12 hours after the procedure and discharged home 4 days later with an arterial oxygen saturation of 95%. Follow-up 1 year later continued to reveal excellent results. The investigators felt that they had ruptured the fused pulmonary valve leaflets, causing the improvement. The authors concluded that "balloon valvotomy," as they described, should be attempted during catheterization in cases with an expected high surgical mortality, but cautioned that this procedure is unlikely to be successful in all cases of organic pulmonary valve obstruction.

Favorable experience with Grüntzig's technique of percutaneous transluminal dilation of atherosclerotic and fibromuscular arterial disease prompted Sos et al. [21] to attempt dilatation of discrete thoracic aortic coarctation postmortem. They introduced a 4 Fr double-lumen balloon catheter into the femoral artery by cut-down, positioned the catheter across the aortic narrowing, and inflated the balloon twice to a diameter of 5 mm with 50/50 mixture of saline and contrast. Following the procedure, they instilled contrast into the aorta and took frontal and lateral radiographs that showed excellent relief of coarctation compared with antemortem angiograms. Pathologic examination of the dilated aortic segment revealed preservation of the structural integrity of the aorta [21]. They expected that there will at least be a temporary relief of coarctation, especially useful in critically ill infants with other associated congenital heart disease, and were not sure if restenosis would occur. They hope that their report will encourage others to do similar experiments and that balloon dilatation will become a clinical reality in live infants [21].

Kan and her associates [22] applied the balloon dilatation technique to relieve congenital pulmonary valve stenosis. They embarked on this clinical application following animal studies on temporary balloon occlusion [23] and balloon valvuloplasty of congenital pulmonary valve stenosis in a bulldog [24]. They positioned a specially prepared 9 Fr catheter with a polyethylene balloon, 14 by 40 mm, across the pulmonic valve in an 8-year-old girl and inflated the balloon by hand with diluted contrast material at a pressure of 45 psi. This resulted in a reduction in peak-to-peak pulmonary valve gradient from 48 to 14 mmHg. At follow-up catheterization, performed 4 months later, the gradient remained low at 20 mmHg. They also mentioned [22] that they performed similar procedures in four other patients, aged 3 months to 14 years, with immediate improvement. No follow-up data were available. They concluded that balloon pulmonary valvuloplasty may become an attractive alternative to open heart surgery for the management of valvar pulmonic stenosis.

The interest in balloon valvuloplasty/angioplasty in children with congenital and acquired heart defects increased exponentially since the publications of Kan and colleagues' report [22]. However, it should be noted that several other investigators have studied balloon dilation techniques in relation to pediatric heart disease [25–30] prior to that.

As shown in the above review, several investigators, beginning in the mid 1950s, have been interested in nonsurgical transcatheter treatment of congenital and acquired heart defects and have advanced the concepts, technology, and methodology such that the techniques achieved significant clinical utility by the mid 1980s. Application of these techniques to other lesions, refinement of the methodology and techniques, and further development of catheter systems have occurred. These will not be reviewed in this chapter, but the reader is referred to each of the ensuing chapters wherein the respective authors have attempted to trace historical aspects related to the particular lesion under discussion in that particular chapter.

REFERENCES

1. Rubio-Alvarez V, Limon-Lason R, Soni J (1953): Valvalotomias intracardiacas por medico de un cateter. Arch Ins Cardiol Mexico 23:183–192.
2. Brock RC (1948): Pulmonary valvulotomy for relief of congenital pulmonary stenosis: Report of three cases. Br Med J 1:1121–1126.
3. Rubio V, Limon-Lason R (1954): Treatment of pulmonary valvular stenosis and of tricuspid stenosis using a modified catheter, abstracted. Second World Congress on Cardiology, Program Abstracts, II:205.
4. Dotter CT, Judkins MP (1964): Transluminal treatment of arteriosclerotic obstruction: Description of a new technique and a preliminary report of its application. Circulation 30:654–670.
5. Dotter CT (1980): Transluminal angioplasty: A long view. Radiology 135:561–564.
6. Rashkind WJ, Miller WW (1966): Creation of an

atrial septal defect without thoracotomy: A palliative approach to complete transposition of the great arteries. J Am Med Assoc 196:173–174.
7. Porstmann W, Wierny L, Warnke H (1967): Der verschluss de Ductus arteriosus persistens ohre Thorakotomie (1 Mitteilung). Thoraxchirgugie 15:199–203.
8. Porstmann W, Wierney L, Warnke H, Gerstberger G, Romaniuk PA (1971): Catheter closure of patent ductus arteriosus: 62 cases treated without thoracotomy. Radiol Clin North Am 9 (2):203–218.
9. Grüntzig A (1976): Die perkutane Rekanalisation chronischer arterieller Verschisse (Dotter-Prinzip) mit einem doppellumigen Dilatations-Katheter. Fortschr Rontgenstr 124:80–86.
10. Grüntzig A (1977): Die perkutane transluminale Rekanalization chronischer Arterien-verschliisse mit einer neuen Dilatation-stechnik. Baden-Baden, G witzstrock Verlag.
11. Grüntzig AR, Kuhlmann V, Vetter W, et al. (1978): Treatment of renovascular hypertension with percutaneous transluminal dilatation of a renal artery stenosis. Lancet 1:801–802.
12. Grüntzig AR (1976): Perkutane Dilatation von Cononarstenosen—Beschreibung eines neuen Kathetersystems. Klin Wochenschr 54:543–545.
13. Grüntzig AR (1978): Transluminal dilatation of coronary-artery stenosis. Lancet 1:263.
14. Grüntzig AR, Senning A, Siegenthaler WE (1979): Nonoperative dilatation of coronary-artery stenosis: Percutaneous transluminary coronary angioplasty. N Engl J Med 301:61–68.
15. King TD, Thompson SL, Steiner C, Mills NL (1976): Secundum atrial septal defect: Nonoperative closure during cardiac catheterization. J Am Med Assoc 235:2506–2509.
16. Mills NL, King TD (1976): Nonoperative closure of left-to-right shunts. J Thorac Cardiovasc Surg 72:371–378.
17. King TD, Mills NL (1974): Nonoperative closure of atrial septal defects. Surg 75:383–388.
18. Park SC, Neches WH, Zuberbuhler JR, Lenox CC, Mathews RA, Fricker FJ, Zoltun RA (1978): Clinical use of blade atrial septostomy. Circulation 58:600–606.
19. Park SC, Zuberbuhler JR, Neches WH, Lenox CC, Zoltun RA (1975): A new atrial septostomy technique. Cathet Cardiovasc Diagn 1:195–201.
20. Semb BKH, Tjonneland S, Stake G, Aabyholm G (1979): "Balloon valvulotomy" of congenital pulmonary valve stenosis with tricuspid valve insufficiency. Cardiovasc Radiol 2:239–241.
21. Sos T, Sniderman KW, Rettek-Sos B, Strupp A, Alonso DR (1979): Percutaneous transluminal dilatation of coarctation of thoracic aorta post mortem. Lancet 2:970–971.

22. Kan JS, White RI Jr, Mitchell SE, Gardner TJ (1982): Percutaneous balloon valvuloplasty: A new method for treating congenital pulmonary valve stenosis. N Engl J Med 307:540–542.

23. Kan JS, Anderson JH, White RI Jr (1982): Experimental basis for balloon valvuloplasty of congenital pulmonary valve stenosis, abstracted. Pediat Res 16:101A.

24. Kan JS, White RJ Jr, Mitchell SE, Anderson JH (1984): Transluminal balloon valvuloplasty for treatment of pulmonary and aortic valvular stenosis. Semin Intervent Radiol 1:217–223.

25. Martin EC, Diamond NG, Casarella WJ (1980): Percutaneous transluminal angioplasty in non-atherosclerotic disease. Radiol 135:27–33.

26. Lock JE, Niemi T, Einzig S, Amplatz K, Burke B, Bass JL (1981): Transvenous angioplasty of experimental branch pulmonary artery stenosis in newborn lambs. Circulation 64:886–893.

27. Singer MI, Rowen M, Dorsey TJ (1982): Transluminal aortic balloon angioplasty for coarctation of the aorta in the newborn. Am Heart J 103:131–132.

28. Driscoll DJ, Hesslein PS, Mullins CE (1982): Congenital stenosis of individual pulmonary veins: Clinical spectrum and unsuccessful treatment by transvenous balloon dilatation. Am J Cardiol 49:1767–1772.

29. Lock JE, Castaneda-Zuniga WR, Bass JL, Foker JE, Amplatz K, Anderson RW (1982): Balloon dilatation of excised aortic coarctations. Radiology 143:689–692.

30. Castaneda-Zuniga WR, Lock JE, Vlodaver Z, Rusnak B, Rysavy JP, Herrera M, Amplatz K (1982): Transluminal dilatation of coarctation of the abdominal aorta: An experimental study in dogs. Radiology 143:693–697.

2

Balloon Atrial Septostomy: Current Perspective

Langford Kidd, M.D., F.R.C.P.

Division of Pediatric Cardiology, The Helen B. Taussig Children's
Cardiac Center, The Johns Hopkins University School of Medicine,
Baltimore, Maryland 21205

INTRODUCTION

Rashkind and Miller's paper in *The Journal of the American Medical Association* in June 1966 announcing that they had successfully created an "Atrial Septal Defect Without Thoracotomy" in three infants with transposition of the great arteries set in motion a train of events similar to that created by Blalock and Taussig's paper [2] in the same journal 21 years earlier. It marked the beginning of a stream of innovative techniques, noninvasive or, rather, minimally invasive in nature, that has come to be called *interventional cardiology* and that continues to grow and develop to this day. For infants born with transposition of the great arteries, this new procedure was life-saving, allowing them to grow to an age when the surgical procedure described 2 years earlier (in 1964) by Mustard [3] could safely be carried out.

The interatrial septum is a structure of complex embryology, but in fetal life there is a flap-covered opening in the septum, the foramen ovale, that is widely patent and allows mostly the relatively oxygen-rich inferior vena caval blood coming from the placenta to cross to the left atrium. With the first few breaths, the increases in volume and pressure in the left atrium close the flap of the foramen ovale and functionally terminate the right-to-left atrial shunting. However, it continues to be "probe" patent for some months, and indeed, in early neonatal life it will again become patent if for

any reason the right atrial pressure were to rise above the left atrial pressure, such as in persistent pulmonary hypertension or right heart obstructive disease. But, in the vast majority of children, the "parallel circulation" of the fetus is superceded by "series circulation" of the normal infant.

There are certain situations in which, however, the maintenance of this route of intracardiac mixing is of vital importance to maintain life, and the foremost of these is *complete transposition of the great arteries*. Earlier studies of the natural history of this condition had shown that 29% of the whole group of patients died before the end of the first week of life, 52% by the end of the first month, and 89% by the end of the first year [4]. Many authors [5–7] demonstrated that early survival was better when there was adequate communication between the two sides of the heart, which was mostly secured through a large ventricular septal defect, present in approximately 50% of cases. In those patients in whom the ventricular septum was intact, death from hypoxia was pervasive and early. In 1950 Blalock and Hanlon [6] introduced an "extracardiac" method for creating an atrial septal defect but mortality was high, often greater than 40% [8,9] although a procedure involving shifting of the atrial septum so that the right pulmonary veins drained into the right atrium [10], thus improving mixing, had better survival rates [9]. Following suggestions by Albert

Transcatheter Therapy in Pediatric Cardiology, pages 7–15
© 1993 Wiley-Liss, Inc.

[11] and unsuccessful attempts at rerouting the systemic and pulmonary venous streams in the atria [12,13], Mustard et al. [14] described the procedure mentioned above, which was generally and widely successful, but could at that time only be carried out when the child was 1–2 years of age. This meant that, at that time, there was no procedure available that could, with low morbidity and mortality, relieve hypoxia and acidosis in the early newborn period to allow children to survive long. The easy applicability of the technique described by Rashkind and Miller carried it to almost immediate widespread use throughout the world and inaugurated a new era in pediatric cardiology.

INDICATIONS

Balloon atrial septostomy is indicated when there is a need to create the opportunity for mixing between the two circulations. This can occur when there are two circulations in parallel as in transposition of the great arteries, or when there is no pulmonary venous return to the left side of the heart, as in total anomalous pulmonary venous return. Balloon atrial septostomy may also be needed when there is obstruction to ventricular inflow or outflow, as on the left side in mitral atresia, aortic atresia, and hypoplastic left heart syndromes and on the right in tricuspid atresia, and pulmonary atresia with intact ventricular septum.

Transposition of the Great Arteries

Balloon atrial septostomy was for many years the procedure of choice in the newborn infant with transposition of the great arteries, particularly those with intact ventricular septum and marked hypoxemia and acidosis. Indeed, as recently as 1985–86 [15], 138 of 187 patients with simple transposition, had balloon atrial septostomy carried out whether they were going for an atrial switch procedure or an arterial switch procedure. As the authors remark, however, the study did "not provide sufficient information as to the need for preliminary balloon atrial septostomy in patients in a treatment protocol leading to arterial switch repair in the first few days of life." Indeed, in many medical centers currently where the arterial switch is the procedure of choice, septostomy is not carried out, and the current practice is to perform balloon atrial septostomy only in those newborn infants who are acidotic and very hypoxic and do not improve on prostaglandin E_1 infusion or in those whose two-dimensional Doppler echocardiography demonstrates poor shunting at atrial level with a small patent foramen ovale. If, however, the management plan is to carry out an atrial switch at 3–4 months of age, it is wise to carry out atrial septostomy early, and some centers follow this up with a Blalock-Hanlon procedure.

When a hypoxic baby diagnosed by echocardiography to have transposition of the great arteries is admitted, it is most commonly our practice to start prostaglandin infusion and to proceed within 24–48 hours to the arterial switch procedure, unless this is contraindicated by anatomic considerations. This means that carrying out balloon atrial septostomy for transposition of the great arteries has become a much rarer procedure in recent years.[1]

Mitral Atresia, Aortic Atresia, Hypoplastic Left Heart Syndromes

In these instances in which the pulmonary blood flow returns to the left atrium, but the forward flow of blood toward the aorta is impeded by mitral or aortic atresia, or a very hypoplastic left ventricle, the pulmonary venous blood has to escape into the right atrium

---

[1]Editor's note: There is some controversy on this issue. In some institutions balloon atrial septostomy is performed routinely in all neonates with transposition of the greater arteries, with intact ventricular septum and arterial switch procedure performed electively during the next few days instead of going for an emergency or urgent arterial switch procedure.

[16,17]. Now that patients can survive with the most severe forms of these left heart obstructive diseases, either by the Norwood procedure or by heart transplantation in the neonatal period, it is important that an adequate circulation by be maintained until the time of surgical intervention; this can be achieved with the ductus maintained open with prostaglandins and an adequate opening in the atrial septum. This need for balloon atrial septostomy can be determined by inspection using two-dimensional Doppler echocardiography, and, if there is evidence that the foramen ovale is obstructive (either by sizing, Doppler measurements, or bowing of the atrial septum), atrial septostomy should be carried out without delay.

Tricuspid Atresia, Pulmonary Atresia With Intact Ventricular Septum, Hypoplastic Right Heart Syndromes

When there is obstruction to the forward flow of blood from the right ventricle, as in pulmonary atresia with intact ventricular septum, or the right atrium, as in tricuspid atresia, or in other hypoplastic right heart syndromes, the circulation is maintained by the systemic venous blood crossing to the left atrium and reaching the pulmonary arteries through a ductus arteriosus, systemic-pulmonary anastomoses, or a surgically created systemic pulmonary shunt. The survival of the infant depends on an adequate opening in the atrial septum [14,18-22] Again, inspection of the size of the interatrial opening, Doppler studies of flow velocity, and bowing of the atrial septum from right to left are indications for urgent balloon septostomy.

Total Anomalous Pulmonary Venous Return

In total anomalous pulmonary venous connection the return is to the right side of the heart; it is important that there be an adequate interatrial communication to allow left heart filling. This is a significant point of risk, especially in those patients who have unobstructed pulmonary venous return, commonly of the supracardiac and cardiac type [23-25]. Again, the indication for balloon atrial septostomy would be in an infant with the signs of obstruction at the atrial septum in whom immediate surgical correction had to be delayed for any reason.

TECHNIQUE

The procedure as originally described by Rashkind and Miller [3] involved cutting down over the femoral vein just above the inguinal ligament, directly introducing a catheter with an inflatable balloon on the tip into the femoral vein, advancing it under fluoroscopic control into the right atrium with the balloon deflated, and then manipulating the catheter across into the left atrium. The balloon was then inflated with 1-2 ml of dilute contrast fluid, and the inflated balloon was swiftly pulled from the left atrium to the right atrial inferior vena cava junction with a sharp jerk of limited extent. The balloon catheter was then advanced again so that the balloon sat in the right atrial cavity, not obstructing the inferior vena cava, and the balloon was deflated. It was recommended that the procedure be repeated two to three times to ensure that an adequate opening had been secured.

There were a number of caveats, the major one being the importance of ensuring that the inflated balloon was, in fact, in the left atrium, since otherwise avulsion of the mitral or tricuspid valves might ensue. This can be done by a number of techniques. If the catheter has passed from the right to the left atrium and clearly out into a pulmonary vein, then when the catheter is gently withdrawn toward the left atrium and inflated slowly it will pop out of the pulmonary vein and into the body of the left atrium. If the inflating balloon tips downward and moves forcibly, it has probably engaged the mitral valve and should be repositioned. Pressure measurement, either by using a double-lumen catheter or by sensing the pressure in the cardiac chamber through a mildly filled balloon, will indicate whether the balloon is in an atrium or a ventricle; rotating either the infant or the x-ray tubes to ensure that the catheter passes backward from the right atrium into the left atrium, rather than forward through the tricuspid valve into the right ventricle, will avoid damage to the tricuspid valve. Rashkind and Miller also emphasized that an important feature of a successful intervention was the sharpness of the initial jerk of the balloon from the left atrium to the right atrium. Slow or gradual withdrawal often resulted in stretching of the foramen ovale without tearing of the membrane, with resultant inadequate mixing.

More recently, some elements of the original technique have been modified somewhat. Difficulties with the femoral approach prompted the use of the umbilical vein to gain access to the right heart [26-30]. The success rate using this approach was reported to be as good as that using the traditional femoral vein cutdown. However, since the early 1970s the *percutaneous approach* to right and left heart catheterization has supplanted all other modes of access, and in the mid-1970s Hurwitz and Girod [31] and Sunderland et al. [32] demonstrated that balloon septostomy could also be carried out successfully percutaneously. The diagnostic procedure is first carried out using a 5 Fr sheath in the femoral vein. The next step is gradual dilation of the femoral vein using dilators and larger sheaths up to 7 or 8 Fr^2 sheath so that a 4 or 5 Fr catheter with the balloon on the tip can be introduced. With these larger sheaths, it is important to ensure that the tip of the sheath be well below the right atrial inferior vena caval junction, since, if it is present in this position, it may rupture the balloon before the atrial septum has been torn. Following the initial Rashkind balloons (USCI), which have an inflation volume of 2–3 ml, and were straight catheters (and were thus sometimes difficult to manip-

ulate through the foramen ovale), larger balloons with a catheter inflected toward the tip and the capacity of being inflated to 6 ml were introduced (Edwards). Since the tear in the atrial septum cannot exceed the foramen ovale, and this does not exceed 1.5 cm in length, it is only necessary to inflate these balloons to 3 ml. Indeed, overinflation to 6 ml may result in tearing the heart and in death [33].

An even more recent modification has been the use of two-dimensional echocardiography, initially to assist in the procedure carried out in a cardiac catheterization lab [34-36]. The logical extension of this was "bedside" balloon atrial septostomy. Here the procedure could be carried out using only echo visualization in neonatal intensive care units without going to the cardiac catheterization laboratory at all [37-41]. This has the advantages of speed and maintenance of a good thermal environment. The balloon can clearly be seen, and the size of the resulting atrial septal opening can be checked instantaneously.

IMMEDIATE AND FOLLOW-UP RESULTS

The immediate consequence of a successful balloon atrial septostomy is improved mixing of flow between the right and left atria. In transposition of the great arteries, there is a rise in PO$_2$ and, because of the shape of the oxygen dissociation curve, an even greater rise in oxygen saturation. This is followed by improvement in pH [3,26,27]. There is an abolition of the pressure gradient between the right and left atria. Occasionally the improvement in oxygen saturation is not immediate following successful balloon septostomy, and this has been attributed to compliance similarities between the right and left ventricles, which will reduce the likelihood of mixing. A successful tear of the atrial septum is followed by maintenance of the improved mixing for up to 2 years [28-32,34]. However, in some cases this improvement is not maintained, and for such patients a Bla-

---

^{2}Editor's note: Currently available septostomy catheters (5 Fr Fogarty Dilatation Atriseptostomy catheters, manufactured by American Edwards Laboratories Baxter, McGow Park, IL) can be introduced via 6 Fr Argon sheaths.

lock-Hanlon procedure or surgical atrial septostomy was performed if delay in definitive surgical repair was still needed. In patients who have obstruction to pulmonary venous return, such as those with mitral atresia, there is, in addition to improvement in systemic blood flow from the right heart, relief of pulmonary venous congestion. Long-term follow-up of the atrial septostomy opening and review at time of surgery [35-42] has shown that the opening created by the balloon septostomy procedure is oval shaped, smooth at the edges, and occupies the site of the foramen ovale.

COMPLICATIONS

Failure to Create Adequate Opening

As mentioned above, if the balloon is not drawn across the atrial septum sharply enough, the flap of the foramen ovale may not tear adequately, but will stretch, and an inadequate opening can result. A second reason for failure to obtain an inadequate opening is increasing age. The flap of the foramen ovale increases in thickness with age [43,44], and it has been our experience that it has been difficult to obtain a good tear if the baby is more than 2-3 months old. Septostomy failed four times, with 1 death out of 26 infants reported by Venables [45] and 4 times out of 65 patients in the series reported by Parsons et al. in 1971 [46].

Arrhythmias

Cardiac arrhythmias are observed commonly during septostomy and include ectopic beats, paroxysmal tachycardia, atrial flutter, atrial fibrillation, partial and complete atrioventricular block, ventricular tachycardia, fibrillation, and standstill [46]. Most of the arrhythmias, however, are transient, and the heart settles back to normal sinus rhythm within a few seconds after the septostomy. Occasionally arrhythmias cause death.

Cardiac Perforation

Perforation of the left atrium or the right atrium has been reported [45-48] and is usu-

ally followed by death. Moore et al. [49] reported aspirating the blood from the pericardial space through a transthoracic needle following such a left atrial laceration and reinfusing it directly into the femoral vein. This maneuver was life saving in one patient [49].

Over-Distension of Balloon

As mentioned, inflation of the balloon to 4-6 ml is rarely necessary and can result in fatal complication [33]. However, others [24,49,50] do not feel that over-distension is a serious problem. Rarely pneumopericardium has been reported [51].

Balloon Embolization

Occasionally, the balloon can rupture as it is drawn back across the atrial septum. In most cases, the balloon material is withdrawn attached to the catheter, but rarely may embolize. If the material remains in the left atrium, it may embolize into the pulmonary circulation, where it rarely causes difficulties. In the right atrium, it may embolize to the systemic circulation. It can then end up at the bifurcation of the aorta, in the right renal artery [52] or in the cerebral circulation.

Balloon Deflation Failure

A rare complication occurs whenever the balloon fails to deflate following septostomy. Rarely does this complication require thoracotomy [53], but the balloon can also be deflated by puncturing it by passing a needle through the chest wall [54] or using a stillette introduced alongside the balloon catheter [55,56].

Laceration of Mitral and Tricuspid Valves

Laceration occurs whenever the balloon is inflated in either the right or left ventricles prior to its forcible withdrawal to the right atrium. A tricuspid valve laceration can result in death [45]. It is important, as mentioned above, to ensure that the catheter is in the left atrium before withdrawal.

Venous Thrombosis

Because of the large size of the balloon catheter, venous thrombosis may result following balloon atrial septostomy [57–60]. This may be limited to the iliac and femoral veins, but can extend into the inferior vena cava. This complication is often asymptomatic and recannalization may later occur.

Failure to Achieve Long-Term Increase in Oxygen Saturation

In some instances, successful balloon septostomy has not been followed by a concomitant increase in oxygen saturation. It is believed in some instances to be due to relative similarities in the compliances of both left and right ventricles with, therefore, lack of mixing at the atrial level, even when an adequate opening occurs [61].

MECHANISM

The mechanism by which the balloon atrial septostomy techniques creates an atrial septal defect is by disruption of the flap of the foramen ovale by the forceful withdrawal of the balloon from the left to right atrium. It appears likely from both angiographic and echocardiographic viewings that the actual tear does not take place until the balloon is forcefully pulled down into the mouth of the inferior vena cava. The tear extends from one margin of the fossa ovalis to the other [62], and its upper and lower limits are defined by the margins of the fossa ovalis.

The improved mixing and rise in arterial oxygen saturation that follows the balloon septostomy is achieved by increased volume of arterialized pulmonary venous blood crossing from the left atrium into the right atrium and hence to the right ventricle and aorta. Rarely, the rise in oxygen saturation will not occur, and this has been attributed to compliance and to the similarities in the two ventricles discouraging mixing at the atrial level. As mentioned above, this situation can sometimes be improved by infusion of prostaglandin E_1.

APPLICABILITY TO ALL AGES

Common experience and the sophisticated statistical analyses of Leanage et al. [44] made it clear that the best results are obtained for balloon atrial septostomy in the first week of life, and, while it can be done at a later age, the chances of success are much less, and these children will usually require the blade septostomy technique of Sang Park to create an adequate atrial opening (see Chapter 3, this volume). This is especially the case in older infants and children with tricuspid or mitral atresia when there has been reduction in size of a functioning atrial septal defect.[3]

NONINVASIVE EVALUATION OF FOLLOW-UP RESULTS

Following the balloon septostomy, the best method for monitoring the size of the atrial septal defect and the shunt across it is by two-dimensional and color Doppler echocardiography. As mentioned above, this has demonstrated improved shunting following the procedure, which will persist without any diminution for at least 6 months. Before arterial switch became the operation of choice for complete transposition, Mustard or Senning repairs were carried out at approximately 3–4 months of age. For the other conditions for which balloon atrial septostomy is the

---

[3]Editor's note: Another alternative, especially if the left atrium is small and hypoplastic, is static balloon dilatation (Shrivatsava S, et al.: Indian Heart J 39:298, 1987; Mullins CE, et al.: Am J Cardiol 65:802, 1990; Hausknecht MJ, et al.: Am J Cardiol 65:1045, 1990; Webber SA, et al.: Br Heart J 65:346, 1991; Rao PS: J Saudi Heart Assoc 4:55, 1992). In this technique, a standard balloon angioplasty catheter is positioned across the interatrial communication and the balloon is inflated. There is a limited but favorable experience with this technique. However, further studies to document safety and efficacy of this technique are necessary prior to recommending it for general use.

initial treatment of choice, the echocardiogram is again the best method of ensuring that the atrial communication is patent until the time of surgical palliation or correction.

COMPARISON WITH SURGICAL THERAPY

The surgical options as alternatives to the balloon atrial septostomy are the Blalock-Hanlon procedure or open atrial septectomy. Both of these procedures had much greater morbidity and mortality rates, particularly in the sick newborn infant, so that balloon atrial septostomy rapidly became the treatment of choice for these children.

SUMMARY AND CONCLUSIONS

Balloon atrial septostomy, introduced by Rashkind and Miller in 1966, rapidly achieved popularity as the treatment of choice for the newborn infant with complete transposition of the great arteries. The usefulness of the technique was further extended and shown to be of value in the management of hypoplastic right and left heart syndromes and in total anomalous pulmonary venous return. The technique is simple and, provided that care was taken to ensure that the balloon was of the appropriate dimension and was in the left atrium, the results were excellent and so much better than the results of the Blalock-Hanlon procedure or open atrial septectomy that the use of these procedures was immediately greatly reduced. The opening created by the procedure was often large enough to maintain adequate mixing for up to 1-2 years, but long-term survival with just a balloon atrial septostomy was rare, and surgical intervention was usually needed.

In the present era, the need for of balloon atrial septostomy has decreased considerably as the arterial switch procedure has become the most frequently used intervention for complete transposition. However, it is still of use for very sick hypoxic and acidotic babies with transpo-

sition before the switch can be carried out and for those in whom the switch is not feasible. It is also a sound and useful therapeutic procedure in newborn patients with mitral and tricuspid atresia and in those with total anomalous pulmonary venous return in whom the atrial septum is obstructive. With the introduction of this technique, Rashkind and Miller opened a new era of catheter intervention in the management of patients with heart disease.

REFERENCES

1. Rashkind WJ, Miller WW (1966): Creation of an atrial septal defect without thoracotomy. JAMA 196:991-992.
2. Blalock A, Taussig HB (1945): The surgical treatment of malformations of the heart in which there is pulmonary stenosis or pulmonary atresia. JAMA 128:189.
3. Mustard WT (1964): Successful two-stage correction of transposition of the great vessels. Surgery 55(3):469-472.
4. Liebman J, Cullum L, Belloc N (1969): Natural history of transposition of the great arteries: Anatomy and birth and death characteristics. Circulation 40:237-262.
5. Noonan JA, Nadas AS, Rudolph AM, Harriss GBC (1960): Transposition of the Great Arteries: A correlation of clinical, physiologic and autopsy data. N Engl J Med 263:592.
6. Blalock A, Hanlon CR (1950): The surgical treatment of complete transposition of the aorta and pulmonary artery. Surg Gynecol Obstet 90:1-15.
7. Shaher RM (1963): Prognosis of transposition of the great vessels with and without atrial septal defect. Br Heart J 25:211-218.
8. Cornell WP, Maxwell RE, Haller JA, Sabiston DC (1966): Results of the Blalock-Hanlon operation in 90 patients with transposition of the great vessels. J Thorac Cardiovasc Surg 52:525-532.
9. Edwards WS, Bargeron LM Jr (1970): Palliative surgery of infants with cyanotic congenital heart disease. Surgery 68:931-941.
10. Trusler GA, Kidd L (1969): Surgical palliation in complete transposition of the great vessels: Experience with Edwards procedure. Can J Surg 12:83.
11. Albert HM (1955): Surgical correction of transposition of the great vessels. Surg Forum 5:74.
12. Merendino KA, Jesseph JE, Herron PW, Thomas GI, Vetto RR (1957): Interatrial venous transposition: A one-stage intracardiac operation for the conversion of complete transposition of the aorta and

pulmonary artery to corrected transposition. Surgery 42:898-909.

13. Senning A (1959): Surgical correction of transposition of the great arteries. Surgery 45:966-980.

14. Mustard WT, Keith JD, Trusler GA, Fowler R, Kidd L (1964): The surgical management of transposition of the great vessels. J Thorac Cardiovasc Surg 48:953-958.

15. Castaneda AR, Trusler GA, Paul MH, Blackstone EH, Kirklin JW (1988): The early results of treatment of simple transposition in the current era. J Thorac Cardiovasc Surg 95:14-28.

16. Starc TJ, Gersony WM (1986): Progressive obstruction of the foramen ovale in patients with left atrioventricular valve atresia. J Am Coll Cardiol 7:1099-1103.

17. Perry SB, Lang P, Keane JF, Jonas RA, Sanders SP, Lock JE (1986): Creation and maintenance of an adequate interatrial communication in left atrioventricular valve atresia or stenosis. Am J Cardiol 58:622-626.

18. Singh SP, Astley R, Parsons CG (1968): Haemodynamic effects of balloon septostomy in tricuspid atresia. Br Med J 1:225-226.

19. Hamill J, Pickering D, Sleight P (1968): Atrial septostomy. Br Med J 2:365.

20. Lenox CC, Zuberbuhler JR (1970): Balloon septostomy in tricuspid atresia after infancy. Am J Cardiol 25:723-726.

21. Sato T, Onoki H, Kano I, Horiuchi T, Ishitoya T (1970): Balloon atrial septostomy in an infant with tricuspid atresia. Tohoku J Exp Med 101:281-288.

22. Rao PS (1985): Comprehensive management of pulmonary atresia with intact ventricular septum. Ann Thorac Surg 40:409-413.

23. Serratto M, Bucheleres HG, Bicoff P, Miller RA, Hastreiter AR (1968): Palliative balloon atrial septostomy for total anomalous pulmonary venous connection in infancy. J Pediatr 73:734-739.

24. Mullins CE, el Said GM, Neches WH, et al. (1973): Balloon atrial septostomy for total anomalous pulmonary venous return. Br Heart J 35:752-757.

25. Ward KE, Mullins CE, Huhta JC, Nihill MR, McNamara DG, Cooley DA (1986): Restrictive interatrial communication in total anomalous pulmonary venous connection. Am J Cardiol 57:1131-1136.

26. Abinader E, Zeltzer M, Riss E (1970): Transumbilical atrial septostomy in the newborn. Am J Dis Child 119:354-355.

27. Romney D, Katzuni E, Aygen MM (1972): Transumbilical balloon atrial septostomy in a case of transposition of the great vessels with situs inversus totalis. Isr J Med Sci 8:529-530.

28. Kaye HH, Tynan M (1974): Balloon atrial septostomy via the umbilical vein. Br Heart J 36:1040-1042.

29. Newfeld EA, Purcell C, Paul MH, Cole RB, Muster AJ (1974): Transumbilical balloon atrial septostomy in 16 infants with transposition of the great arteries. Pediatrics 54:495-497.

30. Roguin N, Sujov P, Montag J, Zeltzer M, Riss E (1984): Transumbilical balloon atrial septostomy for transposition of the great arteries in infants under the age of 60 hours. Am Heart J 107:174-176.

31. Hurwitz RA, Girod DA (1976): Percutaneous balloon atrial septostomy in infants with transposition of the great arteries. Am Heart J 91:618-622.

32. Sunderland CO, Nichols GM, Henken DP, Linstone F, Menashe VD, Lees MH (1976): Percutaneous cardiac catheterization and atrial balloon septostomy in pediatrics. J Pediatr 89:584-587.

33. Sondheimer HM, Cavey RW, Blackman MS (1982): Fatal overdistension of an atrioseptostomy catheter. Pediatr Cardiol 2:255-257.

34. Allan LD, Leanage R, Wainwright R, Joseph MC, Tynan M (1982): Balloon atrial septostomy under two dimensional echocardiographic control. Br Heart J 47:41-43.

35. Perry LW, Ruckman RN, Galioto FM Jr, Shapiro SR, Potter BM, Scott LP, III (1982): Echocardiographically assisted balloon atrial septostomy. Pediatrics 70:403-408.

36. Levin SE, Dansky R (1983): Echocardiographically assisted balloon atrial septostomy for transposition of the great arteries. S Afr Med J 63:836-837.

37. Baker EJ, Allan LD, Tynan MJ, Jones OD, Joseph MC, Deverall PB (1984): Balloon atrial septostomy in the neonatal intensive care unit. Br Heart J 51:377-378.

38. Bullaboy CA, Jennings RB Jr, Johnson DH (1984): 53:971. Bedside balloon atrial septostomy using echocardiographic monitoring. Am J Cardiol 53:971.

39. Steeg CN, Bierman FZ, Hordof AJ, Hayes CJ, Krongrad E, Barst RJ (1985): "Bedside" balloon septostomy in infants with transposition of the great arteries: new concepts using two-dimensional echocardiographic techniques. J Pediatr 107:944-946.

40. Lin AE, Di Sessa TG, Williams RG (1986): Balloon and blade atrial septostomy facilitated by two-dimensional echocardiography. Am J Cardiol 57:273-277.

41. D'Orsogna L, Lam J, Sandor GG, Patterson MW (1989): Assessment of bedside umbilical vein balloon septostomy using two-dimensional echocardiographic guidance in transposition of great arteries. Int J Cardiol 25:271-277.

42. Ozkutlu S, Ozme S, Saraclar M, Baysal K (1988): Balloon atrial septostomy using echocardiographic monitoring. Jpn Heart J 29:415-419.

43. Korns ME, Garabedian HA, Lauer RM (1972):

Anatomic limitations of balloon atrial septostomy. Hum Pathol 3:345–349.

44. Leanage R, Agnetti A, Graham G, Taylor J, Macartney FJ (1981): Factors influencing survival after balloon atrial septostomy for complete transposition of great arteries. Br Heart J 45:559–572.

45. Venables AW (1970): Balloon atrial septostomy in complete transposition of great arteries in infancy. Br Heart J 32:61–65.

46. Parsons CG, Astley R, Burrows FG, Singh SP (1971): Transposition of great arteries. A study of 65 infants followed for 1 to 4 years after balloon septostomy. Br Heart J 33:725–731.

47. Gutgesell HP, McNamara DG (1975): Transposition of the great arteries: Results of treatment with early palliation and late intracardiac repair. Circulation 51:32–38.

48. Blanchard WB, Knauf DG, Victorica BE (1983): Interatrial groove tear: An unusual complication of balloon atrial septostomy. Pediatr Cardiol 4:149–150.

49. Moore JW, Bricker JT, Mullins CE, Ott DA (1985): Infusion of blood from pericardial sac into femoral vein: A technique for survival until operative closure of a cardiac perforation during balloon septostomy. Am J Cardiol 56:494–495.

50. Powell TG, Dewey M, West CR, Arnold R (1984): Fate of infants with transposition of the great arteries in relation to balloon atrial septostomy. Br Heart J 51:371–376.

51. Crosson J, Ringel RE, Haney PJ, Brenner JI (1987): Pneumopericardium as a complication of balloon atrial septostomy. Pediatr Cardiol 8:135–137.

52. Vogel JH (1970): Balloon embolization during atrial septostomy. Circulation 42:155–156.

53. Williams GD, Ahrend TR, Dungan WT (1970): An unusual complication of balloon-catheter atrial septostomy. Ann Thorac Surg 10:556–559.

54. Scott O (1970): A new complication of Rashkind balloon septostomy. Arch Dis Child 45:716–717.

55. Ellison RC, Plauth WH Jr. Gazzaniga AB, Fyler DC (1970): Inability to deflate catheter balloon: A complication of balloon atrial septostomy. J Pediatr 76:604–606.

56. Hohn AR, Webb HM (1972): Balloon deflation failure: A hazard of "medical" atrial septostomy. Am Heart J 83:389–391.

57. Fellows KE Jr (1984): Therapeutic catheter procedures in congenital heart disease: Current status and future prospects. Cardiovasc Intervent Radiol 7:170–177.

58. Hawker RE, Celermajer JM, Cartmill TB, Bowdler JD (1971): Thrombosis of the inferior vena cava following balloon septostomy in transposition of the great arteries. Am Heart J 82:593–595.

59. Mathews RA, Park SC, Neches WH, Fricker FJ, Lenox CC, Zuberbuhler JR (1979): Iliac venous thrombosis in infants and children after cardiac catheterization. Cathet Cardiovasc Diagn 5:67–74.

60. Laurin S, Lundstrom NR (1987): Venous thrombosis after cardiac catheterization in infants. Acta Radiol 28:241–246.

61. Turley K, Ebert PA (1985): Transposition of the great arteries in the neonate: Failed balloon atrial septostomy. J Cardiovasc Surg 26:564–567.

62. Kidd L (1978): Complete transposition of the great arteries. In Keith JD, Rowe RD, Vlad P (eds): "Heart Disease in Infancy and Childhood," 3rd ed. New York: Macmillan, pp 590–611.

3

Blade Atrial Septostomy

Sang C. Park, M.D., and William H. Neches, M.D.

Cardiology Division, Children's Hospital of Pittsburgh,
Pittsburgh, Pennsylvania 15213

INTRODUCTION

In certain cardiac malformations, an adequate interatrial communication either is essential for survival or can be beneficial from a hemodynamic standpoint. As described in the previous chapter on balloon atrial septostomy, nonsurgical enlargement of an interatrial opening became possible by the introduction of the Rashkind and Miller [1] procedure in 1966. The success rate of balloon septostomy was reported to be from 62% to 89% [2,3]. Failure to create an adequate interatrial opening has been largely related to the presence of a thickened atrial septum, which cannot be torn effectively by a balloon catheter. When this is present, the atrial septum is simply stretched, rather than torn, by the balloon catheter. To overcome this limitation of balloon catheters, we reported the blade atrial septostomy technique in 1975, following animal experimentation [4]. Our initial clinical trials, as well as subsequent collaborative studies, have established this technique as an effective modality to enlarge a restrictive interatrial opening in a thickened septum or even to create an interatrial opening in the presence of an intact atrial septum by means of a transseptal approach [5,6]. The blade atrial septostomy procedure has been widely utilized in pediatric patients [7–13] as well as in adults [14].

INDICATIONS

The indications for blade atrial septostomy are the same as for balloon atrial septostomy.

The procedure is used where an interatrial opening is hemodynamically important to promote mixing at atrial level or to decompress an atrial chamber. In most cases, this results in improved systemic oxygen saturation. These cardiac anomalies include transposition of the great arteries, tricuspid atresia, pulmonary atresia with intact ventricular septum, double outlet right ventricle with restrictive ventricular septal defect, mitral atresia, hypoplastic left heart syndrome, and total anomalous pulmonary venous return.

In the newborn, balloon atrial septostomy is still the procedure of choice for enlarging the interatrial opening. However, beyond the newborn period, the atrial septum is generally thickened and balloon atrial septostomy is usually not successful. In particular, this occurs in patients with left-sided atrioventricular valve atresia (e.g., mitral atresia) who tend to have a progressively restrictive interatrial communication even if there is no pressure gradient in the newborn period [15]. In these patients, balloon atrial septostomy is usually not effective [9], and blade atrial septostomy is advisable as an initial procedure. Other patients who require consideration for blade atrial septostomy are those fail to improve after initial balloon atrial septostomy, those who develop recurrent stenosis after an apparently successful initial balloon atrial septostomy, and even those with residual stenosis after surgical septectomy. In these patients, repeat balloon atrial septostomy is usually ineffective [16].

In addition to the use of blade atrial septos-

Transcatheter Therapy in Pediatric Cardiology, pages 17–27

tomy in patients with congenital heart defects, this procedure has also been used in patients with primary pulmonary hypertension. These patients, who usually have an intact atrial septum, have undergone this procedure by transseptal technique in an attempt to provide a means of improving systemic blood flow [14]. Although this palliation has had limited short-term success, the indications and long-term efficacy of blade septostomy in this condition are yet to be determined.

TECHNIQUE

Specifications and Construction of the Blade Atrial Septostomy Catheter

At present, three different sizes of blade atrial septostomy catheters are available (Cook, Inc., Bloomington, IN; see Table I). Effective blade lengths are 9.4, 13.4 and 20 mm. The small and medium sizes are contained in catheters that are 6 Fr in outer diameter, while the largest one is 7.3 Fr. The overall length of these catheters is 65–85 cm. The blade catheter consists of a distal metal tubing that contains the blade component, a longer polyethylene tube, and a "Y" connector at the proximal portion of the catheter (Fig. 1). A slit-like opening is provided along the distal one-half of the metal tube. A tiny blade that is linked to a lever is contained within the metal tube. The blade pivots at the distal tip, and the proximal end is linked to a solid guidewire that passes through the entire catheter and exits at the catheter hub. As the wire is advanced into the catheter, the blade pivots at its distal end and

protrudes through the slit to form a triangular shape. The Y connector at the proximal end of the catheter (Fig. 1A) is for fluid infusion through a side branch (C), as well as for the control of the blade by a wire (F) through the straight branch. There are several accessory devices attached to the Y connector. As shown in Figure 1, a rubber gasket (B) is attached to the Y connector to prevent leakage due to the mismatch between the blade control wire and lumen of the connector. In addition, a wire holder (E) and its threaded locking nut (D) are attached to the distal part of the blade control wire (F). Tightening the locking device (D) on the wire holder (E) will fasten it to the wire. This will eliminate any gap between the gasket (B), and the locking device (D) will prevent inadvertent protrusion of the blade component during the manipulation of the catheter.

To extend the blade component, the locking device is loosened from the blade control wire (F) and pulled backward until the gap between the gasket (B) and the locking device (D) is the same distance as the length of the blade (i.e., 10 mm for small-, 13 mm for medium-, and 20 mm for large-sized blade catheters). The wire holder (E) and the locking device (D) are then tightened on the wire. The blade is extended by advancing the blade control wire holder (E) toward the catheter tip.

Preparation

Patients who undergo blade atrial septostomy do *not* require general anesthesia. The usual sedation for cardiac catheterization is generally sufficient. In our institution, no med-

TABLE I. Blade Septostomy Catheters

	Catheter		Blade length (mm)	Recommended sheath size (Fr)
Selection	Size (Fr)	Length (cm)		
Small	5.7	65	9.4	7
Medium	5.7	65	13.4	7
Large	7.3	85	20.0	9

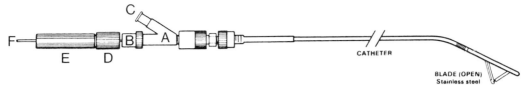

Fig. 1. Diagrammatic illustration of the blade septostomy catheter and its assembly components. See text for a description of the components.

ication is usually given to an infant under 6 months of age. Infants between 6 months and 1 year receive 0.1 mg/kg of morphine sulfate or meperidine 1 mg/kg and promethazine 0.5 mg/kg intramuscularly. Children over 1 year of age receive a combination of meperidine 2 mg/kg, promethazine 0.5 mg/kg, and chlorpromazine 0.5 mg/kg intramuscularly. If routine premedication is not sufficient sedation to immobilize the patient adequately for the procedure, then ketamine 1 mg/kg is given intravenously, particularly for those patients who require the transseptal technique. Atropine sulfate is also given routinely prior to administration of ketamine to prevent possible laryngospasm, which may be associated with the latter medication.

Selection of the Blade Atrial Septostomy Catheter

Since there are three different-sized blade catheters available (Fig. 2), the appropriate-sized catheter can be determined by the size of the interatrial opening as well as by the thickness of the atrial septum. The size of the interatrial communication can be determined by either a two-dimensional echocardiographic study in the subcostal view or by a selective left atrial angiogram in the four-chamber view or lateral view. In patients with an interatrial communication of less than 5 mm, or in newborn infants, the small blade catheter generally will be sufficient. In those patients with an interatrial opening between 5 and 8 mm, a medium-sized blade catheter is recommended. In children weighing over 10 kg or in adults with an atrial defect of greater than 8 mm or an unusually thickened atrial septum, the larg-

est catheter with a 20 mm blade component is suggested. In addition to the size of the existing interatrial communication, the size of the left atrium is an important factor in determining the selection of the blade catheter, since the left atrium must be large enough to accommodate the metal component of the blade catheter.

Procedure

Once the desired blade catheter is selected, an introducer sheath with a bleeding control device is chosen that is 1 Fr size larger than the

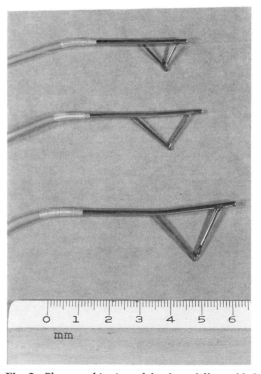

Fig. 2. Photographic view of the three different blade septostomy catheters with the blade extended.

catheter diameter (refer to Table I). Prior to insertion of the blade catheter into the patient, the catheter system should be carefully inspected to ensure smooth movement of each component as outlined above. The catheter also should be inserted through the sheath to be certain that an appropriate match has been selected. The catheter system is then thoroughly flushed with heparinized solution. A flexible plastic tube is connected between the side port (C) and the pressure transducer or intravenous flushing solution. The catheter is then introduced into the left atrium with biplane fluoroscopic guidance. The locking device (Fig. 1D) is then loosened from the blade control wire (F) and pulled backward to the desired gap length between the gasket (B) and the locking device (D). After the device is tightened, the blade is extended by advancing the blade control wire (F) gently toward the catheter tip (see Fig. 3A). If resistance is met or if the blade cannot be fully extended, the catheter tip may have been positioned in the left atrial appendage or in a pulmonary vein. After withdrawing the blade component back into the catheter, the catheter is repositioned by slight withdrawal and a similar maneuver is again attempted. Once the blade has been extended easily, the gasket and locking devices are held together with the thumb and index finger to prevent the blade component from folding back into the catheter during the maneuver.

The catheter is now slightly rotated in a counterclockwise direction until the blade is facing anteriorly, as shown on lateral fluoroscopy in Figure 3B. The entire catheter then is slowly withdrawn to the right atrium using both hands to maintain the same catheter orientation (Fig. 3C) one hand on the locking device and the other hand positioned on the catheter closest to the introducer sheath hub. As the catheter is withdrawn from the left to the right atrium, resistance of the atrial septum is usually encountered in the middle or lower portion of the heart. Gentle but steady and firm withdrawal force is maintained until a sudden loss of resistance is noticed. In partic-

ular, when the septum is unusually thick and tough, resistance to withdrawal of the catheter through the atrial septum can be felt even though the blade has reached the position, fluoroscopically, of the lower level of the diaphragm. As long as the resistance was met in the usual position in the midatrium and there was no loss of resistance or sudden change of catheter position during the withdrawal process, it is safe to maintain traction. Two-dimensional echocardiographic imaging also may be particularly useful to document the engagement of the extended blade component against the atrial septum during the procedure. It should be emphasized that under *no circumstances* should *rapid withdrawal* or a *jerky motion* be attempted as is required by balloon atrial septostomy. For those patients with a thickened atrial septum and small interatrial opening, in particular when using transseptal approach, the blade component only should be partially extended at the initial withdrawal of the blade across the septum. This measure will not only prevent undue stress to the delicate components of the blade assembly but also help to make subsequent cuts in different directions.

Once the blade component has passed through the atrial septum, the catheter is advanced into the mid-right atrium and the blade control wire is withdrawn, thus folding the blade component back into the catheter lumen. Several passages of the blade catheter with a different angulation each time are recommended to ensure multiple cuts. Finally, after confirming that the blade component is within the catheter lumen, the catheter is withdrawn. Intermittent or slow infusion of heparinized solution through the side port of the blade catheter during the procedure will prevent clot formation within the catheter system. Balloon atrial septostomy, using a Rashkind septostomy catheter (USCI product) or a Fogarty septostomy catheter (product of Edwards Laboratories), is usually performed immediately after blade septostomy to promote further enlargement of interatrial opening. In-

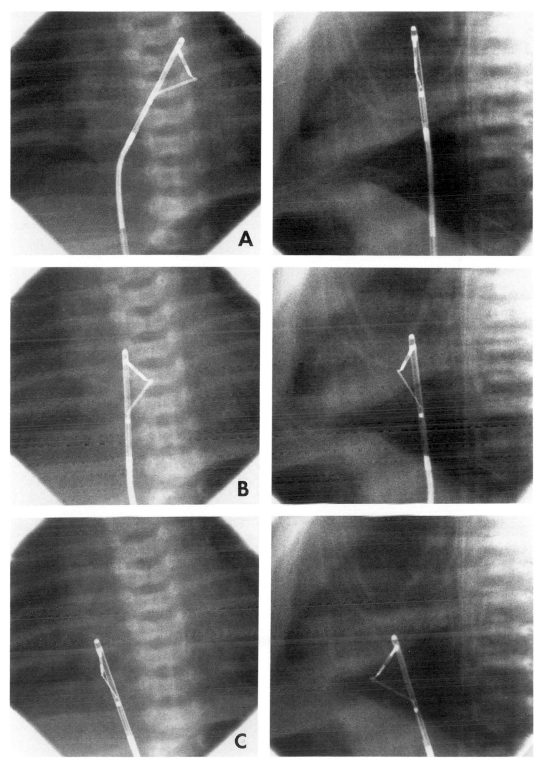

Fig. 3. Sequence of the blade atrial septostomy procedure. (The anteroposterior views are on the left-side column and the lateral views are on the right-side column). **A:** The catheter tip is positioned in the left atrium with the blade extended. **B:** The blade is facing anteriorly and to the left as the blade catheter is withdrawn from the left atrium to the right atrium. **C:** The blade catheter has been withdrawn to the right atrium.

stead of balloon atrial septostomy, balloon dilation using an angioplasty catheter,[1] or even a double balloon technique, has been used to enlarge the interatrial opening (Dr. Charles E. Mullins, personal communication).

Procedure in Patients With Intact Atrial Septum

The transseptal approach has been used to perform blade atrial septostomy in patients with an intact atrial septum or when there is an unusual location of an interatrial opening that is not safe for blade atrial septostomy. We have been using two-dimensional echocardiographic imaging for guidance during the transseptal procedure on a routine basis, as well as occasionally during blade and balloon septostomy (Fig. 4). This is particularly useful in patients with an unusual cardiac orientation such as dextrocardia or even in patients with normal cardiac position to ensure that the puncture site is in the fossa ovalis area. To use this transseptal approach, a Brockenbrough transseptal needle and a long transseptal sheath with a side port and bleeding control device are required. This special sheath not only helps to prevent blood loss resulting from the mismatch between the sheath and the catheter but also facilitates the intermittent or continuous flushing through the side port, which prevents clot formation and possible air embolization during catheter exchange. The long introducer sheath also has been utilized in situations in which it is difficult to maneuver the stiff blade catheter into the left atrium. The long sheath is initially introduced into the left atrium over a more flexible regular catheter. Once the tip of the long sheath is in the left atrium, the regular catheter is exchanged for the blade septostomy catheter. The sheath then should be withdrawn to the level of the midportion of the inferior vena cava before the blade is extended. Once the blade is extended, the sheath is then

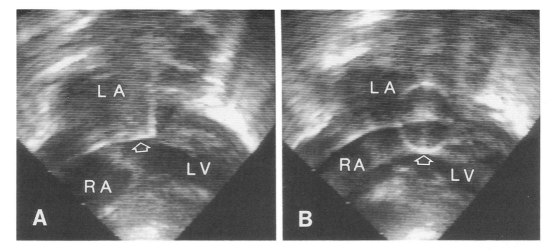

Fig. 4. Two-dimensional echocardiograms in the subcostal view in a patient with transposition of the great arteries. **A:** The blade septostomy catheter is in the left atrium (LA) with extension of the blade component (arrow). **B:** Following the blade septostomy procedure, a Fogarty balloon septostomy catheter with an inflated balloon (arrow) is positioned in the left atrium for further enlargement of the interatrial opening. RA, right atrium; LV, left ventricle.

---

[1]Editor's note: As a matter of fact, static balloon dilatation of restrictive interatrial communication can be performed instead of blade atrial septostomy. However, there are not adequate data to advocate it to replace blade septostomy. For further detail, see Chapter 2, footnote 3, p.12.

withdrawn simultaneously with the blade catheter to prevent inadvertent cutting of the sheath by the blade. For the subsequent balloon atrial septostomy, a similar precaution must be undertaken to prevent damage to the sheath by the balloon. A balloon septostomy catheter such as a Rashkind septostomy catheter (USCI) or a Fogarty septostomy catheter (Edwards Laboratories) is rather short to use in conjunction with a long introducer sheath. Therefore, careful measurement of balloon catheter and the long sheath should be made prior to the procedure. If the balloon catheter is too short to use through the long sheath, then the sheath must be replaced with a shorter one prior to the balloon septostomy procedure.

IMMEDIATE RESULTS

In our early collaborative study among several centers, the overall success rate of blade septostomy was 79% for all types of congenital heart malformations [6]. The success rate varied depending on the type of lesion: 74% for transposition of the great arteries, 70% for mitral atresia complex, and 100% for tricuspid atresia and other miscellaneous groups. In that report, some of the patients with transposition of the great arteries did not have good mixing despite an adequate interatrial communication, and these were regarded as unsuccessful cases. Some other failures were in a few newborns with hypoplastic left heart syndrome or mitral atresia in whom the left atrium was too small to extend the blade component, and thus it was not possible to perform adequate blade septostomy. As we have gained experience with this procedure and several different sizes of blade catheters, as well as the long introducer sheath, have become available, the success rate of blade atrial septostomy has improved substantially to over 90%.

COMPLICATIONS

In our early experience with the blade septostomy procedure, a major complication was perforation of the left atrial wall in a 12-year-old patient with mitral atresia who had an unusually superiorly and posteriorly positioned interatrial opening. In retrospect, this patient was not an ideal candidate for the procedure due to the unusual location of the interatrial opening. Perforation of the right atrium and right ventricle were also reported to have occurred during prolonged manipulation of the blade catheter [6,10]. One incident occurred when biplane fluoroscopy was not used. The difficulty of traversing the atrial septum with the stiff blade catheter has been largely eliminated by the use of a long sheath. The long sheath with a bleeding control device has also eliminated the complication of excessive blood loss that occurred as a result of mismatch between the percutaneous sheath size and the smaller shaft of the blade catheter. Neurologic complications such as seizures or hemiparesis have also occurred following blade septostomy. It is likely that these complications were related to embolism of air or blood clots during the procedure. Therefore, in addition to the use of a sheath with a bleeding control device to prevent inadvertent air embolism, intermittent or slow continuous infusion of heparinized solution through the side ports of the blade catheter, as well as the percutaneous sheath, is mandatory, particularly when the long sheath is used.

Others have reported difficulty in retracting the blade component back into the catheter lumen after the blade septostomy procedure. These incidents are likely related to extending the blade component beyond the recommended level, with resulting disengagement or malalignment of the blade component as a result of undue stress during the procedure. As indicated previously in the procedure section, in patients with an unusually thickened or intact atrial septum, the blade only should be partially opened to minimize the stress to this component. Thus over the years serious complications have been virtually eliminated as we have gained additional experience with the blade septostomy procedure.

MECHANISM

Our earlier experiments in newborn lambs showed that the blade septostomy procedure actually incises the atrial septum in the desired direction, as shown in Figure 5A. Subsequent balloon atrial septostomy will further enlarge the interatrial communication, as shown in Figure 5B. This particularly occurs when the atrial septum is thick and tough and could not have been torn by the balloon catheter alone (Fig. 6A). Figure 6B illustrates an intermediate term result of blade septostomy in a 9-month-old infant with mitral atresia. The patient died of a pulmonary complication 2 months after the procedure. At postmortem examination the atrial septum had an adequate interatrial opening with a thickened and rolled rim (Fig. 6B). It would not have been possible to create such a defect by a balloon catheter alone. Thus the initial cut with the blade catheter facilitates subsequent effective tearing of the atrial septum by balloon septostomy.

APPLICABILITY TO ALL AGE GROUPS AND LIMITATIONS

Blade atrial septostomy has been widely used in all age groups. The main limiting factor is the size of the femoral vein, which must be large enough to accommodate a 7 Fr sheath. The smallest patient in whom we have performed blade septostomy was a premature infant with transposition of the great arteries who weighed 1,900 g. Since the femoral vein approach is essential to perform this procedure, absence of the hepatic segment of the inferior vena cava, or bilateral thrombosis of the ileofemoral venous system, would preclude its use. Although the jugular venous approach has been used to perform the transseptal procedure in adults, to our knowledge blade septostomy has not been done via this route. Occasionally, in some patients with mitral atresia or with the hypoplastic left heart syndrome, the left atrium can be too small to accommodate the blade component. As indicated earlier, left

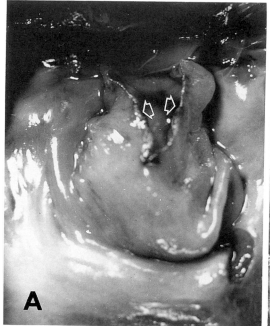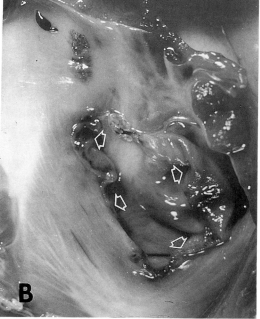

Fig. 5. The left atrial aspect of the atrial septum in newborn lambs following blade atrial septostomy. **A:** An incision in the septum (arrows). **B:** After additional balloon septostomy. The incision is further extended to a sizable defect (arrows).

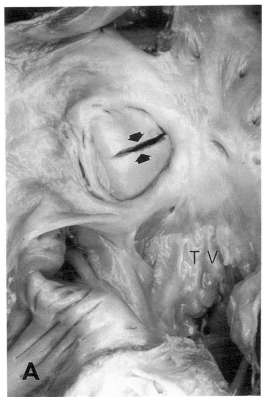 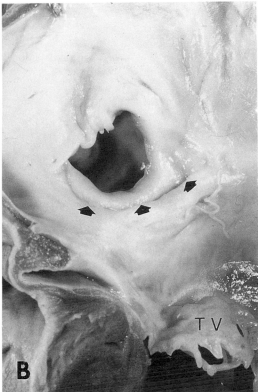

Fig. 6. Right atrial aspect of the atrial septum in human postmortem specimens. **A:** A heart specimen without congenital heart disease. A clean linear cut is made in the fossa ovalis area by the blade septostomy catheter in a thickened atrial septum. **B:** A heart specimen with mitral atresia 2 months after blade septostomy, showing a sizable interatrial defect with a thickened rolled rim (arrow) (See text for details.)

atrial size should be carefully evaluated by echocardiographic as well as angiographic study before initiation of the procedure.

CAUSE OF RESTENOSIS OF AN INTERATRIAL OPENING

Based on our experience as well as those of others, restenosis of an interatrial communication after successful blade atrial septostomy is uncommon [9]. When this does occur, it is usually related to an inadequate initial tear of the atrial septum by the blade catheter and/or by subsequent balloon atrial septostomy. In these cases it is likely that the initial procedure resulted in simply stretching the interatrial communication rather than an actual cut or tear of

the atrial septum. On the other hand, some patients with a thick atrial septum may tend to have gradual narrowing of the interatrial communication over a period of time—months or years. This can be due to growth of the patient in the presence of a fixed interatrial opening, or can be an actual reduction of the opening due to proliferation of the tissue adjacent to the defect as a result of increased flow through the defect. This phenomenon has been also observed even after surgical septectomy [9].

NONINVASIVE EVALUATION OF FOLLOW-UP RESULTS

Two-dimensional echocardiography has been effectively used to evaluate the status of the interatrial opening both before and after blade and balloon septostomy. The subcostal four-chamber view is the most ideal approach for visualization of the atrial septum. In older children or in adults with a poor subcostal window, the parasternal short axis may be a reasonable substitute view to visualize the inter-atrial opening. Color flow mapping and Dopp-ler studies have been valuable additional mo-dalities to assess the size of the interatrial communication as well as the flow direction through the defect. In infants, an 8 mm inter-atrial communication by echocardiographic measurement is regarded as an adequate open-ing, whereas a less than 5 mm opening is usually inadequate. In older children or adults, an interatrial communication larger than 10–12 mm is ideal. Patients with obligatory left to right atrial shunting lesions, such as those with mitral atresia or hypoplastic left heart syn-drome, may show increased flow velocity up to 2 m/sec across the atrial septum despite an adequate interatrial opening. This may be due to torrential pulmonary blood flow with the increased shunt through the defect. Thus var-ious factors that may influence the hemo-dynamics should be taken into consideration carefully at the time of evaluation.

COMPARISON WITH SURGICAL THERAPY

Although the morbidity and mortality of surgical atrial septectomy has steadily im-proved [17], blade atrial septostomy has the obvious advantage of avoiding thoracotomy. Blade septostomy not only has much lower morbidity and mortality rates than surgical septectomy, particularly in a sick infant, but also eliminates the problem of scaring or adhesions of the cardiovascular system that can interfere with subsequent surgery. The blade septostomy technique provides reason-ably good palliation and even may be repeated to enlarge the interatrial communication at a later time. Despite the clear advantage of blade septostomy, there remains a fundamental dif-ference between surgical septectomy and blade septostomy. The blade septostomy procedure does not remove the atrial septal tissue but simply incises the septum. Thus, in patients in whom an adequate interatrial communica-tion is essential for lifelong palliation, open surgical septectomy at the time of any other necessary surgical intervention may be bene-ficial.

SUMMARY AND CONCLUSIONS

The blade atrial septostomy technique was designed to enlarge an existing interatrial com-munication or to create an interatrial defect by the transseptal technique. It is particularly use-ful when the atrial septum is too thick to be torn by a balloon catheter alone. Prior to performing the procedure, a comprehensive review of each component and of the mechan-ics of the blade catheter is essential for the safety, as well as the success, of the procedure. Each step of the procedure should carefully adhere to the details of the recommended instructions. The blade septostomy procedure has been found to be safe and predictably effective in more than 15 years of use.

REFERENCES

1. Rashkind WJ, Miller WW (1966): Creation of an atrial septal defect without thoracotomy: Palliative approach to complete transposition of the great arteries. JAMA 196:991–992.
2. Hawker RE, Krovetz LJ, Rowe RD (1974): An anal-ysis of prognostic factors in the outcome of balloon atrial septostomy for transposition of the great arter-ies. Hopkins Med J 134:95–106.
3. Neches WH, Mullins CE, McNamara DG (1973): Balloon atrial septostomy in congenital heart disease in infancy. Am J Dis Child 125:371–375.
4. Park SC, Zuberbuhler JR, Neches WH, Lenox CC, Zoltun RA (1975): A new atrial septostomy tech-nique. Cathet Cardiovasc Diagn 1:195–201.
5. Park SC, Neches WH, Zuberbuhler JR, Lenox CC, Mathews RA, Fricker FJ, Zoltun RA (1978): Clinical use of blade atrial septostomy. Circulation 58:600–606.
6. Park SC, Neches WH, Mullins CE, Girod DA, Olley PM, Falkowski G, Garibjan VA, Mathews RA,

Fricker FJ, Beerman LB, Lenox CC, Zuberbuhler JR (1982): Blade atrial septostomy: Collaborative study. Circulation 66:258–266.

7. Lin AE, De Sesa TG, Williams RG (1986): Balloon and blade atrial septostomy facilitated by two-dimensional echocardiography. Am J Cardiol 57:273–277.

8. Rao PS. (1984): Transcatheter blade atrial septostomy. Cathet Cardiovasc Diagn 10:335–342.

9. Perry SB, Lang P, Keane JF, Jonas RA, Sanders PS, Lock JE (1986): Creation and maintenance of an adequate interatrial communication in left atrioventricular valve atresia or stenosis. Am J Cardiol 58:622–626.

10. Ward KE, Mullins CE, Huhta JC, Nihill MR, McNamara DG, Cooley DA (1986): Restrictive intratrial communication in total anomalous pulmonary venous connection. Am J Cardiol 57:1131–1136.

11. Vick GW, Mullins CE, Nihill MR, Bricker JT (1986): Blade and balloon atrial septostomy transseptal atrial puncture, abstracted. J Am Coll Cardiol 7:117A.

12. Ledesma Velasco M, Nunez Garduno D, Salgado Escobar JL, Munayer Calderon J, Rodriguez Hernandez L, Rangel Abdundis A (1987): Blade auricular septostomy. Arch Inst Cardiol Mex 57:155–158.

13. Herraiz JI, Bermudez-Caneta R, Acerete F, Alonso MJ, Firpo C, Quero M (1988): Result and perspectives of atrial septostomy using a balloon and blade catheter. An Esp Pediatr 32:227–229.

14. Rich S, Lam W (1988): Atrial septostomy as palliative therapy for refractory primary pulmonary hypertension. Am J Cardiol 51:1560–1561.

15. Mickell JJ, Mathews RA, Park SC, Lenox CC, Fricker FJ, Neches WH, Zuberbuhler JR (1980): Left atrioventricular valve atresia: Clinical management. Circulation 61:123–127.

16. Baker F, Baker L, Zoltun R, Zuberbuhler JR (1971): Effectiveness of the Rashkind procedure in transposition of the great arteries in infants. Circulation 43(Suppl I): 1–6.

17. Hermann V, Laks H, Kaiser BC, Barner HB, Williams VL (1975): The Blalock-Hanlon procedure: Simple transposition of the great arteries. Arch Surg 110:1387–1390.

4

Technique of Balloon Valvuloplasty/Angioplasty

P. Syamasundar Rao, M.D.

Department of Pediatrics, Division of Pediatric Cardiology, University of Wisconsin Medical School, University of Wisconsin Children's Hospital, Madison, Wisconsin 53792-4108

INTRODUCTION

Although the initial descriptions of transcatheter relief of stenotic lesions of the heart were by dynamic techniques, either by pulling back a wire across the stenotic valve to cut it, as suggested by Rubio-Alvarez and Limon-Lason [1,2] or by withdrawing an inflated balloon across the stenotic valve as performed by Semb et al. [3], a static dilation technique, as described by Grüntzig et al. [4] and by Kan et al. [5], is commonly used. In this chapter, I review the technique of balloon dilatation that we have used but also refer liberally to the works of other investigators.

INDICATIONS

The diagnosis and assessment of obstructive lesions of the heart and great vessels are made by the usual clinical, roentgenographic, electrocardiographic, and echo Doppler studies. Once a moderate-to-severe obstruction is diagnosed, cardiac catheterization and cineangiography are performed to confirm the clinical diagnosis and to consider balloon dilatation of the stenotic lesion. By and large, the indications for balloon dilatation are essentially similar to those used for surgical intervention [6,7]. Although some workers have used balloon dilatation for milder obstructions (as detailed elsewhere [8]), I would at the present time suggest that we use the same criteria for

balloon therapy as are used for surgical treatment. Moderate-to-severe gradients in isolated pulmonic and aortic valvar obstructions, congestive heart failure and/or hypertension with aortic coarctation, and right ventricular peak systolic pressure in excess of half of the systemic pressure with branch pulmonary artery stenosis are indications for balloon dilatation. In an infant with a cyanotic heart defect, balloon pulmonary valvuloplasty may be employed to augment pulmonary blood flow. Balloon dilatation has been used to treat infants and children with other congenital, acquired, or postoperative stenotic lesions, including mitral and tricuspid valve stenosis, aortic recoarctation following previous surgery, discrete subaortic membranous stenosis, pulmonary vein stenosis, superior vena caval stenosis, inferior vena caval obstructive lesions, vena caval or interatrial baffle obstruction after Mustard or Senning operations for transposition of the great arteries, supravalvar pulmonary stenosis following arterial switch procedure for transposition of the great arteries, supravalvar aortic stenosis, stenosed Blalock-Taussig shunts, and obstructed bioprosthetic valves. The technique of balloon angioplasty/valvuloplasty has many applications and should now be added to the therapeutic armamentarium available to the pediatric cardiologist in the management of children with heart disease. The specific criteria and indications for each of the lesions are listed and discussed

Transcatheter Therapy in Pediatric Cardiology, pages 29–44
© 1993 Wiley-Liss, Inc.

in their respective chapters and are not detailed here.

PREDILATATION PREPARATION

Informed Consent

Despite usage for almost a decade, the balloon dilation procedures are relatively new and sometimes considered experimental. It is important that a full explanation of the balloon dilatation procedure be given to the parents and to the patients who are old enough to understand. Potential complications associated with the procedure should also be explained. The advantages and disadvantages of both surgical and balloon therapy should be mentioned. Such informed consent is essential, especially in view of the fact that acute complications [9,10] can occur and long-term effects of the balloon procedure are not yet known.

Patient Preparation

In neonates and infants, a neutral thermal environment, a normal acid–base state, normoglycemia, and normocalcemia should be maintained [11–13] by appropriate monitoring and correction if needed. In the neonate with ductal-dependent pulmonary blood flow (e.g., critical pulmonary stenosis), the ductus arteriosus should be kept patent by infusion of prostaglandin E_1 (PGE$_1$); 0.05–0.1 μg/kg/min is the recommended dose. PGE$_1$ is also helpful in ductal-dependent systemic circulations such as critical aortic stenosis. In both of the above situations, PGE$_1$ may be quite helpful in stabilizing the infant and restoring normal metabolic status. In addition, complete occlusion of circulation during balloon inflation may be better tolerated in the face of an open ductus. In neonates with severe aortic coarctation, PGE$_1$ may also be helpful; however, the infants should undergo balloon angioplasty of aortic coarctation not too long after starting PGE$_1$ infusion. If much time has elapsed after starting PGE$_1$, the ductus may be widely dilated, and balloon coarctation angioplasty may not be fea-

sible but, if feasible, not effective. Perhaps no more than a couple of hours of PGE$_1$ infusion should lapse prior to initiation of balloon angioplasty of aortic coarctation.

All infants and children should have blood available prior to initiating the balloon dilatation procedure so that blood transfusion may be given for significant blood loss or for use during surgery, if required. An intravenous line should be established prior to the procedure to serve as access for infusion of fluids and medications should they be required during or after the procedure. Surgical standby is no longer recommended.

Sedation and Anesthesia

We usually perform balloon dilatation with the patient sedated with a mixture of meperidine (1.0 mg/kg, maximum 50 mg), promethazine (0.6 mg/kg, maximum 15 mg), and chlorpromazine (0.6 mg/kg, maximum 15 mg), given intramuscularly [14–20]. If necessary, this can be supplemented with intermittent doses of midazolam (0.1 mg/kg, given intravenously). Other workers use ketamine [21] or general anesthesia [22–25]. Although there is no consensus with regard to the type of analgesia/anesthesia, we have not encountered significant problems with the use of sedative mixture for angioplasty/valvuloplasty procedures in children. We have performed in excess of 300 such procedures, and only two of these children required additional sedation with ketamine. However, institutional practices should be respected with regard to the type of sedation used and whether general anesthesia is employed.

PROCEDURE

General Description

Complete hemodynamic and angiographic studies should be performed first. Once balloon dilatation is decided upon, the following is undertaken: 1) A 4 Fr to 7 Fr end-hole (or multi-A2, Cordis) catheter is introduced percutaneously into either the femoral vein or the femoral artery and advanced across the stenotic lesion. 2) A 0.014–0.038-inch guidewire is passed through the catheter into the vessel or cardiac chamber beyond the stenotic lesion. Whenever feasible, I use an extra-stiff Amplatz exchange guidewire (Cook). Use of this extra-stiff wire facilitates easy insertion of the balloon catheter into the groin area and positioning of the balloon across the stenotic lesion without bending or looping of the wire. 3) A 4 Fr to 9 Fr balloon dilation catheter is advanced over the guidewire and positioned across the stenotic lesion. It is important to ensure that the balloon is positioned such that the obstructive lesion is in the center of the balloon. This can easily be done by superimposing a fluoroscopic view of the balloon onto the frozen video or digital frame of predilatation cineangiographic view of the stenotic lesion. With the currently available digital cineangiography systems, this is relatively easy. 4) The balloon is inflated with diluted contrast material (3 parts saline and 1 part contrast) to approximately 3–5 atm of pressure. Because of the availability of a large variety of balloons with a wide range of inflation pressures that could be safely used, the manufacturer's recommendation should be followed. However, more often than not the manufacturer lists a far less inflation pressure than the balloon material can tolerate. It should also be noted that there is no specific advantage in using an extremely high inflation pressure, since these balloons do not expand significantly at higher inflation pressures. It is important to prevent balloon rupture by avoiding high inflation pressures. It is obvious from this discussion that pressure of inflation should be monitored; this can be done by a commercially available pressure gauge, although some workers [26] have not monitored the pressure of inflation in the past. The recommended duration of inflation is 5 seconds. I do not believe that longer duration of balloon inflation has any advantage and, indeed, may be harmful by producing longer periods of hypotension. I feel that the effect of balloon dilatation occurs at the time point of complete

balloon inflation, abolishing the balloon "waisting." In pediatric dilatations (congenital stenotic lesions), the duration of balloon inflation is unlikely to have a bearing on the effect of angioplasty, in contradistinction to angioplasty of atherosclerotic lesions, where longer duration of inflation is thought to have some favorable effect. Usually, a total of three or four balloon inflations are performed five minutes apart. If the first balloon inflation is successful in relieving the obstruction, there is less or no "waisting" of the balloon during the second and subsequent balloon inflation. Radiographic images of balloon inflation characteristics are helpful adjuncts in the evaluation of effectiveness of success of balloon dilatation (in addition to residual pressure gradient and angiographic appearance). 5) The balloon catheter is exchanged with a 5 Fr or 6 Fr end-hole or multi-A2 catheter over an exchange guidewire to avoid any injury to the freshly dilated site by catheter manipulation. 6) Measurement of pressure gradient across the stenotic lesion and angiographic demonstration of relief of obstruction are recommended. Recording of heart rate, systemic arterial pressure, and cardiac index prior to and 15 minutes following balloon dilatation are made to ensure that any change in pressure gradient is not related to a change in cardiac index, but is, indeed, related to the procedure.

Catheter Insertion Site

Percutaneous insertion of the catheter into the right femoral vein or artery is the method of choice. Rarely, it may be difficult to cannulate the femoral vein or artery, as the case may be. This is most often related to previous catheterization, balloon dilatation, or cut-down in the groin. If percutaneous entry in the left groin is also unsuccessful, a cut-down may be performed and saphenous vein–femoral vein junction isolated. Balloon valvuloplasty can be accomplished via the saphenous venous bulb [27]. When femoral venous access is not possible, balloon dilatation may be performed via axillary venous [28,29] or internal jugular venous [30] approach. These approaches are also useful in the presence of infrahepatic interruption of inferior vena cava with azygous or hemiazygous continuation.

When femoral artery cannot be cannulated percutaneously, it may be isolated and used for left heart dilatation [31,32]. Alternatively, axillary artery cut-down for dilating aortic valve stenosis [33] or aortic coarctation [32] may be used. As a matter of fact, other routes of catheter entry should be sought for left heart dilatation in neonates and young infants because of potential for injury to the femoral arteries. In patients in whom the aorta can be entered from the right ventricle either directly e.g., transposition of the great arteries and double-outlet right ventricle) or via a large ventricular septal defect, such an approach should be utilized for dilation of aortic coarctation [34,35] or even for aortic or truncal [35a] valve stenosis. Other approaches used are carotid artery by cut-down [36] and the umbilical artery [37,38]. These latter methods should be employed preferentially in neonates and infants because of the advantage of sparing the femoral artery.

Positioning the Catheter Across the Stenotic Lesion

In some patients, particularly in neonates and young children, it may be difficult to advance the catheter across the stenotic lesion. In such instances, the following maneuvers may be helpful: 1) Use an end-hole catheter (we use a 5 Fr multi-A2 catheter, Cordis) and position it close to the stenotic lesion and advance a floppy end of a straight guidewire through the tip of the catheter. In case of significant difficulty, angiography should be performed and the stenotic lesion visualized. This will serve as a guide to manipulating the catheter and guidewire. It is important to position the guidewire immediately proximal (or distal) to the stenotic orifice. We usually use a Benson wire (Cook) with a long, soft, floppy end. 2) Use a balloon-wedge catheter, position it just beneath the pulmonic valve, quickly

deflate the balloon, and advance the catheter into the main pulmonary artery. Several rapid inflation/deflation cycles with varying degrees of balloon inflation should be used. Failing this, use a guidewire, as described above. 3) Use a flexible, steerable coronary guidewire (0.014 inch) through the end-hole catheter; this is particularly useful in neonates and young infants. 4) We have encountered one child in whom we could not advance any catheter across the right ventricular infundibulum because of severe infundibular constriction [39]. In this child, administration of propranolol (0.1 mg/kg IV, slowly) had made it possible to pass a catheter across the pulmonary valve and eventually to perform balloon pulmonary valvuloplasty [39]. 5) Entry of Blalock-Taussig shunts is tricky. It may not be possible to catheterize these shunts with conventional catheters. We have used right coronary artery catheters (Cordis); the curve at the tip of the catheter facilitates the entry of the guidewire and subsequently the catheter into the Blalock-Taussig shunt [20]. We use either a Benson or coronary (0.014 inch) guidewire when a regular straight guidewire is unsuccessful in catheterizing the shunt. Others use Cook Cobra and Headhunter catheters successfully [40]. 6) Positioning a balloon catheter across the stenotic lesion is sometimes difficult. Use of an extra-stiff (e.g., Amplatz extra-stiff exchange wire, Cook) guidewire and low-profile catheters eliminate this problem to a great extent. If it is still not feasible to position an appropriate-sized balloon dilatation catheter across the stenotic lesion, a smaller-sized, 4–8 mm diameter, low-profile balloon on a No. 4 or 5 Fr catheter may initially be used to predilate and then to use more appropriate-sized balloons [27,41]. This technique is particularly helpful when dilating very severely stenotic pulmonary valves and in small infants.

Heparinization

We do not routinely heparinize right heart balloon dilatations. However, heparinization is advisable if there is evidence for intracardiac right-to-left shunting. We routinely heparinize all left heart dilatations. We use a single intravenous dose of heparin, 100 units/kg (maximum, 2,500 units). This is administered immediately prior to introduction of balloon dilatation catheter. If the procedure is prolonged (> 1 hour) after introduction of balloon dilatation catheter, an additional amount of heparin (one-half the above dose) is administered. The heparin is not continued, and its effect is not reversed after the procedure. The exception to the rule is balloon angioplasty of narrowed Blalock-Taussig shunts in which we continue heparinization for 24 hours following the procedure.

The major reason for heparin administration is to prevent clot formation on the balloon. Thrombus formation on the deflated balloon is a potential hazard in all balloon dilatation procedures; such thrombus could dislodge and produce cerebrovascular embolism in left heart balloon dilatations [42]. Therefore, it is prudent to anticoagulate these children adequately [43]. Also, attempts should be made to leave the balloon catheter in the ascending aorta for the shortest duration possible. If for some reason the procedure has to be delayed after insertion of the balloon catheter, the catheter should be withdrawn into the descending aorta. Meticulous attention to the details of the technique is necessary to prevent thromboembolic complications [43].

Balloon Choice

Balloon diameter. The diameter of the balloon (inflated) should be carefully chosen; it varies with the type of stenotic lesion to be dilated. Only general guidelines are given in this chapter, and the reader is referred to the respective chapters for details of the reasoning behind the recommendations.

For pulmonary valve dilatation, a balloon that is 1.2–1.4 times the size of the pulmonary valve annulus is recommended [44–47]. These recommendations are based on immediate [44] and follow-up [45–47] results of balloon pulmonary valvuloplasty. Balloons larger than

1.5 times the size of the pulmonary valve annulus should not be used because of potential damage to the right ventricular outflow tract when large balloons are used [48]. However, balloons large enough to produce a balloon: annulus ratio of 1.4–1.5 may be necessary to produce adequate results if the pulmonary valve is dysplastic [49].

When dilating stenotic aortic valves, the size of the balloon chosen should be within 1 to 2 mm of the size of the aortic valve annulus. It is generally recommended that the size of the balloon not exceed the size of the aortic valve annulus for fear of producing aortic valve insufficiency. However, it should be pointed out that while there is a general impression that balloons larger than aortic valve annulus produce more severe aortic insufficiency, some of the available data [50] did not show a correlation between balloon: annulus ratio and subsequent development of aortic valve insufficiency.

Balloon size for balloon dilatation of subaortic membranous stenosis has initially been limited to the size of the aortic valve annulus; this is based on the experience with balloon valvuloplasty in aortic valve stenosis. In agreement with this concept, we also have initially used small balloons so that the mean balloon: annulus ratio was 1.01 [19]. Because of inadequate reduction in the pressure gradient, we had to go to larger balloons (balloon: annulus ratios, 1.14 ± 0.14; range, 0.98–1.39). Despite the use of balloons larger than the valve annulus, we did not observe any increase in aortic insufficiency. Suarez de Lezo et al. [51] and Arora et al. [52] also used balloons that were slightly larger than the aortic annulus, but the aortic insufficiency did not increase significantly. Although the reason for this is not clear, we surmise that nonstenotic aortic valve leaflets are simply compressed against the aortic wall without any damage to the valve mechanism in contradistinction to valvar aortic stenosis, in which the valve mechanism may be distorted when balloon(s) larger than aortic valve annulus are used [19]. However, when both subvalvar and valvar stenoses coexist, balloons larger than the aortic valve annulus should not be used [53].

For aortic coarctation (both native and postsurgical), the balloon size should be two or more times the size of the coarcted aortic segment, but no larger than the descending aorta at the level of the diaphragm [14,54–57]. We usually select a balloon size that is midway between the size of the aortic isthmus (or transverse aortic arch) and the size of the descending aorta at the level of the diaphragm. If there is not an adequate improvement (Fig. 1), a balloon as large as the descending aorta (at the level of the diaphragm) is chosen for additional dilatation. Careful selection of balloon size is important in preventing or reducing the incidence of aneurysms at the site of balloon dilatation.

The balloon diameter should be three to four times the size of the pulmonary arterial [57] or venous stenotic lesions. When dilating a stenosed Blalock-Taussig shunt, the balloon diameter should be 2.5–3.0 times the narrowest site and should probably be as large as the subclavian artery proximal to the shunt [20,58].

For dilatation of stenosed porcine heterografts, the balloon diameter should be similar to the size of the metallic ring into which the porcine valve had been mounted. Using balloons larger than the heterograft ring have produced transverse balloon ruptures [59–61]. Based on theoretical considerations [59–62], it appears that in the presence of a rigid metallic ring the shearing stress on the balloon along its circumference is high and may result in transverse rupture. Consequently, the possible benefits of an oversized balloon are unlikely to be realized because of a rigid metallic ring [62].

The size of the valve annulus (Fig. 2) or the vessel can be measured by echocardiographic techniques and remeasured from the frozen video images of the cineangiograms just before balloon dilatation. Attention should be paid to avoiding parallax error, to identifying and measuring the valve annulus correctly, and to correcting for magnification accurately, especially when the valve or vessel size is small. We generally average the values from two cineangiographic projections (usually the anteroposterior and lateral views). Although

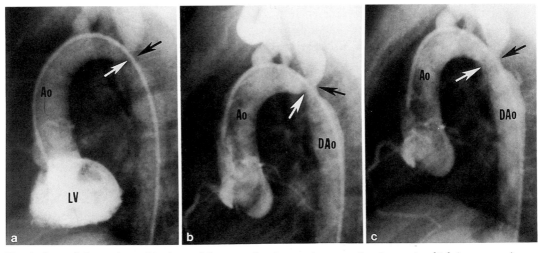

Fig. 1. Lateral cineangiographic views of the aorta showing aortic coarctation (arrows), which is severe prior to balloon angioplasty (**a**). This improved following balloon dilatation with an 8 mm balloon (**b**) but is still narrowed with a residual peak systolic pressure gradient. Balloon angioplasty with a 10 mm balloon showed wide open coarcted segment (**c**) with significant pressure gradient reduction. Ao, aorta; DAo, descending aorta; LV, left ventricle.

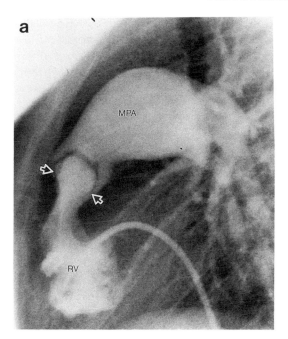 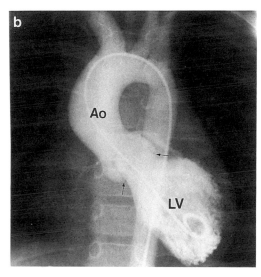

Fig. 2. Selected cineangiographic frames from right ventricular (**a**) and left ventricular (**b**) injections showing the attachments of valve leaflets (arrows) indicating valve annulus. This may not represent valve annulus histologically, but it can be used as a guide to selection of balloon size. Ao, aorta; LV, left ventricle; MPA, main pulmonary artery; RV, right ventricle.

there is reasonable agreement between echocardiographic and angiocardiographic measurements of these structures, we rely more on the angiographically measured sizes.

Balloon length. Most workers use 3 cm long balloons for pulmonary valvuloplasty. There are no data either from our own series or from the literature to assess whether shorter (2 cm) or longer (at least 4 cm) balloons have any advantages or disadvantages over the conventional 3 cm long balloons. The 2 cm long balloons are too short to maintain the balloon center over the pulmonary valve annulus during balloon inflation and therefore are not advisable in children and adolescents. The 2 cm long balloons are appropriate for the neonates and young infants. Four centimeter and longer balloons may impinge on the tricuspid valve mechanism and may injure it. Two recent experiences, one causing avulsion of the papillary muscle [63] and the other causing heart

block [64] when 6 and 4 cm long balloons, respectively, were used, suggest that these long balloons should not be used for balloon pulmonary valvuloplasty. Based on this information, it can be concluded that 3 cm long balloons should be used in children until data to the contrary become available. For aortic valvuloplasty, because of difficulty in maintaining the balloon center over the aortic valve during balloon inflation in children when 3 to 4 cm long balloons are used, it is generally considered that 5.5 cm long balloons are better for aortic valvuloplasty in children and adolescents; these longer balloons ensure adequate positioning of the balloon during valvuloplasty. The 3–4 cm long balloons are adequate in neonates and young infants.

For aortic coarctation, 3 cm long balloons are adequate. Much longer balloons are not advisable because of potential injury to the aortic arch associated with straightening of the longer balloon during inflation. Having said the above, it should be noted that appropriate length of the balloon in the desired balloon diameter may not be available for use on occasion because such a balloon is either not manufactured or not stocked in the catheterization laboratory.

Two balloons. When the valve annulus is too large to dilate with a commercially available single balloon, a double-balloon technique, in which two balloons are simultaneously inflated across the stenotic valve, may be used. Effective balloon size (diameter) is calculated by using the simple formula [45]:

$$\frac{D_1 + D_2 + \pi\left(\dfrac{D_1}{2} + \dfrac{D_2}{2}\right)}{\pi}$$

where D_1 and D_2 are diameters of the balloons used.

However, some workers advocate use of double-balloon technique as a procedure of choice for pulmonic [65] and aortic [66] valve stenosis. To evaluate this issue in pulmonic stenosis, we compared the immediate and follow-up results of 12 patients with single-balloon valvuloplasty (who were matched with the double-balloon group for the balloon: annulus ratio) with those of 12 patients undergoing double-balloon valvuloplasty [67]. The study showed that immediate and follow-up results are excellent in both groups. The results of double-balloon valvuloplasty were similar to those seen with equivalent-sized single-balloon valvuloplasty and did not offer additional advantage over single-balloon results. It was concluded that there are no data to support the contention that the double-balloon technique is superior to the single-balloon pulmonary valvuloplasty when equivalent balloon: annulus ratios are used [67].

With regard to Beekman's claim [66] of superiority of double-balloon aortic valvuloplasty over the single-balloon technique, we scrutinized their results [68] and determined that 1) there was more severe aortic valve obstruc-

tion in the single-balloon group; 2) there were differences in balloon sizes (balloon: annulus ratios); 3) they did not examine valve morphology differences between groups; and 4) they did not use follow-up results in their assessment. Therefore we concluded that there is no evidence to suggest that double-balloon technique is superior to single-balloon aortic valvuloplasty when similar balloon: annulus ratios are used [68]. The results of Shaddy et al. [50] also support our contention. They found a slightly higher percent gradient reduction immediately after valvuloplasty when two balloons were used than when one balloon was used. However, when early and late follow-up results are examined, there were no differences in residual gradients or percent gradient reduction between the single- and double-balloon groups. We feel that balloon:annulus ratio is more important than whether a single- or double-balloon technique is used [68].

Therefore we would recommend that a double-balloon technique be used when the pulmonary or aortic valve annulus is too large to dilate with a commercially available single balloon or when a single balloon cannot be safely passed across the femoral vessels [69] and not because the double-balloon technique gives a better result [67,68].

While a double-balloon technique is required in a significant number of patients with pulmonic and aortic stenoses [18,66,67,69], such a technique is usually not required in aortic coarctation. However, the double-balloon technique can be successfully used with coarctation of the aorta [70]. Double-balloon technique may be quite useful in dilatation of atrioventricular valve stenosis. Their role in and the advantages of the double-balloon technique have been well-documented [71–74] in adults and adolescents. In younger patients, the single-balloon technique may be adequate.

Trefoil and bifoil balloons. Some workers have advocated the use of bifoil and trefoil balloons for pulmonic [75–78] and aortic [77,79] valvuloplasty with the idea that there will be forward flow around the balloon during balloon inflation. Both animal and clinical experimentation shows that there is less fall in systemic arterial pressure with trefoil balloons than with conventional balloons. We have limited experience with this technique (Fig. 3). Because the size of the balloon used is larger than (for pulmonary valve dilatation) or equal to (for aortic) the valve annulus, the amount of forward flow allowed may be limited. In addition, these balloons are bulky and somewhat more difficult to position across the area of obstruction. At the present time, we use single (or double) balloons with short inflation times (5 seconds). With this approach, the degree of circulatory compromise is minimal and results appear good. Until more data are available with regard to the safety and efficacy of the trefoil and bifoil balloons, we continue to use a conventional single- or double-balloon technique.

Monitoring

During a balloon dilatation procedure, there is complete or almost complete obstruction to blood flow. This causes a fall in the systemic pressure. Reflex bradycardia during balloon inflation is also common. Premature beats are also commonly seen, presumable related to ventricular stimulation. In patients with intracardiac right-to-left shunting, hypoxemia may result from right heart dilatation procedures. The majority of effects described above are transient and revert back to normal following balloon deflation. However, monitoring the patients is generally recommended to document the transient nature of the side effects and to intervene if the abnormalities are severe or do not return to normal. Monitoring of 1) heart rate by electrocardiogram, 2) systemic pressure via an arterial line, and 3) arterial oxygen saturation by pulse oximetry is generally performed. If there is persistence of these abnormalities, the balloon should be withdrawn from the site of balloon dilatation. Short duration of balloon inflation (5 seconds) is likely to result in transient effects and prompt recovery. Out of our total experience with balloon dilatation in excess of 300 patients, we

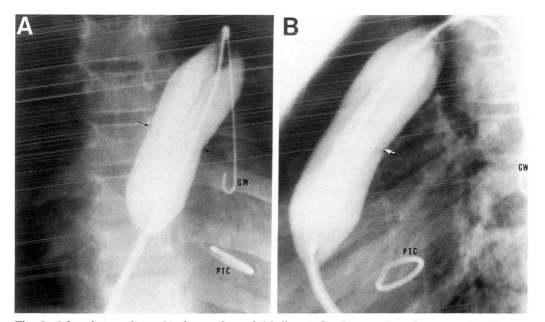

Fig. 3. Selected cineradiographic frame of a trefoil balloon inflated across the pulmonary valve. The arrows show the indentation of the valve annulus on the inflated balloon. GW, guidewire; PTC, pigtail catheter in the left ventricle.

had only two patients requiring institution of brief cardiac massage. One was a child with severe pulmonary stenosis in whom, because of technical difficulties, the balloon could not be rapidly deflated. Extreme bradycardia ensued. Brief cardiac massage and withdrawal of balloon into the inferior vena cava resulted in prompt restoration to normal. Another was an infant with aortic stenosis who sustained ventricular fibrillation. Removal of the balloon from across the aortic valve, brief cardiac massage and administration of xylocaine were rapidly undertaken. The rhythm reverted to normal prior to considering countershock. Meticulous attention to the details of the technique is necessary during the procedure to minimize the complication rate. Limited monitoring, as described above, is adequate to carry out the balloon dilatation procedure successfully.

Following balloon angioplasty/valvuloplasty, we monitor the patient in an intermediate care setting; the electrocardiogram is continuously monitored; vital signs (temperature, pulses, respiration, and blood pressure) are measured intermittently, and perfusion of the extremity used for arterial entry is checked. The intravenous line that was started prior to the procedure is maintained. An echo-Doppler study is performed several hours after the procedure to assess the adequacy of the dilatation procedure. The patient is gradually allowed to recover from sedation and feeding is initiated, starting with clear liquids. The patients are monitored overnight and discharged home on the morning following the balloon dilatation procedure.

OTHER ISSUES
Substances Used for Balloon Inflation

Most workers use diluted contrast material so that the viscosity is low and the balloon can be easily deflated. We use three parts of saline and one part of Conray 400. Balloon inflation with CO_2 has been attempted [80] and successful results reported in pulmonary valve steno-

sis patients. I do not believe that there is any specific advantage of using CO_2 instead of diluted contrast material. Accidental rupture and release of massive amounts of CO_2, causing embolization, is a potential danger and therefore is not recommended.

Pressure, Number, and Duration of Balloon Inflation

The recommendations for pressure of balloon inflation varied from 2.0 to 8.5 atm of pressure [7], and duration of each inflation was suggested to be 5–20 seconds. Between one to four balloon inflations, 2–5 minutes apart, has been suggested. Clearly, no data are available for deciding which is the best method of inflation. We have examined these issues in three commonly used dilatations, namely, pulmonic stenosis [81], aortic stenosis [18], and aortic coarctation [82]. The balloon inflation characteristics in the group with good results were compared with those of the group with poor results in each of the three lesions [18,81,82]. There were no significant differences between the groups, suggesting that the outcome of valvuloplasty is not related to these balloon inflation characteristics. We have also looked at the data with arbitrary division of maximum pressure, number of balloon inflations, and total duration of balloon inflation and found that higher pressure, larger number, and longer duration of balloon inflation did not favorably influence residual gradients at follow-up, especially when the influence of balloon:annulus (or balloon:coarctation) ratio was removed. For further details of these data, the reader is referred to the original papers [18,81,82] and chapters on pulmonic stenosis, aortic stenosis, and aortic coarctation in this book.

Based on the above data and our personal experience with a large number of balloon dilatations, we recommend the following: Perform balloon dilatation sequentially at 3, 4, and 5 atm of pressure inflation using a commercially available pressure gauge. The "waisting" usually disappears at 3 or 4 atm of pressure. With some of the new balloons, higher pressure of inflation is tolerated without balloon rupture. With these balloons, we use higher inflation pressures, as recommended by the manufacturer. With this approach, we have not observed balloon ruptures. It should be realized that extremely high inflation pressures do not have any advantage, because the balloon size does not increase significantly with higher pressure.

Initially, we used a 10 second inflation, and now we use 5 second inflation. With the latter there is less hypotension, and blood pressure returns to normal a few seconds after balloon deflation. After successful dilatation (*i.e.*, "waisting" is abolished), we usually repeat the procedure once or twice. The repeat balloon inflation shows less "waisting" of the balloon if the initial balloon inflation has been successful.

In summary, we recommend sequential balloon inflation with 3, 4, and 5 atm of pressure of 5 second duration, 5 minutes apart. Higher inflation pressures may be used if the manufacturer states that higher pressures are tolerated by the balloon.

Acute Ventricular Obstruction During Valvuloplasty

During balloon pulmonary and aortic valvuloplasty, there is acute obstruction to the respective ventricular outflow tracts with consequent distention of the ventricle, increased transmyocardial pressure, and potential compromise to myocardial perfusion, particularly in the left ventricle. To circumvent this problem, double balloons [65,69], bifoil and trefoil balloons [75–79], Y-connector to create left-ventricle-to-right-atrial shunt [83], and inflow caval balloon occlusion [84] have been advocated. It is not clear if the ventricular distension for short periods of time, as required during balloon valvuloplasty, is truly harmful, nor is it clearly shown that the above-proposed methods cause significant relief of ventricular distension. I have advocated [7] short periods (5 seconds) of inflation and do not believe that

the above-described methods [65,69,75–79,83,84] have significant advantages. Indeed, some of these procedures increase the complexity of the procedure and may prolong the duration of the procedure.

Multiple Obstructions

Some patients may have several obstructive lesions. It is feasible to balloon dilate several stenotic lesions at the same sitting. The criteria used for balloon dilatation for each of the stenotic lesions should be similar to those used for isolated obstruction. But, the evaluation of degree of obstruction becomes more difficult; in the presence of multiple obstructions in series, the pressure gradient across the proximal obstruction may be diminished or abolished [85,86]. This atypical pressure gradient manifestation was thought to be due to "forced vibration" with greater energy transfer into the cardiovascular segment upstream from the distal obstruction [85,86]. The elastic and pulsatile properties of the cardiovascular system are important in the expression of this phenomenon [85,86]. Once the distal obstruction is relieved, proximal gradient manifests; for example, when both aortic valvar stenosis and aortic coarctation coexist, relief of aortic coarctation by balloon angioplasty may actually increase aortic valve gradient. Whether balloon aortic valvuloplasty should be performed should be decided on the basis of measured aortic valve gradient following successful relief of aortic coarctation.

In the presence of intracardiac communications, shunting of blood away from the obstructive lesions may make the detection of distal obstructions more difficult. For example, in a patient with a large ventricular septal defect, severe valvar pulmonary stenosis and branch pulmonary artery stenosis, the distal obstruction may not be evident until valvar obstruction is relieved. The blood is shunted away from the pulmonary circuit through the ventricular septal defect. Because of the small amount of flow, there may not be significant gradient across the branch pulmonary steno-

sis. Relief of valvar pulmonic stenosis by balloon angioplasty increases pulmonary flow,
with consequent appearance of pressure gradient across the branch pulmonary artery narrowing. The above considerations should be
taken into account when evaluating multiple
cardiovascular obstructions.

Several groups of investigators [87–94] and
and those in the author's laboratory have been
able to dilate multiple obstructions at the same
sitting and have attested to the safety and
efficacy of such procedures. It is important to
note that severity of obstruction should be
assessed, taking into account the principles
outlined above. It is also important to retain a
guidewire across the area of freshly dilated
stenotic lesion (especially aortic coarctation) so
that tips of guidewires and catheters are not
manipulated in the region of freshly dilated
lesion.

OTHER TRANSCATHETER METHODS

Yang and associates [95] developed a double-blade valvotomy catheter to treat valvar
pulmonic stenosis. The catheter consists of a
retractable, rhomboid-shaped metal structure
mounted at the tip of the catheter. The proximal half of each side has a blade. The catheter
is positioned in the main pulmonary artery, the
blades are extended and pulled back across the
stenotic pulmonary valve, thus cutting the stenotic leaflets. The authors attempted this technique in three children with pulmonary valve
stenosis after having tested its feasibility and
safety in dogs. Peak systolic right ventricular
pressures were reduced from 85, 100, and 120
to 42, 60, and 90 mmHg, respectively, by
catheter valvotomy. The third patient, with 90
mmHg residual right ventricular pressure, later
underwent balloon valvuloplasty with reduction of right ventricular pressure to 42 mmHg.
Although this is an ingenious method, there
are difficulties in advancing the catheter across
the right ventricle into the pulmonary artery,
and the results appear marginal. Furthermore,
currently used static balloon dilatation appears

safe and effective. Because of these reasons, it
is unlikely that transcatheter blade valvotomy
[95] will be adopted by other workers in the
field.

Laser technology has been applied to treat
cardiac disease. Lee et al. [96,97] demonstrated
feasibility of dissolution of atherosclerotic lesions in human cadavers. Riemenschneider
et al. [98] have used this technique to perform
atrial septostomy in neonatal postmortem
hearts and in dogs. They applied this method
to relieve obstruction in postmortem specimens with valvar pulmonic and aortic stenosis,
coarctation of the aorta, pulmonary atresia,
and pulmonary valve dysplasia. Two-dimensional echocardiographic monitoring, or
visualization, either by a flexible fiberoptic
scope [97] or by a dual fiberoptic/laser catheter
[99], may be necessary to target the area for
vaporization. Because of reasonably good results with balloon dilatation and the difficulty
in introducing, positioning, and operating
these large-sized catheters, it is unlikely that
these methods will be suitable for use in
children. However, Quershi and associates
(100) have successfully used laser technique
(without the use of fiberoptic catheter visualization) to open atretic pulmonary valve. Further clinical trials are necessary prior to their
general use.

Atherectomy catheter devices have been
used to remove atheromatous material from
the peripheral and coronary arteries [101,102]
Qureshi et al. [103] used a Simpson coronary
atherectomy catheter to remove right ventricular infundibular muscle in a 14-month-old
child with tetralogy of Fallot. The systemic
arterial oxygen saturation improved and the
right ventricular outflow tract became wider.
They suggested that this type of transcatheter
resection of infundibular muscle may be important in the palliative management of tetralogy of Fallot [103]. Further clinical trials of this
method in selected patients are warranted, and
this method may serve as a useful adjunct to
balloon pulmonary valvuloplasty [58,104] in
the management of tetralogy of Fallot.

CONCLUSIONS

Balloon dilatation techniques to relieve obstructive lesions of the heart and great vessels is feasible and safe. The method is reasonably well standardized. The indications for use of these techniques are similar to those for surgical intervention. Appropriate choice of balloon size remains critical to achieve good results and to prevent complications. Further miniaturization of balloon/catheter systems and meticulous attention to the details of the technique are necessary for successful relief of the obstruction and to reduce the complication rate.

REFERENCES

1. Rubio-Alvarez V, Limon-Lason R, Soni J (1953): Valvulotomias intracardiacas por medio de un cateter. Arch Inst Cardiol Mex 23:183-192.
2. Rubio V, Limon-Lason R (1954): Treatment of pulmonary valvular stenosis and tricuspid stenosis using a modified catheter, abstracted. Second World Congress on Cardiology, Washington, DC, Program Abstracts II, p 205.
3. Semb BKH, Tijonneland S, Stake G, Aabyholm G (1979): "Balloon valvulotomy" of congenital pulmonary valve stenosis with tricuspid valve insufficiency. Cardiovasc Radiol 2:239-241.
4. Grüntzig AR, Senning A, Siegothaler WE (1979): Non-operative dilatation of coronary artery stenosis: percutaneous transluminal coronary angioplasty. N Engl J Med 301:61-68.
5. Kan JS, White RI Jr, Mitchell SE, Gardner TJ (1982): Percutaneous balloon valvuloplasty: a new method for treating congenital pulmonary valve stenosis. N Engl J Med 307:540-542.
6. Rao PS (1989): Medical progress: balloon valvuloplasty and angioplasty in infants and children. J Pediatr 114:907-914.
7. Rao PS (1989): Balloon angioplasty and valvuloplasty in infants, children and adolescents. Curr Probl Cardiol 14:417-500.
8. Rao PS (1988): Indications for balloon pulmonary valvuloplasty. Am Heart J 116:1661-1662.
9. Fellows KE, Radtke W, Keane JF, Lock JE (1987): Acute complications of catheter therapy for congenital heart disease. Am J Cardiol 60:679-683.
10. Booth P, Redington AN, Shinebourne EA, Rigby ML (1991): Early complications of interventional balloon catheterization in infants and children. Br Heart J 65:109-112.
11. Vincent WR, Rao PS (1973): Early identification of the neonate with suspected serious heart disease. Paediatrician 2:229-250.
12. Rigby JJ, Rao PS (1975): Cardiac catheterization in infancy and childhood. Paediatrician 4:343-355.
13. Rao PS, Stong WB (1981): Congenital heart disease. In Conn HB (ed): "Current Therapy." Philadelphia: W.B. Saunders, pp 185-209.
14. Rao PS (1986): Transcatheter treatment of pulmonary stenosis and coarctation of the aorta. Experience with percutaneous balloon dilatation. Br Heart J 56:250-258.
15. Rao PS (1987): Balloon angioplasty for coarctation of the aorta in infancy. J Pediatr 110:713-718.
16. Rao PS, Brais M (1988): Balloon pulmonary valvuloplasty for congenital cyanotic heart defects. Am Heart J 115:1105-1110
17. Rao PS, Fawzy ME, Solymar L, Mardini MK (1988): Long-term results of balloon pulmonary valvuloplasty. Am Heart J 115:1291-1296.
18. Rao PS, Thapar MK, Wilson AD, Levy JM, Chopra PS (1989): Intermediate-term follow-up results of balloon aortic valvuloplasty in infants and children with special reference to causes of restenosis. Am J Cardiol 64:1356-1360.
19. Rao PS, Wilson AD, Chopra PS (1990): Balloon dilatation of discrete subaortic stenosis: immediate and intermediate-term results. J Invasive Cardiol 2:65-71.
20. Rao PS, Levy JM, Chopra PS (1990): Balloon angioplasty of stenosed Blalock-Taussig anastomosis: role of balloon-on-a-wire in dilating occluded shunts. Am Heart J 120:1173-1178.
21. Robertson M, Benson LN, Smallhorn JF, Musewe N, Freedom RM, Moes CAF, Burrows P, Johnston AE, Burrows FA, Rowe RD (1987): The morphology of the right ventricular outflow tract after percutaneous pulmonary valvotomy: long-term follow-up. Br Heart J 58:239-244.
22. Tynan M, Baker EJ, Rohmer J, Jones ODH, Reidy JF, Joseph MC, Ottenkamp J (1985): Percutaneous balloon pulmonary valvuloplasty. Br Heart J 53:520-524.
23. Chaffe A, Fairbrass MJ, Chatrath RR (1988): Anaesthesia for valvuloplasty. Anaesthesia 43:359-361.
24. Sullivan ID, Wren C, Bain H, Hunter S, Rees PG, Taylor JFN, Bull C, Deanfield JE (1989): Balloon dilatation of the aortic valve for congenital aortic stenosis in childhood. Br Heart J 61:186-191.
25. Wren C, Peart I, Bain H, Hunter S (1987): Balloon dilatation of unoperated aortic coarctation: immediate results and one year follow-up. Br Heart J 58:369-373.
26. Balaji S, Oommen R, Rees PG (1991): Fatal rup-

ture during balloon dilatation of recoarctation. Br Heart J 65:100-101.

27. Rao PS (1993): Balloon pulmonary valvuloplasty for isolated pulmonic stenosis. In Rao PS (ed): "Transcatheter Therapy in Pediatric Cardiology." New York: Wiley-Liss, pp. 59-104.

28. Sullivan ID, Robinson PJ, Macartney FJ, Taylor JFN, Rees PG, Bull C, Deanfield JE (1986): Percutaneous balloon valvuloplasty for pulmonary stenosis in infants and children. Br Heart J 54:435-441.

29. Sideris EB, Baay JE, Bradshaw RL, Jones JE (1988): Axillary vein approach for pulmonic valvuloplasty in infants with iliac vein obstruction. Cathet Cardiovasc Diagn 15:61-63.

30. Chaara A, Zniber L, El Haitem N, Benomar M (1989): Percutaneous balloon valvuloplasty via the right internal jugular vein for valvar pulmonic stenosis with severe right ventricular failure. Am Heart J 117:684-685.

31. Finley JP, Beaulieu RG, Nanton MA, Roy DL (1983): Balloon catheter dilatation of coarctation of the aorta in young infants. Br Heart J 50:411-415.

32. Fontes VF, Esteves CA, Brago SLM, da Silva MVD, e Silva MAP, Sousa EMK, d Souza AM (1990): It is valid to dilate native aortic coarctation with a balloon catheter. Int J Cardiol 27:311-316.

33. Austoni P, Figini A, Vignati G, Donatelli F (1990): Emergency aortic balloon valvotomy in critical aortic stenosis of the neonate. Pediatr Cardiol 11:59-60.

34. Al Yousef S, Khan A, Nihill M, Lababidi Z, Mullins C (1988): Perkutane transvenose antegrade ballonangioplastie bie aortenisthmusstenose. Herz 13:36-40.

35. Wren C (1993): Balloon valvuloplasty/angioplasty: The British experience. In Rao PS (ed): "Transcatheter Therapy in Pediatric Cardiology." New York: Wiley-Liss pp. 421-432.

35a. Ballerini L, Cifarelli A, Di Carlo D (1989): Percutaneous balloon dilatation of stenotic truncal valve in a newborn. Int J Cardiol 23:270-272.

36. Fischer DR, Ettedgui JA, Park SC, Siewers RD, del Nido P (1990): Carotid artery approach for balloon dilatation of aortic valve stenosis in the neonate: A preliminary report. J Am Coll Cardiol 15:1633-1636.

37. Beekman RH, Rocchini AP, Andes A (1991): Balloon valvuloplasty for critical aortic stenosis in the newborn: influence of new catheter technology. J Am Coll Cardiol 17:1172-1176.

38. Rao PS, Wilson AD, Brazy J (1992): Transumbilical balloon coarctation angioplasty in a neonate with critical aortic coarctation. Am Heart J 124:1622-1624.

39. Thapar MK, Rao PS (1990): Use of propranolol for severe dynamic infundibular obstruction prior to balloon pulmonary valvuloplasty. Cathet Cardiovasc Diagn 19:240-242.

40. Marx GR, Allen HD, Ovitt TW, Hanson W, Keiter-Marek J (1988): Balloon dilation angioplasty of Blalock-Taussig shunts. Am J Cardiol 62:824-827.

41. Ali Khan MA, Al Yousef S, Huhta JC, Bricker JT, Mullins CE, Sawyer W (1989): Critical pulmonary valve stenosis in patients less than 1 year of age: Treatment with percutaneous gradational balloon pulmonary valvuloplasty. Am Heart J 117:1008-1114.

42. Treacy EP, Duncan WJ, Tyrrell MJ, Lowry NJ (1991): Neurological complications of balloon angioplasty in children. Pediatr Cardiol 12:98-101.

43. Rao PS: Neurologic complications following balloon angioplasty. Pediatr Cardiol (in press).

44. Radtke W, Keane JF, Fellows KE, Lang P, Lock JE (1986): Percutaneous balloon valvotomy of congenital pulmonary stenosis using oversized balloons. J Am Coll Cardiol 8:909-915.

45. Rao PS (1987): Influence of balloon size on the short-term and long-term results of balloon pulmonary valvuloplasty. Texas Heart Inst J 14:57-61.

46. Rao PS (1988): How big a balloon and how many balloons for pulmonary valvuloplasty. Am Heart J 116:577-580.

47. Rao PS (1988): Further observations on the role of balloon size on the short-term and intermediate-term results of balloon pulmonary valvuloplasty. Br Heart J 60:507-511.

48. Ring JC, Kulik TJ, Burke BA (1986): Morphologic changes induced by dilatation of pulmonary valve annulus with over-large balloons in normal newborn lamb. Am J Cardiol 55:210-214.

49. Rao PS (1988): Balloon dilatation in infants and children with dysplastic pulmonary valves: short-term and intermediate-term results. Am Heart J 116:1168-1176.

50. Shaddy RE, Boucek MM, Sturtevant JE, Ruttenberg HD, Orsmond GS (1990): Gradient reduction, aortic valve regurgitation and prolapse after balloon aortic valvuloplasty in 32 consecutive patients with congenital aortic stenosis. J Am Coll Cardiol 16:451-456.

51. Suarez de Lezo J, Pan M, Sancho M, Herrera N, Arizen J, Franko M, Concha M, Valles F, Romanos A (1986): Percutaneous transluminal balloon dilatation for discrete subaortic stenosis. Am J Cardiol 58:619-621.

52. Arora R, Goel PK, Lochan R, Mohan JC, Khalilullah M (1988): Percutaneous transluminal balloon dilatation in discrete subaortic stenosis. Am Heart J 116:1041-1042.

53. Biancaniello TM (1989): Balloon dilatation in discrete subaortic stenosis. Am Heart J 117:1397.

54. Rao PS, Najjar HN, Mardini MK, Solymar L, Thapar MK (1988): Balloon angioplasty for coarctation of the aorta: Immediate and long-term results. Am Heart J 115:657-665.

55. Lock JE, Bass JL, Amplatz K, Fuhrman BP, Castaneda-Zuniga W (1983): Balloon dilatation angioplasty of aortic coarctation in infants and children. Circulation 68:109-116.

56. Rao PS, Wilson AD, Chopra PS (1990): Immediate and follow-up results of balloon angioplasty of postoperative recoarctation in infants and children. Am Heart J 120:1315-1320.

57. Lock JE, Castaneda-Zuniga WR, Fuhrman BP, Bass JL (1983): Balloon dilatation angioplasty of hypoplastic and stenotic pulmonary arteries. Circulation 67:962-967.

58. Rao PS (1992): Transcatheter management of cyanotic congenital heart defects: A review. Clin Cardiol 15:483-496.

59. Dev V, Shrivastava S (1989): Transverse balloon tear in valvuloplasty. Am Heart J 117:1397-1398.

60. Lloyd TR, Marvin WJ Jr, Mahoney LT, Lauer RM (1987): Balloon dilatation valvuloplasty of bioprosthetic valves in extracardiac conduits. Am Heart J 114:268-274.

61. Waldman JD, Schoen FJ, Kirkpatrick SE, Matthewson JW, George L, Lamberti JJ (1987): Balloon dilatation of porcine bioprosthetic valves in pulmonary position. Circulation 76:109-114.

62. Rao PS (1990): Balloon rupture during valvuloplasty. Am Heart J 119:144.

63. Attia I, Weinhaus L, Walls JT, Lababidi Z (1987): Rupture of tricuspid valve papillary muscle during balloon pulmonary valvuloplasty. Am Heart J 113:1233-1234.

64. Lo RNS, Lau KC, Leung MP (1988): Complete heart block after balloon dilatation of congenital pulmonary stenosis. Br Heart J 59:384-386.

65. Al Kasab S, Ribeiro P, Al Zaibag M (1987): Use of double balloon technique for percutaneous balloon pulmonary valvotomy in adults. Br Heart J 58:136-141.

66. Beekman RH, Rocchini AP, Crowley DC, Snider AR, Serwer GA, Dick M II, Rosenthal A (1988): Comparison of single and double balloon valvuloplasty in children with aortic stenosis. J Am Coll Cardiol 12:480-485.

67. Rao PS, Fawzy ME (1988): Double balloon technique for percutaneous balloon pulmonary valvuloplasty: comparison with single balloon technique. J Interventional Cardiol 1:257-262.

68. Rao PS (1989): Double balloon aortic valvuloplasty in children. J Am Coll Cardiol 13:1216.

69. Mullins CE, Nihill MR, Vick GW III, Ludomirsky A, O'Laughlin MP, Bricker JT, Judd VE (1987): Double balloon technique for dilation of valvular or vessel stenosis in congenital and acquired heart disease. J Am Coll Cardiol 10:107-114.

70. D'Souza VJ, Velasquez G, Weesner KM, Prabhu S (1984): Transluminal angioplasty of aortic coarctation with a two-balloon technique. Am J Cardiol 54:457-458.

71. Al Zaibag M, Ribeiro PA, Al Kasab S, Al Fagih MR (1986): Percutaneous double balloon valvuloplasty for rheumatic mitral valve stenosis. Lancet 1:757-761.

72. Al Zaibag M, Ribeiro PA, Al Kasab S, Halim M, Idris MT, Habbab M, Shahed M, Sawyer W (1988): One year follow-up after percutaneous double balloon mitral valvotomy. Am J Cardiol 63:126-127.

73. Al Kasab S, Ribeiro PA, Al Zaibag M, Al Bitar I, Idris MT, Shahed M, Sawyer W (1989): Comparison of results of percutaneous mitral valvotomy using single- and double-balloon techniques. Am J Cardiol 63:135-136.

74. Ribeiro PA, Al Zaibag M, Al Kasab S, Idris M, Halim M, Abdullah M, Shahed M (1988): Percutaneous double balloon valvotomy for rheumatic tricuspid stenosis. Am J Cardiol 61:660-662.

75. Meier B, Friedli B, Oberhaensli I, Belenger J, Finci L (1986): Trefoil balloon for percutaneous valvuloplasty. Cathet Cardiovasc Diagn 12:227-281.

76. Van den Berg EJM, Niemeyer MG, Plokker TWM, Ernst SMPG, de Korte J (1986): New triple-lumen balloon catheter for percutaneous (pulmonary) valvuloplasty. Cathet Cardiovasc Diagn 12:352-356.

77. Meier B, Friedli B, von Segesser L (1988): Valvuloplasty with trefoil and bifoil balloons and long sheath technique. Herz 13:1-13.

78. Thanopoulos BD, Margetakis A, Papadopoulos G, Kefalakis E, Rokas S (1989): Valvuloplasty with large trefoil balloons for the treatment of congenital pulmonary stenosis. Acta Paediatr Scand 78:742-746.

79. Meier B, Friedli B, Oberhänsli I (1986): Trefoil balloon for aortic valvuloplasty. Br Heart J 56:292-293.

80. Sreeram N, Walsh K, Arnold R (1991): Balloon valvuloplasty in children using carbon dioxide, abstracted. Circulation 84(Suppl II):513.

81. Rao PS, Thapar MK, Kutayli F (1988): Causes of restenosis following balloon valvuloplasty for valvar pulmonic stenosis. Am J Cardiol 62:979-982.

82. Rao PS, Thapar MK, Kutayli F, Carey P (1989): Causes of recoarctation after balloon angioplasty of unoperated aortic coarctation. J Am Coll Cardiol 13:109-115.

83. Lababidi Z, Wu J, Walls JT (1984): Percutaneous balloon aortic valvuloplasty: results in 23 patients. Am J Cardiol 54:194–197.

84. Kiel AA, Devanter V, Readinger RI, Dungan WT, Norton JB (1986): Aortic balloon valvuloplasty with transluminal venous balloon inflow occlusion (case report). Pediatr Cardiol 7:103–105.

85. Silove ED, Vogel JHK, Grover RF (1968): The pressure gradient in ventricular outflow obstruction: influence of peripheral resistance. Cardiovasc Res 3:234–242.

86. Rao PS, Linde LM (1974): Pressure and energy in the cardiovascular chambers. Chest 66:176–178.

87. Pan M, Suárez de Lezo J, Herrera N, Sancho M, Arizón J, Romero M, Franco M, Concha M, Vallés F, Romanos A (1987): Two-level left ventricular outflow balloon dilation: Sequential therapeutic approach. Am Heart J 114:162–165.

88. Chen CR, Lo ZX, Huang ZD, Mei J (1988): Percutaneous double balloon valvuloplasty for a patient with mitral and tricuspid stenosis. Quangdong Med J 9:29–30.

89. Shrivastava S, Radhakrishnan S, Dev V (1988): Concurrent balloon dilatation of tricuspid and calcific mitral valve in a patient with rheumatic heart disease. Int J Cardiol 20:133–137.

90. Chen CR, Lo ZX, Huang ZD, Chen TO (1988): Concurrent percutaneous balloon valvuloplasty for combined tricuspid and pulmonic stenosis. Cathet Cardiovasc Diagn 15:55–60.

91. Cheng TO (1989): Multivalve percutaneous balloon valvuloplasty. Cathet Cardiovasc Diagn 16:109–112.

92. Konugres GS, Lau FYK, Ruiz C (1990): Successive percutaneous double-balloon mitral, aortic and tricuspid valvotomy in rheumatic trivalvar stenosis. Am Heart J 119:663–666.

93. Kritzer G, Block P, Palacios I (1987): Simultaneous percutaneous mitral and aortic balloon valvotomy in an elderly patient. Am Heart J 114:420–423.

94. Savas V, Grines CL, O'Neill WW (1991): Percutaneous triple-valve balloon valvuloplasty in a pregnant woman. Cathet Cardiovasc Diagn 24:288–294.

95. Yang SY, Qian CC, Hsia YF, Hwa YT, Qian TC, Xu DD, Chao SC, Wu TF (1991): Transcatheter double-blade valvotomy for the treatment of valvar pulmonic stenosis. Pediatr Cardiol 12:224–226.

96. Lee G, Ikeda RM, Kozina J, Mason DT (1981): Laser dissolution of coronary atherosclerotic obstruction. Am Heart J 102:1074–1076.

97. Lee G, Ikeda RM, Dwyer RM (1982): Feasibility of intravascular laser irradiation for in vivo visualization and therapy of cardiovascular disease. Am Heart J 103:1070–1072.

98. Riemenschneider TA, Lee G, Ikeda RM, Bommer WJ, Stobbe D, Ogata C, Rebeck K, Reis RL, Mason DT (1983): Laser irradiation of congenital heart disease: Potential for palliation and correction of intracardiac and intravascular defects. Am Heart J 106:1389–1393.

99. Lee G, Ikeda RM, Stobbe D (1983): Laser irradiation of human atherosclerotic obstructive disease: Simultaneous visualization and vaporization achieved by a dual fiberoptic catheter. Am Heart J 105:163–165.

100. Qureshi SA, Rosenthal E, Tynan M, Anjos R, Baker EJ (1991): Transcatheter laser-assisted balloon pulmonary valve dilatation in pulmonic valve atresia. Am J Cardiol 67:428–431.

101. Simpson JB, Matthew RS, Robertson GC, Cipriano PR, Hayden WG, Johnson DE, Fogarty TJ (1988): Transluminal atherectomy for occlusive peripheral vascular disease. Am J Cardiol 61:96G–101G.

102. Simpson JB, Robertson GC, Selmen MR (1988): Percutaneous coronary atherectomy, abstracted. J Am Coll Cardiol 11(Suppl A):110A.

103. Qureshi SA, Parsons JM, Tynan M (1990): Percutaneous transcatheter myectomy of subvalvar pulmonary stenosis in tetralogy of Fallot: A new palliative technique with an atherectomy catheter. Br Heart J 64:163–165.

104. Rao PS, Wilson AD, Thapar MK, Brais M (1992): Balloon pulmonary valvuloplasty in the management of cyanotic congenital heart defects. Cathet Cardiovasc Diagn 25:16–24.

5

Mechanism of Balloon Valvuloplasty/Angioplasty

Mohinder K. Thapar, M.D., and P. Syamasundar Rao, M.D.

Department of Pediatrics, Division of Pediatric Cardiology,
University of Texas Medical School, Houston, Texas 77030 (M.K.T.),
and Department of Pediatrics, Division of Pediatric Cardiology,
University of Wisconsin Medical School, University of Wisconsin
Children's Hospital, Madison, Wisconsin 53792-4108 (P.S.R.)

INTRODUCTION

In the era of balloon mania, the understanding of the mechanics of balloon dilatation, characteristics of the balloon material and the shaft that carries the balloon, and the response of the tissue to be dilated can help the operator to select the appropriate type of catheter to achieve the best results. It can also enhance the understanding of when and where to use a larger or smaller balloon, single or multiple balloons, and the appropriate balloon material. In this chapter we highlight these and other aspects of balloon dilatation.

BALLOON MATERIAL

Ideally, the material of the balloon should be noncompliant; in reality, though, this is not completely so. All of the balloon materials do stretch to a varying degree under pressure. Therefore, the diameter will continue to increase slightly, with increasing pressure. This change in diameter depends on the type of material and on the temperature. Moreover, repeated dilatations also increase the stretching and thus the diameter of the balloon. Most commercially available balloons are made from four basic materials. There are hundreds of resins within each polymer type, and each manufacturer has his own proprietary. The four basic material types are:

1. Polyvinyl chloride (PVC)—used by USCI and Cook
2. Polyethylene (PE)—used by ACS and Mansfield
3. Polyolefin copolymer (POC)—used by SciMed and ACS
4. Polyethylene terephthalate (PET)—used by USCI and Medi Tech

The physical properties of the balloon depend not only on the resin but also on the method of processing the material. All of these materials are biocompatible. For appropriate selection of the balloon, the interventionalist should be aware of yield strength, ultimate tensile strength, distensibility, pressure capability, profile, heat characteristics, and failure mode of the balloon material [1–4].

Yield Strength

Yield strength is the force or pressure required to cause permanent deformation of the material. Therefore, if the pressure used is more than the yield strength of the balloon material, it would result in deformity of the balloon, and consequently its insertion or retrieval may become difficult.

Ultimate Tensile Strength

Ultimate tensile strength is the force or pressure required to break (rupture) the mate-

Transcatheter Therapy in Pediatric Cardiology, pages 45–58
© 1993 Wiley-Liss, Inc.

rial. During dilatation, applied pressure should not exceed ultimate tensile strength in order to avoid rupture of the balloon. However, if the yield strength and ultimate tensile strength are approximately the same, then the diameter of the balloon will change very little under pressure before it ruptures. This is true for most of the materials used in the currently available balloons.

Balloon Distention

The change in diameter with increasing pressure is known as *balloon distention*. Different materials have different rates of distention. Most manufacturers publish this information. However, this is not important when balloons are used in places with large areas and when tissues are compliant. The importance lies when the balloon is applied in vessels of small diameter, such as coronary arteries. For example, a 3 mm balloon at 4 atm of pressure may become 3.5 mm in diameter at 8 atm, resulting in the overdistention of the vessel and consequent complications (*e.g.,* dissection).

Moreover, balloons that do not significantly change in diameter with increasing pressure will be able to produce a higher dilating force. Even repeated inflations will result in resuming the same diameter of the balloon that will retain its shape. Therefore such material produces less trauma at the site of entry during removal.

Balloon Strength

Balloon strength is maximum pressure above which 99.9% of balloons will rupture. This is related to the type of the material and method of its processing. Some materials, such as PET, can be fabricated to produce very thin-walled balloons that can withstand high pressures. The benefit of thin-walled balloons is that the balloons become more flexible and have low profiles. Thin-walled balloons, however, can be easily damaged during manipulation, resulting in low burst pressure. The PVC balloons are thicker and stiffer than PE and POC balloons. A variety of extra-strength balloons are now available for specific applications, which are very good for tract dilatation, tough calcified lesions, and surgical strictures. However, they become more wrinkled after deflation and thus have a higher rate of vascular complications.

Balloon Profile

The balloon profile indicates the ease with which a balloon can be negotiated through a narrow tortuous course. It is well recognized that thin-walled balloons have a lower profile value than thick-walled balloons. The ability of the balloon to negotiate its way through a lesion is also dependent on pushability, trackability, and the balloon wrap. The profile can be measured by attempting to push the distal portion of the balloon through progressively smaller holes with no extra effort. The smallest hole passed by the balloon is the profile value. In marketing tactics, balloon profile is being overemphasized. As pointed out before, other factors are also important for negotiating the small hole. Because of thinner balloon walls, PET balloons have a lower profile value than PVC, PE, and POC balloons.

Heat Characteristics

The ideal balloon should return to a folded, low-profile wrap around the shaft after repeated inflations and deflations. This heat setting characteristic is better with balloons made from PE and POC than those from other materials [4]. Some materials retain this memory for a longer time than others. If they lose this memory, their advancement or removal may be difficult and may result in tissue damage.

Failure Mode

For a variety of reasons, such as manufacturing or packaging damage, handling in the catheterization laboratory, or the need to apply pressure beyond the balloon strength to open a lesion, balloons occasionally fail. In such events, the balloon usually ruptures longitudinally rather than circumferentially. Circumferentially ruptured balloons can cause excessive damage during their removal. Some materials, such as PVC, PE, and POC, are more prone to rupture in a longitudinal manner than is PET.

Balloons tolerating high inflation pressures are also available. These balloons are either reinforced or made from a high-strength polymer. These types of balloons are good for tract dilatation or dilatation of lesions caused by surgical strictures and tough lesions due to calcification. However, these balloons wrinkle more on deflation. This may result in a higher incidence of vascular complications. Cases in which high-pressure balloons are used should be monitored more closely.

DILATING FORCES

During the inflation of the balloon, various forces are responsible for dilating the stenotic segment. Hydrostatic pressure in a cylinder exerts force in a radial manner. This force depends on the following:

Force = pressure × area of the cylinder (1)

Area = length × circumference (2)

Circumference = $2\pi r$ (3)

Thus the hydrostatic force is directly related to the pressure applied and to the length and radius of the cylinder. With the same pressure, therefore, more hydrostatic force will act on the lesion with a larger diameter balloon. Hydrostatic force may play a significant role in dilating long-segment lesions. This force may play a negligible role in localized and narrower lesions. The circumferential force is also known as the *hoop stress* and is based on LaPlace's law [5]. The larger the balloon, the higher is the pressure exerted (Fig. 1). Therefore, to achieve the same amount of force in a small-diameter balloon, a higher pressure is required.

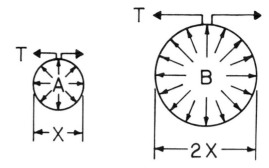

Fig. 1. Hoop stress (T) at the same pressure is twice as great as in a larger balloon. (Reproduced from Abele [2], with permission of the publisher.)

As can be seen by the above equations, force is also affected by the balloon length. This effect depends on the balloon material. With materials that stretch (*e.g.*, PVC), shorter balloons exert more force than longer balloons. However, with balloons that do not stretch (low compliance, *e.g.*, treated PE), the dilating force does not decrease with increasing length of the balloon.

The radial force caused by hydrostatic pressure will be least in the region where the diameter is the smallest. Therefore, to achieve an adequate hydrostatic force, higher pressure is required to stretch the narrow segment of the tube. Because the material of these balloons has a very low compliance, the diameter of the balloon does not change significantly with the increase in hydrostatic force. Once the balloon has achieved its maximum diameter, the increase in pressure results in increased tensile force. The diameter of the balloon does change along the length of the balloon when it is across a localized, stenotic lesion. Thus the hoop stress or tensile force changes at various points along the length of the balloon. This creates vectorial forces that act on the narrow segment. This phenomenon has been compared by Abele [2,3] to the act of trying to lift the weight in the center of a sagging clothesline by pulling on the ends of the string (Fig. 2). These vectorial forces are indirectly related to the angle created by the depressed segment.

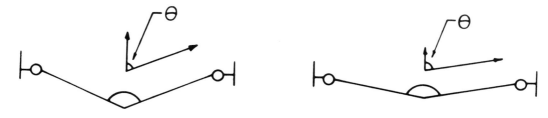

Fig. 2. Clothesline effect. As the line straightens out (balloon surface becomes round), force vector angle (θ) increases and component of force pushing upward (outward on balloon) decreases. (Reproduced from Abele [2], with permission of the publisher.

The smaller the angle along the surface of the membrane, the greater is the vectorial or tensile force acting on the segment.

Thus, based on this principle, a shorter-length balloon will have a deeper indentation or smaller angle than a longer balloon. Therefore a shorter balloon will create a higher dilating force. A deeper indentation or an acute angle can also be achieved by using a larger diameter for the balloon. Thus a short-length, large-diameter balloon will be more effective than a long balloon with a small diameter for the same lesion, and the total dilating force is the sum of hydrostatic pressure and mechanical vector force at the balloon indentation caused by the stenotic lesion (clothesline effect).

Based on the above discussions and on observations made elsewhere [1-4], the following inferences can be drawn:

1. For the same pressure, there is a greater dilating force for a larger-diameter balloon than for a smaller-diameter balloon.

2. For the same pressure, a tighter stenotic area will receive a greater dilating force than a less tight stenotic lesion.

3. For the same pressure, a larger stenotic area will receive a higher dilating force than a smaller stenotic area.

4. For the same size balloon and lesion, the higher the inflation pressure, the greater the dilating force; these are related in a linear fashion.

5. Compliant balloon material stretches under pressure and prevents the force to act on the stenotic lesion. The balloon may expand around the lesion rather than exerting pressure on it. By contrast, a low (or non-) compliance balloon material will allow the balloon to exert the dilating force on the stenotic lesion with less damage to the tissues around the lesion.

6. Higher inflation pressures will not significantly increase the diameter of the balloon because the commonly used balloon materials (especially treated polyethylene) do not expand due to the fact that the yield strength (the force at which permanent deformation of the material occurs) and the ultimate tensile strength (the force necessary to break the balloon material) of the balloon material are very close to each other.

7. Longer durations of balloon inflation at higher pressures can weaken the balloon material. Consequently, a balloon subjected to a longer period of pressure inflation will have a lower burst pressure than when the balloon is fresh.

OTHER ELEMENTS OF BALLOONS AND CATHETERS

1. The catheter tip should be short and smooth for easy entry into the vessel and for positioning the balloon catheter across the stenotic lesion.

2. The transition point between the catheter and balloon should be gradual and smooth.

3. The catheter shaft should have high torque with optimum stiffness to follow the

guidewire. When the catheters are too soft or too stiff, it may be difficult to advance them through a tortuous course.

4. Although automated balloon inflation devices are available, most workers use a simple syringe for balloon inflation because of simplicity and tactile feedback. During inflation of the balloon, the smaller the diameter of syringe, the greater is the pressure that can be applied. However, during deflation of the balloon, a large-diameter syringe should be used because it produces a greater volume displacement and a greater suction force to facilitate rapid deflation of the balloon. Ideally, a three-way stopcock should be attached to the balloon. Inflation should be carried out with a 10 ml syringe, and deflation should be carried out with a 20 or 30 ml syringe. Pressures of inflation and suction that can be achieved with various syringes are listed in Table I.

5. Use of diluted contrast material is advisable to reduce the viscosity of the balloon-inflating fluid. We generally use three parts saline and one part contrast material (Conray 400).

6. It is advisable to have a pressure monitoring device so that pressure of balloon inflation could be limited to the inflation pressure recommended by the manufacturer. This would avoid balloon rupture. However, it should be noted that most manufacturers specify a far lower inflation pressure than the balloon can tolerate; this observation is based on clinical experience of the authors and not on in vivo or in vitro studies. As stated above,

maintaining a high pressure over a period of time will weaken the balloon material and lower the burst pressure compared with a fresh balloon. This varies with the type of balloon material.

7. Rapid inflation and deflation are beneficial when valvar dilatations are performed, because the entire cardiac output is obstructed during the balloon inflation. Improved catheter design to increase the size of balloon-filling lumen and decrease the distal (guidewire-carrying) lumen can be achieved. Some efforts in this direction have already been made [6], and further changes to decrease inflation/deflation time without compromising the ability of positioning the catheter over a guidewire across the stenotic lesion is, in the opinion of the authors, feasible.

8. Under certain circumstances, such as large diameter of the valve annulus, a single balloon may be inadequate to dilate the valve. This may necessitate the use of two balloons. The effective diameter of the two balloons is not the total sum of the diameters of the two balloons. The effective diameter of the two balloons should be calculated based on the following formula [7]:

$$\frac{D_1 + D_2 + \pi\left(\dfrac{D_1}{2} + \dfrac{D_2}{2}\right)}{\pi}$$

where D_1 and D_2 are diameters of the balloons used. Another advantage of the use of two

TABLE I. Syringe Pressure and Suction[a]

Syringe size (ml)	Inside diameter syringe barrel (cm)[b]	Maximum practical pressure generated (atm)[c]	Maximum practical suction generated (atm)
50	2.5	5.2	0.98
10	1.4	9.4	0.90
6	1.23	11.0	0.83
3	0.78	21.0	0.67
1	0.48	40.0	0.50

[a]Reproduced from Abele [2], with permission of the publisher.
[b]Not all manufacturers produce syringes with same diameter for particular volume, so these numbers are approximate.
[c]Pressure generated by hard squeeze of thumb on plunger of syringe.

balloons is that the lumen of valve or vessel is not completely occluded [8]. This may minimize the adverse hemodynamic effects during inflation/deflation. However, the use of two balloons will result in an oblong configuration [8,9] of the valve and may increase the risk of complications. However, in clinical practice, two balloons have been quite frequently used, and serious complications have not been reported [9-16].

9. Due to the concern for the oblong configuration with double-balloon technique, a technique of balloon dilatation with triple balloons attached to the same catheter (trefoil balloons) or three different balloons has been developed [17-22]. The advantage of triple balloons is that it results in a rounded or triangular configuration of the valve or vessel to be dilated. This may result in less damage to the tissues. Based on a mathematical model, Gaylord et al. [22] suggested the following formula to calculate the diameter of the balloons for an undistorted circular lumen:

$$D = 2.154 \, d$$

where D = diameter of the circular lumen, and d = diameter of each balloon. Conversely, the diameter of the balloon to be chosen for dilatation can be calculated [22] if the diameter of the vessel or valve to be dilated is known:

$$d = 0.46 \, D$$

If a larger effective diameter than the actual size of the vascular or valvar lumen is desired, the lumen will be distorted to a triangular shape, and the calculations are somewhat different. The respective formulas for distorted lumen are

$$D' = 1.955d$$

and

$$d = 0.51 \, D'$$

where D' is diameter of the distorted lumen, and d is the diameter of the equal-sized balloons.

The above formulas are based on usage of equal-sized balloons. When unequal-sized balloons are used, the derivations of the formula are more complex [22]. Based on these and other considerations, Gaylord et al. [22] developed tables from which diameters of the balloon sizes needed for a given diameter lumen can be found. The need for use of triple balloons in pediatric cardiology practice is limited. Should such a need arise, the reader is referred to the tables developed by Gaylord and associates [22] for determining the balloon sizes that are needed for balloon dilatation.

These authors also suggested that biplane measurement of the lumen size be performed to ensure the circular nature of the lumen to be dilated. If the lumen is oblong, dilatation with two balloons is suggested. While dilatation with triple balloons has theoretical advantages, including the use of smaller-sized balloons, thus avoiding excessive injury to the entry vessel and increasing pressure of balloon inflation, the major disadvantage is that of finding three sites of balloon entry, which may be difficult and cumbersome.

PHYSIOLOGY OF INTRACARDIAC OCCLUSION DURING BALLOON DILATATION

By technical necessity, balloon dilatation of stenotic lesions of the heart produces complete but transient obstruction to blood flow. This results in development of acute hypertension in the cardiac chamber proximal to the obstruction and hypotension and decreased perfusion in the structures distal to the obstruction. Several workers investigated these issues in intact animal preparations with non-hypertrophied [23-26] and hypertrophied [26] ventricles, as well as in human subjects undergoing balloon valvuloplasty [27,28]. Both animal and human studies suggest that complete ventricular obstruction for brief periods of time is well tolerated and that the hypertrophied ventricle is not at a greater risk for development of severe dysrhythmia or irreversible failure than a normal ventricle [26].

With right ventricular (RV) outflow obstruction, the RV myocardial blood flow increases with increasing RV hypertension, but this fails to increase in proportion to demand [24]. With the onset of RV failure, defined as an increase in RV end-diastolic pressure and decreased aortic pressure and cardiac output, coronary flow reserve decreases. Also, RV free-wall ischemia, as demonstrated by biochemical markers (decreased creatine phosphate and ATP), develops. These changes reverse by raising the aortic pressure following infusion of phenylephrine [24].

During balloon occlusion, the ventricular systolic pressure increases to above the systemic level [26] and may reach 58% (for left ventricle) to 95% (for RV) of predilatation values [27]. The ventricular end-diastolic pressure also increases; the longer the duration of outflow occlusion, the higher is the elevation of end-diastolic pressure. Attempts to relieve high intracardiac pressure seem to take place both by atrioventricular valve regurgitation and shunting across the patent foramen ovale [27,29] and by development of disynergic and hypokinetic ventricular contractions [27]. Following balloon deflation, the pressures return toward preocclusion values, with a slight increase in cardiac output in the postocclusion period.

Suárez de Lezo et al. [28] studied the effects of balloon valvuloplasty (mitral and aortic) on the plasma levels of renin, atrial natriuretic factor (ANF), and vasopressin. They detected no change in renin activity. An abrupt increase in ANF and vasopressin occurred. As expected, the ANF elevation is directly proportional to the increase in left atrial or pulmonary arterial wedge pressure, while vasopressin levels are inversely (exponentially) related to the peak aortic pressure.

Acute ventricular obstruction, as discussed above, causes distention of the ventricle, increased transmyocardial pressure, and potential compromise to myocardial perfusion, particularly in the left ventricle. To circumvent this problem, double balloons [10,13], bifoil and trefoil balloons [17-21], Y-connector to create left-ventricle-to-right-atrial shunt [30], and inflow caval balloon occlusion [31] have been advocated. It is not clear if the ventricular distension for short periods of time, as required during balloon valvuloplasty, is truly harmful, nor is it clearly shown that the above-proposed methods cause significant relief of ventricular distension. We have advocated short periods (5 seconds) of inflation and do not believe that the above-described methods [10,13,17-21,30,31] have significant advantages [32]. Indeed, some of these procedures may increase the complexity of valvuloplasty and prolong the duration of the procedure.

The effect of descending aortic occlusion was studied in animal models by Stokland et al. [33]; this is similar to the situation during balloon coarctation angioplasty. During complete occlusion of the descending aorta, left ventricular systolic pressure increased, as did the end-diastolic and end-systolic volumes. The blood flow more than doubled in the superior vena cava, while that in the inferior vena cava fell by 90%. When both the aorta and inferior vena cava were simultaneously occluded, increases in left ventricular systolic pressure and in superior vena caval flow did not occur, and left ventricular end-diastolic volume actually decreased. Infusion of 25 ml/kg body weight of blood into the jugular vein during combined descending aortic and inferior vena caval obstruction reproduced the effects of isolated descending aortic occlusion. These data suggested that transfer of blood from the inferior vena caval draining areas takes place during descending aortic occlusion and that this transfer of blood accounts for increased left ventricular end-diastolic volume, activation of the Frank-Starling mechanism, and increased stroke volume and, consequently, elevated left ventricular pressure [33]. While these are important and interesting studies, we are not sure that we have, as yet, an adequate basis to institute simultaneous inferior caval occlusion during routine balloon coarctation angioplasty. However, one wonders if the cerebrovascular accidents following balloon angioplasty of aortic coarctation reported in the literature [34–39] could possibly be related to the increased systolic left ventricular and cerebral arterial pressures.

PROPERTIES OF THE TISSUE

The response of the tissue to balloon dilatation varies, depending on the morphology and pathologic process. There have been several studies in which morphology of the tissue has been studied, in animal models, postmortem specimens, or during surgery after the balloon dilatation. These studies suggest that the response depends on the tissue involved and on its basic pathology.

Pulmonary Valve

The morphology of the stenotic pulmonary valve is variable [40,41]. The valve structure may be dome-shaped, bicuspid, tricuspid, or unicuspid. Commissural fusion is frequently present with bicuspid or tricuspid valve leaflets. Even with dome-shaped deformity, which appears to be the most common pathologic type [40], valve commissures are usually recognizable [41] and are fused. In addition, valve ring hypoplasia and dysplastic pulmonary valve leaflets may also be present in some patients.

Several workers examined morphologic changes of the pulmonary valve following balloon pulmonary valvuloplasty in an attempt to determine the mechanism of balloon dilatation. Visual observation during either surgery [42–49] or post mortem examination [45] and assessment by echocardiographic [44,50] and angiographic [32,51] studies have been made.

The majority of the studies suggest that commissural splitting is the most common mechanism by which balloon dilatation works. It is estimated that 90% of the patients have commissural splitting [52]. In one study, 27 of the 29 patients studied echocardiographically

were found to have commissural tears, resulting in improved pulmonary valve gradients following balloon pulmonary valvuloplasty. Increased valve excursion and/or straightening of valve leaflets with increased width of the jet of contrast flow across the pulmonary valve may be noted angiographically [32,51,53]. Partial tears of valve commissures or tearing of some of the commissures [44,45] may occur with partial relief of valve obstruction. It is likely that partial tears may be related to use of balloons smaller than the valve annulus, although no such direct correlation has been documented. The circumferential dilating force exerted by balloon inflation is likely to split (tear) the weakest part of the valve mechanism. It is likely that the fused commissures are the weakest links that can be torn with balloon dilatation. Tearing of the valve leaflets and avulsion of the valve leaflets have also been observed [43,54] following balloon valvuloplasty. Such an effect may be related to either strong, fibrotic, fused commissures that could not be torn or associated subvalvar stenosis [43]. The latter type of valve damage may cause more pulmonary valve regurgitation, although the obstruction may have been relieved.

In patients with annular hypoplasia and severe valve dysplasia, balloon valvuloplasty may not successfully relieve pulmonary valve obstruction. However, if significant valve leaflet fusion is associated with pulmonary valve dysplasia [55,56], balloon pulmonary valvuloplasty can be successful.

With regard to adverse effects of balloon pulmonary valvuloplasty, development of pulmonary insufficiency has already been noted. This appears to be more related to valve morphology in that valve leaflet tear or evulsion can occur when valve commissures are too tough to be torn by balloon force. This does not seem to be related to the size of the balloon. However, focal damage to the right ventricular outflow tract seems to be related to the diameter of the balloon used for balloon valvuloplasty. This issue was examined by Ring et al. [57] in normal newborn lambs. These investigators dilated normal pulmonary valves of newborn lambs with balloons 20% smaller to 90% larger than the valve annuli. Although no damage to the pulmonary valve annulus is noted, mural hemorrhages of varying sizes were noted in the right ventricular outflow tract when balloons larger than 50% of pulmonary valve annulus are used for balloon dilatation. The damage is minimal if the balloon is no larger than 30% of the annulus diameter. Trauma, when present, appears to be pronounced adjacent to the proximal end of the balloon. Therefore, longer balloons are likely to produce damage more than shorter balloons. These hemorrhages later may result in patchy areas of fibrosis. Moreover, in cases in which infundibular stenosis is also present, the balloon may produce damage to the myocardium. These patchy areas of fibrosis may explain some of the changes in the electrocardiogram and may form a substrate for arrhythmias in the future.

Aortic Valve

The morphology of the stenotic congenital aortic valve is also variable [41,58,59]. The majority of these valves are bicuspid in nature, although such ones appear to be formed on a trifoliate template [60]. Infrequently, clearly discernible tricuspid valve leaflet patterns and unicuspid valves may be seen; the latter are more common in symptomatic neonates and infants. Commissural fusion with eccentrically placed orifice is seen. Varying degrees of doming of the valve leaflets and thickening of the leaflets are present. Annular hypoplasia and dysplasia of the valve leaflets may be present, and again, more commonly in neonates and young infants.

The mechanism of balloon aortic valvuloplasty has been evaluated by observation of valve morphology at surgery [43,61] or by echocardiography [62]. These observations suggest that commissural splitting, and sometimes tearing of the valve leaflets, may occur following balloon aortic valvuloplasty. The degree of aortic insufficiency does not increase

and at times may improve [30,63,64]; the latter may be attributed to better co-option of the valve leaflets after valvuloplasty [63]. However, development of aortic insufficiency is a significant risk when unicommissural valves are dilated. Sholler et al. [62] observed large increases in aortic insufficiency in three of eight (38%) unicommissural aortic valves. Sometimes the aortic insufficiency may be due to technical problems; in one instance, the valve leaflet was accidentally traversed with a guidewire, a balloon catheter was positioned across it, and the balloon inflated, causing aortic insufficiency [62].

Balloons that are similar in size to the aortic valve annulus are generally recommended for balloon aortic valvuloplasty for fear of developing aortic insufficiency. Helgason et al. [65] used varying sizes of balloons to dilate aortic valves in normal lambs. When balloon: annulus ratios were <1.1, there was no significant damage to the left ventricular outflow tract or to the aortic valve leaflets. However, when balloons >1.2 times the aortic valve annulus were used, significant aortic insufficiency by aortography and tears in aortic valve cusp, interventricular septum, and ascending aorta were observed on pathologic examination [65]. These data suggest that balloons >1.1 times aortic valve annulus should not be used for balloon aortic valvuloplasty. However, more recent clinical studies in children with valvar and subvalvar aortic stenoses did not substantiate the relationship between balloon:annulus ratio and degree of aortic insufficiency [66,67]. Perhaps the valve morphology of the stenotic aortic valve is more important than the size of the balloon used.

Acquired aortic stenosis, more frequently seen in adult patients, is caused either by degenerative changes or by a rheumatic disease process [41,68,69]. The former, frequently referred to as *calcific aortic stenosis*, may occur in a congenital bicuspid aortic valve, but tricuspid valves are more common [68–71]. The pathogenesis is "wear and tear," with resultant fibrosis and calcification [68–71]. Commissural fusion is minimal and infrequent [70]. With rheumatic disease, commissural fusion is present in addition to degenerative calcific changes. Relief of aortic obstruction by balloon valvuloplasty in calcific aortic stenosis appears to be secondary to fracture of calcified nodules, decreased cusp rigidity, and increased mobility of valve leaflets [69,71]. Separation of fused commissures has also been observed [71]. Liberation and embolization of calcific debris, valve leaflet tears, and disruptions of valve ring have not been observed [69,71].

Atrioventricular Valves

Atrioventricular valve stenosis may be congenital or acquired (most commonly rheumatic) in origin. Balloon valvuloplasty may be beneficial in congenital stenosis of mitral or tricuspid valve if valve fusion is the major pathologic feature. Rheumatic obstructions are more frequently secondary to valve fusion and are amenable to balloon valvuloplasty. For further details of the pathology and mechanisms of balloon dilation in atrioventricular stenosis, the reader is referred to Chapters 8 and 15.

Aortic Coarctation

Native aortic coarctations are most usually located distal to the left subclavian artery at the level of ductus arteriosus. The shelf-like coarcted segment consists of localized hyperplasia of the media and intima and is composed of fibrous and fibroelastic tissue. In addition, Isner et al. [72] described disarray and depletion of elastic tissue (changes akin to cystic medial necrosis) in all specimen studies; severe changes were present in two-thirds of the coarctation segments examined. However, similar histologic studies by Ho et al. [73] revealed cystic medial necrosis type of changes in only one-half of the specimens examined.

Postmortem balloon dilatation of aortic coarctation [74], in vitro dilatation of excised human coarcted aortic segments [73,75], and in vivo dilatation of surgically created aortic

coarctations in animal models [76,77] were performed in an attempt to determine the feasibility of dilating aortic coarctation and to detect the mechanism and effect of balloon dilatation. Linear and oblique intimal and medial tears without disruption of adventitia were noted by most workers. In some, the tears may be limited to the intimal layers; in most, these extend into the media, and rarely the tears may reach adventitial layers. Subsequently, the presence of intimal and medial tears following balloon dilatation of human aortic coarctations was confirmed [39,78–84]. As a matter of fact, Suárez de Lezo et al. [39] suggested that there is less gradient at follow-up in patients with intimal tears immediately after angioplasty than those without intimal tears.

Multiple types of angiographic and pathologic appearances of aortic coarctation exist. It is not clear which type is more amenable to balloon angioplasty. It is generally thought that only discrete short-segment coarctations are "dilatable" whereas diffuse or long-segment coarctations are not amenable to balloon angioplasty. While this may generally be true, we have had success with long-segment coarctations as well [85]. Centrally located coarctations are thought to have better results than eccentric coarctations [83].

Although the cause of aneurysmal formation in a small percentage of patients following balloon angioplasty is not clearly known, use of large-sized balloons and inadvertent manipulation of tips of guidewires/catheters in the area of a recently dilated lesion is likely to increase the incidence of aneurysms. Complete avoidance of manipulation of catheter/guidewire tips in the region of freshly dilated coarctation and limiting the size of balloons to the size of the descending aorta at the level of the diaphragm are likely to be useful in reducing the incidence of aneurysms.

In aortic recoarctations, in addition to the pathologic changes described above, mural and periaortic fibrosis is present. Although the initial impression [76] was that the aortic recoarctations are not "dilatable," subsequent work [77] suggested that surgically created co-arctations are indeed amenable to balloon angioplasty. Intimal tears were noted in the animal experimental model, and these tears extended into the media. The tears are generally located in the nonoperated aortic wall and are thought to be responsible for relief of aortic recoarctations.

Dense fibrous tissue surrounding the suture site was thought to be protective and to prevent rupture of the aorta or aneurysmal formation. But experience reported by the Valvuloplasty and Angioplasty of Congenital Anomalies Registry [35] of aortic rupture in a recoarcted patient negates the theorized advantage of protective periaortic scar tissues.

Spasm of the arterial wall following balloon angioplasty is well documented in coronary and renal artery angioplasty [86,88]. Multiple theories have been advanced to explain the mechanism of vasoconstriction. Recent studies suggest that the arterial spasm may be caused by stretch- or pressure-induced endothelium-dependent vasoconstriction [89]. This phenomenon appears to be independent of platelet aggregation and neurogenic effect and is not prevented by calcium channel blockers, antiplatelet agents, heparin, or a combination thereof, and it appears to be mediated by endothelium-derived cyclooxygenase products [89]. While this vasoconstrictor effect following balloon angioplasty appears to have adverse effects in small-vessel angioplasty, it is not known whether such a vasoconstrictor effect is present following balloon coarctation angioplasty and, if present, whether it has any adverse consequences.

Other Lesions

There are several other types of stenotic lesions of the heart that are amenable to balloon dilatation procedures. The pathology of the lesions and the mechanisms of relief of obstruction by balloon dilatation of these lesions are discussed in Chapters 9, 12, 13, 14, and 15, (this volume) and thus are not reviewed here.

ACKNOWLEDGMENTS

The authors thank Mr. J.E. Abele for his review and critique of the manuscript.

REFERENCES

1. Athansoulis CA (1980): Percutaneous transluminal angioplasty: General principles. Am J Roentgenol 135:893–900.
2. Abele JE (1980): Balloon catheters and transluminal dilatation: Technical considerations. Am J Roentgenol 135:901–906.
3. Abele JE (1985): Balloon catheter: Materials and mechanics. Categorical Course on Interventional Radiology, American Roentgen Ray Society Meeting, Boston, MA, pp 9–12.
4. Adams DO (1984): PTCA Balloon Materials, Their Characteristics and Impact on Catheter Selection. Maple Grove, MN: SCIMED Internal Publication, pp 1–5.
5. Burton AC (1972): "Physiology and Biophysics of Circulation." Chicago: Year Book, pp 67–91.
6. Mitchell SE, White RI Jr, Kan J, Tolkoff J (1984): Improved balloon catheters for large-vessel and valvular angioplasty. Am J Roentgenol 142:571–572.
7. Rao PS (1987): Influence of balloon size on the short-term and long-term results of balloon pulmonary valvuloplasty. Texas Heart Inst J 14:57–61.
8. Butto F, Amplatz K, Bass JL (1986): Geometry of the proximal pulmonary trunk during dilation with two balloons. Am J Cardiol 58:380–381.
9. Park JH, Yoon YS, Yeon KM, Han MC, Kim C, Oh BH, Lee YW (1987): Percutaneous pulmonary valvuloplasty with a double balloon technique. Radiology 164: 715–718.
10. Al Kasab S, Ribeiro P, Al Zaibag M (1987): Use of double balloon technique for percutaneous balloon pulmonary valvotomy in adults. Br Heart J 58:136–141.
11. Beekman RH, Rocchini AP, Crowley DC, Snider AR, Serwer GA, Dick M II, Rosenthal A (1988): Comparison of single and double balloon valvuloplasty in children with aortic stenosis. J Am Coll Cardiol 12:480–485.
12. Rao PS, Fawzy ME (1988): Double balloon technique for percutaneous balloon pulmonary valvuloplasty: Comparison with single balloon technique. J Intervent Cardiol 1:257–262.
13. Mullins CE, Nihill MR, Vick GW III, Ludomirsky A, O'Laughlin MP, Bricker JT, Judd VE (1987): Double balloon technique for dilation of valvular or vessel stenosis in congenital and acquired heart disease. J Am Coll Cardiol 10:107–114.
14. D'Souza VJ, Velasquez G, Weesner KM, Prabhu S

(1984): Transluminal angioplasty of aortic coarctation with a two balloon technique. Am J Cardiol
54:457-458.

15. Al Zaibag M, Ribeiro PA, Al Kasab S, Al Fagih MR
(1986): Percutaneous double balloon valvuloplasty
for rheumatic mitral valve stenosis. Lancet 1:757-
761.

16. Ribiero PA, Al Zaibag M, Al Kasab S, Idris M,
Halim M, Abdullah M, Shahed M (1988): Percutaneous double balloon valvotomy for rheumatic tricuspid stenosis. Am J Cardiol 61:660-662.

17. Meier B, Friedli B, Oberhaensli I, Belenger J, Finci L
(1986): Trefoil balloon for percutaneous valvuloplasty. Cathet Cardiovasc Diagn 12:227-231.

18. Van den Berg EJM, Niemeyer MG, Plokker TWM,
Ernst SMPG, de Korte J (1986): New triple-lumen
balloon catheter for percutaneous (pulmonary)
valvuloplasty. Cathet Cardiovasc Diagn 12:352-
356.

19. Meier B, Friedli B, Von Segesser L (1988):
Valvuloplasty with trefoil and bifoil balloons and
long sheath technique. Herz 13:1-13.

20. Meier B, Friedli B, Oberhänsli I (1986): Trefoil balloon for aortic valvuloplasty. Br Heart J 56:292-293.

21. Thanopoulos BD, Margetakis A, Papadopoulos G,
Kefalakis E, Rokas S (1989): Valvuloplasty with large
trefoil balloons for the treatment of congenital pulmonary stenosis. Acta Paediatr Scand 78:742-746.

22. Gaylord GM, Pitchard WF, Chuang VP, Casarella
WJ, Sprawls P (1988): The geometry of triple-bal-
loon dilatation. Radiology 166:541-545.

23. Taquini AC, Fermoso JD, Aramendia P (1960): Behavior of the right ventricle following acute constriction of the pulmonary artery. Circ Res 8:315-318.

24. Vlahakes GJ, Turley K, Hoffman JIE (1981): The
pathology of failure in acute right ventricular hypertension: Hemodynamic and biochemical considerations. Circulation 63:87-95.

25. Suárez de Lezo J, Casey P, Casey A, Carrasco JL,
Arizón JM, Cantalapiedra IA, Gattikor HF (1987):
Effects of acute changes in load and inotropic state
on the exponential rate of fibre shortening and other
indices of myocardial contractability in the an-
esthesized intact dog. Can J Physiol Pharmacol
65:46-53.

26. Kan JS, White JS Jr, Mitchell SE, Andersen JH
(1984): Transluminal balloon valvuloplasty for the
treatment of pulmonary and aortic valvar stenosis.
Semin Intervent Radiol 1:217-223.

27. Suárez de Lezo J, Pan M, Romero M, Sancho M,
Carrasco JL, Rejano A, Martinez C, Costa A (1988):
Pathophysiology of transient ventricular occlusion
during balloon valvuloplasty for pulmonic or aortic
stenosis. Am J Cardiol 61:436-440.

28. Suárez de Lezo J, Montilla P, Pan M, Romero M,
Sancho M, de Castroviejo JR, Tejero I, Arizón J,

Carrasco JL, Rejano A, Martinez C (1989): Abrupt
homeostatic response to transient intracardiac occlusion during balloon valvuloplasty. Am J Cardiol
64:491-497.

29. Shuck JW, McCormick DJ, Cohen IS, Oetgen WJ,
Brinker JA (1984): Percutaneous balloon valvuloplasty of the pulmonary valve: role of right-to-left shunt
through a patent foramen ovale. J Am Coll Cardiol
4:132-135.

30. Lababidi Z, Wu J, Walls JT (1984): Percutaneous
balloon aortic valvuloplasty: Results in 23 patients.
Am J Cardiol 54:194-197.

31. Kiel AA, Devanter V, Readinger RI, Dungan WT,
Norton JB (1986): Aortic balloon valvuloplasty with
transluminal venous balloon inflow occlusion (case
report). Pediatr Cardiol 7:103-105.

32. Rao PS: (1989) Balloon angioplasty and valvuloppla-
sty in infants, children, and adolescents. Curr Probl
Cardiol 14:417-500.

33. Stokland O, Miller MM, Ilebekk A, Kill F (1980):
Mechanism of hemodynamic response to occlusion
of the descending thoracic aorta. Am J Physiol 238
(Heart Circ Physiol 7): H423-H429.

34. Benson LN, Freedom RM, Wilson GJ, Halliday
WC (1986): Cerebral complications following balloon angioplasty of coarctation of the aorta. Cardiovasc Intervent Radiol 9:184-186.

35. Hellenbrand WE, Allen HD, Golinko RJ, Hagler
DJ, Lutin W, Kan J (1990): Balloon angioplasty for
aortic recoarctation: Results of Valvuloplasty and
Angioplasty of Congenital Anomalies Registry. Am
J Cardiol 65:793-797.

36. Treacy EP, Duncan WJ, Tyrrell MJ, Lowry NJ
(1991): Neurological complications of balloon angioplasty in children. Pediatr Cardiol 12:98-101.

37. Booth P, Redington AN, Shinebourne EA, Rigby
ML (1991): Early complications of interventional
balloon catheterization in infants and children. Br
Heart J 65:109-112.

38. Beekman RH, Rocchini AP, Dick M II, Snider AR,
Crowley DC, Serwer GA, Spicer RL, Rosenthal A
(1987): Percutaneous balloon angioplasty for native
coarctation of the aorta. J Am Coll Cardiol
10:1078-1084.

39. Suárez de Lezo J, Sancho M, Pan M, Romero M,
Olivera C, Luque M (1989): Angiographic follow-up
after balloon angioplasty for coarctation of the aorta.
J Am Coll Cardiol 13:689-695.

40. Gikonyo BM, Lucas RV, Edwards JE (1987): Anatomic features of congenital pulmonary valvar stenosis. Pediatr Cardiol 8:109-115.

41. Becker AE, Hoedemaker G (1987): Balloon
valvuloplasty in congenital and acquired heart disease: Morphologic considerations. Zeistsch Kardiol
76(Suppl 6):73-79.

42. Lababidi Z, Wu J (1983): Percutaneous balloon

pulmonary valvuloplasty. Am J Cardiol 52:560–562.

43. Walls JT, Lababidi Z, Curtis JJ, Silver D (1984): Assessment of percutaneous balloon pulmonary and aortic valvuloplasty. J Thorac Cardiovasc Surg 88:352–356.

44. Benson LN, Smallhorn JS, Freedom RM, Trusler GA, Rowe RD (1985): Pulmonary valve morphology after balloon dilatation of pulmonary valve stenosis. Cathet Cardiovasc Diagn 11:161–166.

45. Ettedgui JA, Ho SY, Tynan M, Jones ODH, Martin RP, Baker EJ, Reidy JF (1987): The pathology of balloon pulmonary valvuloplasty. Int J Cardiol 16:285–293.

46. Rao PS, Brais M (1988): Balloon pulmonary valvuloplasty for congenital cyanotic heart defects. Am Heart J 115:1105–1113.

47. Tynan M, Baker EJ, Rohmer J, Jone ODH, Reidy JF, Joseph MC, Ottenkamp J (1985): Percutaneous balloon pulmonary valvuloplasty. Br Heart J 53:520–524.

48. Kan JS, White RI Jr, Mitchel SE, Anderson JH, Gardner TJ (1984): Percutaneous transluminal balloon valvuloplasty for pulmonary valve stenosis. Circulation 69:554–560.

49. Ben-Shachar G, Cohen MH, Sivakoff MC, Portman MA, Riemenschneider TA, Van Heeckeren DW (1985): Development of infundibular obstruction after percutaneous pulmonary balloon valvuloplasty. J Am Coll Cardiol 5:754–756.

50. Robertson M, Benson LN, Smallhorn JS, Musewe N, Freedom RM, Moes CAF, Burrows P, Johnston AE, Burrows FA, Rowe RD (1987): The morphology of the right ventricular outflow tract after percutaneous pulmonary valvotomy: Long-term follow-up. Br Heart J 58:239–244.

51. Burrows PE, Benson LN, Smallhorn JS, Moes CAF, Freedom RM, Burrows FA, Rowe RD (1988): Angiographic features associated with percutaneous balloon valvotomy for pulmonary valve stenosis. Cardiovasc Intervent Radiol 11:111–116.

52. Radtke W, Lock JE (1990): Balloon dilatation. Pediatr Clin North Am 37(1):193–213.

53. Rao PS (1992): Pulmonic stenosis. In Cheng TO (ed): "Percutaneous Balloon Valvuloplasty." New York: Igaku-Shoin Medical Publishers, pp 365–420.

54. Lucas RV Jr, Burke BA, Edwards JE (1984): Anatomic sequelae of balloon angioplasty in congenital heart disease. Semin Intervent Radiol 1:225–235.

55. Linde LM, Turner SW, Sparks RS (1973): Pulmonary valve dysplasia: A cardiofacial syndrome. Br Heart J 35:301–304.

56. Rao PS (1988): Balloon dilatation in infants and children with dysplastic pulmonary valves: short-term and intermediate-term results. Am Heart J 116:1168–1176.

57. Ring JC, Kulik TJ, Burke BA, Lock JE (1986): Morphologic changes induced by dilation of pulmonary valve annulus with overlarge balloons in normal newborn lambs. Am J Cardiol 55:210–214.

58. Keith JD, Rowe RD, Vlad P (1978): "Heart Disease in Infancy and Childhood," 3rd ed. New York: Macmillan Co, pp 4–6, 698–727.

59. Van Praagh R, Bano-Rodrigo A, Smolinsky A, Schultz TJ, Fyler DC, Van Praagh S (1986): Anatomic variations in congenital valvar, subvalvar, and supravalvar aortic stenosis: A study of 64 postmortem cases. In Takahasi M (ed): "Challenges in the Treatment of Congenital Cardiac Anomalies." New York: Futura, p 13.

60. Angelini A, Ho SY, Anderson RH (1989): The morphology of the normal aortic valve as compared with the aortic valve having two leaflets. J Thorac Cardiovasc Surg 98:362–367.

61. Fischer DR, Ettedgui JA, Park SC, Siewers RD, del Nido P (1990): Carotid artery approach for balloon dilatation of aortic valve stenosis in the neonate: a preliminary report. J Am Coll Cardiol 15:1633–1636.

62. Sholler GF, Keane JF, Perry SB, Sanders SP, Lock JE (1988): Balloon dilation of congenital aortic valve stenosis: Results and influence of technical and morphological features on outcome. Circulation 78:351–360.

63. Lababidi Z (1992): Congenital obstruction of the left ventricular outflow tract. In Cheng TO (ed): "Percutaneous Balloon Valvuloplasty." New York: Igaku-Shoin, pp 305–337.

64. Rao PS, Thapar MK, Wilson AD, Levy JM, Chopra PS (1989): Intermediate-term follow-up results of balloon aortic valvuloplasty in infants and children with special reference to causes of restenosis. Am J Cardiol 64:1356–1360.

65. Helgason H, Keane JF, Fellows KE, Kulik TJ, Lock JE (1987): Balloon dilation of the aortic valve: Studies in normal lambs and in children with aortic stenosis. J Am Coll Cardiol 9:816–822.

66. Shaddy RE, Boucek MM, Sturtevant JE, Ruttenberg HD, Orsmond GS (1990): Gradient reduction, aortic valve regurgitation, and prolapse after balloon aortic valvuloplasty in 32 consecutive patients with congenital aortic stenosis. J Am Coll Cardiol 16:451–456.

67. Rao PS, Wilson AD, Chopra PS (1990): Balloon dilatation for discrete subaortic stenosis: Immediate and intermediate-term results. J Invasive Cardiol 2:65–71.

68. Subramanian R. Olson LJ, Edwards WD (1984): Surgical pathology of pure aortic stenosis: A study of 374 cases. Mayo Clin Proc 59:683–690.

69. McKay RG, Safian RD, Lock JE, Mandell VS, Thurer RL, Schnitt SJ, Grossman W (1986): Bal-

loon dilatation of calcific aortic stenosis in elderly patients: Postmortem, intraoperative, and percutaneous valvuloplasty studies. Circulation 74:119-125.

70. Roberts WC, Perloff WK, Costantino T (1971): Severe valvular aortic stenosis in patients over 65 years of age: A clinicopathologic study. Am J Cardiol 27:497-506.

71. Safian RD, Mandell VS, Thurer RE, Hutchins GM, Schnitt SJ. Grossman W, McKay RG (1987): Postmortem and intraoperative balloon valvuloplasty of calcific aortic stenosis in elderly patients: mechanisms of successful dilatation. J Am Coll Cardiol 9:655-660.

72. Isner JM, Donaldson RF, Fulton D, Bhan I, Payne DD, Cleveland RJ (1987): Cystic medial necrosis in coarctation of the aorta: A potential factor contributing to adverse consequences observed after percutaneous balloon angioplasty of coarctation sites. Circulation 75:689-695.

73. Ho SY, Somerville J, Yip, WCL, Anderson RH (1988): Transluminal balloon dilatation of resected coarcted segments of thoracic aorta: Histological study and clinical implications. Int J Cardiol 19:99-105.

74. Sos T, Sniderman KW, Rettek-Sos B, Strupp A, Alonso DR (1979): Percutaneous transluminal dilatation of coarctation of thoracic aorta post mortem. Lancet 2: 970-971.

75. Lock JE, Castaneda-Zuniga WR, Bass JL, Foker JE, Amplatz K, Anderson RW (1982): Balloon dilatation of excised aortic coarctations. Radiology 143:689-691.

76. Castaneda-Zuniga WR, Lock JE, Vlodaver Z, Rusnak B, Rysavy JP, Herrera M, Amplatz K (1982): Transluminal dilatation of coarctation of the abdominal aorta: an experimental study in dogs. Radiology 143:693-697.

77. Lock JE, Niemi T, Burke BA, Einzig S, Castaneda-Zuniga WR (1982): Transcutaneous angioplasty of experimental aortic coarctation. Circulation 66:1280-1286.

78. Finley JP, Beaulieu RG, Nanton MA, Roy DL (1983): Balloon catheter dilatation of coarctation of the aorta in young infants. Br Heart J 50:411-415.

79. Rao PS (1986): Transcatheter treatment of pulmonary stenosis and coarctation of the aorta. Experi-

ence with percutaneous balloon dilatation. Br Heart J 56:250-258.

80. Allen HD, Marx GR, Ovitt TW, Goldberg SJ: (1986) Balloon dilatation angioplasty for coarctation of the aorta. Am J Cardiol 57:828-832.

81. Morrow WR, Vick GW III, Nihill MR, Rokey R, Johnston DL, Hedrick TD, Mullins CE (1988): Balloon dilatation of unoperated coarctation of the aorta: Short-term and intermediate-term results. J Am Coll Cardiol 11:133-138.

82. Hagemo PS, Birnstad PG, Smevik B, Foerster A (1988): Aortic wall lesion in balloon dilatation of coarctation of the aorta. Eur Heart J 9:1271-1273.

83. Fontes VF, Esteves CA, Braga SLM, da Silva MVD, E Silva MAP, Sousa EMK, de Souza AM (1990): It is valid to dilate native aortic coarctation with a balloon catheter. Int J Cardiol 27:311-316.

84. Erbel R, Bednarczyk I, Pop T, Todt M, Henrichs KJ, Brunier A, Thelen M, Meyer J (1990): Detection of dissection of the aortic intima and media after angioplasty of coarctation of the aorta: An angiographic, computer tomographic, and echocardiographic comparative study. Circulation 81:805-814.

85. Rao PS (1993): Balloon angioplasty of native aortic coarctation. In Rao PS (ed): "Transcatheter Therapy in Pediatric Cardiology." New York: Wiley-Liss, pp. 153-196.

86. Hollman J, Austin GE, Grüntzig AR, Douglas JS, King SB (1983): Coronary artery spasm at the site of angioplasty in the first two months after successful percutaneous transluminal coronary angioplasty. J Am Coll Cardiol 1:1039-1045.

87. Beinart C, Sos TA, Saddekni S, Weiner MA, Sniderman K (1983): Arterial spasm during renal angioplasty. Radiology 149:97-100.

88. Fischell TA, Derby G, Tse TM, Stadius ML (1988): Coronary artery spasm routinely occurs following percutaneous transluminal angioplasty (PTCA): A quantitative arteriographic analysis. Circulation 78:1323-1334.

89. Fischell TA, Nellessen U, Johnson DE, Ginsburg R (1989): Endothelium dependent arterial vasoconstriction after balloon angioplasty. Circulation 79:899-910.

6

Balloon Pulmonary Valvuloplasty for Isolated Pulmonic Stenosis

P. Syamasundar Rao, M.D.

Department of Pediatrics, Division of Pediatric Cardiology,
University of Wisconsin Medical School, University of Wisconsin
Children's Hospital, Madison, Wisconsin 53792-4108

INTRODUCTION

Valvular pulmonary stenosis constitutes 7.5%–9.0% of all congenital heart defects [1,2]. The pathologic features of pulmonary stenosis vary [3–5], but the most commonly found pathology is what is described as "dome-shaped" pulmonary valve. The "fused" pulmonary valve leaflets protrude from their attachment into the pulmonary artery as a conical or dome-shaped structure. The size of the orifice of the pulmonary valve may vary from a pinhole to several millimeters, most commonly central in location but can be eccentric. Raphae, presumably representing fused valve leaflet commissures, extend from the stenotic valve orifice to a varying extent down into the base of the dome-shaped valve. The number of raphae vary from none to seven. Other, less common pathologic variants include unicommisural, bicuspid, and tricuspid pulmonary valves [5]. Hypoplastic pulmonary annulus and valve leaflets and dysplastic pulmonary valves are also present in a small but definite number of cases of pulmonic stenosis. Thickening of valve leaflets is seen in all types described above, and this may be due to an increase in valve spongiosa or due to excessive fibrous, collagen, myxomatous, and elastic tissue. There is also abnormality of the valve annulus in that there is partial or complete lack of fibrous backbone in most pulmonic stenosis specimens studied [5].

Children with pulmonic stenosis usually present with asymptomatic murmurs, although they can present with signs of systemic venous congestion (usually interpreted as congestive heart failure) due to severe right ventricular dysfunction or cyanosis because of right-to-left shunt across the atrial septum. Clinical findings of ejection systolic click and ejection systolic murmur at the left upper sternal border, right ventricular hypertrophy on an electrocardiogram, prominent main pulmonary artery segment on a chest roentgenogram, and increased Doppler flow velocity in the main pulmonary artery are characteristic of this anomaly. When the pulmonary valvar obstruction is moderate to severe, relief of the obstruction is recommended to treat symptoms, if present, or to prevent right ventricular fibrosis and dysfunction. Until recently, surgical valvotomy was the only treatment available, but at the present time relief of pulmonary valve obstruction can be accomplished by balloon valvuloplasty.

Rubio-Alvarez et al. [6,7] in the early 1950s described a technique by which pulmonic valve stenosis could be relieved via a catheter; they used a ureteral catheter with a wire. Twenty-five years later, Semb et al. [8] used a Berman balloon angiographic catheter to produce rupture of the pulmonary valve (commissures); they withdrew an inflated balloon from the main pulmonary artery to the right ventricle and reduced the pulmonary valve

Transcatheter Therapy in Pediatric Cardiology, pages 59–104
© 1993 Wiley-Liss, Inc.

gradient. More recently, Kan et al. [9] used a static dilatation technique [similar to that used by Dotter and Judkins [10] and Grüntzig et al. [11,12] in which they introduced a deflated balloon across the pulmonic valve and inflated the balloon; the radial forces of balloon inflation produced relief of pulmonary valve obstruction. This static dilatation technique is what is currently used. The purpose of this chapter is to present the current state of the art of balloon pulmonary valvuloplasty; personal experience with this procedure, including that reported previously [13–31], and the experiences reported in the literature are used as supportive material. Issues related to transcatheter therapy of pulmonic stenosis associated with complex heart defects and valvar pulmonary atresia will be included in the chapter on cyanotic congenital heart defects.

INDICATIONS

By and large, the indications for balloon dilatation of pulmonic stenosis are essentially the same as those used for surgical intervention. The indications for surgical pulmonary valvotomy are reasonably clear; patients with moderate to severe degree of stenosis irrespective of the symptoms are candidates for surgical relief of the obstruction [32,33]. The indications for balloon valvuloplasty appear less clear and are rarely defined [34,35]. Careful examination in 1988 [22] of all the studies available at that time [9,34,36–44] revealed that many patients with what may be considered mild pulmonic stenosis (natural history study definition [33]: gradient <25 mmHg = trivial, 25–49 mmHg = mild, 50–79 mmHg = moderate, and ≥80 mmHg = severe) underwent balloon valvuloplasty. Review of the results of balloon valvuloplasty in these patients with mild stenosis revealed that 59 patients from 11 studies [9,34,36–44] underwent the procedure for a peak pulmonary valve gradient less than 50 mmHg. Valve gradient data were not available for analysis in six of these patients [44].

In the remaining 53 patients, the peak-to-peak systolic pressure gradient across the pulmonary valve was reduced from 38 ± 6 (mean ± SD) mmHg to 20 ± 11 mmHg ($P < 0.01$) immediately after valvuloplasty. The reduction in the right ventricular peak systolic pressure was from 60 ± 9 to 43 ± 11 mmHg ($P < 0.01$). At follow-up several months after balloon valvuloplasty, the pulmonary valve gradients (24 ± 12 mmHg) and the right ventricular pressure (45 ± 12 mmHg) remained improved ($P < 0.01$) compared with prevalvuloplasty values. The residual pulmonary valvar gradients and right ventricular peak systolic pressures at follow-up, respectively, were 60 ± 25% and 75 ± 18% of prevalvuloplasty values [22]. These data indicate that there was a statistically significant reduction in pulmonary valvar gradients even in patients with mild pulmonary stenosis. However, the mean residual right ventricular peak systolic pressure at follow-up was 75% of prevalvuloplasty measurements. The question to be asked is whether this modest reduction in the right ventricular pressure is worth the risk, morbidity, and expense associated with cardiac catheterization and balloon pulmonary valvuloplasty? The answer (my answer) is "no," especially in view of a benign natural course of the disease process. Natural history studies of pulmonic stenosis [33,45–47] indicated that mild pulmonary stenosis remains mild on follow-up. Therefore the advisability of balloon valvuloplasty for mild obstruction can be questioned. My recommendations are to consider the indications for balloon valvuloplasty to be the same as those used for surgical valvuloplasty and that balloon dilatation should not be performed in patients with gradients less than 50 mmHg. Because noninvasive Doppler estimates of pulmonary valve gradients are reasonably accurate [48–51], patients with mild stenosis can be followed, and, once the Doppler estimate of the gradient is in excess of 50 mmHg, they can undergo balloon valvuloplasty. Although there is some wisdom in using valve areas for setting criteria for intervention, gradients are adequate for the pulmonary valve provided cardiac indices are measured during prevalvuloplasty catheterization and are shown to be within normal range.

Some investigators [35] suggested that balloon valvuloplasty should not be performed in severe stenosis if the peak systolic pressure in the right ventricle is approximately twice that in the left ventricle. While their concern is understandable, balloon valvuloplasty can be performed safely (see Technique) in such patients. There were 16 patients of a total of 71 infants and children [52] who had right ventricular pressures approximately twice that in the left ventricle in whom we were able to perform balloon valvuloplasty successfully.

Some investigators consider dysplastic pulmonary valves as a relative contraindication for balloon valvuloplasty [53,54], but, based on the results of others [42,55] and our data [21], balloon valvuloplasty is the initial treatment of choice; perhaps large balloons to produce balloon: annulus ratios of 1.4–1.5 should be used [21]. Our experience [13,14] and that in the Registry [56] indicate that the procedure is also successful in patients with Noonan syndrome. Patients whose pulmonary valves restenosed following a previous surgical pulmonary valvotomy also respond favorably to balloon pulmonary valvuloplasty. In conclusion, moderate to severe valvar pulmonic stenosis (gradient > 50 mmHg) irrespective of previous surgical intervention and pulmonary valve dysplasia is an indication for percutaneous balloon pulmonary valvuloplasty.

TECHNIQUE

The diagnosis and assessment of the pulmonary valve obstruction are made by the usual clinical, roentgenographic, electrocardiographic, and echo-Doppler data. Once a moderate to severe obstruction is diagnosed, cardiac catheterization and cineangiography are performed percutaneously to confirm the clinical impression and to consider for balloon dilatation of the pulmonic valve. The indications for

catheter intervention (described above) are usually those prescribed for surgical intervention. Once balloon dilatation is decided upon, 1) a 5 to 7 Fr multi-A-2 (Cordis) catheter is introduced percutaneously into the femoral vein and advanced across the pulmonic valve and then into the left pulmonary artery; 2) a 0.014 to 0.035 inch J-shaped guidewire is passed through the catheter into the distal left pulmonary artery; 3) a 4 to 9 Fr balloon dilatation catheter is advanced over the guidewire, and the balloon is positioned across the pulmonary valve; 4) the balloon is inflated with diluted contrast material to approximately 3–5 atm of pressure (Fig. 1). I recommend monitoring pressure of inflation with the help of any of the commercially available pressure gauges. The recommended duration of inflation is 5 seconds. Usually a total of three to four balloon inflations are performed, 5 minutes apart. We use a double-balloon technique (two balloons simultaneously inflated across the stenotic region) when the valve annulus is too large to dilate with a commercially available single balloon; and 5) measurement of pressure gradients across the pulmonic valve and angiographic demonstration of the relief of obstruction are performed. Recordings of heart rate, systemic pressure, and cardiac index prior to and after balloon dilatation are made to ensure that change in pressure gradient is not related to change in cardiac index but is indeed related to the procedure.

We generally perform this procedure with the patient sedated (usually with a mixture of meperidine, promethazine, and chlorpromazine, intramuscular), although others use ketamine [43] or general anesthesia [34,57]. Other aspects of importance for successfully accomplishing balloon angioplasty are as follows:

1. Difficult femoral venous access. Sometimes it can be difficult to cannulate the femoral vein percutaneously either because of technical problems or because of femoral vein thrombosis secondary to previous catheterization and/or surgery. Cut-down and isolation of saphenous vein–femoral vein junction may be

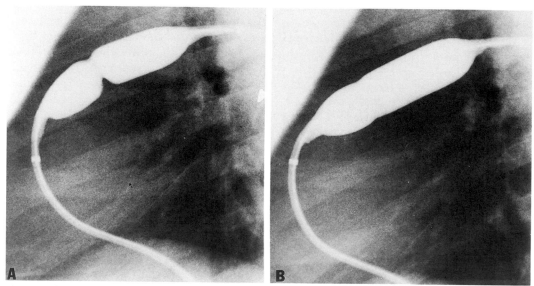

Fig. 1. Selected cineradiographic frames of a balloon dilatation catheter placed across the pulmonic valve. Note "waisting" of the balloon during the initial phases of balloon inflation **(A),** which is almost completely abolished during the later phases of balloon inflation **(B).**

performed, and catheterization and balloon valvuloplasty can be accomplished via saphenous venous bulb. When femoral venous access is not possible, balloon pulmonary valvuloplasty may be performed via axillary venous [40,58] or internal jugular venous [59] approach. The latter two approaches are also useful in the presence of infrahepatic interruption of the inferior vena cava with azygos or hemiazygos continuation.

2. Passing an end-hole catheter across the pulmonic valve. This can be difficult in some patients, particularly in young children and neonates. On such occasions, we employ several maneuvers: a) position an end-hole catheter (usually a multi-A-2) just underneath the pulmonary valve and advance the floppy end of a straight guidewire through the tip of the catheter into the main pulmonary artery; b) position a balloon-wedge catheter just beneath the pulmonic valve and quickly deflate the balloon and advance the catheter into the main pulmonary artery. Failing this, use a guidewire, as described earlier; c) use a flexi-

ble, steerable coronary guidewire through an end-hole catheter. We have encountered one child in whom we could not advance any catheter across the right ventricular infundibulum because of severe infundibular constriction. In this child, administration of propranolol (0.1 mg/kg IV slowly) had made it possible to pass a catheter across the pulmonary valve and eventually balloon pulmonary valvuloplasty [29].

3. Choice of size of balloon dilatation catheter. The current recommendations are to use a balloon that is 1.2–1.4 times the size of the pulmonary valve annulus. These recommendations are formulated on the basis of immediate [41] and follow-up [16,19,24] results [For further discussion of reasoning behind such recommendations, the reader is referred to these publications 16,19,24,26]. Balloons larger than 1.5 times the size of the pulmonary valve annulus are not recommended because of potential damage to the right ventricular outflow tract caused by use of large balloons [60]. However, it may be advisable to use a

large balloon to produce a balloon: annulus ratio of 1.5 when pulmonary valve dysplasia is present [21].

When the pulmonary valve annulus is too large to dilate with a single balloon, valvuloplasty with simultaneous inflation of two balloons across the pulmonary valve annulus (Fig. 2) should be performed. When two balloons are used, the following formula is used to calculate the effective balloon size [16]:

$$\frac{D_1 + D_2 + \pi \left(\dfrac{D_1}{2} + \dfrac{D_2}{2} \right)}{\pi}$$

where D_1 and D_2 are diameters of the balloons used.

Although we do not believe that the double-balloon technique is superior to the single-balloon technique [19,25,61], it does reduce injury to the femoral veins because smaller-sized catheters can be used.

Some workers [62–65] have advocated bifoil and trefoil balloons with the idea that there will be forward flow around the balloon during balloon inflation. While such attempts to allow forward flow during balloon inflation are laudable, I do not believe that there will be any significant forward flow in view of the fact that the balloons used for pulmonary valve dilatation are larger than the valve annulus.

4. On occasion, it may be difficult to advance the balloon angioplasty catheter across the pulmonic valve. It is important to avoid kinking or looping of the guidewire to prevent such a problem. Replacement of the guidewire with an extra-stiff Amplatz guide may circumvent the problem.

5. Sometimes it may not be feasible to advance an appropriate-sized balloon dilatation catheter across the pulmonic valve even after having a guidewire across it. In such situations, we use a smaller-sized 4–6 mm balloon on a 4 or 5 Fr catheter initially to predilate and then use larger, more appropri-

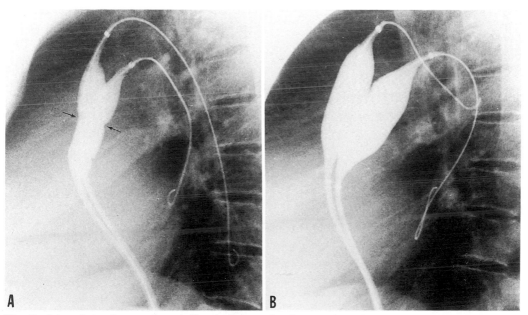

Fig. 2. Selected cine frames of two balloon catheters placed across the pulmonary valve showing "waisting" of the balloons (arrows) during the initial phases of balloon inflation **(A)**, which is completely abolished after complete inflation of the balloons **(B)**.

ate-sized balloons. This technique is also help-ful when dilating very severely stenotic pulmo-nary valves and in small infants.

ACUTE RESULTS

Since the description of balloon pulmonary valvuloplasty by Kan *et al.* [9], several pediatric cardiology centers across the world have uti-lized this technique [13,14,34–42,54,55,62–81]. Most groups of investigators [34–42,56,62–81], including mine [13,14,18,24, 26,52,61], have reported excellent immediate relief of pulmonic valve obstruction following balloon valvuloplasty. From our group, 73 infants and children, aged 2 days to 20 years (median 5 years), underwent balloon dilatation of valvar pulmonic stenosis during a 7 year 8 month period ending May 1991. Following valvuloplasty, the peak systolic pressure in the right ventricle decreased (108 ± 41 [mean ± SD] *vs.* 53 ± 22 mmHg, $P < 0.001$) as did the peak systolic gradient across the pul-monic valve (91 ± 41 *vs.* 26 ± 19 mmHg, $P < 0.001$) (Fig. 3). The pulmonary artery pressure (17 ± 5 *vs.* 23 ± 6, $P < 0.001$) increased. The cardiac index did not change ($P > 0.1$). Width of the jet of the contrast material through the pulmonary valve as vi-sualized in the cineangiograms (Figs. 4,5)

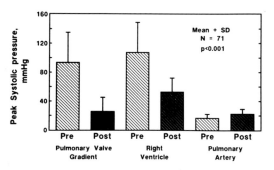

Fig. 3. Bar graph showing acute results of balloon pulmonary valvuloplasty in 73 patients showing a significant ($P<0.001$) decrease in the peak-to-peak sys-tolic pressure gradient across the pulmonic valve and peak systolic pressures in the right ventricle. Also, note a significant ($P<0.001$) increase in the peak systolic pressure in the pulmonary artery.

increased. Less doming and much more "free" movement of the pulmonary valve leaflets [82] occurred following the valvuloplasty in each case. Improvement of the right ventricular function and decrease in right-to-left atrial shunting [31,31a] also occurred. Though not studied by us, improvement in the function of the left ventricle [83] is expected. Surgical intervention is avoided in all cases. Most patients are discharged home within 24–48 hours following the procedure.

FOLLOW-UP RESULTS

Several investigators [34,37–40,66,68,69, 73,81a] recatheterized 6–53 patients 1 week to 18 months (mean) following balloon valvu-loplasty and reported significant residual gra-dients (> 30 mmHg) in 14%–100% of patients (Table I). We recatheterized 45 children 6–34 months (mean, 11.0 months) following bal-loon valvuloplasty. For the group of children in whom follow-up catheterization data were available, the peak systolic pressure gradient across the pulmonic valve (92 ± 43 *vs.* 29 ± 23 mmHg, $P < 0.001$) and the peak systolic pressure in the right ventricle (109 ± 41 *vs.* 56 ± 22 mmHg, $P < 0.001$) decreased im-mediately after balloon dilatation. The cardiac index (3.3 ± 0.9 *vs.* 3.2 ± 0.7 1/min/m², $P > 0.1$) remained unchanged. Upon follow-up approximately 11 months later, systolic pres-sure gradient across the pulmonic valve (29 ± 23 mmHg, $P < 0.001$) remains improved com-pared with the predilation value (Fig. 6). The cardiac index (3.5 ± 0.8 1/min/m²) did not significantly]$P > 0.1$) change. Despite improve-ment as a group, several children had signifi-cant residual gradients (Fig. 7) across the pul-monic valve, hereafter referred to as *restenosis*. Nine of 45 children who were restudied had pulmonary valve gradients in excess of 30 mmHg. Six of these children underwent repeat balloon valvuloplasty with larger balloons (Fig. 7), and the pulmonary valve gradients were reduced from 96 ± 40 to 40 ± 22 mmHg ($P < 0.01$). The other three children, with residual

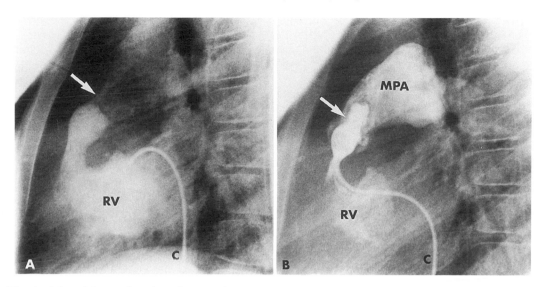

Fig. 4. Selected frames from lateral views of a right ventricular (RV) cineangiogram before **(A)** and after **(B)** balloon pulmonary valvuloplasty. Note extremely thin jet (arrow) prior to balloon dilatation (A), which increased to a much wider jet (arrow) after valvuloplasty (B) opacifying the main pulmonary artery (MPA). C, catheter. (Reproduced from Rao [61], with permission of the publisher.)

gradients of 45, 50, and 60 mmHg, are being followed clinically. Repeat follow-up catheterization data (in four) or Doppler studies (in four) were available in eight children (24 months after first balloon valvuloplasty), and the residual pulmonary valve gradients were 28 ± 12 mmHg.

The restenosis rate (9 of 45; 20%) in our group, though high, is comparable to the 14%–100% reported by other workers (Table I).

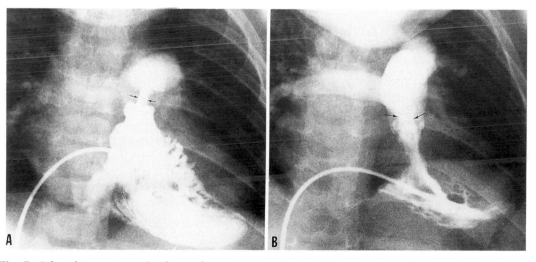

Fig. 5. Selected cineangiographic frames from a "sitting-up" view (40° cranial and 15° left anterior oblique) of a right ventricular angiogram prior to **(A)** and 15 minutes following **(B)** balloon pulmonary valvuloplasty. The thin jet of passage of contrast across the pulmonic valve (arrows) in A has markedly increased (arrows) in B.

TABLE I. Intermediate-Term Follow-Up Catherization Results of Balloon Pulmonary Valvuloplasty (BPV) From the Literature

Author and year	No. of patients undergoing BPV	No. of patients with follow-up	Duration of follow-up, mean (range) months	Poor results[a] on follow-up, No. (%)	Comments
Kan et al., 1984 [37]	20	11	7	(2-12)	2(18)	The failure was in patients with dysplastic valve or after previous Brock
Tynan et al., 1985 [34]	27	6	–	(2-6)	2(33)	Both patients underwent surgery
Kveselis et al., 1985 [38]	19	7	12	(9-13)	7(100)[b]	Repeat BPV in one patient with 52 mmHg gradient with reduction to 34 mmHg
Miller, 1985 [39]	16	7	4	(3-6)	1(14)	Two patients with gradients of 24 and 22 mmHg at follow-up underwent repeat BPV with excellent results.
Sullivan et al., 1985 [40]	23	12	5.5	(0.25-6)	6(50)	Repeat valvuloplasty in four patients with good results
Ali Khan et al., 1986 [68]	32	14	10	(6-14)	2(14)	–
Srivastava et al., 1987 [66]	32	21	–	(3-18)	9(43)	–
Rey et al., 1988 [42]	51	23	–	(1-17)	5(22)	Repeat BPV in five patients with satisfactory results
Fontes et al., 1988 [69]	100	44	12	(3-14)	10(23)	–
Schmaltz et al., 1989 [73]	273	53	11	(–)	14(26)[c]	Repeat BPV in 14 patients; successful in 10; remaining 4 with dysplastic valves required surgery
Melgaret et al., 1991 [81a]	21	19	5	(3-10)	4(20)	Repeat BPV in 1 & surgery in 1.
Rao, 1991	73	45	11	(6-34)	9(20)	Repeat BPV in six patients with good results

[a]Poor result is defined as pulmonary valve gradient in excess of 30 mm Hg at follow-up.
[b]The pulmonary valve gradient ranged between 31 and 52 mm Hg, with a mean of 38 mm Hg.
[c]Poor result is defined as gradient ≥40 mm Hg.

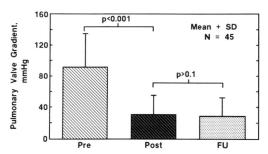

Fig. 6. Bar graph showing acute and follow-up results of the 45 unselected patients (from among 73 patients undergoing balloon valvuloplasty—Fig. 2) who underwent cardiac catheterization 11 months (mean) following balloon pulmonary valvuloplasty. Note significant ($P<0.001$) fall in the peak systolic pressure gradient across the pulmonary valve immediately after the procedure, which remained unchanged ($P>0.1$) at follow-up; the later continues to be significantly ($P<0.001$) lower than the prevalvuloplasty gradient. The gradients represented are valvar gradients without any regard to infundibular gradients.

However, it should be noted that we initially recommended recatheterization 6–12 months following valvuloplasty, but now routine post-operative catheterization is not recommended unless the Doppler estimate of the residual gra-

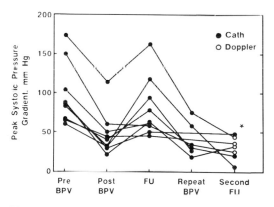

Fig. 7. Sequential pulmonary valvar gradients are shown for each of the nine patients who had gradients in excess of 30 mmHg at follow-up catheterization. Repeat balloon dilatation at the time of follow-up (FU) catheterization in six of these children produced a fall in the gradient in each patient. At a second follow-up study (catheterization or Doppler), the gradients remained low. Solid circles, gradients measured at cardiac catheterization; open circles, Doppler estimated peak instantaneous gradients [49].

dient is high. Therefore it is concluded that restenosis occurred in 9 of 70 patients for whom catheterization and/or Doppler follow-up data are available, i.e., 12.9% recurrence rate. In the recently compiled VACA Registry data [84], suboptimal long-term result, defined as need for surgery or repeat balloon valvuloplasty or a pulmonary valve gradient in excess of 36 mmHg, was noted in 89 of 433 (21%) patients who were followed-up at a median interval of 31 months after balloon valvuloplasty. Thus our data compare favorably with the VACA Registry data from 17 institutions. Electrocardiographic and echo-Doppler follow-up studies are also reflective of the pressure gradient relief [15,20] and are discussed later in this chapter.

Apart from the pressure gradient relief, there are other benefits. The Right-to-left interatrial shunt that was present prior to valvuloplasty has completely disappeared in most patients [31,31a]. Right ventricular dysfunction and tricuspid insufficiency improved. Figures 8 and 9 illustrate improvement in the cardiac size and tricuspid insufficiency following balloon valvuloplasty.

Based on these data, the intermediate-term follow-up results appear encouraging and lead me to recommend balloon valvuloplasty as a procedure of choice for treatment of isolated valvar pulmonic stenosis. Further refinement of the catheter technology and a better understanding of the use of balloon catheters with appropriate choices for specific situations may decrease or abolish the recurrence rate. Despite these good results, much longer-term (10 year) follow-up data are necessary to confirm the long-term effectiveness of balloon pulmonary valvuloplasty for relief of valvar pulmonic stenosis.

APPLICABILITY TO ALL AGE GROUPS

Although balloon pulmonary valvuloplasty is used most frequently in children, it has also been used in neonates [17,31,42,56,85–93] and in adults [37,66,69,72,94–102].

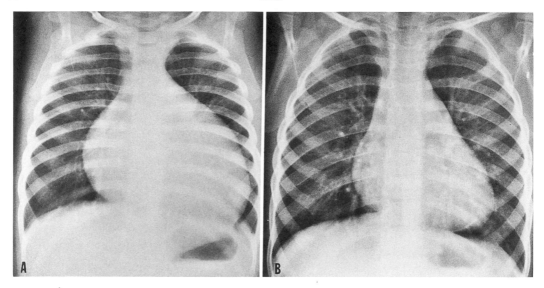

Fig. 8. Posteroanterior view of a chest roentgenogram showing cardiomegaly **(A)** prior to balloon pulmonary valvuloplasty. The cardiomegaly has improved on a chest x-ray taken 1 year following balloon valvuloplasty **(B)**.

Neonates

The experience with balloon pulmonary valvuloplasty in the neonate with critical pulmonary stenosis is limited, and the series with the largest numbers contain five [86], eight [42], and 11 [91,93] patients (Table II). The procedure is more technically difficult but can be accomplished by the use of end-hole balloon-wedge catheters, small-sized, hi-torque guidewires, low-profile balloon catheters, and

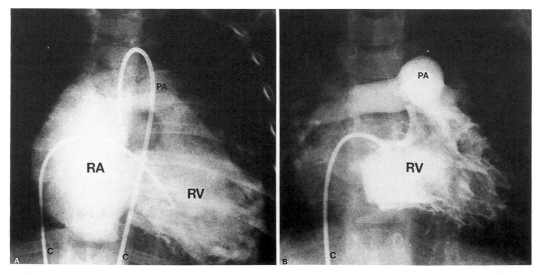

Fig. 9. Posteroanterior views of the right ventricular (RV) cineangiogram prior to **(A)** and 1 year following **(B)** balloon pulmonary valvuloplasty. Note difference of tricuspid insufficiency at follow-up **(B)**. The right ventricular cineangiograms correspond to Figure 8A, B. C, catheter; PA, pulmonary artery; RA, right atrium.

TABLE II. Results of Balloon Pulmonary Valvuloplasty in Neonates From the Literature[a]

Author and year	No. of patients undergoing BPV	Pulmonary valve gradient (mean ± SD; mm Hg)			Follow-up No. duration (months)	Poor result No. (%)	Comments
		Before	After	Follow-up			
Rey et al, 1988 [42]	8	107 ± 22	59 ± 90	25 ± 10	−/1-17	2(25)	Pressure data were from 8 neonates and 11 infants <1.0 year. Repeat valvuloplasty in both neonates
Zeevi et at, 1988 [86]	5	123 ± 7[b]	59 ± 8[b]	35 ± 27	5/11	1(20)	Before and after pressures were RV peak systolic pressures
Ali Khan et al, 1989 [87]	4	61 ± 45	6 ± 10	69 ± 47	3/8	2(66)	Repeat valvuloplasty in 2 children reduced gradient to 10 and 30 mmHg, respectively
Qureshi et al, 1989 [88]	3	125,135[b]	15,0[c]	13,16	2/8	0(0)	One patient died after unsuccessful attempt at balloon dilatation
Caspi et al, 1990 [91]	11[d]	68 ± 4 (mean ± SEM)	20 ± 4 (mean ± SEM)	−	11/19	–	FU results were not given but stated to be not changed
Ladusans et al, 1990 [93]	11[e]	81 ± 30	33 ± 28	39 ± 23	10/22	4(40)	One patient died 7 days after BPV; 4 patients required repeat intervention
Rao et al, 1991	3	69 ± 50	11 ± 11	25 ± 32	3/14	1(33)	Repeat balloon valvuloplasty reduced gradient from 61 to 18 mmHg

[a]Single case reports and abstracts are not included.
[b]Right ventricular peak systolic pressures.
[c]Infundibular gradient was 100, which subsequently disappeared.
[d]Attempts for balloon valvuloplasty were made in 20 patients; the procedure was accomplished in 11 neonates.
[e]Attempts for balloon valvuloplasty were made in 15 patients; the procedure was accomplished in 11 neonates. BPV, balloon pulmonary valvuloplasty; FU, follow-up; No., number.

progressive dilatation starting with small balloons.

The pulmonary outflow tract occlusion during valvuloplasty is well tolerated by continuous administration of prostaglandins to maintain ductal patency. Once the ductus is closed,
progressive dilatation of the stenotic pulmonary valve [88] may be of benefit. The complication rates [56] and failure rates to accomplish
balloon valvuloplasty are higher than those
seen with older children. The overall result is
also perhaps not as favorable as in children.
Right ventricular hypoplasia, severe infundibular obstruction, pulmonary valve ring hypoplasia, and pulmonary valve dysplasia may
adversely affect the results of valvuloplasty in
the neonate with critical pulmonary stenosis.

Adults

Relief of pulmonary stenosis in adult patients has been accomplished by balloon
valvuloplasty [37,66,69,72,94–102,103,a,b,c].
Because of the physical size of the pulmonary
valve ring, many of them may require balloon
valvuloplasty using two balloons [97,98]. However, as pointed out elsewhere [19,25], the
double-balloon technique is comparable with
but not superior to the single-balloon technique when equivalent balloon: annulus ratios
are compared.

Acute results (Table III) of balloon
valvuloplasty [94–102,102,a,b,c] are similar
to those reported for children. Success has
been documented even in the sixth and
seventh decades of life [96,100,101]. Based
on our own experience with teenagers [18,27]
and on that of others in adult patients
[94,97,99], infundibular obstruction following
balloon valvuloplasty appears to be more
common in older patients than in young
patients. The reason for this is probably
long-standing right ventricular hypertension
and consequent right ventricular hypertrophy
in older patients. Follow-up results (Table
III), though documented in few studies
[98,99], do indicate persistent relief after a
mean follow-up of 1–2 years. In summary, it

appears that successful balloon valvuloplasty
is feasible in all age groups.

APPLICABILITY TO PATIENTS WITH RESTENOSIS FOLLOWING PREVIOUS SURGICAL PULMONARY VALVOTOMY

Some authors [34,39] observed poor results
of balloon valvuloplasty in patients with previous surgical pulmonary valvotomy; in some of
these[34], pulmonary valve dysplasia is associated with a lack of success. Others [42,43,99]
did not specifically comment on the results of
balloon valvuloplasty in patients with previous
surgery. Poor results of balloon valvuloplasty
have also been reported in patients with previous surgical pulmonary valvotomy for pulmonary atresia with intact ventricular system
[37,40], while others [74,103] achieved significant reduction in the gradient. Indeed, balloon
valvuloplasty was incorporated into the overall
management of patients with pulmonary atresia with intact ventricular septum [103].

In our patient population, only two children, aged 3 and 14 years, had previous surgical pulmonary valvotomy, respectively 1 and 4
years prior to balloon valvuloplasty. The pulmonary valvar gradients were 120 and 146
mmHg and were reduced, respectively, to 48
and 34 mmHg immediately after valvuloplasty.
In the first patient, the pulmonary valve gradient fell further to 25 mmHg at a 10 month
follow-up catheterization. Based on the available data, successful balloon valvuloplasty can
be expected even after recurrence following
previous surgical valvotomy, and therefore I
believe balloon valvuloplasty is the treatment
of choice for restenosed pulmonary valve following previous surgery.

COMPARISON WITH SURGICAL RESULTS

Over the years, the risk from surgical correction of cardiac defects has diminished markedly. Despite this, there are many disadvantages to the surgical repair of cardiac defects,

TABLE III. Results of Balloon Pulmonary Valvuloplasty in Adults Reported in the Literature[a]

Author and year	No. of patients undergoing BPV	Pulmonary valve gradient (mean ± SD; mmHg)			FU No. duration (months)	Poor result[b] No. (%)	Comments
		Before	After	FU			
Pepine et al., 1982 [94]	1	140	42	38	1/10 days	1(100)	Infundibular gradient developed
Kan et al., 1984 [37]	2	83,70	30,24	22 –	1/–	–	–
Shuck et al., 1984 [102]	1	30	32	2	1/14 days	–	Gradients after exercise were higher (69,28, and 20, before, after, and FU, respectively)
Khalilullah et al., 1985 [95]	1	107	52	36	1/1 months	1(100)	–
Gibbs et al., 1986 [96]	1	95	25	–	–	–	Only clinical follow-up
Cooke et al., 1987 [101]	1	105	13	–	–	–	No follow-up
Al Kasab et al., 1988 [99]	21	93 ± 22	26 ± 12	17 ± 5	14/17 months	5(36)	Double-balloon in all patients
Mashru et al., 1988 [72]	3	70 ± 28	10 ± 3	–	–	–	No follow-up
Flugelman et al., 1988 [100]	1	260	90	90	1/3 weeks	1(100)	–
Fawzy et al., 1988 [98]	18	105 ± 30	32 ± 14	26 ± 11	11/6 months	4(36)	Repeat balloon valvuloplasty in two patients reduced the gradient from 59 and 52, respectively, to 24 and 22 mmHg at last follow-up
Silvert et al., 1989 [102a]	24	92 ± 36	43 ± 19	30 ± 5	23/0.3-3 years	7(30)	None of the patient had gradients >50 mmHg at last follow-up
Sherman et al., 1990 [102b]	4	92 ± 36	31 ± 8	27 ± 8	3/0.5-1 year	1(33)	–
Herrann et al., 1991 [102c]	8	62 ± 8	22 ± 6	20 ± 3	6/25 ± 5 mo	0(0)	One patient died of sepsis 10 days after BPV

[a]Shrivastava et al., [66] and Fontes et al., [69] reported successful balloon valvuloplasty in adults, but the data were not separately given for adult patients.
[b]Poor result is defined as a residual pulmonary valvar gradient > 30 mmHg at follow-up.
BPV, balloon pulmonary valvuloplasty; FU, follow-up.

including prolonged hospitalization, scary postoperative appearance (especially to the parents), residual scars, possible psychological trauma to the child and/or parents, and expense. For these reasons, it is better if these defects can be treated by catheter techniques, provided morbidity and mortality figures and recurrence rates are better than, or at least comparable with, those of surgical therapy. However, comparison of immediate and follow-up results of surgical versus balloon therapy is fraught with problems because of 1) the small number of balloon valvuloplasty patients available for follow-up; 2) the shorter duration of balloon follow-up; and 3) possible inaccuracy of comparing "older" surgical studies with "current" balloon dilatation.

Surgical treatment for valvar pulmonic stenosis has been available for 40 years since the first description by Brock [104]. Nine representative surgical pulmonary valvuloplasty papers [33,105–112] were chosen for comparison with balloon valvuloplasty. These authors [33,105–112] followed 46–234 patients for months to 30 years after surgical relief of pulmonary valve obstruction. Operative mortality varied between 3% and 14%; the cooperative study involving several institutions had only 3% mortality in 304 patients presented [33]. Poor results at follow-up were noted in 0%–8% [33,105–112]. Again, the cooperative study had 4% poor results at follow-up; *poor result at follow-up* is defined as a pulmonary valvar gradient in excess of 50 mmHg. Pulmonary valve insufficiency was reported in all studies. Follow-up catheterization studies following balloon valvuloplasty [34,37–40,42,66, 68,69,73], including the current study, involved recatheterization in 6–53 patients 1 week to 34 months after valvuloplasty (Table I) and reported varying degrees of recurrence. No significant mortality has been reported following balloon valvuloplasty [56]. The mortality and morbidity figures appear higher following surgery; however, the recurrence rate appears higher following the balloon procedure. With refinement of balloon techniques,

as indicated elsewhere [19,24,25], recurrence rates can be brought down to extremely low levels; of the 32 dilatations with balloons larger than 1.2 times the size of the pulmonary valve annulus [24], none required repeat valvuloplasty and none had pressure gradients in excess of 30 mmHg at follow-up. Based on the available information, it is likely that both immediate and follow-up results are better with balloon than with surgical pulmonary valvuloplasty, and such a categoric statement can be substantiated when 5 and 10 year follow-up studies of balloon valvuloplasty confirm the current intermediate-term follow-up results.

MECHANISM OF VALVULOPLASTY

Inflation of a balloon placed across an obstructive lesion exerts radial forces upon the stenotic lesion without any axial component [113]. Several physical principles of the "dilating force" are important in the mechanism of action and should be understood for successful application of the balloon dilatation technique [113]: 1) for the same pressure, there is a greater dilating force for a larger diameter balloon than a smaller diameter balloon; 2) for the same pressure, longer balloons have a greater dilating force than shorter balloons; 3) for the same size balloon, the higher the inflation pressure, the greater is dilating force (these are related in a linear fashion); 4) for the same pressure, a tighter stenotic area will receive a greater dilating force than a less tight stenosis; 5) for the same pressure, a large stenotic area will receive a higher dilating force compared with a small stenotic area; and 6) high inflation pressures will not significantly increase the diameter of the balloon because the balloon material (especially treated polyethylene in most pediatric dilatation balloons) does not expand due to the fact that "yield strength" (the force at which permanent deformation of the material occurs) and "ultimate tensile strength" (the force necessary to break the material) of the balloon material are very close to each other.

Based on these principles and our experience with balloon dilatations in children, we now routinely perform sequential balloon inflation with 3, 4, and 5 atm of pressure of 5 second duration, 5 minutes apart. If "wasting" of the balloon cannot be abolished, then we sequentially increase the pressure of inflation to 6, 7, and 8 atm of pressure; this was required on only two occasions (both native coarctations) of a total experience in excess of 300 balloon dilatations in children.

The mechanism of valvuloplasty was assessed by Walls [114] by inspection of valve mechanism by direct vision at surgery. They found tearing of valve raphae, tearing of the valve leaflets, and avulsion of the valve leaflets; all are conceivably the mechanisms by which relief of pulmonary or aortic valve obstruction can occur. Direct visual observations by others [17,34,36,37,115], though limited in numbers, and echocardiographic observations [43,115] also indicate a similar mechanism. The circumferential dilating force exerted by balloon inflation is likely to rupture (tear) the weakest part of the valve mechanism. It is likely that the fused commissures are the weakest links that can be broken with balloon dilatation. However, in a given patient, when the fused commissures are strong and cannot be torn, tears in the valve cups [116] or avulsion of the valve leaflets [114] can occur. The latter events may cause more severe semilunar valve insufficiency. Morphologic studies [5,117] of postmortem specimens with valvar pulmonic stenosis suggest that commissural splitting is feasible. However, abnormality of valve annulus and pulmonary valve leaflet dysplasia have been identified in these studies [5,117] that, if severe, may preclude successful balloon pulmonary valvuloplasty.

COMPLICATIONS

Acute

Complications during and immediately after balloon pulmonary valvuloplasty have been remarkably minimal. Transient bradycardia,

premature beats, and fall in systemic pressure during balloon inflation have been uniformly noted by all workers, particularly with valvar dilatations. These return rapidly back to normal following balloon deflation (Fig. 10). Systemic hypotension may be minimal during balloon inflation in the presence of a patent foramen ovale because of the right-to-left shunt across it, filling the left ventricle [102]. Use of double balloons [97] and of a trefoil or a bifoil balloon [62–65], to allow blood egress from the ventricle during balloon inflation and shorter periods (5 seconds) of inflation (19,25), have been advocated to reduce the systemic hypotension. Having had experience with each of these techniques, the author's opinion is that short periods of balloon inflation (5 seconds or less) are most efficacious without compromising immediate or follow-up results.

Blood loss requiring transfusion has been reported in many studies. Complete right bundle branch block [86], transient or permanent complete heart block [34,118,881a][1], cerebrovascular accident [42], loss of consciousness [34], cardiac arrest [119], convulsions [34], balloon rupture at high inflation pressures [36,42,68,120], tricuspid valve papillary muscle rupture [121], pulmonary artery tears [122], perforation of the right ventricular outflow tract [89], transient pulmonary hypertension [121a], right-sided endocarditis [123], and severe infundibular obstruction requiring propranolol administration [18,27,29,42,68] and/or surgical intervention [68,124], though rare, have been reported. Some of these complications may be unavoidable. However, meticulous attention to the details of the technique, use of an appropriate length of the balloon, avoiding extremely high inflation pressures, and short inflation–deflation cycles may prevent or reduce the complications.

---

[1]Steinberg et al. [118a] used a short course (<2 weeks) of systemic corticosteroid to treat a complete heart block that developed after balloon pulmonary valvuloplasty in a 5-year-old child and advocated steroid use in similar situations.

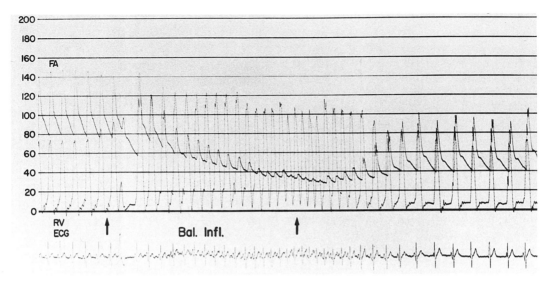

Fig. 10. Simultaneous recording of the right ventricular (RV) and femoral artery (FA) pressures during balloon dilatation of the stenotic pulmonary valve. Note a marked increase in the RV pressure, presumably related to complete obstruction of the RV. There is a simultaneous fall in the FA pressure, again related to complete obstruction to flow during balloon valvuloplasty. Following deflation of the balloon, the FA pressure returns toward normal. The 10 second period of balloon inflation (Bal. Infl.) is marked with arrows. (Reproduced from Rao and Mardini [13], with permission of the publisher.)

Holter monitoring for 24 hours following balloon valvuloplasty [38] revealed premature ventricular contractions (grade 1, Lown criteria) in one-third of the 12 patients so studied. It is not clear from this study [38] whether the premature beats were present prior to valvuloplasty and for how long after valvuloplasty they persisted.

Transient prolongation of the QTc interval following balloon angioplasty valvuloplasty [125,126] may be a potential hazard for developing R-on-T phenomenon in children with ventricular ectopy. The Holter findings [38] of premature beats following valvuloplasty may have significance in the light of prolongation of QTc interval [125]. However, no patients from our series or many other studies have been known to develop ventricular arrhythmias, although two cases of sudden death from ventricular fibrillation shortly after balloon angioplasty of aortic coarctation [127,128] were reported. Whether these arrhythmias are related to QTc prolongation is not known. How-

ever, patient monitoring following balloon valvuloplasty–angioplasty is warranted [125].

Although multiple complications were listed, the VACA Registry reported only a 0.24% death rate and a 0.35% major complication rate from the 822 balloon pulmonary valvuloplasty procedures from 26 member institutions [56] attesting to the safety of the procedure.

Complication at Follow-Up

With regard to the complications at the intermediate-term follow-up, femoral venous occlusion, pulmonary valve insufficiency, and pulmonary valve restenosis have been noted. Restenosis will be discussed in the next section. Anywhere between 10% to 29% [18,38,42] of femoral veins through which balloon valvuloplasty have been performed were noted to be occluded at follow-up. In the present series, 3 out of 45 patients (7%) whom we restudied following pulmonary valvuloplasty had blocked femoral vein. It is the consensus that the femoral venous occlusion is more common in small infants [38,42,119].

Auscultatory evidence for pulmonary valve insufficiency has not been thoroughly scrutinized. Doppler evidence for pulmonary insufficiency appears sensitive but was studied by only a few investigators [18,38,43,70,76,129]. Rocchini and Beekman [129] reported pulmonary insufficiency in 31 of 37 (84%) patients, whereas Robertson et al. [43] found mild pulmonary insufficiency in all 29 patients studied. When we reviewed this last from our group, 50 out of 54 (93%) patients had Doppler-demonstrable pulmonary insufficiency. However, the pulmonary insufficiency is minimal as evidenced by lack of right ventricular overloading (normal-sized right ventricle and no paradoxical septal motion) in this group of patients as well as by equilibrium-gated radionuclide angiograms reported by Tynan [34]. Although the long-term follow-up studies should be scrutinized for progressive right ventricular volume

overloading, the current data suggest that the pulmonary insufficiency produced by balloon valvuloplasty is unlikely to be problematic.

CAUSES OF RESTENOSIS

Recurrence of valve stenosis following balloon pulmonary valvuloplasty has been reported by most investigators (Table I), but the reasons for the restenosis at intermediate-term follow-up have been studied only to a limited degree [34,37–40,81b,84]. We have systemically investigated the cause of recurrence of pulmonic stenosis following balloon valvuloplasty [23,28]. On the basis of results of 6–34 month follow-up catheterization data in 40 children, they were divided into: group I with good results (pulmonary valve gradient of 30 mmHg or less), 33 patients; group II with poor results (gradient greater than 30 mmHg), seven patients (Table IV). Fourteen biographic, anatomic, physiologic, and technical factors

TABLE IV. Various Groupings Used in the Text[a]

Group	Characteristics
I	Good results group (at follow-up), with catheterization pulmonary valve gradients ≤30 mmHg; 33 children
II	Poor results group (at follow-up) with catheterization pulmonary valve gradients >30 mmHg; 7 patients
III	Balloon dilatations in which balloon:annulus ratio was 1.0 or less (0.89 ± 0.08; range 0.76–1.0); 12 dilatations
IV	Balloon dilatations in which balloon:annulus ratio was more than 1.0 (1.31 ± 0.19; range 1.01–1.8); 44 dilatations
V	Balloon dilatations in which balloon:annulus ratio was 1.2 or less (1.03 ± 0.13; range 0.76–1.2), 32 dilatations
VI	Balloon dilatations in which balloon:annulus ratio was more than 1.2 (1.43 ± 0.13; range 1.21–1.8); 32 dilatations
VII	Balloon valvuloplasties in which balloon:annulus ratio was between 1.21 and 1.5 (1.36 ± 0.08); 23 dilatations
VIII	Balloon valvuloplasties in which balloon:annulus ratio was between 1.51 and 1.8 (1.6 ± 0.09); 9 dilatations
IX	Double-balloon valvuloplasty (balloon:annulus ratio, 1.19 ± 0.14; range 1.01–1.53) ; 12 patients
X	Single-balloon valvuloplasty, matched with group IX for balloon: annulus ratio (1.19 ± 0.15; range 1.0–1.53); 12 patients
XI	Good results group with catheterization and/or Doppler gradients ≤30 mmHg at follow-up; 54 children
XII	Poor results group with catheterization and/or Doppler gradients >30 mmHg at follow-up; 9 children
XIII	Dysplastic pulmonary valves; 13 patients
XIV	Nondysplastic pulmonary valves; 43 patients

[a]Modified from Rao [26], with permission of the publisher.

TABLE V. Variables Examined by Multivariate Logistic Regression Analysis to Identify Factors Responsible for Pulmonary Valve Restenosis Following Balloon Valvuloplasty[a]

1. Age at valvuloplasty
2. Duration of follow-up
3. Pulmonary valve dysplasia, severe or mild
4. Pulmonary valve ring hypoplasia
5. Right ventricular hypoplasia
6. Angiographic infundibular stenosis
7. Right ventricular peak systolic pressure prior to valvuloplasty
8. Pulmonary valve peak systolic pressure gradient prior to valvuloplasty
9. Right ventricular infundibular pressure gradient prior to valvuloplasty
10. Pulmonary valve peak systolic pressure gradient immediately after valvuloplasty
11. Balloon: pulmonary valve annulus ratio
12. Maximum pressure achieved in the balloon
13. Number of balloon dilations
14. Total duration of balloon inflation

[a]Reproduced from Rao [26], with permission of the publisher.

(Table V) were examined by multivariate logistic regression analysis to identify factors associated with restenosis. The identified risk factors were 1) residual pulmonary valve gradient in excess of 30 mmHg immediately following balloon valvuloplasty and 2) a balloon-to-pulmonary valve annulus ratio less than 1.2. Dysplastic pulmonary valves did not seem to play a role in recurrence, and this may have been due to use of large balloons with dysplastic valves. The influence of these factors on the restenosis is examined in Figures 11 and 12.

The smaller balloon: annulus ratios are associated with a higher chance for recurrence, as are the higher residual gradients immediately following balloon pulmonary valvuloplasty. The data suggested that a balloon: annulus ratio of less than 1.2 is the cause for pulmonary valve restenosis at intermediate-term follow-up, and such recurrences can be predicted in patients with immediate postvalvuloplasty pulmonary valve gradient in excess of 30 mmHg. We suggested use of progressively larger balloons and reduce the valve gradient to less than 30 mmHg [23,28,61].

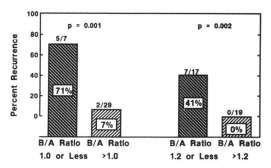

Fig. 11. Rates of recurrence of pulmonary valve stenosis after balloon valvuloplasty as it relates to balloon:annulus ratio are shown. Note that the rates of restenosis increase as the balloon:annulus ratio decreases. Percentages are marked within the bars, and actual numbers are shown on the top of each bar.

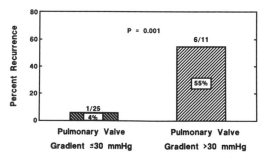

Fig. 12. Similar to Figure 11 except that the immediate postballoon valvuloplasty peak-to-peak pulmonary valve gradients are used instead of the balloon:annulus ratio. Note a higher rate of recurrence at follow-up when the gradient is >30 mmHg immediately after valvuloplasty.

Pulmonary valve dysplasia and pulmonary valve annular hypoplasia may well play a significant role in the recurrence of pulmonary valve obstruction but did not seem to have an adverse effect in our study group. Perhaps this is related to the narrow ranges of such abnormalities in our study group.

A recent analysis of VACA Registry data [84] on 433 patients followed up to a median interval of 31 months also identified the balloon:annulus ratio and an immediate postvalvuloplasty gradient of ≥ 36 mmHg as factors predicting suboptimal follow-up result, very similar to our study [23,28]. The Registry data, in addition, identified dysplastic pulmonary valve morphology and age less than two years as factors predisposing to recurrence. A patient's age of less than 2 years at the time of balloon dilatation was also found to be a significant risk factor in the study my McCrindle and Kan [81b].

INFLUENCE OF TECHNICAL FACTORS ON VALVULOPLASTY
How Large a Balloon Should Be Used?

Radtke [41] and Rao [16] evaluated the influence of balloon size on the results of pulmonary valvuloplasty and recommended a balloon-to-pulmonary valve annulus ratio of 1.2–1.4. Such recommendations are arbitrary and were based on 1) small number of patients [16,11], 2) no follow-up results [41], or 3) follow-up results on only a few patients [16]. Our experience with 64 consecutive balloon dilatation procedures performed in 56 patients with isolated valvar pulmonic stenosis and 39 follow-up catheterizations in 36 patients was reviewed to examine this issue [19,24,26]. Five repeat valvuloplasty procedures were performed at follow-up catheterization, and three patients had valvuloplasty sequentially with balloons resulting in increasingly larger balloon:annulus ratios. Thus there were 64 valvuloplasty procedures in 56 patients. These were divided into two groups: group III, those in which the balloon:annulus ratio was 1.0 or less, 12 dilatations; and group IV, those in

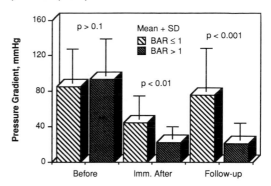

Fig. 13. Peak-to-peak pulmonary valvar gradients were compared between two groups of patients. The groups with balloon:annulus (B/A) ratios of ≤ 1.0 and >1.0 had similar prevalvuloplasty gradients, while higher gradients were found in the smaller balloon group both immediately following balloon valvuloplasty ($P<0.01$) and at follow-up ($P<0.001$).

which the ratio was more than 1.0, 52 dilatations (Table IV). The two groups had similar ($P > 0.1$) prevalvuloplasty valvar gradients (84.3 $\pm$ 39.2 vs. 92.8 $\pm$ 42.1 mmHg; Fig. 13). Immediately after valvuloplasty, there was a significant reduction pulmonary valve gradient (Fig. 14) in both group III (84.3 $\pm$ 29.2 vs. 43.6 $\pm$ 26.8 mmHg, $P < 0.02$) and group IV (92.8 $\pm$

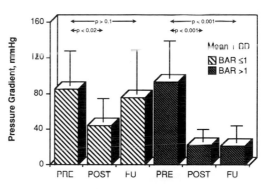

Fig. 14. Results of balloon pulmonary valvuloplasty in patient groups with balloon:annulus (B/A) ratios of ≤ 1.0 and >1.0. Note statistically significant ($P<0.002$ and <0.01) falls in peak-to-peak gradients immediately after valvuloplasty in both groups. In the group with B:A ratios ≤ 1.0, the gradient returned toward prevalvuloplasty values ($P>0.1$), whereas in the group with B:A ratios of >1.0 the gradients remained low ($P<0.001$).

42.1 *vs.* 22.4 ± 13.6 mmHg, $P < 0.001$), although there was a greater fall in the gradient in group IV with larger balloons (Fig. 13). On intermediate-term follow-up (which ranged between 6 and 34 months), residual pulmonary valve gradients were significantly lower ($P < 0.001$) in group IV (20.8 ± 18.5 mmHg) than in group III (75.0 ± 49.4 mmHg), suggesting restenosis in group III with small balloons (Fig. 13). At follow-up, repeat balloon valvuloplasty was required in four group III patients and only one from group IV ($P < 0.005$; Table VI). Similarly, a higher ($P < 0.005$) number of patients with a residual pulmonary valve gradient in excess of 30 mmHg were present in group III than in group IV (Table VI). These data suggest that, although good immediate results are seen with either small or large balloons, balloons larger than the pulmonary valve annulus produce more sustained relief from pulmonary stenosis.

Second, the balloon:annulus ratio cut-off point was increased to 1.2 and balloon valvuloplasties were divided into another two groups (Table IV): group V, those in which the ratio was 1.2 or less; and group VI, those in which the ratio was more than 1.2. In group V, consisting of 32 dilatations, the mean ratio was 1.03 ± 0.13, while in group VI, which also consisted of 32 balloon dilatations, the ratio was 1.43 ± 0.13. Both of these groups had similar ($P > 0.1$) prevalvuloplasty gradients (Fig. 15). Both groups had significant ($P < 0.001$) reduction in pulmonary valve gradients

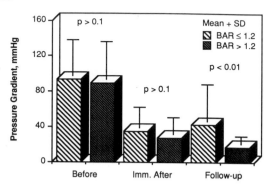

Fig. 15. Comparison of gradients similar to those in Figure 13 but the balloon:annulus (B/A) ratios were ≤1.2 and >1.2. Note similar gradients ($P>0.1$) prior to and immediately after valvuloplasty. However, at follow-up the gradients were higher ($P<0.01$) in the group with B:A ratios of ≤1.2 than the group with B:A ratios of >1.2.

both immediately after valvuloplasty and on follow-up (Fig. 16). However, the follow-up gradients in group VI with larger balloons were lower ($P < 0.01$ than those in group V with small balloons (Fig. 15). Five patients in group V required repeat balloon dilatation at follow-up while none in group VI required repeat valvuloplasty ($P < 0.001$; Table VI). Also, seven patients in group V had gradients in excess of 30 mmHg while none in Group VI had that high a gradient on follow-up ($P < 0.001$; Table VI). Based on these data, balloons smaller than 1.2 times the pulmonary valve annulus have a significant chance for having residual pulmonary stenosis on follow-up and as such are not recommended.

TABLE VI. Prevalence of Repeat Valvuloplasty and Significant Residual Gradients in Various Groups[a]

Groups	No. of patients needing repeat valvuloplasty	p value[b]	No. of patients wit pulmonary valve gradient >30mmHg	p value[b]
III (n = 7)[c]	4	0.002	5	0.001
IV (N = 32)	1		2	
V (N = 21)	5	0.005	7	0.002
VI (N = 18)	0		0	

[a]Modified from Rao [19], with permission of the publisher.
[b]Fisher's exact test.
[c]Number of patients with intermediate-term follow-up catheterization.

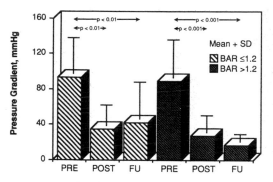

Fig. 16. Results of valvuloplasty depicted similarly to those in Figure 14 but with balloon:annulus (B/A) ratio groups of ≤1.2 and >1.2. Note significant (P<0.001) fall in the gradients in both groups immediately following valvuloplasty and at follow-up. The residual gradients were higher in the smaller B:A ratio group (Fig. 11).

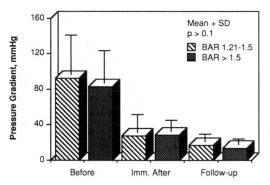

Fig. 17. Comparison of peak-to-peak systolic pressure gradients across the pulmonic valve in a manner similar to that in Figures 13 and 15 but for balloon:annulus (B/A) ratio groups of 1.21–1.5 vs. >1.5. Note that the gradients are similar (P>0.1) prior to and immediately after valvuloplasty and at follow-up, signifying that the group with a B:A ratio of >1.5 is not better off than the group with ratios of 1.21–1.5 with regard to residual gradients.

Finally, the results of balloon valvuloplasty with a balloon:annulus ratio of 1.21–1.5 (group VII) were compared with those in which the ratio was in excess of 1.5 (group VIII), because balloons larger than 1.5 times the size of the valve annulus are reported to produce damage to the right ventricular outflow tract [60]. Group VII with a mean balloon:annulus ratio of 1.36 ± 0.08 consisted of 23 patients, while group VIII with a mean balloon:annulus ratio of 1.6 ± 0.09 consisted of 9 patients (Table IV). The pulmonary valve gradients were similar (P > 0.1; Fig. 17) prior to valvuloplasty in both groups. Significant (P < 0.001) reduction of gradient occurred in both groups immediately after valvuloplasty as well as at follow-up catheterization (Fig. 18). Residual pulmonary valvar gradients immediately after balloon dilatation and on follow-up (Fig. 17) were similar (P > 0.1). None of the patients in either group required repeat balloon dilatation, nor was there any patient with residual pulmonary valvar gradient in excess of 30 mmHg. These data signify that balloons larger than 1.5 times the size of the pulmonary valve annulus do not offer any advantage over the balloons with a ratio of 1.2–1.5.

Thus the data presented in this section indicate that balloons larger than 1.2 times the diameter of the pulmonary valve annulus should be used for pulmonary valvuloplasty if restenosis is to be prevented and that there is no advantage to the use of balloons larger than 1.5 times the size of the pulmonary valve annulus. Therefore balloons that are 1.2–1.5 times the diameter of the pulmonary valve

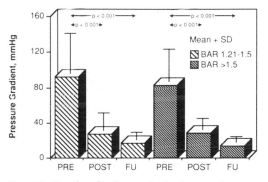

Fig. 18. Results of balloon valvuloplasty in the groups with balloon:annulus ratios of 1.21–1.5 and >1.5. Note the excellent fall in gradients (P<0.001) both immediately after and at follow-up in both groups.

annulus are most ideal for relief of pulmonary stenosis and are recommended.

How Long a Balloon?

The majority of workers use 30 mm long balloons for pulmonary valvuloplasty. There are no data either from our own series or from the literature to assess whether shorter (20 mm) or longer (≥40 mm) balloons have any advantages or disadvantages over the conventional 30 mm length balloons. The 20 mm long balloons are too short to maintain the balloon center over the pulmonary valve annulus during balloon inflation and therefore are not advisable in children and adolescents. The 20 mm long balloons are appropriate for the neonates and infants. Forty millimeter and longer balloons may impinge upon the tricuspid valve mechanism and may injure it. Two recent experiences, one causing avulsion of the papillary muscle [121] and another causing complete heart block [118] when 60 and 40 mm long balloons, respectively, were used, suggest that these long balloons should not be used for balloon pulmonary valvuloplasty. Based on this discussion, it can be concluded that 30 mm long balloons should be used in children for valvuloplasty until data to the contrary become available.

How Many Balloons?

Although single balloons are used in the majority of cases, valvuloplasty with simultaneous inflation of two balloons placed across the stenotic pulmonary valve (Fig. 2) when the pulmonary valve annulus is too large to dilate with a single balloon has also been reported [14,16,18,24,41,44,68,97]. Indeed, some authors [97] advocate use of double-balloon valvuloplasty as the procedure of choice, especially in adults. To evaluate this issue, 12 patients from our series who underwent double-balloon valvuloplasty (group IX) were compared with 12 patients with single-balloon valvuloplasty who were matched for the balloon:annulus ratio (group X; Table IV) [25]. Effective balloon diameter with double bal-

loons was calculated by using a formula that we previously proposed [16]; this formula was given in the section on technique.

The balloon:annulus ratio in group IX with double balloons, 1.19 ± 0.14, was similar ($P >$ 0.1) to that (1.19 ± 0.15) in group X with single balloon (Table IV, Fig. 19). The two groups had similar ($P > 0.1$) prevalvuloplasty pulmonary valvar gradients (100.5 ± 28.0 vs. 96.3 ± 40.1 mmHg) and peak right ventricular systolic pressures (Fig. 19). Immediately following valvuloplasty, there was a significant reduction ($P < 0.001$) in pulmonary valvar gradients in both groups, which remained improved ($P < 0.001$) at 6 to 14 month follow-up catheterizations (Fig. 20). Residual pulmonary valvar gradients immediately after valvuloplasty and at follow-up catheterization were similar ($P > 0.1$) in both groups (Fig. 21). These data indicate that double-balloon valvuloplasty success is comparable to and not superior to that observed with single-balloon valvuloplasty. The balloon-to-pulmonary valve annulus ratio, as presented in the earlier part of this discussion, is perhaps a better determinant of relief of pulmonary valve stenosis than whether a single- or

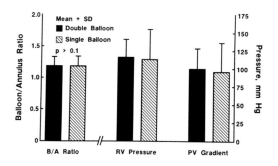

Fig. 19. Bar graphs showing prevalvuloplasty comparison of double- and single-balloon groups. Balloon to pulmonary valve annulus (B:A) ratios of the double-balloon group are similar (P>0.1) to those of the single-balloon group. The right ventricular (RV) peak systolic pressure and pulmonary valve (PV) peak systolic pressure gradients in both groups were similar prior to balloon valvuloplasty; these data suggest that severity of pulmonary valve stenosis is similar in both groups. (Reproduced from Rao and Fawzy [25], with permission of the publisher.)

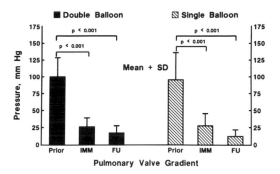

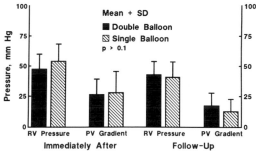

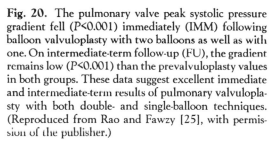

Fig. 20. The pulmonary valve peak systolic pressure gradient fell (P<0.001) immediately (IMM) following balloon valvuloplasty with two balloons as well as with one. On intermediate-term follow-up (FU), the gradient remains low (P<0.001) than the prevalvuloplasty values in both groups. These data suggest excellent immediate and intermediate-term results of pulmonary valvuloplasty with both double- and single-balloon techniques. (Reproduced from Rao and Fawzy [25], with permission of the publisher.)

Fig. 21. Residual right ventricular (RV) pressures and pulmonary valvar (PV) peak systolic pressure gradients immediately after balloon pulmonary valvuloplasty and at intermediate-term follow-up were similar (P>0.1) in both double- and single-balloon groups. The data suggest good results whether a double- or a single-balloon technique was used for pulmonary valvuloplasty provided that balloon:annulus ratios are similar. (Reproduced from Rao and Fawzy [25], with permission of the publisher.)

double-balloon technique is used. The choice of the specific formula that we used for calculation of balloon size and balloon:annulus ratio may be criticized, but this formula was simultaneously and independently advocated by us [16] and others [41,130,131] and fits the best available geometric model. Therefore, despite the age difference between the groups, I feel that the comparison of double-balloon data with single-balloon data is justified.

The suggestion by Al Kasab and his associates [97] that a double-balloon technique is preferable is based on immediate and short-term 6-week follow-up only) results (but without single-balloon controls) and less systemic hypotension and bradycardia during balloon inflation. Initially, we inflated the balloon(s) for 10 seconds [13] for valvuloplasty, and we also noticed hypotension [13] during balloon inflation, but the blood pressure promptly returned to normal after balloon deflation (Fig. 10). More recently [19,22], we have used 5 second inflation with less hypotension (Fig. 22) not too different from that reported with double-balloon technique [44,97] and without sacrificing the results. Although we

and others [44] did not find a significantly higher complication rate with the double-balloon technique, it does indeed prolong the procedure and involves use of additional femoral venous site and the attended potential complications. Therefore we would recommend that the double-balloon technique be used when the pulmonary valve annulus is too large to dilate with a commercially available single balloon or when a single balloon cannot be safely passed across the femoral vein [44], not because the double-balloon technique gives a better result. Bifoil and trefoil balloon catheters [62–65] may help to resolve the problem, but our limited personal experience (Fig. 23) suggests that these catheters are too bulky, and the advantage of less hypotension during valvuloplasty is minimal.

In conclusion, the immediate and follow-up results of pulmonary valvuloplasty with two balloons are excellent. These results are similar to those achieved with equivalent-sized single-balloon valvuloplasty and did not offer additional advantage over single-balloon results. There are no data to support the contention that double-balloon technique is superior to

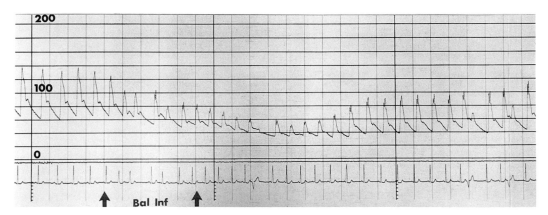

Fig. 22. Femoral artery pressure recorded during balloon valvuloplasty in which a 5 second balloon inflation is used. Note fall in femoral artery pressure but the decrease in pressure is not as severe (peak pressure of 60 mmHg). The return toward normal is not as slow as with 10 second inflation (see Fig. 10). The 5 second balloon inflation (Bal Infl) is marked with arrows.

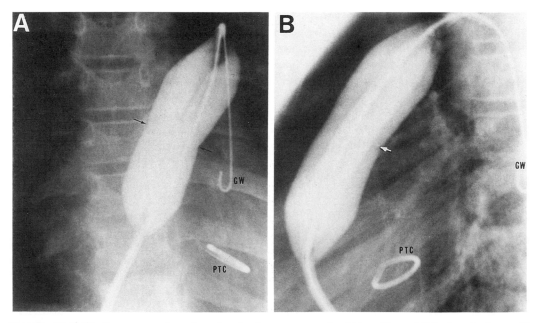

Fig. 23. Trefoil balloon across the pulmonic valve in posteroanterior **(A)** and lateral **(B)** views is shown. Note the indentation of the balloons (arrows) produced by pulmonary valve annulus. Guidewire (GW) in the left pulmonary artery and pigtail catheter (PTC) in the left ventricle are shown.

TABLE VII. Balloon Inflation Characteristics in Group I With Good Results and Group II With Poor Results[a]

Inflation characteristic	Group I (Mean ± SD)	Group II (Mean ± SD)	P value
Maximum pressure in the balloon (atm)	4.6 ± 0.2	4.0 ± 1.4	>0.1
Number of balloon inflations	4.4 ± 1.1	4.0 ± 1.0	>0.1
Total duration of balloon (seconds)	36.2 ± 13.5	37.9 ± 13.5	>0.1

[a]Reproduced from Rao [26], with permission of the publisher.

single-balloon pulmonary valvuloplasty. It is suggested that a double-balloon technique be used when the pulmonary valve annulus is too large to dilate with a commercially available single balloon.

Pressure, Number, and Duration of Balloon Inflation

The recommendations for pressure of inflation of the balloon varied between 2 and 8.5 atmo [9,13,18,36,37,40–42,44,87], and duration of each inflation was suggested to be 5–20 seconds. Anywhere between one to four balloon inflations, two to five minutes apart has been suggested. Clearly, no data are available for determining which is the best method of inflation. We examined these issues from our data. The inflation characteristics of group I, with good results (Table IV), were compared with those of the group II with poor results

(Table VII). There were no significant differences between the groups, suggesting that the outcome of valvuloplasty is not related to these balloon inflation characteristics. We have also looked at the data with arbitrary division of maximum pressure, number of balloon inflations, and total duration of balloon inflation (Tables VIII–X) and found that higher pressure, larger number, and longer duration of balloon inflation did not favorably influence residual gradients at follow-up, especially when the influence of balloon: annulus ratio was removed.

Some investigators [36] recommend 7–8.5 atmo of pressure, which in our opinion has a good chance for balloon rupture and potential problems associated with rupture. In our own experience, the "waisting" of the balloon was noted to disappear even at 2 atm of pressure with resultant good valvuloplasty [13]. Now, we routinely perform valvuloplasty sequen-

TABLE VIII. Influence of Maximal Pressure of Balloon Inflation on the Immediate and Follow-Up Residual Pulmonary Valve Gradients[a]

	Maximum pressure of balloon inflation (Atm)			
	≤3	4–5	>5	P value[b]
Pre-BPV gradient (mmHg, mean ± SD)	94.8 ± 51.8	90.1 ± 29.5	97.6 ± 45.6	>0.1
Post-BPV gradient (mmHg, mean ± SD)	24.9 ± 19.8	26.8 ± 15.6	33.3 ± 26.2	>0.1
FU gradient (mmHg, mean ± SD)	43.0 ± 46.5	18.1 ± 15.5	30.1 ± 36.4	>0.1
FU gradient (mmHg; B:A ratio >1.0; mean ± SD)	24.6 ± 35.4	18.3 ± 16.1	20.6 ± 13.4	>0.1

[a]Reproduced from Rao [26], with permission of the publisher.
[b]The P value was derived by comparing groups ≤3 with 4–5, 4–5 with >5.0, and > 5 with ≤3 atm.
B:A, balloon: annulus ratio; BPV, balloon pulmonary valvuloplasty; FU, follow-up.

TABLE IX. Influence of Number of Balloon Dilatations on the Immediate and Follow-Up Residual Pulmonary Valve Gradients[a]

	No. of balloon dilatations			
	3	4	5-7	P value[b]
Pre-BPV gradient (mm Hg, mean ± SD)	77.9 ± 20.1	101.0 ± 52.4	97.0 ± 36.0	>0.05
Post-BPV gradient (mm Hg, mean ± SD)	22.0 ± 9.0	33.2 ± 25.6	29.6 ± 19.7	>0.05
FU gradient (mm Hg, mean ± SD)	42.3 ± 50.3	32.9 ± 37.1	19.1 ± 15.3	>0.1
FU gradient (mm Hg; B:A ratio >1.0; mean ± SD)	27.2 ± 38.0	20.7 ± 13.5	19.1 ± 15.3	>0.1

[a]Reproduced from Rao [26], with permission of the publisher.
[b]The P value was derived by comparing dilatation groups 3 with 4, 4 with 5-7, and 5-7 with 3.
B:A, balloon/annulus ratio; BPV, balloon pulmonary valvuloplasty; FU, follow-up.

tially at 3, 4, and 5 atm of pressure inflation. The "waisting" usually abolishes at 3 or 4 atm of pressure. With this protocol, we have not found any balloon ruptures. Initially, we used 10 second inflation, and now we use 5 second inflation. With the latter, there is less hypotension (Fig. 22), which returns to normal a few seconds after deflation. After a successful valvuloplasty, we usually repeat the procedure for two additional times. We agree with Yeager's suggestion [132] that pressures much higher than those required to abolish "waisting" of the balloon offer no advantage, especially because the polyethylene balloons are designed to maintain a relatively uniform diameter even at high pressures. Furthermore, high pressures tend to produce balloon rupture. Shorter inflation–deflation cycles produce minimal hemodynamic disturbances durng valvuloplasty.

Based on the data presented and on our own experience, we recommend sequential balloon inflation with 3, 4, and 5 atm of presure of 5 second duration, 5 minutes apart.

NONINVASIVE FOLLOW-UP EVALUATION
Electrocardiographic Studies

Kveselis et al. [38], Fontes et al. [69], Lloyd and Donnerstein [133], and we [20] previously reported electrocardiographic changes following valvuloplasty. Kveselis et al. [38] observed a significant decrease in R-wave voltage in lead

TABLE X. Influence of Total Duration of Balloon Inflation on the Immediate and Follow-Up Residual Pulmonary Valve Gradient[a]

	Total duration of balloon inflation (seconds)			
	≤25	26-40	>40	P value[b]
Pre-BPV gradient (mm Hg, mean ± SD)	87.3 ± 47.6	99.4 ± 40.5	96.2 ± 35.2	>0.1
Post-BPV gradient (mm Hg, mean ± SD)	25.7 ± 18.0	29.5 ± 23.9	36.0 ± 20.2	>0.1
FU gradient (mm Hg, mean ± SD)	25.5 ± 25.3	34.4 ± 42.2	22.7 ± 16.7	>0.1
FU gradient (mm Hg, B:A ration >1.0; mean ± SD)	25.4 ± 25.3	16.9 ± 15.0	22.7 ± 16.7	>0.1

[a]Reproduced from Rao [26], with permission of the publisher.
[b]The P value was derived by comparing groups ≤25 with 26-40, 26-40 with >40, and >40 with ≤25.
B:A, balloon/annulus ratio; BPV, balloon pulmonary valvuloplasty; FU, follow-up.

V_1 and leftward shift of frontal plane mean QRS vector in 13 patients, 16 ± 9 months following valvuloplasty. Fontes *et al.* [69] reported a shift of frontal plane mean vector (axis) from $118 \pm 31°$ to $86 \pm 31°$ in 56 patients during follow ups from 6 to 52 months following balloon pulmonary valvuloplasty. They also found regression of right ventricular hypertrophy in 16 (29%) cases, whereas mild to moderate hypertrophy persisted in 29 (52%) cases. Lloyd and Donnerstein [133] noted reversion to normal (inversion) of T waves in lead V_1 in 17 of 19 (89%) patients under 12 years of age, which had been upright prior to balloon valvuloplasty. They attributed this change in T-wave polarity to favorable alteration of the relationship between myocardial oxygen consumption and coronary blood flow following pressure gradient relief produced by balloon valvuloplasty.

In a detailed study [20] of 35 patients with electrocardiogram follow-up 3 to 34 (mean 11) months following valvuloplasty, we made the following observations. When electrocardiograms immediately prior to and following balloon valvuloplasty were compared, there was practically no change in mean vectors, QRS voltages, and T waves in any patient. In our study, we did not find any T-wave changes, in contradistinction to the findings of Lloyd and Donnerstein [133]; however, most of our electrocardiograms were obtained within a few hours of valvuloplasty and probably did not allow sufficient time for regression of T waves. In 30 children with excellent relief of pulmonic stenosis at follow-up, the frontal plane mean QRS vector moved toward the left ($P < 0.001$) from $127 \pm 25°$ to $81 \pm 47°$, as did the horizontal plane mean QRS vector from $88 \pm 36°$ to $27 \pm 51°$ ($P < 0.001$). The QRS vector loop in the horizontal plane rotated clockwise in the vast majority (25 of 30; 83%) of patients prior to valvuloplasty (Fig. 24) but only a small percentage (8 of 30; 27%) had clockwise rotation at follow-up. The T waves were upright in the right chest leads in 21 patients and biphasic in three patients prior to valvuloplasty, but, at follow-up, upright T waves were present in only seven patients ($P < 0.001$) and biphasic T in four patients. The amplitude of R waves in V_1 (19.0 ± 11.6 mm) and V_2 (19.7 ± 12.2 mm) decreased ($P < 0.001$), respectively, to 9.5 ± 5.9 mm and 11.3 ± 6.1 mm. S-wave amplitudes in V_5 and V_6, 10.5 ± 6.5 and 6.7 ± 4.7 mm, respectively, decreased ($P < 0.01$) to 5.9 ± 3.9 and 2.9 ± 2.6 mm (Fig. 25). An

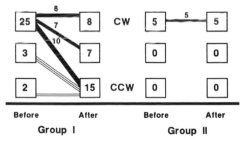

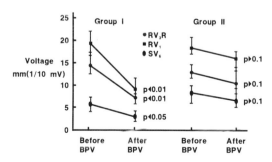

Fig. 24. Pictorial depiction of changes of the horizontal plane QRS vector loop rotation following balloon valvuloplasty. Note that the QRS loop in 17 of the group I good result patients changed from clockwise to either a figure of 8 or a counterclockwise configuration, while none of the five group II poor result patients changed their QRS loop configuration. (Reproduced from Rao and Solymar [20], with permission of the publisher.)

Fig. 25. Precordial voltage magnitudes before and after (intermediate-term follow-up) balloon pulmonary valvuloplasty (BPV). Note significant ($P<0.01–<0.001$) decrease in voltages in group I with good results, while there was no statistically significant fall ($P>0.1$) in group II with poor results. Mean $\pm$ standard deviation for each precordial lead are shown. (Reproduced from Rao [61], with permission of the publisher.)

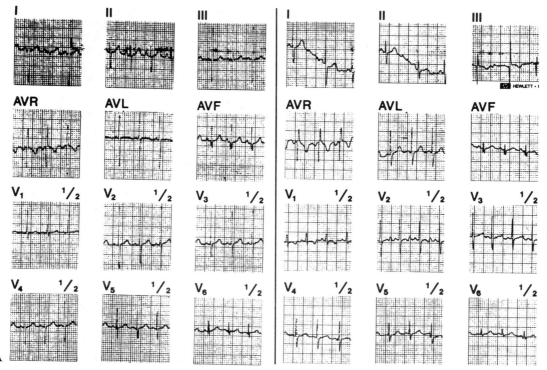

Fig. 26. Note that right ventricular hypertrophy prior to valvuloplasty (**A**) has disappeared in the ECG obtained 12 months after valvuloplasty (**B**).

example is shown in Figure 26. The improvement in the electrocardiogram is associated with a decrease in pulmonary valve gradient from 95 ± 50 to 29 ± 23 mmHg. In five children with significant residual gradient, the electrocardiogram did not show any significant change (Fig. 24 and 25).

Evaluation of the time course of the electrocardiographic changes in the group with good results revealed that there was minimal or no improvement in electrocardiographic parameters at the 3 month follow-up visit (P > 0.05–0.2), whereas at 6, 12, and 18 month follow-up visits there were significant improvements (P < 0.05 to 0.001) (Fig. 27).

Having concluded that the electrocardiogram improves following successful balloon pulmonary valvuloplasty, it was attempted to determine if each individual postvalvuloplasty electrocardiogram reflected significant residual valve gradient at follow-up. Thirty pairs of

electrocardiographic and pulmonary valve pressure gradient data obtained within 24 hours of each other were available for analysis. Fifteen electrocardiograms were interpreted to be normal, and their pulmonary valve gradients were low, 18.3 ± 8.2 mmHg (range 4–30 mmHg) (Fig. 28). These electrocardiograms and catheterization-measured gradients were obtained 7–28 months (12.0 ± 5.5 months) following balloon valvuloplasty. Ten electrocardiograms were found to have right ventricular hypertrophy and were not significantly different from prevalvuloplasty tracings. These were obtained 6–23 months (10 ± 5 months) following valvuloplasty, and their right ventricular outflow gradients (valvar plus infundibular) ranged between 32 and 118 mmHg (55.8 ± 26.4 mmHg) and were higher (P < 0.01) than those seen in a normal electrocardiographic group (Fig. 28). The remaining five electrocardiograms, obtained within 6 months

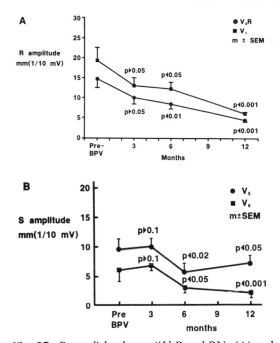

A

R amplitude
mm(1/10 mV)

● V_3R
■ V_1
m ± SEM

p>0.05

p<0.05

p<0.001

p>0.05

p<0.01

p<0.001

Pre-BPV   3   6   9   12
Months

B

S amplitude
mm(1/10 mV)

● V_5
■ V_6
m±SEM

p>0.1

p>0.1

p<0.02

p<0.05

p<0.05

p<0.001

Pre BPV   3   6   9   12
months

Fig. 27. Precordial voltages, RV_3R and RV_1 **(A)** and SV_5 and SV_6 **(B)** prior to and 3, 6, and 12 months following balloon pulmonary valvuloplasty (BPV) in group I with good results. Note that precordial voltages did not significantly change ($P>0.05$->0.1) at 3-month follow-up while 6 and 12 months following BPV there was a significant decrease ($P<0.05$-<0.001) in the right ventricular voltages. Electrocardiograms were available in all 30 group I patients prior to valvuloplasty. The follow-up data are based on electrocardiograms in 20, 24, and 22 patients, respectively, at 3, 6, and 12 month follow-up. SEM, standard error of mean. (Reproduced from Rao and Solymar [20], with permission of the publisher.)

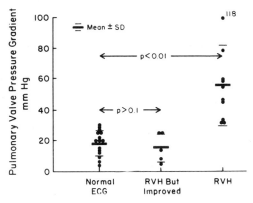

Pulmonary Valve Pressure Gradient
mm Hg

Mean ± SD

●118

p<0.01

p>0.1

Normal
ECG

RVH But
Improved

RVH

Fig. 28. Relationship of postvalvuloplasty electrocardiograms with the residual pulmonary outflow tract (valvar plus infundibular) gradients. Note that in the presence of normal electrocardiogram (ECG) the pulmonary valve gradients were low, less than 30 mmHg (left-hand column). The electrocardiograms shown in the RVH (right ventricular hypertrophy) column were obtained 6 months or more after balloon valvuloplasty and all had right ventricular outflow tract gradients in excess of 30 mmHg. The electrocardiograms shown in the "RVH but improved" column were obtained less than 6 months after balloon valvuloplasty and had right ventricular outflow gradients less than 30 mmHg. These data would suggest that normal ECG would indicate right ventricular outflow gradient ≤30 mmHg, whereas RVH would indicate significant (>30 mmHg) right ventricular outflow gradients unless the ECG was obtained less than 6 months after valvuloplasty. (Reproduced from Rao and Solymar [20], with permission of the publisher.)

following balloon valvuloplasty, were interpreted to have right ventricular hypertrophy but were markedly improved compared with pre-valvuloplasty electrocardiograms. Their pulmonary valve gradients at catheterization were 5-25 mmHg (15.2 ± 9.4 mmHg) and were not significantly different ($P > 0.1$) from the normal electrocardiogram group (Fig. 28). Three of these patients had repeat electrocardiograms 6 months later (1 year after valvuloplasty) and were found to be normal. Thus pulmonary gradients less than 30 mmHg are likely to be present in patients with normal

electrocardiograms. If right ventricular hypertrophy is present and the electrocardiogram was obtained later than 6 months after valvuloplasty, significant residual gradient could be expected. Right ventricular hypertrophy in an electrocardiogram obtained at or before 6 months following valvuloplasty does not accurately predict pulmonary valve gradient.

In conclusion, electrocardiograms improve after successful pulmonary valvuloplasty, and the electrocardiogram is a useful adjunct in the evaluation of intermediate-term result of balloon pulmonary valvuloplasty. However, electrocardiographic evidence for hemodynamic improvement does not become apparent until after 6 months following balloon valvuloplasty.

Echo-Doppler Evaluation

Kveselis *et al.* [38], Rocchini and Beekman [129], Robertson and his associates [43], Mullins and colleagues [70], and we [14,15,18,26] as well as others [76,84] previously reported echo-Doppler follow-up studies after balloon valvuloplasty. Kveselis *et al.* [38] reported results in 11 patients 15 ± 19 months following valvuloplasty; calculated right ventricular outflow gradient was reduced from 86 ± 29 to 38 ± 9 mmHg immediately after valvuloplasty, which decreased, though, to an insignificant degree, to 33 ± 7 mmHg at follow-up. Doppler evidence for pulmonary insufficiency was present in 8 of 11 patients. Similar improvements were noted in a subsequent publication [129] involving 28 patients with successful valvuloplasty. Robertson *et al.* [43], while analyzing the morphology of right ventricular outflow tract following balloon valvuloplasty, reported follow-up (10.2 ± 5.6 months) Doppler studies in 18 patients. The calculated pulmonary valvar gradient, having been reduced to 37 ± 23 from 72 ± 31 mmHg immediately following valvuloplasty, decreased further to 31 ± 21 mmHg at follow-up.

Mullins *et al.* [70] obtained continuous-wave Doppler flow measurements in 30 (of 63) children who underwent balloon pulmonary valvuloplasty at a mean of 13 months following valvuloplasty; the estimated residual gradient was 20 ± 8 mmHg.

We performed echo-Doppler follow-up studies in 63 children for 3 to 36 months (15 ± 6 months) following valvuloplasty. Two D-derived, M-mode tracings of the right ventricle and left ventricle and pulsed- and continuous-wave Doppler flow velocity recordings from the right ventricular outflow tract and the main pulmonary artery were recorded, as previously reported [15,18,49], initially at 3 to 6 month intervals and subsequently at 12 month inter-

vals. Pulmonary valvar gradient was calculated using a modified Bernoulli equation (gradient $= 4\ V_2^2$, where V_2 is peak Doppler flow velocity in the main pulmonary artery). When the right ventricular outflow tract Doppler flow velocity (V_1) was in excess of 1.0 m/sec, V_1 was incorporated into the Bernoulli equation [gradient $= 4\ (V_2^2 - V_1^2)$]. The echo-Doppler results were analyzed separately for group XI (with good results) and group XII (with poor results; Table IV). In group XI patients with good results, the right ventricular end-diastolic dimension decreased, but not significantly ($P > 0.05$), from 18.3 ± 5.6 to 16.2 ± 5.3 mm immediately after valvuloplasty, which decreased further to 15.4 ± 5.0 mm ($P < 0.01$) at the last available follow-up (Fig. 29). The left ventricular end-diastolic dimension did not change immediately following valvuloplasty (30.8 ± 8.3 vs. 29.6 ± 7.8 mm, $P > 0.1$), but at follow-up there was a significant increase (34.1 ± 8.1 mm $P < 0.02$; Fig. 30). The Doppler flow velocity in the main pulmonary artery decreased ($P < 0.001$) from 4.3 ± 0.8 to 2.8 ± 0.64 m/sec immediately following valvuloplasty, which on follow-up was 2.4 ± 0.6 m/sec ($P < 0.001$ Fig. 31); when pressure

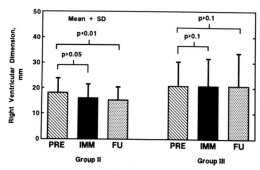

Fig. 29. Right ventricular end-diastolic dimensions prior to (PRE), and immediately after (IMM) valvuloplasty and at follow-up (FU). Note that there was an insignificant ($P>0.05$) fall in right ventricular size immediately after valvuloplasty, which diminished significantly ($P<0.01$) at follow-up in the group XI good result patients, while no change ($P>0.1$) was noted in the group XII poor result patients. SD, standard deviation.

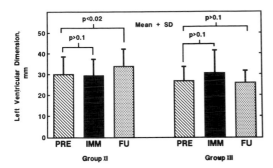

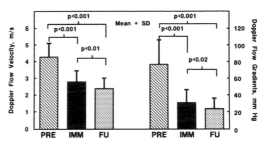

Fig. 30. Similar to Figure 29 but left ventricular end-diastolic dimensions are shown. Note that there was no change immediately after valvuloplasty, but a significant (P <0.02) increase was seen at follow-up in group XI good result patients. No change (P>0.1) was noted in the group XII poor result group.

Fig. 31. Peak Doppler flow velocities across the pulmonic valve prior to (PRE) and immediately after (IMM) pulmonary valvuloplasty and at follow-up (FU) are shown in the left-hand panel, and peak instantaneous Doppler-calculated gradients are shown in the right-hand panel for group XI patients with good results. Note significant (P<0.001) falls in Doppler velocities and gradients immediately after valvuloplasty. There was further fall (P<0.01–0.02) at follow-up, presumably related to resolution of infundibular obstruction.

gradient was calculated, these values respectively corresponded to 77 ± 29 (before), 31 ± 15 (after), and 24 ± 12 (at follow-up) mmHg. An example is shown in Figure 32. Doppler evidence for mild pulmonary insufficiency was present in 50 of 54 patients in whom data was available. Longitudinal follow-up Doppler flow velocities in the pulmonary artery and calculated gradients are shown in Figures 33 and 34. These data show that there is rapid reduction of flow velocities immediately following

valvuloplasty with further reduction at 6 months follow-up. Subsequently there was minimal fall, if any.

By contrast, in group XII with poor results, the right ventricular, end-diastolic dimension (21.0 ± 9.4 mm) did not change (P > 0.1) either immediately after valvuloplasty (21.0 ± 10.6 mm) or at follow-up (21.0 ± 12.7 mm) (Fig.

Main Pulmonary Artery Doppler Flow Velocity

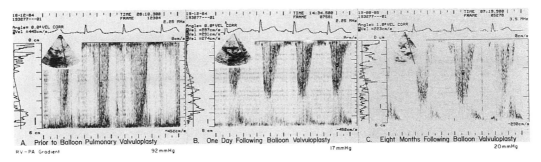

Fig. 32. Doppler flow velocities across the pulmonic valve in a patient prior to, on the day following, and 8 months after balloon pulmonary valvuloplasty. Note the significant fall in velocity after valvuloplasty. (Reproduced from Rao [49], with permission of the publisher.)

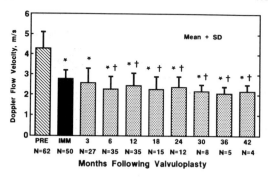

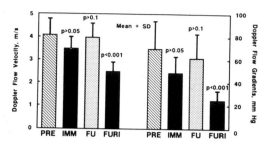

Fig. 33. Peak Doppler flow velocities in the main pulmonary artery prior to (PRE) and immediately after (IMM) balloon valvuloplasty and at follow-up are shown. N indicates the number of patients in whom the data were available at that particular interval. Note that a fall in the flow velocity occurred immediately after valvuloplasty with further reduction at 6 month follow-up. There was minimal, if any, change subsequent to 6-month follow-up. *$P<0.01$ compared with pre-valvuloplasty values. †$P<0.05$ compared with immediate postvalvuloplasty values. SD, standard deviation.

Fig. 35. Doppler flow velocity and instantaneous Doppler gradients across the pulmonic valve in the group II children with poor results. Note that there was no fall in the gradient either immediately after (IMM) or at follow-up (FU). Repeat balloon valvuloplasty (RI) has resulted in a fall in gradients ($P<0.001$).

29). Similarly, left ventricular, end-diastolic dimension (27.0 ± 6.7 mm) did not change ($P > 0.1$) immediately following (30.8 ± 10.8 mm) or several months after (26.1 ± 5.6 mm) valvuloplasty (Fig. 30). Peak Doppler flow velocity in the pulmonary artery prior to valvuloplasty was 4.1 ± 0.7 m/sec in group XII, which remained essentially unchanged ($P > 0.05$) after valvuloplasty (3.5 ± 0.5) and on follow-up (4.0 ± 0.6) (Fig. 35). Doppler evidence for pulmonary insufficiency was present

in two of the nine patients on follow-up. Six of the nine group XII patients underwent repeat valvuloplasty; 7–12 months following repeat valvuloplasty the Doppler flow velocity decreased to 2.5 ± 0.4 m/sec ($P < 0.001$) (Fig. 35). The corresponding instantaneous Doppler flow gradients are also displayed in Figure 35.

Doppler's ability to predict pulmonary valvar gradients after valvuloplasty was then evaluated. There were 37 pairs of Doppler and catheterization data obtained within 24 hours of each other immediately following pulmonary valvuloplasty. There were 30 pairs of Doppler and catheterization also obtained within 24 hours of each other 6–36 months following valvuloplasty. There was excellent correlation between Doppler-calculated and catheterization-measured pulmonary valvar gradients at follow-up ($r = 0.9$), while there was not such a good correlation ($r = 0.6$) immediately following valvuloplasty. These results are similar to those reported by us in a smaller number of subjects [49]. No technical or fixed anatomic reason was found [49]. The reason appears to be hyperreactive, right ventricular outflow tract immediately following balloon valvuloplasty; this was shown in the right ventricular angiography immediately following valvuloplasty, but sometimes without demonstrable pressure gradient on pressure pullback tracings.

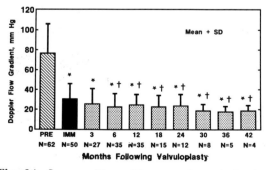

Fig. 34. Same as Figure 33 except that calculated instantaneous Doppler gradients are shown.

No significant changes in the ventricular sizes were observed immediately following valvuloplasty. Whether or not the results of valvuloplasty were good, the Doppler-flow velocity recordings often overestimated the residual gradient; this is probably related to infundibular hyperreactivity (Fig. 36). Therefore, echo-Doppler studies immediately following valvuloplasty may not be reflective of the favorable hemodynamic changes immediately following valvuloplasty in a substantial number of patients.

At follow-up, improvement in the echocardiographic size of the right ventricle, Doppler flow velocity in the main pulmonary artery, and calculated, pulmonary valve gradient occurred in patients with successful balloon valvuloplasty, while no such change was observed in the group of patients with significant residual pulmonary stenosis. The data indicate that intermediate-term, follow-up echo-Doppler studies are reflective of the hemodynamic improvement. These studies suggest that repeat cardiac catheterization to evaluate intermediate-term and long-term results of balloon pulmonary valvuloplasty may not be necessary.

Although our initial impression was that there was a low incidence of pulmonary valve insufficiency following balloon valvuloplasty [14,15], the results of this larger study showed that 50 of 54 (93%) patients with successful balloon valvuloplasty developed pulmonary insufficiency on intermediate-term follow-up. This is understandable, because the balloon valvuloplasty produces commissural splitting and tearing or avulsion of valve leaflets [114]. However, the pulmonary insufficiency is minimal and unlikely to be problematic; there was no evidence for right-ventricular volume overloading (near-normal, right ventricle size and no paradoxical septal motion) in our echocardiographic studies and by equilibrium-gated radionuclide angiograms reported by Tynan and associates [34]. Although the long-term follow-up studies should be scrutinized for progressive, right-ventricular volume overload, the current data suggest that pulmonary insufficiency produced by balloon dilatation is unlikely to be problematic.

OTHER ISSUES
Dysplastic Pulmonary Valve

Dysplastic pulmonary valves have been implicated as a cause of failure following balloon pulmonary valvuloplasty [34,37,40,42,74,

Main Pulmonary Artery Doppler Flow Velocity

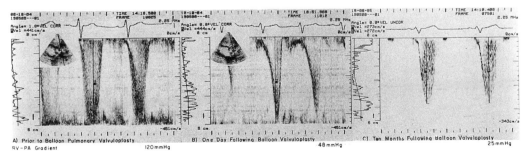

Fig. 36. Doppler flow velocity recordings from the main pulmonary artery prior to (left) and 1 day (center) and 10 months (right) following balloon pulmonary valvuloplasty are shown. Note that there is no significant fall in the peak flow velocity immediately after valvuloplasty, but there is a characteristic triangular pattern, indicative of infundibular obstruction. At 10-month follow-up, the flow velocity markedly diminished, suggestive of resolution of infundibular obstruction. (Reproduced from Thapar and Rao [27], with permission of the publisher.)

129]. More recently, detailed reports of balloon valvuloplasty in patients with dysplastic pulmonary valves [53,54] suggested that poor results may be expected with dysplastic pulmonary valves. A summary of experience reported in the literature is provided in Table XI. Our experience with dysplastic pulmonary valves is contrary to that reported in these papers. Therefore we previously reviewed [21] the results of balloon valvuloplasty in 13 patients with dysplastic pulmonary valves (group XIII) from our total experience with 56 patients (Table IV) to assess the outcome of balloon valvuloplasty in dysplastic valves. These results were compared with valvuloplasty results of 43 nondysplastic pulmonary valves (group XIV). Dysplasia of the pulmonary valve was assessed based on the criteria outlined by Jeffery, Koretzky, and their associates [134,135]. When all criteria—namely, 1) angiographic appearance of nodular and uneven thickening and poor doming of the valve leaflets (Fig. 37); 2) valve ring hypoplasia (less than the mean value for the given body surface area as defined by Rowlatt et al. [136]; and 3) no poststenotic dilatation—were present, the pulmonary valve was considered dysplastic. When valve leaflets appeared dysplastic without the presence of one or both of the other criteria, the valve was considered mildly dysplastic. A total of 13 dysplastic pulmonary valves were identified; seven were severely dysplastic, and six were mildly dysplastic.

Balloon valvuloplasty in 13 patients, aged 6 days to 12 years (median 1 year), with dysplastic pulmonary valves (group XIII) reduced the pulmonary valve gradient from 77.2 ± 44.2 to 26.8 ± 17.0 mmHg ($P < 0.001$), which remained improved 34.9 ± 34.6 mmHg ($P < 0.02$) at 6 to 19 month (mean, 10 months) follow-up (Table XII). The results of individual patients are depicted in Figure 38. Valvuloplasty in 43 patients without dysplastic pulmonary valves (group XIV) reduced the valve gradient from 94.3 ± 41.0 to 31.1 ± 22.4 mmHg ($P < 0.001$) immediately following the procedure, which at 6–34 month follow-up in 23 patients was 29.2 ± 33.5 mmHg ($P < 0.001$) (Table XII). The pulmonary valvar gradients (77.2 ± 44.2 vs. 94.3 ± 41.0 mmHg) prior to valvuloplasty, residual pulmonary valvar gradient (26.8 ± 17.0 vs. 31.1 ± 22.4 mmHg) immediately after valvuloplasty, and residual gradient (34.9 ± 34.6 vs. 29.2 ± 33.5 mmHg) at follow-up catheterization were similar ($P > 0.1$) in both groups (Table XII). However, the balloon:annulus ratio used in dysplastic pulmonary valve patients (1.3 ± 0.25) was slightly

TABLE XI. Summary of Results From the Literature Regarding Balloon Valvuloplasty in Patients With Pulmonary Valve Dysplasia (DPV)

Author, Year	No. of patients with DPV	Immediate success (%)		Follow-up success (%)	
Kan et al., 1984 [37]	1	0	(0)	0	(0)
Tynan et al., 1985 [34]	3	0	(0)	0	(0)
Miller, 1986 [39]	1	0	(0)	—	
Sullivan et al., 1986 [40]	2	1	(50)	0	(0)
Rocchini and Beekman, 1986 [129]	7	0	(0)	3	(43)
Musewe et al., 1987 [53]	5	1	(20)	1	(20)
DiSessa et al., 1987 [54]	3	0	(0)	—	
Rey et al., 1988 [42]	4	3	(75)	3	(75)
Marantz et al., 1988 [55]	4	3	(75)	2	(50)
Rao et al., 1988 [21]	13	9	(69)	10	(77)
Ballerini et al., 1990 [74]	9	2	(22)	3	(33)
Total	52	19	(37)	22	(47)[a]

[a]Patients without follow-up were excluded for the purpose of calculation of percent success.

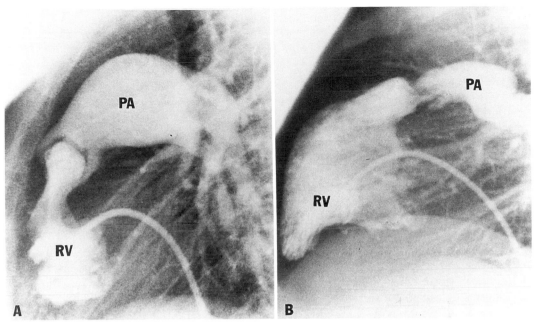

Fig. 37. Selected frames from right ventricular (RV) cineangiograms of patients without (A) and with (B) dysplastic pulmonary valves. A: Thickened and domed pulmonary valve leaflets are seen. Note poststenotic dilation of the pulmonary artery (PA). B: Pulmonary valve leaflets are markedly and unevenly thickened without doming. There was no jet formation and no poststenotic dilatation of the PA. The pulmonary valve ring is smaller than the norms described by Rowlatt et al. [10]. (Reproduced from Rao [21], with permission of the publisher.)

higher than that used in nondysplastic pulmonary valve patients (1.2 ± 0.24), although this difference did not attain statistical significance ($P > 0.1$). Two of the 13 dysplastic pulmonary valve patients (Fig. 38) and 3 of the 23 nondysplastic pulmonary valve patients required repeat valvuloplasty ($P > 0.1$) at follow-up catheterization. Residual pulmonary valvar gradients in excess of 30 mmHg at follow-up were present in 3 of 13 and 4 of the 23 ($P > 0.1$) patients, respectively, with and without dysplastic valves.

When all valvuloplasties were divided into those with good results (gradient $\leq$ 30 mmHg at follow-up), 29 patients (group I), and poor results (gradient > 30 mmHg at follow-up), 7 patients (group II) (Table IV), the prevalence of dysplastic pulmonary valves, respectively, in these two groups was 10 and 3 and was similar ($P > 0.1$). In 10 patients with dysplastic pulmonary valves with good results, the balloon:an-

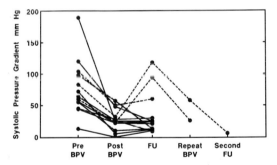

Fig. 38. Peak-to-peak pulmonary valve systolic pressure gradients in 13 patients with dysplastic pulmonary valves are shown. Note a significant fall in pressure gradient immediately after balloon pulmonary valvuloplasty (BPV) in all patients. Gradients in excess of 30 mmHg were present in four patients. At follow-up (FU) study, gradients remained low or fell further in 10 patients (solid lines), whereas the gradient increased in three patients (broken lines). Two of these children underwent repeat valvuloplasty with larger balloons at follow-up study with resultant decrease in gradients. One of these children underwent a second follow-up study, and residual gradient was low. (Reproduced from Rao [21], with permission of the publisher.)

TABLE XII. Comparison of Group XIII With Dysplastic Pulmonary Valves With Group XIV With No Pulmonary Valve Dysplasia[a]

	Group XI (Mean ± SD)	Group XII (Mean ± SD)	P value
Pulonary valve gradient prevalvuloplasty (mmHg)	77.2 ± 44.2	94.3 ± 41.0	>0.1
Pulmonary valve gradient immediately after valvuloplasty (mmHg)	26.8 ± 17.0*	31.3 ± 22.4*	>0.1
Pulmonary valve gradient at follow-up (mm Hg)	34.9 ± 34.6**	29.2 ± 33.5*	>0.1

[a]Reproduced from Rao [21], with permission of the publisher.
*P <0.0001 compared with the prevalvuloplasty gradient.
**P <0.02 when compared with the prevalvuloplasty gradient.

nulus ratio (1.37 ± 0.22) used for valvuloplasty was larger (P < 0.01) than that (1.04 ± 0.17) used in three patients with poor results.

These data suggest that 1) the results of balloon valvuloplasty in patients with dysplastic valves are comparable to those without; 2) the dysplastic valves were not responsible for recurrence of valve stenosis; and 3) use of large balloons in patients with dysplastic valves may have reduced the chance for recurrence.

Marantz et al. [55] compared immediate and follow-up results of balloon valvuloplasty in four patients with dysplastic pulmonary valves with those of 32 patients without dysplastic valves and concluded that significant palliation or relief of gradient occurred following valvuloplasty and suggested that dysplastic pulmonary valves should not be excluded from an attempt at balloon valvuloplasty. McCrindle and Kan [81b] did not detect pulmonary valve dysplasia as a cause of the poor result of balloon pulmonary valvuloplasty.

In the VACA Registry study [84], examining the causes of suboptimal follow-up result, dysplastic valve morphology was identified as one of the factors predisposing to poor outcome. However, this group included complex pulmonary stenosis (for example, tetralogy of Fallot).

The reason for the discrepancies between studies [21,53–55,81b,84] in the results of valvuloplasty in patients with dysplastic pulmonary valves is not clear; it may be related to interpretation of clinical and angiographic data in labeling a given patient as having dysplastic pulmonary valves, to variable degrees of pulmonary valve dysplasia [53,137, 138], or to the presence of commissural fusion mixed with dysplasia [53,54,137]. It is generally considered that splitting of commissural fusion [114] is one of the major mechanisms of relief of valvar stenosis by balloon dilatation. Therefore, it is somewhat surprising that some patients with dysplastic valves would have good results. However, variability of extent of dysplasia and dysplasia mixed with commissural fusion [53,54, 135,137,138] can to some extent explain these results. Musewe et al. [53] suggested that if echocardiographic features of commissural fusion are present, catheterization and angiography should be performed to confirm commissural fusion, and if so balloon valvuloplasty should be performed. We agree with this approach. However, based on these results [21] and on those observed by Marantz et al. [55], we would recommend balloon valvuloplasty for relief of pulmonary valve obstruction even with angiographic features of pulmonary valve dysplasia. Also, it seems reasonable to use larger balloons than is recommended for nondysplastic pulmonary valves; we personally tend to use balloons large enough to produce balloon:annulus ratios of 1.4–1.5 and tend to avoid ratios in excess of 1.5 for fear of damage to the right ventricular outflow tract [60].

Infundibular Obstruction

Several reports identify infundibular obstruction as a complicating feature immediately following balloon valvuloplasty [13,14,18,40–43,68–70,94,99,102,124,139,140]. We studied this problem further in order to define the prevalence and significance of infundibular obstruction in patients undergoing balloon valvuloplasty for valvar pulmonic stenosis [27]; we used the data from 62 children who had undergone balloon angioplasty during a 55 month period ending May 1988.

Thirteen of the 62 (21%) children had infundibular pressure gradients prior to valvuloplasty; these ranged between 10 and 137 mmHg (49 ± 42 mmHg). Following valvuloplasty, infundibular gradients disappeared in five patients (Fig. 39). The infundibular gradient in the remaining eight patients was 33 ± 26 mmHg, with a range of 5–80 mmHg. In six of these eight patients, the infundibular gradients diminished compared with the prevalvuloplasty gradients. In one child, the gradient remained unchanged at 20 mmHg and in the final patient the infundibular gradient increased form 40 to 45 mmHg. In five additional patients without infundibular gradi-

ents but with angiographic infundibular narrowing, an infundibular gradient appeared after valvuloplasty; new infundibular gradients were 15,30,34,50, and 69 mmHg (40 ± 21 mmHg; Fig. 39). Thus 18 of 62 (29%) patients had infundibular gradients prior to or immediately after valvuloplasty. Examples of severe infundibular reaction demonstrated by Doppler echocardiography and cineangiography are shown in Figures 36 and 40.

One child received propranolol prior to valvuloplasty [29]. Two other children, with what was thought to be successful balloon valvuloplasty, developed systemic-level pressures in the right ventricle because of severe infundibular reaction. Propranolol, 0.1 mg/kg, was slowly administered intravenously with a decrease in the right ventricular pressures and infundibular gradients. These three and three other patients with infundibular stenosis were prescribed oral propranolol, 2–3 mg/kg/day in three to four divided doses, for approximately 3 months. None of our patients required surgical infundibular resection.

Out of the total of 13 patients with infundibular gradients at the end of balloon valvuloplasty, the gradients disappeared at follow-up in seven patients. No follow-up data were available in one child. In the remaining five patients with persistent infundibular gradients at follow-up, the gradients were low (range 10–47 mmHg; mean 29 mmHg); in each patient, the gradient at follow-up was lower than the immediate postvalvuloplasty gradient (Fig. 39).

The influences of severity of pulmonary valve obstruction and of age of patient on the development of infundibular obstruction were examined. The patients with infundibular obstruction (n = 18) had higher (P < 0.01) pulmonary valve gradient (119 ± 51 mmHg) than those (n = 44) without infundibular gradient (83 ± 35 mmHg). When the prevalence of infundibular obstruction was scrutinized (Table XIII), patients with higher degrees of obstruction had a greater prevalence of infundibular stenosis. The age distribution of

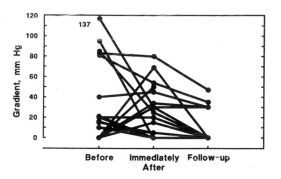

Fig. 39. Sequential infundibular gradients before and immediately after balloon pulmonary valvuloplasty and at follow-up are shown. Thirteen children had initial gradients, five disappeared following valvuloplasty. New gradients appeared in five other patients. The gradients either disappeared or improved at follow-up. (Reproduced from Thapar and Rao [27], with permission of the publisher.)

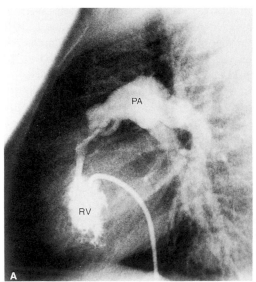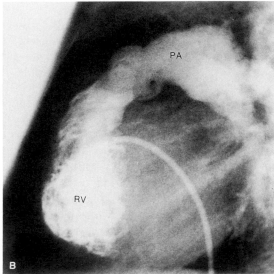

Fig. 40. Selected frames from lateral view of the right ventricular (RV) cineangiogram showing severe infundibular reaction (**A**) immediately following balloon valvuloplasty (corresponding to Fig. 36, center). Note wide-open right ventricular outflow tract (**B**) at 10 month postvalvuloplasty catheterization (corresponds to Fig. 36, right). The peak-to-peak pulmonary valvar pressure gradient at follow-up catheterization was 20 mmHg; there was no infundibular gradient. PA, pulmonary artery. (Reproduced from Thapar and Rao [27], with permission of the publisher.)

patients with and without infundibular gradients (9.8 ± 7.1 vs. 8.2 ± 6.4 years) was similar (P > 0.1). However, the prevalence of infundibular gradient was higher (P < 0.01) in older patients than in younger patients (Table XIII).

Several authors reported either persistence of right ventricular infundibular gradients or appearance of such gradients following balloon pulmonary valvuloplasty [13,18,40–43,68,74,94,102,124,139,140]. When such infundibular obstruction was severe, propranolol was administered by several groups of workers [18,42,68,99,139] with variable result. Infundibular resection by surgery was

TABLE XIII. Relationship Between Severity of Pulmonary Valvar Stenosis and Age With the Prevalence of Infundibular Gradients[a]

	No. of patients in the specified group	No. with infundibular gradients	P value[b]
Pulmonary valve gradient ≥ 100 mmHg	21	9	< 0.01
Pulmonary valve gradient < 100 mmHg	41	9	
Pulmonary valve gradient ≥ 80 mmHg	32	12	< 0.01
Pulmonary valve gradient < 80 mmHg	30	6	
Age ≥5 years	40	14	< 0.01
Age <5 years	22	4	

[a]Reproduced from Thapar and Rao [27], with permission of the publisher.
[b]Chi-squared.

required in three patients [68,124,140]. In a few studies with follow-up catheterization, the infundibular obstruction improved [18,40–42,94,139].

The absence of pressure gradient across angiographically narrow right ventricular infundibulum in the presence of a more severe distal obstruction (valve stenosis) is well known [141–143]; this atypical behavior of multiple obstructions may be due to "forced vibration" with greater energy transfer into the cardiovascular segment upstream to the proximal obstruction than into the segment upstream to the distal obstruction [142,143]. The elastic and pulsatile characteristics of the cardiovascular system are important for expressing this property [142,143]. Once the valvar (distal) gradient was relieved, infundibular (proximal) gradient appeared.

Infundibular gradients immediately following valvuloplasty appear to be related to infundibular hyperreactivity and, if severe (producing near systemic pressure in the right ventricle), may need treatment with propranolol. We, indeed, observed significant improvement in the gradient following intravenous propranolol. This response is similar to that observed in patients with surgical pulmonary valvotomy [144]. Although we were able to manage all our patients without surgical resection of the infundibular obstruction, an occasional patient may require infundibular resection [68,124]. Oral propranolol therapy may be required in some patients with significant infundibular obstruction; patients with an infundibular gradient in excess of 50 mmHg, as suggested by Fontes et al. [139], may be candidates for such therapy. The infundibular obstruction is expected to regress with time, as has been observed following surgical pulmonary valvotomy [45,145–149] and balloon valvuloplasty [14,18,27,40,94]. Whether propranolol has any effect in enhancing regression of infundibular obstruction cannot be answered by this study.

Al Kasab and associates [99] observed that five patients receiving propranolol prior to balloon dilatation developed insignificant infundibular gradients (12 ± 4 mmHg) following valvuloplasty, while six other patients not receiving propranolol developed more severe infundibular gradients (45 ± 27 mmHg). The latter gradient diminished (9 ± 4 mmHg) following propranolol. Although these authors did not recommend routine use of propranolol therapy prior to valvuloplasty, they implied the potential use of β-blockage. At this time there is not, in my opinion, sufficient evidence to advocate routine use of β-blocking agent prior to valvuloplasty.

Based on our own observation and those reported in the literature, the following considerations might help in the management of infundibular obstruction in patients with pulmonic stenosis following balloon valvuloplasty [30].

1. Consider the possibility of development of infundibular obstruction after valvuloplasty in all patients with severe valvar pulmonic stenosis.

2. Perform careful pressure pullback recordings across the pulmonic valve and right ventricular outflow tract both prior to and 15 minutes following balloon pulmonary valvuloplasty.

3. Right ventricular cineangiograms should be performed and scrutinized for infundibular obstruction both prior to and 15 minutes following valvuloplasty.

4. Use adequate-sized balloon(s) so as to have a balloon:annulus ratio of 1.2–1.5 so that adequate relief of valvar obstruction occurs, which in turn encourages resolution of infundibular obstruction.

5. Balloons that produce balloon:annulus ratios in excess of 1.5 should be avoided for fear of damage to right ventricular outflow tract muscle and precipitating infundibular reaction.

6. If angiographic and pressure data suggest significant residual infundibular obstruction, β-blocker drug therapy may be necessary; I recommend it if the residual gradient is in excess of 50 mmHg.

7. If follow-up echo-Doppler or catheterization and angiographic studies performed 6 months to 1 year after balloon valvuloplasty reveal residual infundibular gradients ≥ 50 mmHg, then a consideration for surgical resection of the infundibular muscle should be given. If there is significant residual valvar obstruction, repeat balloon valvuloplasty with adequate-sized balloon(s) would be our therapeutic choice. With this approach, surgical resection of infundibular obstruction can be avoided in most, if not all, cases.

In summary, infundibular gradients in association with balloon pulmonary valvuloplasty were documented in 29% (18 of 62) of patients. The prevalence of such gradients appears to be more frequent with increasing age and severity of valve stenosis. Some of these children may develop systemic or suprasystemic pressures in the right ventricle because of hyperreactivity of the right ventricular infundibulum and may need β blockage. The infundibular stenosis does regress to a great degree at follow-up. The potential for development of infundibular gradient after balloon valvuloplasty should not deter physicians from use of this technique in the treatment of valvar pulmonic stenosis.

SUMMARY AND CONCLUSIONS

The technique of balloon dilatation of stenotic pulmonary valve has been available since 1982. Balloon pulmonary valvuloplasty has been used successfully over the last few years for the relief of moderate to severe valvar pulmonic stenosis in neonates, infants, children, and adults. Both immediate and intermediate-term follow-up results have been well documented by cardiac catheterization and Doppler studies. Electrocardiographic and echo-Doppler evaluation at follow-up is reflective of the results and may avoid the need for recatheterization. The results of balloon valvuloplasty are either comparable to or better than those reported with surgical valvuloplasty.

Complications of the procedure have been minimal. The causes of restenosis have been identified, and appropriate modifications in the technique, particularly use of balloon:annulus ratio of 1.2–1.5, should result in better results than previously documented. Further refinement of the catheters and technique may further reduce the complication rate and prevalence of restenosis.

The major mechanism by which relief of pulmonary obstruction is relieved by balloon valvuloplasty appears to be commissural splitting, although occasional tearing or avulsion of valve leaflets may be present.

The indications for balloon valvuloplasty have not been clearly defined but should probably be similar to those used for surgical valvotomy; only patients with moderate to severe valvar pulmonic stenosis are candidates for balloon valvuloplasty. Previous surgery, pulmonary valve dysplasia, and Noonan syndrome are not contraindications for balloon valvuloplasty.

Infundibular reaction may be present in older patients and in patients with severe obstruction and can most often be managed with adequate valvuloplasty and β-blocking drugs, with rare need for surgery.

Miniaturization of the balloon/catheter systems, further refinement of the procedure, and meticulous attention to details of the technique may further reduce the complication rate and increase the safety. Documentation of the favorable results at 5–10 year follow-up is necessary. Transcatheter techniques are excellent alternatives to open or closed heart surgery in most, if not all, patients with pulmonary stenosis.

ACKNOWLEDGEMENTS

The author wishes to acknowledge with thanks the contributions to this material by past and present colleagues in pediatric cardiology and cardiovascular surgery, including Drs. M. Brais, P.S. Chopra, M.E. Fawzy, F. Kutayli, J. Levy, M.K. Mardini, L. Solymar,

M.K. Thapar, and A.D. Wilson. Thanks are also due to Nanette Kelsey for her assistance in the preparation of the manuscript.

This work was supported in part by a grant from the Oscar Rennebohm Foundation, Inc., Madison, WI.

REFERENCES

1. Nadas AS, Fyler DC (1972): "Pediatric Cardiology," 3rd ed. Philadelphia: W.B. Saunders Co., p 683.
2. Keith JD, Rowe RD, Vlad P (1978): "Heart Disease in Infancy and Childhood," 3rd ed. New York: Macmillan Co., pp 4–6.
3. Edwards JE (1953): Congenital malformation of the heart and great vessels. In Gould SE (ed): "Pathology of the Heart." Springfield, IL: Charles C. Thomas, pp 319–324.
4. Brock RC (1957): "The Anatomy of Congenital Pulmonic Stenosis." New York: Paul B. Hoeber, pp 1–114.
5. Gikonyo BM, Lucas RV, Edwards JE (1987): Anatomic features of congenital pulmonary valvar stenosis. Pediatr Cardiol 8-109–115.
6. Rubio-Alvarez V, Limon-Lason R, Soni J (1953). Valvulotomias intracardiacas por medio de un cateter. Arch Inst Cardiol Mexico 23:183–192.
7. Rubio V, Limon-Lason R (1954): Treatment of pulmonary valvular stenosis and tricuspid stenosis using a modified catheter. Second World Congress on Cardiology, Washington DC, Program Abstracts II, p 205.
8. Semb BKH, Tijonneland S, Stake G, et al. (1979): "Balloon valvulotomy" of congenital pulmonary valve stenosis with tricuspid valve insufficiency. Cardiovasc Radiol 2:239–241.
9. Kan SJ, White RI, Jr, Mitchell SE, et al (1982): Percutaneous balloon valvuloplasty: a new method for treating congenital pulmonary valve stenosis. N Engl J Med 307:540–542.
10. Dotter CT, Judkins MP (1964): Transluminal treatment of arteriosclerotic obstruction: Description of a new technique and a preliminary report of its application. Circulation 30:654–670.
11. Zeitler E, Grüntzig A, Schoop W (1978): "Percutaneous Vascular Recanalization: Technique, Application, Clinical Results." Berlin: Springer-Verlag.
12. Grüntzig AR, Senning A, Siegothaler WE (1979): Non-operative dilatation of coronary artery stenosis: Percutaneous transluminal coronary angioplasty. N Engl J Med 301:61–68.
13. Rao PS, Mardini MK (1985): Pulmonary valvotomy without thoracotomy: The experience with percutaneous balloon pulmonary valvuloplasty. Ann Saudi Med 5:149–155.
14. Rao PS (1986): Transcatheter treatment of pulmonic stenosis and coarctation of the aorta: The experience with percutaneous balloon dilatation. Br Heart J 56:250–258.
15. Rao PS (1986): Value of echo-Doppler studies in the evaluation of the results of balloon pulmonary valvuloplasty. J Cardiovasc Ultrasonogr 5:309–312.
16. Rao PS (1987): Influence of balloon size on the short-term and long-term results of pulmonary valvuloplasty. Texas Heart Inst J 14:57–61.
17. Rao PS, Brais M (1988): Balloon pulmonary valvuloplasty for congenital cyanotic heart defects. Am Heart J 115:1105–1113.
18. Rao PS, Fawzy ME, Solymar L, et al. (1988): Long-term results of balloon pulmonary valvuloplasty. Am Heart J 115:1291–1296.
19. Rao PS (1989): How big a balloon and how many balloons for pulmonary valvuloplasty. Am Heart J 116:577–580.
20. Rao PS, Solymar L (1988): Electrocardiographic changes following balloon dilatation of valvar pulmonic stenosis. J Intervent Cardiol 1:189–197.
21. Rao PS (1988): Balloon dilatation in infants and children with dysplastic pulmonary valves: Short-term and intermediate-term results. Am Heart J 116:1168–1176.
22. Rao PS (1989): Indications for balloon pulmonary valvuloplasty. Am Heart J 116:1661–1662.
23. Rao PS, Thapar MK, Kutayli F (1988): Causes of restenosis following balloon valvuloplasty for valvar pulmonic stenosis. Am J Cardiol 62:979–982.
24. Rao PS (1988): Further observations on the role of balloon size on the short-term and intermediate-term results of balloon pulmonary valvuloplasty. Br Heart J 60:507–511.
25. Rao PS, Fawzy ME (1988): Double balloon technique for percutaneous balloon pulmonary valvuloplasty: Comparison with single balloon technique. J Intervent Cardiol 1:257–262.
26. Rao PS (1989): Balloon pulmonary valvuloplasty: A review. Clin Cardiol 12:55–74.
27. Thapar MK, Rao PS (1989): Significance of infundibular obstruction following balloon valvuloplasty for valvar pulmonic stenosis. Am Heart J 118:99–103.
28. Rao PS (1990): Causes of restenosis following balloon angioplasty/valvuloplasty: A review. Pediatr Rev Comm 4:157–172.
29. Thapar MK, Rao PS (1990): Use of propranolol for severe dynamic infundibular obstruction

prior to balloon pulmonary valvuloplasty. Cathet Cardiovasc Diagn 19:240–242.

30. Rao PS, Thapar MK (1991): Development of infundibular obstruction following balloon pulmonary valvuloplasty. Am Heart J 121:1839–1840.

31. Rao PS, Wilson AD, Thapar MK, Brais M (1992): Balloon pulmonary valvuloplasty in the management of cyanotic congenital heart defects. Cathet Cardiovasc Diagn 25:16–24.

31a. Rao PS (1992): Right ventricular filling following balloon pulmonary valvuloplasty. Am Heart J 123:1084–1086.

32. Nadas AS (1972): Pulmonary stenosis: Indications for surgery in children and adults. N Engl J Med 287:1196–1197.

33. Nugent EW, Freedom RM, Nora JJ, et al (1977): Clinical course of pulmonic stenosis. Circulation 56(Suppl I):I-18–I-47.

34. Tynan M, Baker EJ, Rohmer J, et al. (1985): Percutaneous balloon pulmonary valvuloplasty. Br Heart J 53:520–524.

35. Yeager SB, Neal WA, Balian AA, et al. (1986): Percutaneous balloon pulmonary valvuloplasty. WV Med J 82:169–171.

36. Lababidi Z, Wu JR (1983): Percutaneous balloon pulmonary valvuloplasty. Am J Cardiol 52:560–562.

37. Kan JS, White RI Jr, Mitchel SE, et al. (1984): Percutaneous transluminal balloon valvuloplasty for pulmonary valve stenosis. Circulation 69:554–560.

38. Kveselis DA, Rocchini AP, Snider AP, et al. (1985): Results of balloon valvuloplasty in the treatment of congenital valvar pulmonary stenosis in children. Am J Cardiol 56:527–532.

39. Miller GAH (1986): Balloon valvuloplasty and angioplasty in congenital heart disease. Br Heart J 54:285–289.

40. Sullivan ID, Robinson PJ, Macartney FJ, et al. (1986): Percutaneous balloon valvuloplasty for pulmonary stenosis in infants and children. Br Heart J 54:435–441.

41. Radtke W, Keane JF, Fellows KE, et al. (1986): Percutaneous balloon valvotomy of congenital pulmonary stenosis using oversized balloons. J Am Coll Cardiol 8:909–915.

42. Rey C, Marche P, Francart C, et al. (1988): Percutaneous transluminal balloon valvuloplasty of congenital pulmonary valve stenosis, with a special report on infants and neonates. J Am Coll Cardiol 11:815–820.

43. Robertson M, Benson LN, Smallhorn JF, et al. (1987): The morphology of the right ventricular outflow tract after percutaneous pulmonary valvotomy: Long-term follow-up. Br Heart J 58:239–244.

44. Mullins CE, Nihill MR, Vick WG III, et al. (1987): Double balloon technique for dilatation of valvar or vessel stenosis in congenital and acquired heart disease. J Am Coll Cardiol 10:107–114.

45. Tinker J, Howitt G, Markman P, et al. (1965): The natural history of isolated pulmonary stenosis. Br Heart J 27:151–160.

46. Moller I, Wennevold A, Lyngborg KE (1973): The natural history of pulmonic stenosis: Long-term follow-up with serial heart catheterizations. Cardiology 58:193–202.

47. Mody MR (1975): The natural history of uncomplicated valvar pulmonic stenosis. Am Heart J 90:317–321.

48. Stevenson JG, Kawabori I (1984): Noninvasive determination of pressure gradients in children: Two methods employing pulsed Doppler echocardiography. J Am Coll Cardiol 3:179–192.

49. Rao PS (1987): Doppler ultrasound in the prediction of transvalvar pressure gradients in patients with valvar pulmonic stenosis. Int J Cardiol 15:195–203.

50. Lima CO, Sahn DJ, Valdes-Cruz LM, et al. (1983): Noninvasive prediction of transvalvar pressure gradient in patients with pulmonic stenosis by quantitative two-dimensional echocardiographic Doppler studies. Circulation 67:866–871.

51. Kasturakis D, Allen HD, Goldberg SJ, et al. (1984): Noninvasive quantitation of stenotic semilunar valve area by Doppler echocardiography. J Am Coll Cardiol 3:1256–1262.

52. Rao PS (1992): Balloon valvuloplasty for pulmonic stenosis. In Cheng TO (ed): "Percutaneous Balloon Valvuloplasty." New York: Igaku-Shoin Medical Publishers, Inc., pp 365–420.

53. Musewe NN, Robertson MA, Benson LN, et al. (1987): The dysplastic pulmonary valve: Echocardiographic features and results of balloon dilatation. Br Heart J 57:364–370.

54. DiSessa TG, Alpert BS, Chase NA, et al. (1987): Balloon valvuloplasty in children with dysplastic pulmonary valves. Am J Cardiol 66:405–407.

55. Marantz PM, Huhta JC, Mullins CE, et al. (1988): Results of balloon valvuloplasty in typical and dysplastic pulmonary valve stenosis: Doppler echocardiographic follow-up. J Am Coll Cardiol 12:476–479.

56. Stanger P, Cassidy SC, Girod DA, et al. (1990): Balloon pulmonary valvuloplasty: Results of the Valvuloplasty and Angioplasty of Congenital Anomalies Registry. Am J Cardiol 65:775–783.

57. Chaffe A, Fairbrass MJ, Chatrath RR (1988): Anaesthesia for valvuloplasty. Anaesthesia 43:359–361.

58. Sideris EB, Baay JE, Bradshaw RL, et al. (1988):

Axillary vein approach for pulmonic valvuloplasty in infants with iliac vein obstruction. Cathet Cardiovasc Diagn 15:61-63.

59. Chaara A, Zniber L, Haitem NE, et al. (1989): Percutaneous balloon valvuloplasty via the right internal jugular vein for valvar pulmonic stenosis with severe right ventricular failure. Am Heart J 117:684-685.

60. Ring JC, Kulik TJ, Burke BA (1986): Morphologic changes induced by dilatation of pulmonary valve annulus with over-large balloons in normal newborn lamb. Am J Cardiol 55:210-214.

61. Rao PS (1989): Balloon angioplasty and valvuloplasty in infants, children, and adolescents. Curr Probl Cardiol 14(8):417-500.

62. Van den Berg N, Niemyeyer MG, Plokker TWM, et al. (1986): New triple-lumen balloon catheter for percutaneous (pulmonary) valvuloplasty. Cathet Cardiovasc Diagn 12:352-356.

63. Meier B, Friedli B, Oberhaensli I, et al. (1986): Trefoil balloon for percutaneous valvuloplasty. Cathet Cardiovasc Diagn 12:227-281.

64. Thanopoulos BD, Margetakis A, Papadopoulos G, et al. (1989): Valvuloplasty with large trefoil balloons for the treatment of congenital pulmonary stenosis. Acta Paediatr Scand 78:742-746.

65. Meier B, Friedli B, Von Segesser L (1988): Valvuloplasty: With trefoil and bifoil balloons and long sheath technique. Herz 13:1-13.

66. Shrivastava S, Sundar AS, Muhkopadyaya S, et al. (1987): Percutaneous transluminal balloon pulmonary valvuloplasty: Long-term results. Int J Cardiol 17:303-314.

67. McCredie RM, Lee CL, Swinburn MJ, et al. (1986): Balloon dilatation pulmonary valvuloplasty in pulmonary stenosis. Aust NZ J Med 16:20-23.

68. Ali Khan MA, Al Yousef S, Mullins CE (1986): Percutaneous transluminal balloon pulmonary valvuloplasty for the relief of pulmonary valve stenosis with special reference to double-balloon technique. Am Heart J 112:158-166.

69. Fontes VF, Sousa JEMR, Esteves CA, et al. (1988): Pulmonary valvuloplasty: Experience of 100 cases. Int J Cardiol 21:335-342.

70. Mullins CE, Ludomirsky A, O'Laughlin MP, et al. (1988): Balloon valvuloplasty for pulmonic valve stenosis: Two year follow-up hemodynamic and Doppler evaluation. Cathet Cardiovasc Diagn 14:76-81.

71. Hsieh K, Ou T, Hwang B, et al. (1987): Percutaneous balloon pulmonary valvuloplasty in children. Chin Med J 39:247-254.

72. Mashru MR, Loya YS, Sharma S (1988): Percutaneous balloon valvuloplasty for pulmonary

valve stenosis using single or double balloon technique. J Assoc Phys India 36:546-550.

73. Schmaltz AA, Bein G, Gravinghoff L, et al. (1989): Balloon valvuloplasty of pulmonary stenosis in infants and children: Cooperative study of the German Society of Pediatric Cardiology. Eur Heart J 10:967-971.

74. Ballerini L, Mullins CE, Cifarelli A, et al. (1990): Percutaneous balloon valvuloplasty of pulmonary valve stenosis, dysplasia, and residual stenosis after surgical valvotomy after surgical valvotomy for pulmonary atresia with intact ventricular septum: Long-term results. Cathet Cardiovasc Diagn 19:165-169.

75. Ng MP, Wong KY, Cheng HK, Tam KA (1990): Percutaneous balloon pulmonary valvuloplasty—The Singapore General Hospital experience. Ann Acad Med 19:54-57.

76. Hsu Y, Lue H, Wang J, Wu M, Wang N (1989): Echocardiographic changes following balloon valvuloplasty in valvular pulmonic and aortic stenosis. Acta Paediatr Sin 30:290-297.

77. Yip WCL, Tay JSH, Chan KY, Wong JCL, Wong HB (1990): Percutaneous transluminal balloon valvuloplasty: The treatment of choice for congenital valvar pulmonic stenosis. Ann Acad Med 19:58-63.

78. Zacharison MC, Friedberg DZ (1991): Percutaneous pulmonary valvuloplasty in children. Wis Med J 9:15-18.

79. Latson LA, Cheatham JP, Gumbiner CH, Hofschire PJ, Kugler JD, Fleming W (1985): Percutaneous valvuloplasty for congenital pulmonary valve stenosis. Nebr Med J 70:76-79.

80. Sutton TM, Carlson R, Bayron H, Griese GG (1986): Balloon pulmonary valvuloplasty for treatment of congenital pulmonary stenosis. Wis Med J 85:30-32.

81. Brodsky SJ (1984): Percutaneous balloon angioplasty: Treatment for congenital coarctation of the aorta and congenital valvar pulmonic stenosis. Am J Dis Child 138:851-854.

81a. Melgares R, Prieto JA, Azpitarte J (1991): Success determining factors in percutaneous transluminal balloon valvuloplasty of pulmonary valve stenosis. Eur Heart J 12:15-13.

81b. McCrindle BW, Kan JS (1991): Long-term results after balloon pulmonary valvuloplasty. Circulation 83:1915-1922.

82. Burrows PE, Benson LN, Smallhorn JS, Moes CAF, Freedom RM, Burrows FA, Rowe RD (1988): Angiographic features associated with percutaneous balloon valvotomy for pulmonary valve stenosis. Cardiovasc Intervent Radiol 11:111-116.

83. Stenberg RG, Fixler DE, Taylor AL, et al. (1988): .

Left ventricular dysfunction due to chronic right ventricular pressure overload: Resolution following percutaneous balloon valvuloplasty for pulmonic stenosis. Am J Med 84:157-161.

84. McCrindle BW, VACA Registry Investigators (1991): Factors affecting long-term results after balloon pulmonary valvuloplasty, abstracted. Circulation 84 (Suppl. II):546.

85. Tynan M, Jones O, Joseph MC, et al. (1984). Relief of pulmonary valve stenosis in the first week of life by percutaneous balloon valvuloplasty. Lancet 1:123.

86. Zeevi B, Keane JF, Fellows KE, et al. (1988): Balloon dilatation of critical pulmonary stenosis in the first week of life. J Am Coll Cardiol 11:821-824.

87. Ali Khan MA, Al Yousef S, Huhta JC, et al. (1989): Critical pulmonary valve stenosis in patients less than 1 year of age: Treatment with percutaneous gradational balloon pulmonary valvuloplasty. Am Heart J 117:1008-1114.

88. Qureshi S, Ladusans EJ, Martin RP (1989): Dilatation with progressively larger balloons for severe stenosis of the pulmonary valve presenting in the late neonatal period and early infancy. Br Heart J 62:311-314.

89. Robida A, Parchik D (1990): Perforation of the heart in a newborn with critical valvar pulmonary stenosis during balloon valvuloplasty. Int J Cardiol 26:111-112.

90. Gordon LS (1990): Neonatal Cardiology Casebook: Emergency pulmonary balloon valvuloplasty of congenital pulmonary valve stenosis. J Perinatol 10:86-88.

91. Caspi J, Coles JG, Benson LN, et al. (1990): Management of neonatal critical pulmonic stenosis in the balloon valvotomy era. Ann Thorac Surg 49:273-278.

92. Latson L, Cheatham J, Kugler J, et al. (1990): Balloon valvuloplasty in pulmonary valve atresia, abstracted. J Am Coll Cardiol 15:241A.

93. Ladusans EJ, Qureshi SA, Parsons JM, Arab S, Baker EJ, Tynan M (1990): Balloon dilatation of critical stenosis of the pulmonary valve in neonates. Br Heart J 63:362-367.

94. Pepine CJ, Gessner IH, Feldman RL (1983): Percutaneous balloon valvuloplasty for pulmonic valve stenosis in the adult. Am J Cardiol 50:1442-1445.

95. Khalilullah M, Bahl VK, Choudhary A, et al. (1985): Pulmonary balloon valvuloplasty for the nonsurgical management of valvar pulmonic stenosis. Indian Heart J 37:150-153.

96. Gibbs, JL, Stanley CP, Dickenson DF (1986): Pulmonary balloon valvuloplasty in late adult life. Int J Cardiol 11:237-239.

97. Al Kasab S, Riberio P, Al Zaibag M (1987): Use of double balloon technique for percutaneous balloon pulmonary valvotomy in adults. Br Heart J 58:136-141.

98. Fawzy ME, Mercer EN, Dunn B (1988): Late results of pulmonary balloon valvuloplasty in adults using double balloon technique. J Intervent Cardiol 1:35-42.

99. Al Kasab S, Ribeiro PA, Al Zaibag M, et al. (1988): Percutaneous double balloon pulmonary valvotomy in adults: One- to two-year follow-up. Am J Cardiol 62:822-825.

100. Feugelman MY, Lewis BS (1988): Pulmonary balloon valvuloplasty in the seventh decade of life. Isr J Med Sci 24:112-113.

101. Cooke JP, Seward JB, Holmes DR, Jr (1987): Transluminal balloon valvotomy for pulmonic stenosis in an adult. Mayo Clin Proc 62:306-311.

102. Shuck JW, McCormick DJ, Cohen IS, et al. (1984): Percutaneous balloon valvuloplasty of the pulmonary valve: Role of right-to-left shunt through a patent foramen ovale. J Am Coll Cardiol 4:132-135.

102a. Silvert H, Kober G, Bussman J, et al. (1989): Long-term results of percutaneous pulmonary valvuloplasty in adults. Eur Heart J 10:712-717.

102b. Sherman W, Hershman R, Alexopoulos D, et al. (1990): Pulmonic balloon valvuloplasty in adults. Am Heart J 119:187-190.

102c. Herrmann HC, Hill JA, Krol J, et al. (1991): Effectiveness of percutaneous balloon valvuloplasty in adults with pulmonary valve stenosis. Am J Cardiol 68:1111-1113.

103. Latson LA, Flemming WH, Hofschire PJ, Kugler JD, Cheatham JD, Moulton AL, Danford DA, Gumbiner CH (1991): Balloon valvuloplasty in pulmonary valve atresia. Am Heart J 121:1567-1569.

104. Brock RC (1948): Pulmonary valvotomy for relief of congenital pulmonary stenosis: Report of three cases. Br Med J 1:1121-1126.

105. Campbell M, Brock R (1954): The results of valvotomy for simple pulmonary stenosis. Br Heart J 17:229-246.

106. Mirowski M, Shah KD, Neill CA, et al. (1963): Long-term (10 to 13 years) follow-up study after transventricular pulmonary valvotomy for pulmonary stenosis with intact ventricular septum. Circulation 28:906-914.

107. Engle MA, Ito T, Goldberg HP (1964): The fate of the patient with pulmonic stenosis. Circulation 30:554-561.

108. Reid JM, Coleman EN, Stevenson JG, et al. (1976): Long-term results of surgical treatment for

pulmonary valve stenosis. Arch Dis Child 51:79–81.

109. Rowe RD (1975): Pulmonary stenosis with normal aortic root. In Keith JD, Rowe RD, Vlad P (eds): "Heart Disease in Infancy and Childhood," 3rd ed. New York: Macmillan Co., pp 761–788.

110. McNamara DG, Latson LA (1982): Long-term follow-up of patient with malformations for which definitive surgical repair has been available for 25 years or more. Am J Cardiol 50:560–568.

111. Kopecky SL, Gersh BJ, McGoon MD, et al. (1988): Long-term outcome of patients undergoing surgical repair of isolated pulmonary valve stenosis: Follow-up at 20-30 years. Circulation 78:1150–1156.

112. Vogel M, Eger R, Klinner W, et al. (1990): Brock transventricular pulmonary valvotomy in patients with pulmonary stenosis: long-term results. Pediatr Cardiol 11:191–194.

113. Abels JE (1980): Balloon catheters and transluminal dilatation: Technical considerations. Am J Roentgenol 135:901–906.

114. Walls JT, Lababidi Z, Curtis JJ, et al. (1984): Assessment of percutaneous balloon pulmonary and aortic valvuloplasty. J Thorac Cardiovasc Surg 88:352–356.

115. Benson LN, Smallhorn JS, Freedom RM, Trusler GA, Rowe RD (1985): Pulmonary valve morphology after balloon dilatation of pulmonary valve stenosis. Cathet Cardiovasc Diagn 11:161–166.

116. Lucas RV Jr, Burke BA, Edwards JE (1984): Anatomic sequelae of balloon angioplasty in congenital heart disease. Semin Intervent Radiol 1:225–235.

117. Becker AE, Hoedemaker G (1987): Balloon valvuloplasty in congenital and acquired heart disease: Morphologic considerations. Zeistsch Kardiol 6:73–79.

118. Lo RNS, Lau KC, Leung MP (1988): Complete heart block after balloon dilatation of congenital pulmonary stenosis. Br Heart J 59:384–386.

118a. Steinberg C, Levin AR, Engle MA (1992): Transiet complete heart block following percutaneous balloon pulmonary valvuloplasty: Treatment with systemic carticosteroids. Pediat Cardiol 13:181–183.

119. Fellows KE, Radtke W, Keane JF, et al. (1987): Acute complications of catheter therapy for congenital heart disease. Am J Cardiol 60:679–683.

120. Weinhaus L, Lababidi Z (1987): Catheter rupture during balloon valvuloplasty. Am Heart J 113:1035–1036.

121. Attia I, Weinhaus L, Walls JT, et al. (1987): Rupture of tricuspid valve papillary muscle during balloon pulmonary valvuloplasty. Am Heart J 113:1233–1234.

121a. Bhagwat AR, Loya YS, Sharma S (1992): Transient pulmonary hypertension following pulmonary balloon valvuloplasty. Am Heart J 123:1397–1398.

122. Burrows PE, Benson LN, Moes F, Freedom RM (1991): Pulmonary artery tears following balloon valvotomy for pulmonary stenosis. Cardiovasc Intervent Radiol 12:38–42.

123. Karla GS, Wander G, Anand IS (1990): Right-side endocarditis after balloon dilatation of the pulmonary valve. Br Heart J 63:368–369.

124. Ben-Shachar G, Cohen MH, Sivakoff MC, et al (1985): Development of infundibular obstruction after percutaneous pulmonary balloon valvuloplasty. J Am Coll Cardiol 5:754–756.

125. Martin GR, Stanger P (1986): Transient prolongation of the QTc interval after balloon valvuloplasty and angioplasty in children. Am J Cardiol 58:1233–1235.

126. Levine JH, Guarnieri T, Kadish AH, Shie RI, Calkins H, Kan JS (1988): Changes in the myocardial repolarization in patients undergoing balloon valvuloplasty for congenital pulmonary stenosis: Evidence for contraction excitation on feedback in humans. Circulation 77:70–77.

127. Kan JS, White RI, Jr, Mitchell SE, et al. (1983): Treatment of restenosis of coarctation by percutaneous transluminal angioplasty. Circulation 68:1087–1094.

128. Suarezde Lezo J, Fernandez R, Sancho M, et al. (1984): Percutaneous transluminal angioplasty for aortic isthemic coarctation in infancy. Am J Cardiol 54:1147–1149.

129. Rocchini AP, Beckman MA (1986): Balloon angioplasty in the treatment of pulmonary valve stenosis and coarctation of the aorta. Texas Heart Inst J 13:377–382.

130. Yeager SB (1987): Balloon selection for double balloon valvulotomy. J Am Coll Cardiol 9:467.

131. Butto F, Amplatz K, Bass JL (1986): Geometry of proximal pulmonary trunk during dilation with two balloons. Am J Cardiol 58:380.

132. Yeager SB (1985): Occlusion time and inflation pressure in pulmonary valvuloplasty. Am J Cardiol 55:619–620.

133. Lloyd TR, Donnerstein RL (1989): Rapid T-wave normalization after balloon pulmonary valvuloplasty in children. Am J Cardiol 64:399–400.

134. Koretzky ED, Moller JH, Korns ME, et al (1969): Congenital pulmonary stenosis resulting from dysplasia of the valve. Circulation 60:43–53.

135. Jeffery RF, Moller JH, Amplatz K (1972): The dysplastic pulmonary valve: A new roentgenographic entity. Am J Roentgenol Ther Radium Nucl Med 114:322–339.

136. Rowlatt UF, Rimoldi HLA, Lev M (1963): The quantitative anatomy of the normal child's heart. Pediatr Clin North Am 10:499-588.

137. Linde LM, Turner SW, Sparks RS (1973): Pulmonary valve dysplasia: A cardiofacial syndrome. Br Heart J 35:301-304.

138. Schneeweiss A, Blisen LC, Shem-Tov A, et al. (1985): Diagnostic angiographic criteria in dysplastic pulmonary valve. Am Heart J 106:761-762.

139. Fontes VF, Esteves CA, Sousa JEMR, et al. (1988): Regression of infundibular hypertrophy after pulmonary valvuloplasty for pulmonic stenosis. Am J Cardiol 62:977-979.

140. Pearl W, Wilkin JH, Bruno FL (1988): Balloon valvuloplasty in an unusually severe case of pulmonic stenosis with direct observation of the valve at subsequent surgery. Milit Med 153:446-448.

141. Brock R (1955): Control mechanisms in the outflow tract of the right ventricle in health and disease. Guy's Hosp Rep 104:356-379.

142. Silove ED, Vogel JHK, Grover RF (1968): The pressure gradient in ventricular outflow obstruction: Influence of peripheral resistance. Cardiovasc Res 3:234-242.

143. Rao PS, Linde LM (1974): Pressure and energy in the cardiovascular chambers. Chest 66:176-178.

144. Moulaert AJ, Buis-Liem TN, Geldof WC, et al. (1976): The postvalvulotomy propranolol test to determine reversibility of residual gradient in pulmonary stenosis. J Thorac Cardiovasc Surg 71:865-868.

145. Engle ME, Holswade GR, Goldberg HP, Lukas DS, Glenn F (1958): Regression after open valvotomy of infundibular stenosis accompanying severe valvar pulmonic stenosis. Circulation 17:862-873.

146. Johnson AM (1959): Hypertonic infundibular stenosis complicating simple pulmonary valve stenosis. Br Heart J 21:429-439.

147. Gilbert JW, Morrow AG, Talbert JL (1963): The surgical significance of hypertrophic infundibular obstruction accompanying valvular pulmonic stenosis. J Thorac Cardiovasc Surg 46:457-467.

148. Danielson GK, Exarhos ND, Wiedman WH, et al. (1971): Pulmonic stenosis with intact ventricular septum: Surgical considerations and results of operation. J Thorac Cardiovasc Surg 61:228-234.

149. Griffith BP, Hardesty RL, Siewers RD, et al. (1982): Pulmonary valvotomy alone for pulmonic stenosis: results in children with and without muscular infundibular hypertrophy. J Thorac Cardiovasc Surg 83:577-583.

7

Balloon Valvuloplasty for Aortic Stenosis

P. Syamasundar Rao, M.D.

Department of Pediatrics, Division of Pediatric Cardiology,
University of Wisconsin Medical School, University of Wisconsin
Children's Hospital, Madison, Wisconsin 53792-4108

INTRODUCTION

The prevalence of congenital valvar aortic stenosis is 5%–6% of patients with congenital heart defects [1,2]. Valvar aortic stenosis has a male preponderance, with a M:F gender ratio of approximately 4:1 [3]. The pathology of the stenotic aortic valve is variable. It is most frequently a bicuspid valve [2]; however, tricuspid valves can be present. Rarely, there may be a unicuspid valve. Thickening and decreased pliability of the valve leaflets are frequent, though variable. Commissural fusion of a variable degree is present and perhaps determines the severity of obstruction in most cases. Commissural fusion usually results in an eccentrically placed valve orifice. The raphae (fused valve leaflet commissures) vary in number, depending on the number of valve leaflets: three with tricuspid, two with bicuspid, and one or none with unicuspid valves. Additional "false" raphae may be present with bicuspid valves. Varying degrees of doming of the valve leaflets may be evident because of restriction of valve opening, which is secondary to commissural fusion. Dysplastic aortic valve leaflets are also seen, particularly more frequent in the neonate. Hypoplasia or underdevelopment of the valve ring may be found in neonates, infants, and young children. Calcification of aortic valve leaflets is uncommon in childhood. Dilatation of the ascending aorta, the so-called poststenotic dilation, is seen in most cases, and the extent of aortic dilatation is independent of severity of aortic obstruction. Hypertrophy of the left ventricular muscle is concentric in nature and is largely proportional to the degree of obstruction. Longstanding, severe obstruction causes myocardial fibrosis, particularly prevalent in the subendocardial region [4].

The majority of children with valvar aortic stenosis are asymptomatic and are detected because of a cardiac murmur heard on routine auscultation. When symptoms are exhibited, dyspnea, easy fatigability, or chest pain are the presenting complaints. Syncope may be a presenting complaint in some children. In contradistinction to children, neonates and young infants usually present with dyspnea and signs of heart failure.

In patients with significant aortic stenosis, increased left ventricular impulse, systolic thrill at the right upper sternal border, a constant ejection systolic click, and an ejection systolic murmur heard best at the right upper sternal border with radiation into both carotid arteries are observed. Prominent ascending aorta on a chest roentgenogram and left ventricular hypertrophy on an electrocardiogram may be present. Estimation of the severity of aortic valve obstruction with the aid of clinical and noninvasive laboratory data has been difficult in the past. With the availability of continuous-wave Doppler this has become easier. Doppler flow velocity measurement of the aortic jet gives a reasonably good estimate of severity of aortic obstruction. The peak instantaneous gradients across the aortic valve can be calculated with the use of a modified Bernouli equation ($\Delta P = 4V^2$, where ΔP is aortic valve gradient and V is peak velocity in the ascending aorta), which reflects the peak-to-peak systolic pressure gradients measured at cardiac catheterization. When the aortic stenosis is moderate to severe, relief of obstruction is recommended to prevent myocardial fibrosis, syncope, and sudden death. In the past, surgical valvotomy was the treatment of choice; however, as will be discussed later in this chapter, balloon aortic valvuloplasty is becoming a viable treatment option.

Following successful application of the balloon dilatation technique in children with pulmonic stenosis by Kan et al. [5], Lababidi [6] and Lababidi: et al. [7] applied this technique in children with aortic stenosis and showed that balloon dilatation can also be effectively used in the relief of aortic valve obstruction. Other reports followed [8–18]. The purpose of this chapter is to present the current state-of-the-art of balloon aortic valvuloplasty in infants and children; personal experience with this procedure, including that reported previously [14,19–21], and the experiences reported in the literature will be used as supportive material. Issues related to balloon angioplasty of subaortic membranous stenosis are discussed in Chapter 9 (this volume).

INDICATIONS

By and large, the indications for balloon dilation of stenotic aortic valve are essentially similar to those for surgical correction [22–25]. A peak-to-peak systolic pressure gradient in excess of 80 mmHg irrespective of the symptoms or a gradient ≥ 50 mmHg with normal cardiac index with either symptoms or electrocardiographic ST–T wave changes is generally considered to be an indication for catheter intervention. Because the aortic valvar gradient appears to decrease to approximately 50%–60% of prevalvuloplasty values (Table I) and

because of lack of long-term follow-up results documenting its effectiveness, one could question routine use of balloon aortic valvuloplasty. However, based on reasonably good intermediate-term results of balloon intervention [7,11,14–16,18] and significant incidence of early and late mortality and need for reoperation following surgical aortic valvotomy [22–30], as discussed in a later section of this chapter, I would recommend balloon aortic valvuloplasty as the initial treatment option in children with moderate to severe valvar aortic stenosis. Previous surgical valvotomy does not affect the result unfavorably [13,14]. Despite a high complication rate, critical aortic stenosis in the neonate and young infant is an indication for balloon therapy because of high morbidity and mortality with surgical intervention.

Presence of significant aortic insufficiency is considered a contraindication for balloon valvuloplasty for fear of increasing aortic insufficiency. Stenotic porcine heterograft in the aortic position is probably a contraindication as well. Balloon dilation has no role in the management of fibromuscular or tunnel-type subaortic stenosis and hypertropic cardiomyopathy with dynamic subaortic obstruction.

TECHNIQUE

Diagnosis and assessment of the aortic valve obstruction are made by the usual clinical, roentgenographic, electrocardiographic, and echo-Doppler data. Once a moderate-to-severe obstruction is diagnosed, cardiac catheterization and cineangiography are performed percutaneously to confirm the clinical impression and to consider for balloon dilatation of the aortic valve. After recording pressure pullback tracings across the aortic valve and cardiac output measurements, cineangiography (aortic root and left ventricle) is performed and a final diagnosis made. Once balloon valvuloplasty is decided upon, 100 units/kg of heparin (maximum 3,000 units) are administered. A 5 to 7 Fr multi-A-2 catheter (Cordis) is introduced from the aorta into the left ventricle across the

TABLE I. Acute Results of Balloon Aortic Valvuloplasty in Children[a]

Authors, year	No. of patients undergoing BAV	Age (Years), mean ± SD [Range]	Pre-BAV gradient (mmHg)[b]	Gradient immediately after BAV (mmHg)[b]	Percent reduction of gradient (Mean ± SD [Range])	Comments
Lababidi et al., 1984 [7]	23	9 ± 5 (2-17)	113 ± 45	32 ± 15	71 ± 11 (51-89)	Two patients required surgery
Walls et al., 1984[c] [40]	27	9 ± 5 (1.7-17)	108 ± 46	32 ± 16	—	—
Choy et al., 1987 [8]	8	7 ± 5 (0.25-12)	74 ± 25	38 ± 14	47 ± 16 (29-67)	—
Helgason et al., 1987 [9]	14[d]	9 ± 5 (0.2-15)	85 ± 23	27 ± 14	68 ± 15 (49-94)	—
Mullins et al., 1987 [10]	14	—	68	24	65	Only double-balloon BAV
Beekman et al., 1988[e] [12]	16	8 ± 2 (0.25-17)	82 ± 24	46 ± 16	43	Only single-balloon BAV
	11	10 ± 2 (0.25-21)	76 ± 16	22 ± 13	67	Only double-balloon BAV
Sholler et al., 1988[f] [11]	68	11 ± 9 (0.2-39)	79 ± 23	34 ± 19	55 ± 21 (0-94)	Three patients required surgery
Rao et al., 1989 [14]	16	7 ± 5 (0.6-16)	72 ± 21	28 ± 13	60 ± 17 (35-92)	—
Meliones et al., 1989 [13]	9	12 ± 5 (0.35-17.5)	88 ± 27	41 ± 18	53 ± 18 (32-81)	Previous surgical aortic valvotomy in all children.
Sullivan et al., 1989 [15]	33	Median ~7 (1.3-17.0)	71 ± 30	28 ± 19	61	—
Vogel et al. 1989 [40a]	25	9 ± 5 (0.5-16.7)	66 ± 26	24 ± 17	63 ± 21 (18-92)	Four patients required surgery
Shrivastava et al., 1990 [16]	25[g]	12 ± 9 (1-36)	112 ± 55	44 ± 21	—	One infant required surgery
Rocchini et al., 1990 [17]	204	10 ± 1 (0 to > 20)	77 ± 28	30 ± 14	61	Results of VACA Registry Includes 22 neonates
Shaddy et al., 1990 [18]	32	8 ± 6 (0.01-28)	77 ± 27	23 ± 16	70	Four were < 1 year of age.
Lababidi 1991 [40c][h]	93	10 ± 6	93 ± 37	25 ± 14	—	At least one of these was a neonate.
Witsenberg et al., 1992 [40b]	21	8	71 ± 25	22 ± 10	65 ± 20 (16-89)	Previous surgical aortic valvotomy in 10 children
Present report[i]	24	7 ± 5 (0.13-16)	71 ± 21	26 ± 12	62 ± 16 (35-92)	—

[a]Excludes neonates and literature reports containing < 3 patients.
[b]Gradient is peak-to-peak systolic pressure gradient across the aortic valve obtained at cardiac catheterization.
[c]Includes the patients previously reported by Lababidi et al., 1984 [7].
[d]Neonates in these series were excluded.
[e]Includes the patients previously reported by Choi et al., 1987 [8]
[f]Includes the patients previously reported by Helgason et al., 1987 [9].
[g]Eighteen of these 25 were younger than 18 years of age.
[h]Includes the patients previously reported by Lababidi et al., 1984 [7] and Walls et al., 1984 [40].
[i]Includes 16 children reported by Rao et al., 1989. [14].

aortic valve. A 0.014–0.035 inch J-shaped exchange guidewire is passed through the catheter into the left ventricular cavity (I prefer an apex, extra-stiff Amplatz exchange guidewire [Cook]) and the catheter removed. A 4 to 9 Fr balloon dilatation catheter is advanced over the guidewire, and the balloon is positioned across the aortic valve. Whenever possible, low-profile 5.5 cm long balloons are used in children and adolescents. Balloons 3–4 cm long are adequate in neonates, infants, and small children. The size of the balloon chosen should be within 1–2 mm of the size of the aortic valve annulus. The balloon is inflated with diluted contrast material to approximately 3–5 atm of pressure (Fig. 1). I recommend monitoring pressure of inflation with the help of a commercially available pressure gauge. The recommended duration of inflation is 5 seconds. Usually, a total of two to four balloon inflations are performed, 5 minutes apart. When the valve annulus is too large to dilate with a commercially available single balloon, I use a

double-balloon technique in which two balloons are simultaneously inflated across the aortic valve (Fig. 2). Effective balloon size is calculated by using a simple formula that we developed in our laboratory [31]:

$$\frac{D_1 + D_2 + \pi\left(\dfrac{D_1}{2} + \dfrac{D_2}{2}\right)}{\pi}$$

Fifteen minutes following the last balloon dilatation, a pressure pullback tracing across the aortic valve is recorded, cardiac output measured, and aortic root cineangiogram repeated.

We generally perform this procedure under sedation, usually with a mixture of meperidine, promethazine, and chlorpromazine given intramuscularly. When needed, this is supplemented with intermittent doses of midazolam. Other workers use ketamine or general anesthesia [15,32,33].

Because of the potential for injury to the femoral artery in the neonate, balloon

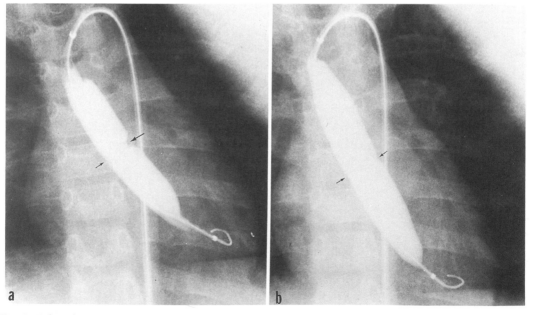

Fig. 1. Selected cineradiographs in posteroanterior view showing the balloon positioned across the aortic valve. Waisting of the balloon (arrow) is shown **(a)** during the initial phases of balloon inflation, which was completely abolished **(b)** after complete balloon inflation.

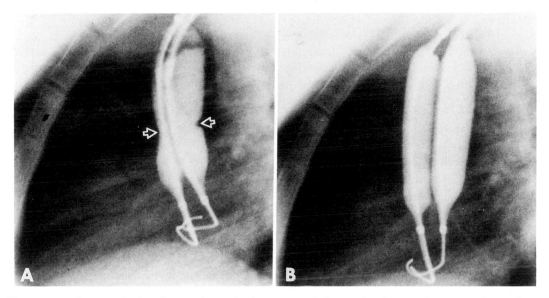

Fig. 2. Lateral views of selected cineradiographs showing two balloons placed across the aortic valve. Balloon waisting (arrows) during the initial phases of balloon inflation is shown **(A)**. The waisting is completely abolished **(B)** after full inflation of the balloon.

valvuloplasty had been performed via carotid artery cut-down [34], the umbilical artery [35], and axillary artery cut-down [36]. These are attractive alternative routes of balloon catheter entry and have the advantage of preserving femoral arteries. The experience with these techniques at our institution is limited but favorable.

To circumvent difficulty in crossing the aortic valve, some workers have utilized a trans-septal route with a femoral vein-femoral artery loop technique [36a] or antegrade sharing of the guidewire [36b].

During balloon aortic valvuloplasty, there is acute obstruction to aortic flow with consequent distention of the left ventricle, increased transmyocardial pressure, and potential compromise to myocardial perfusion. To circumvent this problem, Y-connectors to create left-ventricle-to-right-atrial shunt [7], double balloons [10], trefoil balloons [37], and inflow caval balloon occlusion [38] have been advocated. It is not clear if the left ventricular distension for short periods of time, as required during balloon valvuloplasty, is truly

harmful, nor is it clearly shown that the above-proposed methods [7,10,37,38] cause significant relief of left ventricular distension. We [39] have advocated short periods (5 seconds) of inflation and do not believe that the above-described methods [7,10,37,38] have significant advantages. They may indeed increase complexity of the procedure and prolong its duration.

ACUTE RESULTS

Balloon aortic valvuloplasty had been performed in children by several groups of workers [7–18,40,40a,b,c], and the results, though acceptable, are not as good as those following pulmonary valvuloplasty; generally, the valvar gradient is reduced to 60% of prevalvuloplasty values. The reported results are shown in Table I [7–18,40,40a,40b,40c]. No significant increase in aortic insufficiency was reported. Our own experience with this lesion [14,19,20] is not as extensive as with the other lesions; we have performed balloon aortic valvuloplasty in 24 children, aged 7 weeks to

16 years (7.4 ± 5.1 years). The peak systolic pressure gradient across the aortic valve was reduced from 71 ± 21 to 26 ± 12 mmHg (P<0.001) (Fig. 3). Reduction in the gradient in one of these children is demonstrated in Figure 4. The percent reduction of aortic valvar gradient ranged between 35% and 92% (62 ± 16%). The left ventricular end-diastolic pressure also decreased (13.3 ± 4.6 vs. 8.9 ± 5.5 mmHg, P<0.01). There was no evidence for increase in aortic insufficiency. None required immediate surgical intervention. All patients were discharged home within 24 hours after the procedure.

FOLLOW-UP RESULTS

Although acute results of balloon aortic valvuloplasty and clinical follow-up are available from many studies [7–18,40,40a-d], follow-up results have not been extensively documented (Table II). Lababidi et al. [7] reported cardiac catheterization results in six patients 3 to 9 months following balloon aortic valvuloplasty; the residual aortic valvar gradient was 38 ± 32 mmHg, with gradients in excess of 60 mmHg in two of six children restudied. In

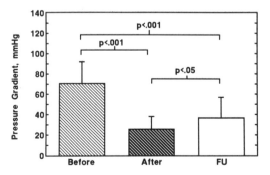

Fig. 3. Bar graphs showing peak-to-peak aortic valvar gradient prior to (before), immediately after (after), and 20 months (mean) following (FU) balloon aortic valvuloplasty. Note significant (P < 0.001) decrease in the gradient immediately after valvuloplasty. There was a slight but significant (P < 0.05) increase in the gradient at follow-up. But the follow-up gradients continue to be lower than those prior to balloon valvuloplasty.

a later publication [40], they reported 3 to 13 month follow-up catheterization data in 14 patients and found residual gradients of 37 ± 22 mmHg. However, the number of patients with moderate to severe stenosis has not been mentioned. In a more recent report [40c], the 1 to 8 year follow-up gradient in 32 (of 93 initial balloon valvuloplasty cases) patients was 30 ± 18 mmHg. Helgason et al. [9] recatheterized 10 patients 6 weeks to 6 months after valvuloplasty and found significant increase in gradient in two, but aortic valve gradients of ≥35 mmHg in eight patients and ≥50 mmHg in four patients were present at follow-up. Later [11] they reported recatheterization results in 16 patients 1–25 months after valvuloplasty and found significant residual aortic valve gradients (45 ± 29 mmHg) at follow-up. They also performed Doppler evaluation in 29 patients 1–24 months after dilatation and found a maximum instantaneous gradient of 40 ± 22 mmHg. However, it is not clear how many patients had residual gradients in excess of 50 mmHg at follow-up.

Meliones and associates [13] restudied eight of nine children who underwent balloon aortic valvuloplasty for relief of recurrent aortic valve obstruction after a previous surgical aortic valvotomy; the residual aortic valvar gradient after a mean follow-up of 1.5 years after aortic balloon valvuloplasty was 37 ± 14 mmHg, which had been reduced from 85 ± 28 to 38 ± 14 mmHg immediately following balloon valvuloplasty. Only one of the eight children had an aortic valvar gradient in excess of 50 mmHg. O'Connor et al. [40d] reported the follow-up results of 33 patients who underwent balloon aortic valvuloplasty between 1985 and 1988. Three children required surgery to relieve left ventricular outflow tract obstruction. In 27 children undergoing repeat catheterization at a mean follow-up time of 1.7 years, the residual gradient was 29 ± 10 mmHg. Thirteen (48%) had residual gradients >30 mmHg while gradient >50 mmHg was present in only 2 (7%) patients. Sullivan and colleagues [15] recatheterized 24 children 9 months following

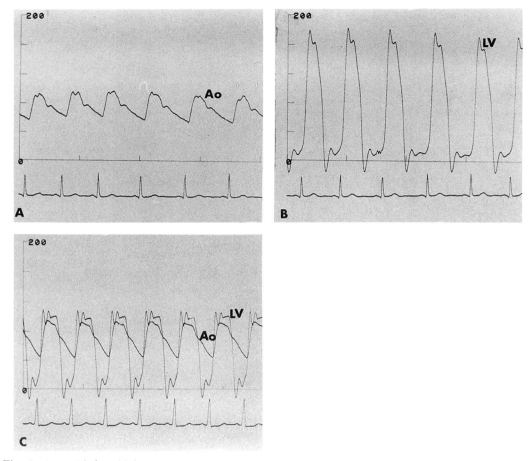

Fig. 1. Aortic (Ao) and left ventricular (LV) pressures prior to balloon aortic valvuloplasty (**A, B**) show that there is a significant peak to-peak aortic valve gradient. Following valvuloplasty (**C**), the gradient was reduced markedly.

balloon valvuloplasty and found residual gradients of 35 ± 20 mmHg, which were similar to immediate postvalvuloplasty gradients of 31 ± 20 mmHg. Five (21%) of the 24 children appear to have residual gradients in excess of 50 mmHg at follow-up; one required surgical intervention and two required repeat balloon valvuloplasty. Vogel et al. [40a] cited Doppler follow-up data in 9 children; the residual peak instantaneous gradient was 30 ± 13 mmHg. Shaddy et al. [18] reported early follow-up (4 months) results in 30 patients and late follow-up (19 months) results in 17 patients. The follow-up results were assessed by peak instan-

taneous Doppler gradients. Early follow-up aortic valvar gradients were 36 ± 12 mmHg, representing a 48% reduction compared with prevalvuloplasty gradients, whereas the late follow-up gradients were 44 ± 19 mmHg, representing a 40% reduction in gradients. Peak-to-peak aortic valve gradients >50 mmHg were present in 3% (1 of 32) of the patients immediately after valvuloplasty, while peak instantaneous gradients >50 mmHg were present in 10% (3 of 30) at early follow-up and in 41% (7 of 17) at late follow-up, indicating progressive restenosis. Shrivastava and associates [16] recatheterized 13 patients 11 ± 4

TABLE II. Intermediate-Term Follow-Up Results of Balloon Aortic Valvuloplasty (BAV) Reported in Literature

Author, year	No. (%) of patients with follow-up data	Duration (months) of follow-up (mean [Range])	Aortic valve gradient (mm Hg)			Poor results[a] at follow-up (No. [%])	Method of data acquisition[b] at follow-up
			Before	After	At follow-up		
Lababidi et al., 1984 [7]	6 (26)	5 (3–9)	127 ± 56	35 ± 25	38 ± 32	2 (33)	Cath
Walls et al., 1984 [40]	14 (52)[c]	7 (3–13)	125 ± 51	35 ± 18	37 ± 22	Not reported	Cath
Helgason et al., 1987 [9]	10 (71)	– (1.5–6)	88 ± 24	29 ± 16	41 ± 25	4 (40)	Cath
Sholler et al., 1988 [11]	16 (24)[d]	8 (1–25)	76 ± 26	30 ± 20	45 ± 29	Not reported	Cath
	29 (43)[d]	7 (1–24)	76 ± 26	30 ± 20	40 ± 22	Not reported	Doppler
Rao et al., 1989 [14]	16 (100)	12 (3–32)	72 ± 21	28 ± 13	37 ± 23	4 (25)	Cath + Doppler
Meliones et al., 1989 [13]	8 (89)	18 (10–30)	85 ± 28	38 ± 14	37 ± 14	1 (13)	Cath
Sullivan et al., 1989 [15]	24 (73)	9 (2–19)	71 ± 30	31 ± 20	35 ± 20	5 (21)	Cath
Vogel et al., 1989 [40a]	9 (31)	9 (3–13)	66 ± 26	24 ± 17	30 ± 17	Not reported	Doppler
Shrivastava et al., 1990 [16]	13 (52)	11 ± 4[e]	112 ± 35[f]	40 ± 18	45 ± 30	3 (23)	Cath
	10 (40)	9 ± 7[e]	106 ± 26	59 ± 26	54 ± 23	Not reported	Doppler
Shaddy et al., 1990 [18]	17 (52)	19 (12–27)	72 ± 18	36 ± 12	44 ± 19	7 (41)	Doppler
O'Connor et al., 1991 [40d]	27 (90)[h]	20 (10–38)	76 ± 22	32 ± 11	29 ± 16	2 (7)	Cath
Lababidi, 1991 [40c]	32 (34)[i]	– (12–96)	93 ± 37	25 ± 14	30 ± 18	Not reported	Not stated
Witseburg et al., 1992 [40b]	21 (100)	34 (20–50)	71 ± 23	22 ± 10	43 ± 13	Not reported	Doppler
Present report	24 (106)[g]	20 (3–42)	71 ± 21	26 ± 12	37 ± 20	5 (23)	Cath + Doppler

[a]Defined as a peak-to-peak or peak or instantaneous aortic valvar gradient ≥50 mmHg.
[b]Cath, peak-to-peak systolic pressure gradient across the aortic valve measured from cardiac catheterization data; Doppler, peak instantaneous Doppler-derived aortic valvar gradients.
[c]Includes the patients reported by Lababidi et al., 1984 [7].
[d]Includes the patients reported by Helgason et al., 1987 [9].
[e]Mean ± standard deviation.
[f]The gradient prior to valvuloplasty is for the entire group of 25 patients.
[g]Includes the patients reported by Rao et al., 1989.
[h]Includes the patients reported by Meliones et al., 1989 [13].
[i]Probably includes the patients reported by Meliones et al., 1989 [13].
[i]Includes the patient reported by Lababidi et al., 1986 [7] and Walls et al., 1984 [40].

months after valvuloplasty and found no significant increase in the peak-to-peak gradient for the group undergoing repeat catheterization (Table II). However, restenosis developed in three patients. An additional 10 patients underwent Doppler studies 9 ± 7 months following balloon valvuloplasty; the residual peak instantaneous gradients were 54 ± 23 mmHg at follow-up, which had been reduced from 106 ± 28 to 59 ± 26 mmHg immediately after valvuloplasty.

The follow-up results in our study were from all 24 children, 3–39 months (mean 20 months) after valvuloplasty; the residual gradients were 37 ± 20 mmHg. These values continue to be lower (P<0.001) than those prior to valvuloplasty and not significantly different (P>0.1) compared with immediate postvalvuloplasty gradients. However, when individual values were examined, 5 of 24 (21%) had gradients in excess of 50 mmHg. Two of these five children had repeat balloon valvuloplasty and three surgical valvotomy, all with good results (Fig. 5). Repeat balloon and surgical intervention was performed 3–13 months (mean 8 months) after the initial balloon valvuloplasty. Late follow-up in 22 pa-

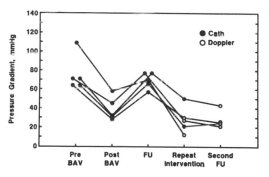

Fig. 5. Peak-to-peak gradients across the aortic valve in the group of patients with poor results. Although the initial gradient (pre) decreased immediately after (post) valvuloplasty, it returned toward prevalvuloplasty values at follow-up (FU). Repeat intervention by surgery in three and repeat balloon valvuloplasty in two has resulted in significant improvement in the gradient. Follow-up Doppler gradients were available in four children, all with good results.

tients, 3–70 months (30 ± 17 months) after valvuloplasty, revealed a peak instantaneous Doppler gradient of 28.5 ± 7.2 mmHg.

It may be concluded that balloon aortic valvuloplasty, despite modest decrease in aortic gradients and potential for arterial complications, may have a place in the treatment of aortic valve stenosis because of the high chance for recurrence following surgical valvuloplasty. Miniaturization of balloon/catheter systems and documentation of long-term follow-up results of balloon valvuloplasty are essential prior to using this technique as a preferred alternative to surgical valvotomy.

APPLICABILITY TO ALL AGES

Neonates

Several authors [11,34–36,41–44] performed balloon aortic valvuloplasty in neonates with severe or critical aortic stenosis (Table III) and found it useful in the management of these sick babies. Lababidi and Weinhaus [41] were the first to report balloon valvuloplasty in the neonate with critical aortic stenosis; reduction of aortic valvar gradient and clinical improvement occurred in both neonates. The improvement persisted at 5 month follow-up. Wren and associates [42] attempted this technique in eight neonates, aged 1–30 days; the procedure could be performed in only seven patients; the aortic valve was not crossed in the eighth patient. Three neonates improved after balloon valvuloplasty, one neonate died during balloon dilatation, and the remaining four infants died following surgical intervention that was required after valvuloplasty. They concluded that, despite the disappointing results, balloon valvuloplasty may provide an alternative to initial surgical management in some patients. Sholler and his colleagues [11] applied this techniques in 12 neonates, aged 1 day to 3 weeks, and reduced the peak systolic pressure gradient across the aortic valve from 56 ± 34 to 29 ± 28 mmHg. However, there were

TABLE III. Results of Balloon Aortic Valvuloplasty in Neonates Reported in the Literature[a]

Authors, year	No. of patients undergoing BAV	Aortic valve gradient (mean±SD; mmHg)[a]			Follow-up (No./months)	Poor result (No. [%])[b]	Comments
		Before	After	FU			
Lababidi and Weinhaus, 1986 [41]	2	75,34	34,–	–[c]	2/5	0 (0)	Aortic coarctation was also dilated in one neonate
Wren et al., 1987 [42]	8	50 ± 26	22 ± 16	13 ± 11	3/2–23	5 (63)	Valve was not crossed in one patient, one died during catheter manipulation, four died after surgery
Sholler et al., 1987 [11]	12	56 ± 34	29 ± 28	–	–	–	Three deaths
Zeevi et al., 1989 [44]	16[d]	55 ± 30	27 ± 24	45 ± 16	9/8 ± 8	13 (81)	Five early deaths, two late deaths, two technical failures
Kasten-Sporter et al., 1989 [43]	10	61 ± 24	20 ± 14	39 ± 6	4/16 ± 5	6 (60)	Three deaths, one transplantation, three open valvotomy
Fischer et al., 1990 [34]	5[e]	76 ± 17	33 ± 15	47 ± 19	3/7 ± 3	4 (80)	One death, one open valvotomy, two repeat balloon
Beekman et al., 1991 [35]	8[f]	69 ± 19	25 ± 7	–	5/2–16	3 (38)	Three technical failures

[a]Single case reports are not included.
[b]Poor result defined as early or late death, gradient ≥50 mmHg or repeat BAV.
[c]Doppler gradients were interpreted as mild gradient, no values given.
[d]Includes patients reported by Sholler.(11)
[e]BAV performed via carotid artery cutdown.
[f]BAV attempted via umbilical artery in seven patients and via femoral artery in one patient.

three deaths in this group. They commented that unfavorable valve morphology, associated left ventricular dysfunction or hypoplasia, and technical difficulties in accomplishing balloon valvuloplasty in these sick babies may, to a great degree, account for the problems in the neonates. In a later paper [44], they extended their observations to 16 neonates and compared them with a surgical group. The results of balloon valvuloplasty are essentially similar to those observed in their initial cohort of 12 patients.

Kasten-Sportes et al. [43] attempted balloon aortic valvuloplasty in 10 neonates aged 3–34 days. The aortic valve could not be crossed in one neonate. The remaining neonates underwent balloon valvuloplasty. Six infants had good immediate and intermediate-term results. Three neonates died, and one required cardiac transplantation. Hypoplasia of the left ventricle, technical difficulties, and development of aortic insufficiency were thought to contribute to the mortality. These authors concluded that balloon aortic valvuloplasty is an acceptable alternative to surgery in the management of neonates with critical aortic stenosis. Our own personal experience [20] was with only two neonates, both of whom did well and continue to do well clinically at follow-up approximately 1 year following valvuloplasty.

Fischer et al. [34] performed balloon aortic valvuloplasty with balloon catheters introduced via right common carotid artery cutdown in five neonates aged 1–20 days and reduced the peak systolic aortic valve gradient from 76 ± 17 to 33 ± 15 mmHg. One patient with left ventricular hypoplasia died, while another patient required open valvotomy. All four survivors did well clinically; two of these required repeat balloon dilatation of the aortic valve at 8 and 10 months of age, respectively. The authors concluded [34] that aortic valvuloplasty with balloon catheters introduced via carotid artery cut-down is feasible and safe for initial palliation of severe aortic stenosis in the neonate and that the risks of using femoral artery catheterization in the ne-

onate are eliminated. Beekman and associates [35] approached via umbilical artery to dilate critically stenosed aortic valves in the neonate. In the initial three patients, the procedure was not successful. In the last four neonates, the peak aortic valvar gradient was reduced from 75 ± 15 to 27 ± 8 mm Hg, and the infants' congestive heart failure improved. No follow-up aortic valvar gradient data were reported. They concluded that transumbilical balloon aortic valvuloplasty can be performed safely and effectively and has the advantage of preserving the femoral arteries.

The issue of whether surgical or balloon therapy is a better option in the treatment of neonatal aortic stenosis is not completely settled [45,46]. Based on the available data, the balloon valvuloplasty technique appears quite attractive, especially because of high surgical mortality at the initial or repeat aortic valvotomy in the neonate with critical aortic stenosis [26,47–53]. The vast majority of balloon failures appear to be related to technical problems or are secondary to poor anatomic substrate, namely, left ventricular hypoplasia, aortic valvar dysplasia, aortic annular hypoplasia, associated abnormalities of the mitral valve, and severe endocardial fibroelastosis. Meticulous attention to the technique and to choosing a balloon no larger than the aortic valve annulus to avoid aortic insufficiency may decrease the complications of the procedure.

Adults

Though the initial application of balloon valvuloplasty technique for valvar aortic stenosis was in children by Lababidi [6] in 1983, this technique is now extensively used in adult patients, particularly in the elderly, with calcific aortic stenosis [54–58]. Despite some reservations on the usefulness of this technique [59,60], most workers [54–58,61] consider this technique to be valuable in the management of the elderly with calcific aortic stenosis. Further discussion on this subject will not be presented in this book.

Other Age Groups

The foregoing discussion covers the role of balloon aortic valvuloplasty in children, neonates, and adults. The reported experience of this technique in other age groups will now be reviewed.

Fetus. Prenatally diagnosed critical aortic stenosis appears to have a poor prognosis [62]; most fetuses suffered intrauterine or neonatal death, and only about one-third of them lived long enough to undergo postnatal balloon or surgical intervention. The reason for the poor prognosis appears to be left ventricular hypoplasia and/or development of endocardial fibroelastosis. With the thesis that relief of aortic valve obstruction *in utero* may prevent left ventricular abnormalities, Maxwell and associates [62] attempted balloon dilatation of the aortic valve in two fetuses. The technique used by Maxwell and associates [62] is similar to that described by Daffos *et al.* [63]. An 18 gauge transabdominal chorionic villus sampling needle is inserted into the maternal abdominal wall under ultrasound guidance after local anesthesia. The needle is advanced into the fetal left ventricular cavity through the left ventricular apex. A flexible guidewire is initially positioned in the needle and advanced into the left ventricle and across the aortic valve into the aorta. The wire is withdrawn and replaced with a balloon dilatation catheter. After positioning the balloon across the aortic valve, the balloon is inflated (two or more times). The catheter and needle are withdrawn. Doppler echocardiography is used to assess the result. In one, the procedure was not successful. In the other, the procedure was successfully carried out with evidence for reduction in aortic valvar gradient. However, this infant required repeat postnatal dilatation of the aortic valve and eventually died. Postmortem examination revealed endocardial fibroelastosis, dysplastic aortic valve leaflets, and commissural split. Although the experience reported by Maxwell *et al.* [62] did not result in salvage of the affected fetuses, they did demonstrate that balloon aortic valvuloplasty can be accom- plished *in utero*. Further clinical trials to test the safety and efficacy of this technique and to determine the characteristics of the subset of patients that are likely to be benefitted by fetal aortic balloon valvuloplasty are in order.

Premature infants. Premature infants can also undergo successful balloon aortic valvuloplasty in a manner similar to that described in a preceding section of this chapter. Indeed, Tometzki *et al.* [64] reported successful balloon aortic valvuloplasty in an 8-day-old, 28-week gestational-age preterm baby weighing 1.08 kg. They used a 5 mm balloon carried on a 4.3 Fr catheter and reduced peak systolic pressure gradient across the aortic valve from 90 to 20 mmHg. However, evulsion of the femoral artery, requiring surgical reconstruction, occurred. It may be concluded that balloon aortic valvuloplasty can be accomplished in the premature infants, although arterial complications may be encountered. Use of carotid or umbilical artery to access the aortic valve may be considered to prevent femoral artery complications.

Infants. The neonates (≤4 weeks) and children (≥1 year) were included in the previous discussions. Infants aged 1–12 months have not been included in the discussions. Several groups of workers [8,9,11–13,16–19,42,65,66] included infants in their reports. The results are generally similar to those seen with children. However, the arterial complications are slightly more frequent. While balloon aortic valvuloplasty can be successfully accomplished in this age group, because of increased arterial complications it may be advisable to be more selective in subjecting infants to balloon aortic valvuloplasty.

APPLICABILITY TO PATIENTS WHO PREVIOUSLY HAD AORTIC VALVE SURGERY

Sholler *et al.* [11], Meliones *et al.* [13], and Rao *et al.* [14] have applied this technique in children with recurrent aortic valve stenosis following previous surgical valvotomy. Although the experience is limited, results appear encouraging and comparable with those obtained in patients without previous surgical valvotomy. Furthermore, immediate [11] or follow-up [14,67] results seem not to be influenced by previous surgical intervention. However, Witsenburg et al. [40b] noted that all three patients requiring valve replacement following balloon aortic valvuloplasty were those that previously had surgical aortic valvotomy.

Calcification and development of stenosis of bioprosthetic valves, particularly in children, is well documented. Such calcification and valve dysfunction may require replacement of the heterograft. However, balloon dilatation of the stenotic porcine valve may avoid or postpone reoperation. Several authors have reported dilatation of the bioprosthetic valves in the pulmonary, aortic, mitral, and tricuspid position. Although reasonably good results have been reported following balloon dilation of stenotic porcine heterografts in pulmonary, tricuspid, and mitral positions [68–71], such attempts to relieve heterograft stenosis in aortic position did not produce favorable results [72]. McKay et al. [72] performed balloon valvuloplasty of the bioprosthetic aortic valve in two patients; in one, there was a good relief of aortic gradient, while in the other no significant gradient reduction occurred. In the patient with gradient relief, severe aortic insufficiency developed, presumably related to a tear in one of the valve cusps. Because of clinically unpredictable results, these authors recommended that balloon valvuloplasty of aortic porcine heterograft be restricted to highly selected patients.

COMPARISON WITH SURGICAL RESULTS

Comparison of follow-up results of surgical versus balloon aortic valvuloplasty is fraught with problems because of 1) small number of balloon valvuloplasty patients available for follow-up, 2) shorter duration of balloon follow-up, and 3) possible inaccuracy of comparing "older" surgical studies with "current" balloon aortic valvuloplasty. Ten representative papers [22–30,73] investigating long-term follow-up results were reviewed to assess the long-term outlook of surgical aortic valvotomy. These authors [22–30,73] followed 41–179 patients for 0.3–26 years following surgical relief of aortic stenosis. Operative mortality varied between 0% and 4% when neonates and young infants were excluded; the cooperative natural history study [27] had a 1.2% mortality rate among 162 children undergoing open aortic valvotomy. Late mortality varied between 4% and 22% [22–30,73], while in the natural history study [27] it was only 1.9%. Restenosis of the aortic valve was noted in 16%–78% of patients, while significant aortic insufficiency developed in 6%–65% of patients. Reoperation either to relieve residual aortic obstruction or to correct aortic insufficiency was required in 16%–39% of patients [22–30,73]. Thus, the significant incidence of early and late mortality, the development of aortic valve restenosis and insufficiency at follow-up, and the need for reoperation associated with surgical aortic valvotomy as reported by several investigators [22–30,73], including the natural history study [27], would make balloon aortic valvuloplasty an attractive alternative to surgical valvotomy. It is likely that balloon valvuloplasty may be used to postpone surgical intervention and that it is a reasonable first approach, although long-term comparative data are not available.

MECHANISM OF VALVULOPLASTY

The mechanism of valvuloplasty in children was assessed by Walls et al. [40] by inspection of valve mechanism at surgery; they found tearing of valve raphae, tearing of the valve leaflets, and avulsion of the valve leaflets, all of which are conceivably the mechanisms by which relief of pulmonary or aortic valve obstruction can occur. Direct visual observations by other authors [34,74–77] in patients undergoing balloon pulmonary and aortic valvuloplasty and echocardiographic observations [78] also indicate a similar mechanism.

The circumferential dilating force exerted by balloon inflation is likely to rupture (tear) the weakest part of the valve mechanism. It is likely that the fused commissures are the weakest links that can be broken with balloon dilatation. However, in a given patient, when the fused commissures are strong and cannot be torn, tears in the valve cusps or avulsion of the valve leaflets [40] can occur. The latter events may cause more severe semilunar valve insufficiency. The mechanism in adult patients with calcific aortic stenosis appears to be fracture of nodular calcification and improved leaflet mobility [54,79].

COMPLICATIONS

Immediate

Complications during and immediately after balloon aortic valvuloplasty have been remarkably minimal. Transient bradycardia, premature beats, and a fall in systemic pressure during balloon inflation have been uniformly noted by all workers. These return rapidly back to normal following balloon deflation. Use of double balloons [10,80] and of a trefoil or a bifoil balloon [37,81] to allow blood egress from the ventricle during balloon inflation and shorter periods (5 seconds) of inflation [39,82,83] have been advocated to reduce the systemic hypotension. Having had experience with each of these techniques, the author is of the opinion that short periods of balloon inflation (≤ 5 seconds) are most efficacious without compromising immediate or follow-up results.

Blood loss requiring transfusion has been reported in many studies. Transient left bundle branch block and other transient electrocardiographic abnormalities [9,84], nonsustained ventricular tachycardia [85], ventricular fibrillation [14,17,84,86], cardiac arrest [16,83], transmural tears with vessel or ventricular wall perforation [17,83,85–87], balloon rupture [7,88], balloon dislodgement [17], aortic insufficiency or mitral valve tears [17,84], cerebrovascular accidents [89], and

development of subvalvar obstruction [90], though rare, have been reported. Femoral artery thrombosis requiring heparin, streptokinase or thrombectomy occurred in 39% (12 of 31) of patients undergoing balloon dilation of aortic coarctation or stenosis, while such a complication occurred in only 2.2% of arterial catheterizations not involving balloon dilatation [91]. Equally impressive incidences of arterial complication have been observed by others [17,92].

Deaths associated with balloon dilatation of the aortic valve have been reported [9,11,17, 42,43,84,86,87]; these were either related to aortic rupture [17,84,87] or occlusion of extremely critical obstruction [42,43,84], perforation or avulsion of aortic valve cusp [17], exanguination from torn iliac/femoral artery [17] or ventricular fibrillation [86].

Aortic insufficiency is a potential serious complication. Most workers reported a mild increase in aortic insufficiency following balloon valvuloplasty [7–12,14,16,40,42]. In one study involving 80 children, the aortic insufficiency grade was 0.7 ± 1 higher after valvuloplasty than before [11]. Our own data from 20 children [20] show that the aortic insufficiency grade increased from 0.6 ± 0.6 to 0.8 ± 0.8 after balloon valvuloplasty. None of the children required immediate surgical intervention because of development of aortic insufficiency after valvuloplasty, although such intervention was required in neonates [11,43].

Rocchini and colleagues [17] carefully analyzed VACA Registry data and reported 5% (11 of 204) life-threatening complications following balloon aortic valvuloplasty. There were five deaths. The other major complications included life-threatening arrhythmias in three and perforation of the left ventricle, dislodgement of balloon portion of the valvuloplasty catheter, and mitral perforation in one each. The complication rate appears to be related to the age of the patient. Younger patients had a higher rate of complication than did older children. The neonates appear to be at a high risk for complications. Some of these complications may be unavoidable. However, meticulous attention to the details of the technique, use of an appropriate length of the balloon, use of low-profile balloon catheters, selection of the smallest available catheter, use of a balloon diameter no larger than the aortic valve annulus, appropriate use of the double-balloon technique, avoiding extremely high inflation pressures, and short inflation/deflation cycles may prevent or reduce the complications.

Transient prolongation of the QTc interval following balloon valvuloplasty [85,93] has been reported, which may be a potential hazard for developing R-on-T phenomenon in children with ventricular ectopy. The Holter findings of premature ventricular beats following balloon pulmonary [94] and aortic [85] valvuloplasty may have a significance in the light of prolongation of QTc interval [93]. However, no patients from our series or many other studies have been known to develop ventricular arrhythmias, although three cases of sudden death from ventricular fibrillation shortly after balloon dilatation of aortic coarctation [95,96] and stenosis [86] were reported. Whether or not these arrhythmias are related to QTc prolongation is not known. However, patient monitoring following balloon valvuloplasty is warranted [85,93].

Complications at Follow-Up

With regard to complications at intermediate-term follow-up, femoral artery occlusion, aortic valve insufficiency, and recurrence of obstruction have been noted. Data with regard to the incidence of femoral artery occlusion at follow-up are not readily available from the literature. Of the 32 infants and children from our study [20] who underwent follow-up catheterization after balloon coarctation angioplasty or aortic valvuloplasty, three femoral arteries were found to be obstructed (complete in two and partial in one), but all of them had good collateral flow.

Doppler evidence for aortic insufficiency appears sensitive, but was studied by only a few investigators. This is discussed in the section

on noninvasive evaluation of follow-up results. The issue of recurrent stenosis following balloon valvuloplasty is also discussed in a later section of this chapter.

INFLUENCE OF TECHNICAL FACTORS ON THE RESULTS

Sholler et al. [11] examined the effect of balloon:annulus ratio and the number of dilating balloons (one vs. two) on the immediate results of balloon aortic valvuloplasty and found that they did not significantly influence the gradient relief. Beekman et al. [12] claimed that double-balloon technique may be superior to single-balloon valvuloplasty. The validity of these results was questioned [21] because of more severe aortic obstruction in the single-balloon group, differences in balloon sizes, and nonexamination of valve morphology. Furthermore, follow-up results have not been used in assessing the results. Shaddy and associates [18] found a slightly higher percent gradient reduction immediately after valvuloplasty when two balloons were used than when one balloon was used. However, when early and late follow-up results are looked at, there were no differences in residual gradients or percent gradient reduction between the single- and double-balloon groups. We feel that balloon:annulus ratio is more important than whether a single-balloon or a double-balloon technique is used [21]. However, we are not opposed to using the double-balloon technique; it may be used when the valve annulus is too large to dilate with a commercially available single balloon or when a single balloon cannot be safely passed across the femoral artery [10,21].

We [14,21] examined the role of technical factors (Table IV) and found that number of balloons used (single vs. double), maximum pressure achieved in the balloon, number of balloon inflations, and total duration of balloon inflation did not appear to influence the outcome at intermediate-term follow-up. The balloon to aortic valve annulus ratio, within

TABLE IV. Influence of Technical Factors on the Outcome of Balloon Aortic Valvuloplasty at Follow-Up[a]

	Group I (n = 12)	Group II(n = 4)	P value
Number of patients in whom double-balloon technique was used (n)	3	1	1.0[b]
Maximum pressure achieved in the balloon, (atm; mean±SD)	5.3±0.6	4.5±1.0	0.71
Number of balloon inflations (mean±SD)	3.8±1.5	3.8±2.9	0.9
Total duration of balloon inflation (seconds mean±SD)	20±7	20±14	1.0
Balloon aortic valve annulus ratio	1.03±0.13	1.02±0.17	0.75

[a]Reproduced from Rao [20], with permission of the publisher.
[b]Fisher's exact.
n, No. of patients. SD, standard deviation.

the range of variability found in the study [14], also did not seem to be responsible for restenosis following balloon valvuloplasty. Because of difficulty in maintaining the balloon center over the aortic valve during balloon inflation in children when 3 to 4 cm long balloons are used, it is generally considered that 5.5 cm long balloons are better for aortic valvuloplasty in children and adolescents; these longer balloons ensure adequate positioning of the balloon during valvuloplasty. Although there is a general impression that balloons larger than the aortic valve annulus produce more severe aortic insufficiency, Shaddy et al. [18] were unable to show correlation between balloon:annulus ratio and subsequent development of aortic insufficiency.

CAUSES OF RESTENOSIS

Although acute results of balloon aortic valvuloplasty have been reported, there are only a few studies [7,9,11,13,15–18,40] with follow-up results and much less with regard to recurrence of stenosis. To our knowledge, the causes for recurrence of aortic valve stenosis at follow-up have not been studied. We have examined this issue [14,67]. On the basis of 3–32 month (mean 12 months) follow-up results in 16 children, they were divided into two groups: group I with good results (gradient ≤49 mmHg), 12 patients; and group II with poor results (gradi-

ents ≥50 mmHg), four patients. All four patients in group II required balloon valvuloplasty or surgical valvotomy; none from group I required these procedures. Seventeen biographic, anatomic, physiologic, and technical variables were examined by a multivariate logistic regression analysis to identify factors associated with restenosis, and these risk factors were 1) age ≤3 years and 2) immediate postvalvuloplasty aortic valvar gradient ≥30 mmHg. Aortic valve morphology [11] and balloon:annulus ratio may play a significant role in the recurrence of aortic stenosis, but within the range of variability found in our study [14,67], however, there did not seem to be a difference. Identification of these risk factors may help in patient selection. Avoiding or minimizing risk factors may help reduce the chance of restenosis after valvuloplasty. Because the immediate postvalvuloplasty aortic valvar gradient in excess of 30 mmHg is an alterable and significant risk factor, one might consider using progressively larger balloons to reduce the gradient to <30 mmHg. The benefit of use of a larger balloon must be weighed against the risk of development of significant aortic insufficiency.

NONINVASIVE EVALUATION OF FOLLOW-UP RESULTS

Wren and his associates [42] studied six surviving infants 2–23 months (12±7 months) following balloon aortic valvuloplasty by Doppler and found that the residual Doppler flow velocity was 3.0 ± 0.7 m/sec (range 1.9–4.0 m/sec), representing a slight increase compared with immediate postvalvuloplasty values. Sholler et al. [11] performed Doppler evaluation in 29 patients 1–26 months after balloon aortic valvuloplasty and found a residual maximum instantaneous aortic gradient of 40 ± 22 mgHg. Shrivastava and associates [16] measured Doppler gradients in 10 patients 9 ± 7 months following valvuloplasty and found no significant change compared with immediate postvalvuloplasty gradients (54 ± 23 mmHg vs. 59 ± 26 mmHg). Voget et al. [40a] performed Doppler studies in nine children at a mean of nine months after valvuloplasty and found Doppler gradients unchanged compared to immediate post-valvuloplasty values. Shaddy et al. [18] reported early (4 ± 3 mo) and late (19 ± 6 months) follow-up Doppler-derived aortic valvar gradients. The aortic valvar gradients decreased from 77 ± 27 to 23 ± 16 mmHg (P < 0.01) immediately after valvuloplasty. At early follow-up evaluation in 30 of the 32 patients, the residual Doppler gradient was 36 ± 12 mmHg, representing significant increase (P < 0.01) compared with immediate postvalvuloplasty gradient of 23 ± 16 mmHg. At late follow-up evaluation of 17 patients, the residual gradient has further increased to 44 ± 19 mmHg. Wistenburg et al. [40b] recorded Doppler flow velocities prior to, immediately after, and at 6, 12, and 24 to 50 months following balloon valvuloplasty, and found that the Doppler-calculated instantaneous gradient decreased from 94 ± 36 to 49 ± 15 mmHg immediately after valvuloplasty and remained unchanged at follow-up.

We [14,21] obtained echo-Doppler studies in 16 children undergoing balloon aortic valvuloplasty. The Doppler flow velocity in the ascending aorta decreased from 4.0 ± 0.5 to 3.0 ± 0.8 m/sec (P < 0.001) immediately following valvuloplasty, indicative of a fall in calculated pressure gradient from 61 ± 17 to 34 ± 20 mmHg. At follow-up 3–32 months

after valvuloplasty, echocardiographic left-ventricular end-diastolic dimension (34 ± 6 vs. 38 ± 5 mm, P < 0.05), left ventricular posterior wall thickness (6.9 ± 2.1 vs. 7.1 ± 1.5 mm, P > 0.1), and left ventricular shortening fraction (48 ± 7% vs. 48 ± 6%, P > 0.1) remain unchanged compared with prevalvuloplasty valves. Peak Doppler flow velocities in the ascending aorta, 3.1 ± 0.7 m/sec, representing a calculated gradient of 35 ± 19 mmHg, remains improved (P < 0.001) compared with prevalvuloplasty values (4.0 ± 0.5 m/sec) but unchanged (P > 0.1) compared with immediate postvalvuloplasty values (3.0 ± 0.8 m/sec). The Doppler studies appear useful in evaluating residual aortic gradients following balloon aortic valvuloplasty. It should be recognized that the Doppler calculated gradient is maximum instantaneous gradient in contrast to the peak-to-peak gradient measured at catheterization. The former usually slightly overestimates the latter. When we compared the Doppler gradient with the catheterization gradient in 10 children in whom both Doppler and catheterization follow-up data were available, we found that in each patient the catheterization gradient was overestimated by the Doppler gradient by 0–15 mmHg (6 ± 6 mmHg). It was not underestimated in any patient [14].

Sholler et al. [11] restudied 12 patients for aortic insufficiency by Doppler and found that in 5 patients the Doppler grade decreased by one grade; in 6, it increased by 1+; and in 1 patient it increased by 2+; the last patient subsequently required aortic valve replacement. Analysis by Shrivastava et al. [16] in nine patients did not reveal an increase in the severity of aortic insufficiency. From our study group, follow-up Doppler studies examining for aortic insufficiency were scrutinized in 16 patients [14]. In seven, we utilized pulsed-Doppler technique, and in the remaining nine patients color Doppler was also used. The severity of aortic regurgitation was judged by the depth of the regurgitan jet into the left ventricular cavity in the pulsed Doppler cases, as described by Ciobanu et al. [97] and by the ratio of the aortic regurgitation jet width to the left ventricular outflow tract width in the color Doppler cases, as described by Perry et al. [98]. The Doppler grade at follow-up was 1+ in three, 2+ in four, 3+ in three, and 0 in six patients. The mean Doppler grade was 1.3 ± 1.2, which was 0.6 ± 0.6 prior to valvuloplasty (Fig. 6). Thus there is no evidence for significant aortic insufficiency at follow-up. However, Shaddy et al. [18] reported an increase in aortic insufficiency by ≥2 grades in 31% of the patients at follow-up. Witsenburg et al. [40b] noted grade 3 aortic regurgitation in 5 of 21 children that they followed for two to 4.2 years. Three of these children required aortic valve replacement.

OTHER ISSUES

Subaortic Stenosis

Subvalvar obstruction, similar to that described following balloon pulmonary valvuloplasty [99,100], can also develop after balloon dilatation of aortic valve stenosis. We observed this in 1 of 24 children who underwent balloon aortic valvuloplasty at our institution; this was a 9-year-old girl whose peak systolic pressure gradient across the aortic valve was reduced from 112 to 36 mmHg. In an echo-Doppler study performed on the morning following balloon aortic valvuloplasty, there was marked subaortic hyperactivity with a

peak Doppler velocity of 5.5 m/sec; there was a characteristic triangular pattern of the Doppler flow curve with a late peak. Similar findings were reported by Ludomirsky et al. [90] in 3 of the 33 (9%) patients undergoing balloon aortic valvuloplasty at their institution. This appears to be due to hyperactive and hypertrophied left ventricular muscle in response to long-standing and severe left ventricular outflow tract obstruction. The subvalvar (proximal) obstruction gets unmasked after the valvar (distal) obstruction is relieved and may be due to the phenomenon of forced vibration [101]. The subvalvar obstruction appears to resolve with time [90].

Transesophageal Echocardiography

Transesophageal echocardiographic (TEE) monitoring during balloon aortic valvuloplasty has the advantage of instantaneous evaluation of the effects of valvuloplasty. Stumper and associates [102] used TEE during balloon aortic valvuloplasty in four children aged 2.4 to 14.6 years and weighing 12.8 to 48.4 kg. In the preballoon studies, documentation of commissural fusion, detection of aortic insufficiency and its origin, and measurement of aortic annulus diameter were accomplished. In one additional patient, prolapse of the right coronary cusp and moderate aortic insufficiency were detected during TEE examination, resulting in cancellation of balloon aortic valvuloplasty. Positioning of the guidewire was determined and detection of a guidewire within the chordal apparatus of the mitral valve in one patient resulted in appropriate repositioning of the guidewire. Immediately after dilatation, documentation of opening of at least one commissure with improved mobility of the aortic valve leaflets, exclusion of prolapse of the aortic valve leaflets, and detection of trivial to mild aortic insufficiency was possible. However, residual gradient across the aortic valve could not be determined because of poor alignment of the Doppler beam with aortic flow. Transgastric imaging following valvuloplasty was helpful

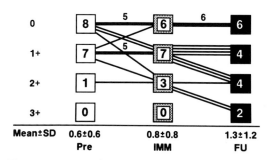

Fig. 6. Degree of aortic insufficiency, graded 1+ through 4+, prior to, immediately after balloon aortic valvuloplasty, and at follow-up are shown. Note that there is no significant worsening of aortic insufficiency.

in assessing shortening fraction and regional wall motion of the left ventricle.

While there are advantages with the use of TEE during balloon aortic valvuloplasty, the procedure is semi-invasive, requiring general anesthesia and endotracheal intubation. This is a definite disadvantage, especially in institutions, such as ours, in which the balloon valvuloplasty procedure is routinely performed under sedation with local anesthesia. Based on the available data [102,103], it is not clear whether TEE has significant advantages over the conventional catheter and angiographic data in view of 1) potential risks of TEE, 2) need for endotracheal intubation and general anesthesia, and 3) prolonging the time taken for interventional procedure. The advantages and disadvantages of TEE monitoring during aortic balloon valvuloplasty should be studied further prior to its routine use during valvuloplasty.

SUMMARY AND CONCLUSIONS

The technique of balloon aortic valvuloplasty has been used in infants, children, and adults since its first description in 1983. Immediate results reported by several investigators and intermediate-term results by a few workers appear encouraging. The technique has been successfully applied in all age groups, starting with neonate to the elderly. It has also been attempted in the fetus. Previous surgical valvuloplasty does not adversely affect the result. Complications are minimal, although potential for arterial complications, especially in younger children, and aortic insufficiency should be recognized. Significant restenosis rates at intermediate-term follow-up have been reported and could be minimized by reducing the risk factors associated with recurrence. Echo-Doppler studies are helpful in follow-up evaluation of balloon valvuloplasty. The results seem to compare favorably with those following surgical valvotomy. The indications are essentially the same as those used for surgery. The procedure is particularly useful in neonates in view of high mortality associated with surgery in these sick neonates.

Thus far, only 1 to 2 year follow-up results are available. Five to 10 year follow-up results to document long-term effectiveness of balloon aortic valvuloplasty are needed. Some reduction in the size of the dilating catheter systems has taken place. Further miniaturization and improving rapidity of inflation/deflation of balloons are necessary for increasing safety and effectiveness of these techniques in infants and children. Meticulous attention to the details of the technique and additional refinement of the procedure may further reduce the complication rate and increase effectiveness.

REFERENCES

1. Nadas AS, Fyler DC (1972): "Pediatric Cardiology," 3rd ed. Philadelphia: W.B. Saunders Co., p 683.
2. Keith JD, Rowe RD, Vlad P (1978): "Heart Disease in Infancy and Childhood," 3rd ed. New York: Macmillan Co., pp 4–6, 698–727.
3. Friedman WF (1989): Aortic stenosis. In Adams FH, Emmanouilides GC, Riemenschneider TA (eds): "Moss Heart Disease in Infants, Children, and Adolescents," 4th ed. Baltimore: William & Wilkins, pp 224–243.
4. Cheitlin MD, Rabinowitz M, McAllister H, Hoffman JIE, Bharati S, Lev M (1980): The distribution of fibrosis in the left ventricle in congenital aortic stenosis and coarctation of the aorta. Circulation 62:823–830.
5. Kan JS, White RI Jr, Mitchell SE, Gardner TJ (1982): Percutaneous balloon valvuloplasty: A new method for treating congenital pulmonary valve stenosis. N Engl J Med 307:540–542.
6. Lababidi Z (1983): Aortic balloon valvuloplasty. Am Heart J 106:751–752.
7. Lababidi Z, Wu J, Walls JT (1984): Percutaneous balloon aortic valvuloplasty: Results in 23 patients. Am J Cardiol 54:194–197.
8. Choy M, Beekman RA, Rocchini AP, Crowley DC, Snider AR, Dick M II, Rosenthal A (1987): Percutaneous balloon valvuloplasty for valvar aortic stenosis in infants and children. Am J Cardiol 59:1010–1013.
9. Helgason H, Keane JF, Fellows KE, Kulik TJ, Lock JE (1987): Balloon dilation of the aortic valve: Studies in normal lambs and in children with aortic stenosis. J Am Coll Cardiol 9:816–822.

10. Mullins CE, Nihill MR, Vick GW III, Ludomirsky A, O'Laughlin MP, Bricker JT, Judd VE (1987): Double balloon technique for dilation of valvular or vessel stenosis in congenital and acquired heart disease. J Am Coll Cardiol 10:107–114.

11. Sholler GF, Keane JF, Perry SB, Sanders SP, Lock JE (1988): Balloon dilation of congenital aortic valve stenosis: Results and influence of technical and morphological features on outcome. Circulation 78:351–360.

12. Beekman RH, Rocchini AP, Crowley DC, Snider AR, Serwer GA, Dick M II, Rosenthal A (1988): Comparison of single and double balloon valvuloplasty in children with aortic stenosis. J Am Coll Cardiol 12:480–485.

13. Meliones JN, Beekman RH, Rocchini AP, Lacina SJ (1989): Balloon valvuloplasty for recurrent aortic stenosis after surgical valvotomy in childhood: Immediate and follow-up results. J Am Coll Cardiol 13:1106–1110.

14. Rao PS, Thapar MK, Wilson AD, Levy JM, Chopra PS (1989): Intermediate-term follow-up results of balloon aortic valvuloplasty in infants and children with special reference to causes of restenosis. Am J Cardiol 64:1356–1360.

15. Sullivan ID, Wren C, Bain H, Hunter S, Rees PG, Taylor JFN, Bull C, Deanfield JE (1989): Balloon dilatation of the aortic valve for congenital aortic stenosis in childhood. Br Heart J 61:186–191.

16. Shrivastava S, Das GS, Dev V, Sharma S, Rajani M (1990): Follow-up after percutaneous balloon valvuloplasty for noncalcific aortic stenosis. Am J Cardiol 65:250–252.

17. Rocchini AP, Beekman RH, Ben Shachar G, Benson L, Schwartz D, Kan JS (1990): Balloon aortic valvuloplasty: Results of the valvuloplasty and angioplasty of congenital anomalies registry. Am J Cardiol 65:784–789.

18. Shaddy RE, Boucek MM, Sturtevant JE, Ruttenberg HD, Orsmond GS (1990): Gradient reduction, aortic valve regurgitation and prolapse after balloon aortic valvuloplasty in 32 consecutive patients with congenital aortic stenosis. J Am Coll Cardiol 16:451–456.

19. Rao PS (1989): Balloon dilatation in infants and children with cardiac defects. Cathet Cardiovasc Diagn 18:136–149.

20. Rao PS (1990): Balloon aortic valvuloplasty: A review. Clin Cardiol 13:458–466.

21. Rao PS (1989): Double balloon aortic valvuloplasty in children. J Am Coll Cardiol 13:1216.

22. Jones J, Barnhart GR, Morrow AG (1982): Late results after operations for left ventricular outflow tract obstruction. Am J Cardiol 50:569–579.

23. Ankeney JL, Tzeng TS, Liebman J (1983): Surgical therapy for congenital aortic valvular stenosis: A 23-year experience. J Thorac Cardiovasc Surg 85:41–48.

24. Jack WD II, Kelly DT (1976): Long-term follow-up of valvuloplasty for congenital aortic stenosis. Am J Cardiol 38:231–234.

25. Hsieh KS, Keane JF, Nadas AS, Bernhard WF, Castaneda AR (1986): Long-term follow-up of valvotomy before 1968 for congenital aortic stenosis. Am J Cardiol 58:338–341.

26. Sandor GGS, Olley PM, Trussler GA, Williams WG, Rowe RD, Morch JE (1980): Long-term follow-up of patients after valvotomy for congenital valvar aortic stenosis in children. J Thorac Cardiovasc Surg 80:171–176.

27. Wagner HR, Ellison RC, Keane JF, Humphries JO, Nadas AS (1987): Clinical course in aortic stenosis. Circulation 56(Suppl I):47–56.

28. Lawson RM, Bonchik LI, Menashe V, Starr A (1976): Late results of surgery for left ventricular outflow tract obstruction in children. J Thorac Cardiovasc Surg 71:334–342.

29. Dobell ARC, Bloss RS, Gibbons JE, Collins GF (1981): Congenital valvular aortic stenosis: surgical management and long-term results. J Thorac Cardiovasc Surg 81:916–920.

30. Presbitero P, Somerville J, Revel-Chion R, Ross D (1982): Open aortic valvotomy for congenital aortic stenosis: Late results. Br Heart J 47:26–34.

31. Rao PS (1987): Influence of balloon size on short-term and long-term results of balloon pulmonary valvuloplasty. Texas Heart Inst J 14:57–61.

32. Rickards AF, Somerville J (1986): Successful balloon aortic valvotomy in a child with a pulmonary hypertensive duct and aortic valve stenosis. Br Heart J 56:185–186.

33. Chaffe A, Fairbrass MJ, Chatrath RR (1988): Anesthesia for valvuloplasty. Anaesthesia 43:359–381.

34. Fischer DR, Ettedgui JA, Park SC, Siewers RD, del Nido P (1990): Carotid artery approach for balloon dilatation of aortic valve stenosis in the neonate: A preliminary report. J Am Coll Cardiol 15:1633–1636.

35. Beekman RH, Rocchini AP, Andes A (1991): Balloon valvuloplasty for critical aortic stenosis in the newborn: influence of new catheter technology. J Am Coll Cardiol 17:1172–1176.

36. Austoni P, Figini A, Vignati G, Donatelli F (1990): Emergency aortic balloon valvotomy in critical aortic stenosis of the neonate. Pediatr Cardiol 11:59–60.

36a. Hosking MCK, Benson LN, Freedom RM (1991): A femoral vein–femoral artery loop technique for aortic dilatation in children. Cathet Cardiovasc Diagn 23:253–256.

36b. Latson LA (1990): Antegrade catheter snare for

retrograde catheterization of left ventricle: A new technique to facilitate balloon aortic valvuloplasty. Cathet Cardiovasc Diagn 19:56-57.

37. Meier B, Freedli B, Oberhansli I (1986): Trefoil balloon for aortic valvuloplasty. Br Heart J 56:292-293.

38. Kiel AA, Devanter V, Readinger RI, Dungan WT, Norton JB (1986): Aortic balloon valvuloplasty with transluminal venous balloon inflow occlusion (case report). Pediatr Cardiol 7:103-105.

39. Rao PS (1989): Balloon angioplasty and valvuloplasty in infants, children and adolescents. Curr Probl Cardiol 14:417-500.

40. Walls JT, Lababidi Z, Curtis JJ, Silver D (1984): Assessment of percutaneous balloon pulmonary and aortic valvuloplasty. J Thorac Cardiovasc Surg 88:352-356.

40a. Vogel M, Benson LN, Burrows P, Smallhorn JF, Freedom RM (1989): Balloon dilatation of congenital aortic valve stenosis in infants and children: Short term and intermediate results. Br Heart J 62:148-153.

40b. Witsenburg M, Cromme-Dijkhuis AH, Frohn-Mulder IME, Hess J (1992): Short- and midterm results of balloon valvuloplasty for valvar aortic stenosis in children. Am J Coll Cardiol 69:945-950.

40c. Lababidi Z (1991): Congenital obstruction of the left ventricular outflow tract. In Cheng TO (ed): "Percutaneous Balloon Valvuloplasty" New York: Igaku-Shoin, pp 305-337.

40d. O'Connor BK, Beekman RH, Rocchini AP, Rosenthal A (1991): Intermediate term effectiveness of balloon valvuloplasty for congenital aortic stenosis: A prospective follow-up study. Circulation 84:732-738.

41. Lababidi Z, Weinhaus L (1986): Successful balloon valvuloplasty for neonatal critical aortic stenosis. Am Heart J 12:913-916.

42. Wren C, Sullivan I, Bull C, Deanfield J (1987): Percutaneous balloon dilation of aortic valve stenosis in neonates and infants. Br Heart J 58:608-612.

43. Kasten-Sportes CH, Piechaud J, Sidi D, Kachaner J (1989): Percutaneous balloon valvuloplasty in neonates with critical aortic stenosis. J Am Coll Cardiol 13:1102-1105.

44. Zeevi B, Keane JF, Castaneda AR, Perry SB, Lock JE (1989): Neonatal critical valvar aortic stenosis: A comparison of surgical and balloon dilation therapy. Circulation 80:831-839.

45. Freedom RM (1989): Balloon therapy of critical aortic stenosis in the neonate: The therapeutic conundrum resolved? Circulation 80:1087-1088.

46. Freedom RM (1990): Neonatal aortic stenosis: the balloon deflated? J Thorac Cardiovasc Surg 100:927-928.

47. Edmunds LH Jr, Wagner HR, Heymann MA (1980): Aortic valvulotomy in neonates. Circulation 61:421-427.

48. Sink JD, Smallhorn JF, Macartney FJ, Taylor JFN, Stark J, de Leval MR (1984): Management of critical aortic stenosis in infancy. J Thorac Cardiovasc Surg 87:82-86.

49. Binet JP (1986): Critical aortic stenosis: Surgical results in infancy. In Doyle EF, Engle MA, Gersony WM, Rashkind WJ, Talner NS (eds): "Pediatric Cardiology." New York: Springer-Verlag, pp 653-656.

50. Duncan K, Sullivan I, Robinson P, Horvath P, de Leval M, Stark J (1987): Transventricular aortic valvotomy for critical aortic stenosis in infants. J Thorac Cardiovasc Surg 93:546-550.

51. Pelich AN, Dyck JD, Trusler GA, Williams WG, Olley PM, Rowe RD, Freedom RM (1987): Critical aortic stenosis. J Thorac Cardiovasc Surg 94:510-517.

52. Turley K, Bove EL, Amato JJ, Iannetoni M, Yeh J, Cotroneo JV, Galdieri RJ (1990): Neonatal aortic stenosis. J Thorac Cardiovasc Surg 99:679-689.

53. Karl TR, Sano S, Brawn WJ, Mee RBB (1990): Critical aortic stenosis in the first months of life: surgical results in 26 infants. Ann Thorac Surg 50:105-109.

54. Cribier A, Saoudi N, Berland J, Savin T, Rocha P, Letac B (1986). Percutaneous transluminal valvuloplasty of acquired aortic stenosis in elderly patients: an alternative to valve replacement? Lancet 1:63-67.

55. Cribier A, Savin T, Berland J, Rocha P, Mechmeche R, Saoudi N, Behar P, Letac P (1987): Percutaneous transluminal balloon valvuloplasty of adult aortic stenosis: Report of 92 cases. J Am Coll Cardiol 9:381-386.

56. McKay RG, Safian RD, Lock JE, Mandell VS, Thurer RL, Schmitt SJ, Grossman W (1986): Balloon dilatation of calcific aortic stenosis in elderly patients: Postmortem, intraoperative and percutaneous valvuloplasty studies. Circulation 74:119-125.

57. Drobinski G, Lechat P, Metzger JP, Lepailleur C, Vacheron A, Grosgogeat Y (1987): Results of percutaneous catheter valvuloplasty for calcified aortic stenosis in the elderly. Eur Heart J 8:322-328.

58. Isner IM, Salem DN, Desnoyers MR, Hougen TJ, Mackey WC, Pandian NG, Eichhorn EJ, Konstam MA, Levine HJ (1987): Treatment of calcific aortic stenosis by balloon valvuloplasty. Am J Cardiol 59:313-317.

59. Robicsek F, Harbold NB, Daugherty HK, Cook JW, Selle JG, Hess PJ, Gallagher JJ (1988): Balloon valvuloplasty in calcified aortic stenosis: A cause

for caution and alarm. Ann Thorac Surg 45:515–525.

60. Robicsek F, Harbold NB Jr (1987): Limited value of balloon dilatation in calcified aortic stenosis in adults: Direct observations during open heart surgery. Am J Cardiol 58:322–202.

61. Roberts WC (1987): Good-bye to thoracotomy for cardiac valvulotomy. Am J Cardiol 59:198–202.

62. Maxwell D, Allan L, Tynan MJ (1991): Balloon dilatation of the aortic valve in the fetus: A report of two cases. Br Heart J 65:256–258.

63. Daffos F, Capella-Parlovsky M, Forestier F (1988): Fetal blood sampling during pregnancy with needle guided by ultrasound: A study of 606 consecutive cases. Am J Obstet Gynecol 153:655–659.

64. Tometzki AJP, Gibbs JL, Weil J (1991): Balloon valvuloplasty of critical aortic and pulmonary stenosis in the premature neonate. Internat J Cardiol 30:248–269.

65. Rupprath G, Neuhaus K (1985): Percutaneous balloon valvuloplasty for aortic valve stenosis in infancy. Am J Cardiol 55:1655–1656.

66. Sanchez GR, Mehta AV, Ewing LL, Brickley SE, Anderson TM, Black IFS (1985): Successful percutaneous balloon valvuloplasty of the aortic valve in an infant. Pediatr Cardiol 6:103–106.

67. Rao PS (1990): Causes of restenosis following balloon angioplasty/valvuloplasty: A review. Pediatr Rev Commun 4:157–172.

68. Waldman JD, Schoen FJ, Kirkpatrick SE, Matthewson JW, George L, Lamberti JJ (1987): Balloon dilatation of porcine bioprosthetic valves in the pulmonary position. Circulation 76:109–114.

69. Lloyd TR, Marvin WJ Jr, Mahoney LT, Lauer RM (1987): Balloon dilatation valvuloplasty of bioprosthetic valves in extra cardiac conduits. Am Heart J 114:268–274.

70. Calvo OL, Sobrino N, Gamallo C, Oliver J, Dominquez F, Iglesias A (1987): Balloon percutaneous valvuloplasty for stenotic bioprosthetic valves in mitral position. Am J Cardiol 60:736–739.

71. Feit F, Stecy PJ, Nachamie MS (1986): Percutaneous balloon valvuloplasty for stenosis of a porcine bioprosthesis in the tricuspid valve position. Am J Cardiol 58:363–364.

72. McKay CR, Waller BF, Hong R, Rubin N, Reid CL, Rahimthoola SH (1988): Problems encountered with catheter balloon valvuloplasty of bioprosthetic aortic valves. Am Heart J 115:463–465.

73. DeBoer DA, Robbins RC, Maron BJ, McIntosh CL, Clark RE (1990): Late results of aortic valvotomy for congenital valvar aortic stenosis. Ann Thorac Surg 50:69–73.

74. Rao PS, Brais M (1988): Balloon pulmonary valvuloplasty for cyanotic congenital heart defects. Am Heart J 115:1105–1113.

75. Tynan M, Baker EJ, Rohmer J, Jone ODH, Reidy JF, Joseph MC, Ottenkamp J (1985): Percutaneous balloon pulmonary valvuloplasty. Br Heart J 53:520–524.

76. Lababidi Z, Wu J (1983): Percutaneous balloon pulmonary valvuloplasty. Am J Cardiol 52:560–562.

77. Kan JS, White RI Jr, Mitchell SE, Anderson JH, Gardner TJ (1984): Percutaneous transluminal balloon valvuloplasty for pulmonary valve stenosis. Circulation 69:554–560.

78. Robertson M, Benson LN, Smallhorn JF, Musewe N, Freedom RM, Moes CAF, Burrows P, Johnston AE, Burrows FA, Rowe RD (1987): The morphology of the right ventricular outflow tract after percutaneous pulmonary valvotomy: Long-term follow-up. Br Heart J 58:239–244.

79. Safian RD, Mandell VS, Thurer RE, Hutchins GM, Schnitt SJ, Grossman W, McKay RG (1987): Postmortem and intraoperative balloon valvuloplasty of calcific aortic stenosis in elderly patients: Mechanisms of successful dilatation. J Am Coll Cardiol 9:655–660.

80. Al Kasab S, Riberio P, Al Zaibag M (1987): Use of double balloon technique for percutaneous balloon pulmonary valvotomy in adults. Br Heart J 58:136–141.

81. Van den Berg E, Niemeyer MG, Plokker TWM, Ernst SMPG, deKorte J (1986): New triple-lumen balloon catheter for percutaneous (pulmonary) valvuloplasty. Cathet Cardiovasc Diagn 12:352–356.

82. Rao PS (1989): Balloon pulmonary valvuloplasty: A review. Clin Cardiol 12:55–74.

83. Rao PS (1988): How big a balloon and how many balloons for pulmonary valvuloplasty. Am Heart J 116:577–580.

84. Fellows KE, Radtke W, Keane JF, Lock JE (1987): Acute complications of catheter therapy for congenital heart disease. Am J Cardiol 60:679–683.

85. Weesner KM (1990): Ventricular arrhythmias after balloon aortic valvuloplasty. Am J Cardiol 66:1534–1535.

86. Booth P, Redington AN, Shinebourne EA, Rigby MI (1991): Early complications of interventional balloon catheterization in infants and children. Br Heart J 65:109–112.

87. Waller BF, Girod DA, Dillon JC (1984): Transverse aortic wall tears in infants after balloon angioplasty for aortic valve stenosis: Relation of aortic valve damage to diameter of inflated angioplasty balloon and aortic lumen in seven necropsy cases. J Am Coll Cardiol 4:1235–1241.

88. Loya Y, Sharma S (1991): Balloon tear during valvuloplasty. Am Heart J 121:1841–1842.

89. Treacy ED, Duncan WJ, Tyrrell MJ, Lowry NJ (1991): Neurological complications of balloon angioplasty in children. Pediatr Cardiol 12:98–101.

90. Ludomirsky A, O'Laughlin MP, Nihill MR, Mullins CE (1991): Left ventricular mid-cavity obstruction after balloon dilatation in isolated aortic valve stenosis in children. Cathat Cardiovasc Diagn 22:89–92.

91. Wessel DL, Keane JF, Fellows KE, Robicharud H, Lock JE (1986): Fibrinolytic therapy for femoral arterial thrombosis after cardiac catheterization in infants and children. Am J Cardiol 58:347–351.

92. Burrows PE, Benson LN, Williams WG, Trusler GA, Coles J, Smallhorn JF, Freedom RM (1990): Iliofemoral arterial complication of balloon angioplasty for systemic obstructions in infants and children. Circulation 82:1697–1706.

93. Martin GR, Stanger P (1986): Transient prolongation of the QTc interval after balloon valvuloplasty and angioplasty in children. Am J Cardiol 58:1233–1235.

94. Kveselis DA, Rocchini AP, Snider AP, Rosenthal A, Crowley DC, Dick M (1985): Results of balloon valvuloplasty in the treatment of congenital valvar pulmonary stenosis in children. Am J Cardiol 56:527–532.

95. Kan JS, White RI, Mitchell SE, Farmiett EJ, Danahoo JS, Gardner TJ (1983): Treatment of restenosis of coarctation by percutaneous transluminal angioplasty. Circulation 68:1087–1094.

96. de Lezo JS, Fernandez R, Sancho M, Concha M, Arizon J, Franco M, Alemany F, Barcones F, Lopez-Rubio F, Vallés F (1984): Percutaneous transluminal angioplasty for aortic isthmic coarctation in infancy. Am J Cardiol 54:1147–1149.

97. Ciobanu M, Abbasi AS, Allen M, Hermer A, Spellberg R (1982): Pulsed Doppler echocardiography in the diagnosis and estimation of severity of aortic insufficiency. Am J Cardiol 49:339–343.

98. Perry GJ, Helmcke F, Nanda NC, Byard O, Soto B (1987): Evaluation of aortic insufficiency by Doppler color flow mapping. J Am Coll Cardiol 9:952–959.

99. Fontes VF, Esteves CA, Sousa JE, Silva MVD, Bembom MCB (1988): Regression of infundibular hypertrophy after pulmonary valvuloplasty for pulmonic stenosis. Am J Cardiol 62:977–979.

100. Thapar MK, Rao PS (1989): Significance of infundibular obstruction following balloon valvuloplasty for valvar pulmonic stenosis. Am Heart J 118:99–103.

101. Rao PS, Linde LM (1974): Pressure and energy in the cardiovascular chambers. Chest 66:176–178.

102. Stumper O, Witsenburg M, Sutherland GR, Cromme-Dijhuis A, Godman MJ, Hess J (1991): Transesophageal echocardiographic monitoring of interventional cardiac catheterization in children. J Am Coll Cardiol 18:1506–1514.

103. Feltes TF (1991): Advances in transesophageal echocardiography: Impact of a changing technology in children with congenital heart disease. J Am Coll Cardiol 18:1515–1516.

8

Balloon Valvotomy in Atrioventricular Valve Stenoses

Muayed Al-Zaibag, M.D., and Mutrada Halim, M.D.

Adult Cardiology Division, Riyadh Armed Forces Hospital,
Riyadh 11159, Saudi Arabia

BALLOON MITRAL VALVOTOMY

Introduction

Inoue reported successful balloon dilatation of the stenotic mitral valve in 1984 using a single-balloon catheter [1]. In 1986 we described an alternative method, the double-balloon technique [2]. Since then, balloon mitral valvotomy has become well established as an accepted alternative to the surgical treatment of symptomatic mitral stenosis, with over 1,000 procedures performed worldwide [3-7].

Patient Selection[1]

Percutaneous balloon mitral valvotomy (PBMV) is offered to patients with symptomatic, severe mitral stenosis. Initially, in our experience, strict criteria were observed for selection of patients for balloon mitral valvotomy [2], namely: a mitral valve area (MVA) ≤ 1.0 cm^2, no history of thromboembolism sinus rhythm, no evidence of left atrial clot by 2-dimensional echocardiography (2-DE), absence of mitral regurgitation and calcification, and no other valvular pathology requiring surgery. However, with greater experience, increased confidence in procedure, and the very low complication rate, the strict criteria

were relaxed. At the present time, the presence of a left atrial thrombus and moderate-to-severe mitral regurgitation are the only contraindications to the procedure. Patients with atrial fibrillation, previous surgical mitral valvotomy [8], and even calcific mitral valves [9,10] have had successful balloon mitral valvotomy. In a few centers the procedure has even been performed in severely symptomatic pregnant women [11,12], though this still remains controversial because of the radiation hazard [7], especially if the alternative closed surgical valvotomy—which carries less risk to the fetus than open valvotomy—can be performed.

Patients with moderate mitral stenosis, (MVA 1.0–1.5 cm^2) are usually offered balloon dilatation if they are symptomatic despite medical therapy, as are women in the child bearing age if cardiac symptoms arose during a previous pregnancy.

Mechanism of Balloon Mitral Valvotomy

Intra-operative observation [1,2] and *in vitro* studies [13,14] have demonstrated that commissural splitting is the mechanism by which MVA increases after successful balloon valvotomy. This has been further supported by postmortem evidence from patients who had previous balloon valvotomy [15]. The commis-

---

[1]Editor's note: This chapter on atrioventricular valve stenosis deals with almost entirely with adult population with rheumatic heart disease. With regard to treatment of this subject in infants and children with congenital mitral and tricuspid valve stenosis, the reader is referred to Chapter 15.

Transcatheter Therapy in Pediatric Cardiology, pages 129–141
© 1993 Wiley-Liss, Inc.

sural splitting occurs through both non-calcific and calcific commissures [14].

Procedure of Balloon Mitral Valvotomy

The basic technique of balloon mitral dilatation relies upon advancing single- or double-balloon catheters over wires, across the stenotic mitral valve orifice, and then inflating the balloons to split the commissures, thus achieving an increase in MVA. Two different routes may be used to position the balloons across the mitral valve orifice, namely antegrade or retrograde.

In the antegrade technique the balloons are advanced from a femoral vein, through an atrial septal puncture into the left atrium, and then placed across the mitral valve orifice. In the retrograde technique the balloon is inserted from a femoral artery and advanced retrogradely from the aorta into the left ventricle and then across the mitral valve orifice. Variations of the antegrade technique concern either the use of a single balloon [1,16,17], the use of two 14 Fr transeptal sheaths through two septal punctures, with two balloons [2,18], two septal punctures with no sheaths [19], or the use of two balloons placed through a single transeptal puncture [4,20]. The retrograde technique was proposed [21], with the suggested theoretical advantage of not creating an atrial septal defect (ASD), since the shaft of the balloon catheter does not have to be advanced through the atrial septum. However, the majority of those performing PBMV prefer the antegrade technique, since the retrograde technique is cumbersome and the potential remains for arterial damage.

With the balloons positioned across the orifice of the stenotic mitral valve, they are inflated a few times until the indentation of the balloon, caused by the stenotic valve, disappears. Successful dilatation is defined as the achievement of a MVA of 1.5 cm^2 or more, in the absence of serious complication.

Patients are kept on oral anticoagulation for 6 weeks after PBMV, regardless of their cardiac rhythm, to reduce the risk of left atrial thrombus and embolization during the procedure [2,4].

Types and sizes of balloons. Several years after the first PBMV, there is still no universal agreement on the criteria for selection of technique, balloon type, and size. However, six points should be considered, namely: 1) a single balloon is technically easier to use than two balloons; 2) the balloon, or combination of balloons, must be of adequate size to produce an optimal MVA, of around 2.0 cm^2; 3) the balloon, or combination, must not be oversized, thus causing significant mitral regurgitation; 4) the size of the residual atrial septal communication after the procedure, possibly atrial septal communication after the procedure, possibly related to the balloon catheter, must be considered; one must also consider 5) balloon length, and 6) balloon technology.

Most centers performing PBMV advocated the use of a double-balloon technique, since the available single-balloon catheters were not satisfactory; they were either not large enough, thus resulting in inadequate dilatation, or so large that they had to be carried on a large shaft and caused a large ASD. *In vitro* [14] and *in vivo* [15,22,23] studies showed that the then-available 20-, 23-, or even 25-mm diameter balloon used singly produced an inadequate mitral valve dilatation. However, the single balloon specially designed by Inoue, 24 to 30 mm in diameter, which is increasingly available in the market, has shown good results, with adequate dilatation and no significant increase in ASD or the incidence of severe mitral regurgitation (MR) [6,24], compared to the double-balloon technique. To date, there is no large series comparing the results obtained from the single Inoue balloon technique and the double-balloon technique from a center that has considerable experience in the use of both; the only published work [25] had such an unacceptably high incidence of complications, from quite a small group of 21 patients undergoing the double-balloon technique, that the comparison was invalid.

There is no standardized formula for the choice of balloon size in balloon mitral valvotomy, in contrast to the balloon dilatation of the stenotic aortic or pulmonary valve, where a simple valve annulus/balloon size ratio is accepted [26,27]. In view of the complexity of the mitral valve pathology in rheumatic mitral stenosis, we were not satisfied by selection of balloon size based simply on the the mitral valve annulus measurement by 2-dimensional echocardiography (2-DE). Knowing that the combination of 15+15-mm diameter balloons achieved a relatively small valve area [2], we prospectively compared the results of various combinations of balloon sizes in 77 patients [7,18,28], concluding that for adult patients a combination of 20+18-mm diameter balloons achieved most effective dilatation, with an acceptable incidence of mild MR. Brandi-Pifano et al. [29], Herman et al. [30], Chen et al. [31], and Ruiz et al. [4] suggested various methods for balloon selection, respectively: effective balloon-dilating area (EBDA), EBDA/BSA ratio, the ratio of the sum of the diameters of the dilating balloons to the mitral valve annulus, and empirical choice followed by analysis of results

Therefore, with no absolute guideline, it can be speculated that an EBDA of 6.47 cm², an EBDA/BSA ratio of 3.9, or a ratio of the sum of the diameters of balloon to the mitral valve annulus of ≤ 1.1 may be used to produce an adequate MVA with acceptable MR. Paradoxically, the balloon size combination that emerges independently by all these different methods is around 20±18 mm, which we have concluded pragmatically!

From our experience with different balloon lengths, we found that the original 3-cm balloon was too short to maintain stability during inflation. The 5.5-cm balloon was unnecessary for good positioning, when one takes into account the potential trauma to the left ventricular apex or atrial septum from such a long balloon. Therefore we preferred to use the 4-cm balloon length with a pigtailed distal end (Mansfield S-21-88 for 20-mm diameter, or 2625 for 18 mm).

Further refinements in material, and even lower profiles, will be required in all existing balloons.

Two-Dimensional Echocardiography/Doppler Studies and Balloon Mitral Valvotomy

A comprehensive 2-DE/Doppler study is mandatory in all patients undergoing balloon mitral valvotomy, to: a) confirm the presence of severe mitral stenosis; b) determine the morphology and suitability of the valve for balloon valvotomy; c) determine the degree of mitral regurgitation; d) verify the presence or absence of left atrial thrombi; e) detect the presence or absence of other valvular lesion; f) assess and assist intra-operatively; g) detect complications; and h) enhance long-term follow-up.

Severe mitral stenosis is confirmed by MVA calculation using 2-DE and Doppler—the pressure half-time formula. Doppler-determined MVA is more reliable in patients who have severely deformed mitral valves or who had previous mitral commissurotomy and in whom delineation of the valve area may be inaccurate by planimetry [32].

A variety of subjective scoring assessments of morphologic features have been utilized to determine the suitability for balloon valvotomy and the likelihood of a good result; these include leaflet mobility, leaflet thickening, the presence or absence of calcification, and subvalvular morphology. A semi-quantitative approach has been proposed for grading each of the above mentioned features on a scale of 0–4 [33]. Patients with high total echo scores, i.e. >8, were found to have less favorable results, with a higher incidence of inadequate dilatation, <1.5 cm², in 56% of patients, and early restenosis of 70% at 9 months follow-up [23]. Other studies, on the contrary, showed that the total echo score was not a predictor of a successful result [31,34]; not only that, there was no agreement between them on which of the individual morphological features, whether leaflet mobility [34] or subvalvular disease [31],

were independent predictors of optimal results. Moreover, the incidence of major subvalvular disease is recorded to be as high as
53% [36] to 64% [37] of patients undergoing
open surgical valvotomy, with a similar figure
of 64% assessed by 2-DE in those who underwent balloon dilatation [34]. If this feature is
the major predictor of optimal success, how
can we explain the high success rate of closed
surgical valvotomy, which is well-documented
in a large series? [38]

Using the same semiquantative scoring system [23], we found no correlation between the
severity of the MR produced by PBMV and
baseline valve morphology [35]. Once again,
there were contrary conclusions, with the severity of subvalvular disease emerging as an
independent factor [31] correlating with the
severity of post-valvotmy MR.

This lack of unanimity in predictability of
success reinforces our experience in the relatively younger age group. Since we know that
patients with high total echo scores can have
successful balloon valvotomy, and that the
risk of complications from the procedure is
very low, undue emphasis should not be
placed on these specific morphological features
of the mitral valve. In fact, we do not reject
patients on the grounds of high total echo
scores, even though optimum success (MVA
around 2.0 cm^2) may not be achieved. Quite
simply, the appropriate balloon size combination selected is of prime importance in the
achievment of optimal success in our patient
population.

It is logical that the presence of a left atrial
clot should remain a contraindication to balloon valvotomy. Since 2-DE cannot visualize
the atrial appendage well, detection of left atrial
clot by this means is usually not very reliable
[39], but transoesophageal echo has greatly
improved the detection of left atrial clot [40];
since we have this facility, all patients in atrial
fibrillation, or patients with a history of systemic embolization undergo this examination.
We anticoagulate all patients for 4–6 weeks
before balloon mitral valvotomy.

2-DE is also used to assess the severity of
MR [41], and the presence and severity of other
valvular lesions. The presence of more than
moderate MR, grade 3 or 4/4, usually excludes
patients from undergoing PBMV.

Inoue has advocated the use of echocardiography during the procedure after each balloon inflation, to assess the MVA by 2-DE and
by Doppler, and also to determine the presence
or absence of commissural splitting and the
degree of MR. Since the accuracy of Doppler
MVA measurement immediately following
balloon dilatation is debatable [42,43], possibly because of sudden changes in left atrial
pressure and left ventricular compliance, this
intraprocedural use of 2-DE may actually mis-
guide the operator into an erroneous belief that
the MVA achieved is optimal. But we agree
with Inoue that if one commissure is split, with
accompanying MR, further dilatation will most
likely produce a greater increase in MR, with
no substantial increase in the MVA and no
split of the other commissure.

Though the use of intra-procedure 2-DE has
also been reported in guiding the manipulation of the dilating catheter [44], finally fluoroscopy was used. We believe that the advantage of using fluoroscopy in PBMV outweighs
any inherent risk.

Echocardiography is of great value in the
detection of complications, mainly tamponade, MR, and ASD. Transoesophageal echocardiography has proved to be more sensitive
than oximetry or angiography in the detection
of ASDs [24], and may be used for follow-up
of this potential complication after balloon
dilatation, obviating the need for repeat cardiac
catheterization.

It has been shown that there is good correlation between the MVA calculated by Doppler and cardiac catheterization in long-term
follow-up studies [43]; thus this noninvasive
investigation can be used in preference for this
purpose.

In summary, Echo-Doppler studies are essential in all patients who undergo balloon
mitral valvotomy.

TABLE I. Patient Characteristics

	Mean age years	AF	Ca^{2+}	Incidence of MR[a] 1/4	2/4	Restenosed valve
Inoue [6] (n=527)	50	58%	–	28%	–	10%
Block [5] (n=311)	54	50%	46%	29%	4%	21%
Ruiz [4] (n=285)	44	30%	38%	36%	12%	16%
Vahanian [3] (n=200)	43	34%	34%	31%	1%	21%
Al-Zaibag[b] (n=179)	30	17%	13%	40%	7%	10%

AF, atrial fibrillation Ca^{2+} mitral valve calcification; MR, mitral regurgitation.
[a] Grossman scale 0-4.
[b] Unpublished series.

Results

The validity of the use of balloon mitral valvotomy to achieve successful mitral valve dilatation has now been well established by reports from various centers [3–7]. Successful balloon mitral valvotomy has been defined as the achievement of MVA of more than 1.5 cm^2, in the absence of serious complication.

All the published reports of PBMV have shown symptomatic improvement in patients after successful valvotomy. This symptomatic improvement tends to be maintained in the immediate and short term follow-up studies [3,4,6,45,46].

Tables I and II shows the patient characteristics and results after PBMV, from five large series of worldwide studies. Note that the baseline characteristics are similar, apart from our unpublished study, in which the mean age was relatively younger, i.e., 30 years, with less incidence of atrial fibrillation and mitral valve calcification.

Excluding bias from early experience and the use of prototype balloon catheters and transseptal sheaths etc., a 2-4% incidence of technical failure has been reported. This is usually due to inability to advance the balloon catheter across the atrial septum or mitral valve. Using the appropriate balloon size, the mean MVA achieved after successful PBMV should be around 1.9–2.1 cm^2. Inadequate dilatation, defined as a final MVA of <1.5 cm^2, has been variously reported as 11% [7], 12% [3], and up to 23% [5]. However, Ruiz et al. [4] reported successful PBMV in 98.5% (281/285) of patients and Inoue and Hung [6] in 96% (505/527); neither of these studies reported the incidence of inadequate dilatation. The cause of inadequate balloon valvotomy is usually related to the size of the selected balloon or [5,7,28,30] and to the complexity of the pathological involvement of the mitral valve [5,31].

Complications. Complications associated with PBMV in a total of approximately 1500

TABLE II. Results After PBMV

	Mean MVA	% MR increase	Inadequate valvotomy
Inoue [6]	1.9 cm^2	21%	–
Block [35]	2.1 cm^2	–	23%
Ruiz [4]	2.4 cm^2	51%	–
Vahanian [3]	2.2 cm^2	35%	11%
Al-Zaibag[a]	1.8 cm^2	–	11%

[a] Unpublished series.

procedures, from five major studies, are shown in Table III.

Though procedure-associated complications are rare, mortality and morbidity do occur. The reported mortality is 0–1%, with most of the deaths occuring in the early learning curve and particularly in the elderly in western countries. Cardiac tamponade from left ventricular perforation and transseptal puncture are the major causes of mortality. Left ventricular perforation, caused either by the guidewire or the tip of balloon, occured in less than 2% [4]. This complication can be avoided by careful manipulation of the heavy duty, stiff guidewire and the use of the newly designed, pigtailed balloon catheter (Mansfield) or the Inoue balloon catheter. In our center, the outmoded balloon catheter with the sharp distal end is no longer used, even though we have had no left ventricular perforation. Cardiac tamponade as a consequence of transseptal puncture has been reported to be less than 3%. In experienced hands, the use of biplane fluoroscopy should reduce this incidence to less than 1%.

The other major complications are MR and systemic embolization After PBMV, the increase in MR has varied from 21% [6], to 35% [3], 45% [35], and 51% [4]. However, in most patients it is mild, with an increase of only one grade (Grossman scale 0–4). An increase of more than two grades occurs in 10% of patients or less [3–5]. Severe MR requiring urgent surgery is a potential complication that has occured in <2.0% [4,5], though up to 4% [3] has been reported; emergency surgery was required in <1%. The cause of severe MR was tearing of the anterior or posterior mitral leaflet [3,4,7]. Contrary to the belief drawn from closed surgical valvotomy, that severe MR is a catastrophe and must be corrected by valve replacement, in our experience of PBMV, 8% had severe MR after dilatation (unpublished data); surgery was performed in only 1.3%. The remainder were controlled by medical therapy including Captopril. Follow-up of patients with mild increase of MR has shown that it is well-tolerated, and most of the patients remained symptom-free [3,4,6,7,45]. Furthermore, follow-up cardiac catheterization demonstrated that the MR may even decrease over time [5]. This decrease is possibly due to improved mobility of the leaflets after PBMV, rather than fibrosis and healing of the split commissures; postmortem studies of 31 patients up to 18 months after closed surgical valvotomy confirmed the absence of endothelialization of the split commissures [47].

The increase in MR has been found to relate to the balloon size used [5,7]. With the double-balloon technique [7], it has been shown that the use of 20+20 mm diameter balloons is associated with an increase in MR of one grade in 36% of patients and two grades or more in 20%. Using 20+18-mm diameter balloons, 30% of patients developed an increase in MR, but this was more than two

TABLE III. Procedure-Related Complications

	Mortality	Cardiac tamponade	Thromboembolism	Severe Mr needed surgery	Oximetry ASD
Inoue [6]	0%	1.5%	0.6%	1.7%	12%
Block [5]	2%	1%	1.2%	1%	19%
Ruiz [4]	1%	3%	1.5%	1.2%	14%
Vahanian [3]	0%	1%	4%	4%	8%
Al-Zaibag[a]	0%	2.5%	0%	1.3%	0%

[a] Unpublished series.

grades in only 7%. With a combination of 20 + 15-mm diameter balloon or less, no patient acquired an increase in MR of two grades, and 30% or less developed only a mild increase. These studies have shown that the MVA achieved after PBMV, using balloon combinations of 20+20-mm or 20+18-mm, was more than 1.5 cm^2 in 86% and 86% of patients respectively. Although it has been shown that there is no relationship between the 2-DE morphological features of mitral valve stenosis and the degree of induced MR after PBMV [35], others [31] have reported findings to the contrary. We believe that the diameter of the balloon catheter selected is of prime importance in determining the incidence and degree of MR following PBMV. However, significant MR may result from incorrect positioning of the balloon catheter through the chordae tendinae, since inflation in such a position is very likely to cause chordae rupture.

Systemic embolization may be caused by dislodgement of left atrial thrombus, by debris from the mitral valve [12], or by small clots forming over wires and catheters. Systemic embolizations occured in ≤ 1.5%, but up to 4% [3] have been reported. To date, more than 200 procedures have been performed in our center without incidence of thromboembolic complication. We believe that this is related to a) the method of patient selection, b) the routine use of oral anticoagulation for 6–8 weeks prior to the procedure, regardless of the cardiac rhythm, c) large doses of heparin, i.e., 150–200 units/kg after completing the transeptal punctures [we monitor the activated clotting time (ACT) throughout the procedure, keeping it above 250–300 seconds], and d) avoidance of manipulation of the guidewire in the left atrial appendage.

The incidence of persistent ASD after PBMV varies according to the procedural technique and the method used for detecting the ASD. The retrograde technique [21] should not produce residual ASD, since no balloon or shaft of a balloon catheter is advanced across the atrial septum, but only the guidewire. During balloon inflation it is possible for the balloon catheter to slip rapidly in either direction across the valve. Thus, theoretically, even with the retrograde technique, the balloon could potentially dilate the atrial septal puncture during inflation.

Using the antegrade technique, the size of the ASD will be determined by a) whether one or two septal punctures are made, b) whether one or two balloons are passed through a single septal puncture, and c) whether a large (14 Fr) transseptal sheath is used to protect the septal puncture from excessive dilatation. Inoue uses his specially designed balloon of 4.7 mm diameter at deflation, introduced through a single transeptal puncture, previously dilated with a 14 Fr dilator. Using oximetry, a 12% incidence of ASD was detected [6]. Using the double-balloon technique through a single transeptal puncture, previously dilated with an 8-mm balloon, the residual ASD detected by oximetry was 8% to 19% [3–5]. In our center, where the double-balloon technique is used, two 14F transseptal sheaths are positioned in the left atrium and will remain in situ throughout the whole procedure. One of the functions of the sheaths is to stop accidental enlargement of the ASD by a) preventing retrograde movement of the inflated balloon (18 mm diameter or more) through the septal puncture, b) preventing the heavy-duty guidewires from cutting through the septum, c) preventing the separation of the two shafts of the balloon catheters across the atrial septum during inflation (this is a potential problem in the double-balloon technique when both balloon catheters are introduced through a single septal puncture), and d) preventing further injury to the septum on withdrawal of these corrugated, bulky balloons, even though they are fully deflated. Using this technique, at 6 weeks follow-up study we found 6% ASD by angiography, and 8% by color transthoracic echocardiography; none was detected by oximetry [7].

Two studies comparing the incidence of ASD detection by various methods have been reported [24,48]. In 15 patients [23] who underwent PBMV with the Inoue technique, studied by color transoesophageal echocardiography, the incidence of ASD immediately after dilatation was 87%. However, this figure decreased rapidly, and by 6 months follow-up only 20% of all patients had an ASD detectable by this method. With transthoracic Doppler, ASD immediately after dilatation could be demonstrated in 14% of the patients, and with oximetry in only 7% (one patient). In another study of 68 patients [48], using oximetry and/or dye dilutional curves, an ASD was present in 62% of patients after PBMV; with oximetry alone, it was detected only in 25%. At the 6-month follow-up study an ASD was detected in 48% of patients, and once again oximetry detected only 9%. In this study, 97% of all the patients who underwent PBMV had had the double-balloon technique through a single transseptal puncture, previously dilated with a 6-mm to 8-mm balloon catheter.

Although no complications have been reported due to post-PBMV atrial septal defect, its importance lies with the fact that it may result in overestimation of the MVA calculated by the Gorlin formula; this may occur in those centers that do not use the large transseptal sheath, keeping it *in situ* during post dilatation calculation of the achieved MVA. Since it has been shown that 46% of the ASDs will close spontaneously within one month, and 77% within six months [24], the reported incidence of early restenosis in such studies will thus be overestimated.

The residual ASDs in most of the studies are too small to be detected by oximetry—a qualitative but not sensitive methodology for small ASDs—in the short-term follow-up study, and their long-term hemodynamic significance will thus be negligable. Therefore, it is not appropriate to equate these findings with either "iatrogenic" Lutembacher's syndrome, the development of pulmonary hypertension, or paradoxical embolization.

Other minor complications include transient conduction problems [4,5] and local vascular injury [3].

Long-term results. Since this procedure started in 1984–1985, as yet there are no published studies on the long-term follow-up. To assess the rate of mitral valve restenosis, we should not repeat the suboptimal method of follow-up studies applied to closed surgical mitral valvotomy, which relied on subjective symptoms rather than serial objective measurements of the valve area.

We observed the apparent discrepancy between the MVA calculation by Doppler and Gorlin immediately after PBMV. This has been confirmed in two studies [42,43]. When we reported our zero restenosis rate at the 1-year follow-up study [45], we regarded the MVA measurement at 6-weeks follow-up assessment as the final MVA achieved—well away from the controversial period. We felt secure in the knowledge that endothelialization of the split commissures and early restenosis after closed surgical valvotomy was not found at postmortem studies in 31 cases within this period of time [31], which corroborates our belief that restenosis does not occur within the first few weeks, or even months, after PBMV. Therefore, caution must be used in the interpretation of studies showing an early rate of restenosis after PBMV. This may be explained by the fact that, because of the ASD, the Gorlin MVA calculation immediately after BMV is limited by the potential inaccuracy in the measurement of cardiac output and mitral valve gradient; the validity of the Doppler MVA calculation is also debatable during this period [42,43]. This may explain the discrepancy between our results [45] and those of other studies, where the "early restenosis" rate was 24% in the 6-months follow-up study [48] and up to 70% in a subgroup of patients with an 2-DE score of more than 8, in the 9-months follow-up study [22].

Comparative Results of Balloon vs Surgical Valvotomy

Two randomized studies [49,50] comparing balloon and closed surgical valvotomy produced not only comparable results, but one study favored balloon valvotomy [50]. The result of PBMV using 20+20-mm balloon diameter was compared retrospectively with those of open surgical valvotomy in 122 consecutive patients [51]. The mean MVA achieved in the PBMV group was 1.9 cm² compared to 2.2 cm² in the surgical group, and inadequate valvotomy occured in 11% and 6% respectively. Mitral valve replacement was required in a comparable number of patients in each group, less than 3%. For other considerations (for example, hospital stay, infection, patient comfort, cosmetics, cost in most countries, and ease of repetition), there is no doubt that the PBMV is preferable.

As yet, insufficient time has elapsed since the introduction of balloon mitral valvotomy to compare the long-term results with closed surgical valvotomy. However, since the mechanism of the increase in MVA is similar to surgical valvotomy, the long-term results of both procedures are expected to be similar.

The Future of Balloon Mitral Valvotomy

PBMV is a valid alternative to surgical commissurotomy for the treatment of the stenotic mitral valve in all age groups. Its future may lie with the use of the single-balloon technique, which is easier to perform, but only when the cost and refinement of the balloon catheters improves. The double-balloon technique may also have a place in a subgroup of patients in whom the single-balloon technique fails to achieve optimum valve area, or in those who have severe subvalvular disease or calcification.

PERCUTANEOUS BALLOON TRICUSPID VALVOTOMY

Introduction

Balloon valvotomy is feasible as an alternative, nonsurgical treatment of pulmonary [52], aortic [26,53], and mitral valve stenosis [1,2]. Tricuspid valve stenosis can also be treated by this methodology [54–56], but since tricuspid stenosis (TS) is rare, there have been only sporadic reports of percutaneous balloon tricuspid valvotomy (PBTV) [26,57–60].

Patient Selection

There are pitfalls in the diagnosis of TS: the symptoms and physical signs of significant TS are not only vague but difficult to detect, and significant tricuspid stenosis produces only a small pressure gradient across the valve. Hence meticulous hemodynamic measurements by cardiac catheterization are essential for the accurate diagnosis of TS [61]. Furthermore, since 12% of patients with severe organic TS showed no diastolic gradient across the valve at rest, provocative hemodynamic studies may be required to expose this occult pressure gradient [61].

Although 2-DE evidence of TS is not a precise indicator for hemodynamically significant stenosis, it is a sensitive methodology to diagnose both significant and mild TS [61]—where the valvular leaflets are thickened, with some degree of commissural fusion, but where mobility is only mildly impaired [61].

Since isolated TS is rare, most of the cases selected for treatment will have other valvular pathology, and this should be taken into consideration when offering PBTV. The possibility of balloon valvotomy of multiple stenosed valves must be considered in the selection of such patients. Thus any patient with significant TS in the absence of severe tricuspid regurgitation (TR), absence of concomitant valvular disease requiring surgery, and absence of intracavity thrombus in the right side of the heart could be selected for PBTV.

Mechanism of Balloon Tricuspid Valvotomy

Splitting of fused commissures was detected by 2-DE after PBTV in four consecutive patients, showing improvement in the mobility of the anterior leaflet of the tricuspid valve in all four, the posterior leaflet in two, and the septal leaflet in one [56]. Subsequently this was corroborated by the *in vitro* study [59] of balloon valvotomy of an excised rheumatic, stenotic tricuspid valve. This demonstrated first that the mechanism by which the tricuspid valve area (TVA) increases after balloon valvotomy is by splitting the fused commissures, and second, that two balloons, each of 20-mm diameter, were required, since two balloons of 15+18-mm diameter failed to produce adequate valve dilatation [59]. Similar commissural findings were demonstrated in a patient who underwent PBTV and subsequently required cardiac surgical intervention 6 months later [59]. In a report on a large series of surgical tricuspid valvotomy, comment was made that splitting of all three commissures is not necessary to achieve adequate valvotomy, since this is also most likely to produce severe TR [62].

Procedure of PBTV

Since the normal TVA is relatively large, measuring at least 7 cm^2 at necropsy, and the annulus of a stenotic valve, measured by 2-DE [59], is approximately 4 cm^2, a double-balloon rather than the single-balloon technique will be required to achieve adequate valvotomy [26,54,56,57]. Two 7 Fr pigtail catheters are introduced through two punctures in the right femoral vein and positioned in the right ventricular apex. The preshaped end of a 0.038″ Teflon-coated, heavy-duty, exchange wire, formed into a large curve, is advanced through each pigtail catheter and positioned in the right ventricular apex. The two balloon catheters, preferably 20+20-mm diameter, are then advanced over these heavy-duty exchange guidewires and positioned across the tricuspid valve. The newly designed Mansfield balloon catheter with a pigtailed end, rather than the outmoded catheter, are used to minimize potentially serious trauma to the apex of the right ventricle. Because of the problem of balloon alignment across the tricuspid valve, we prefer balloons of 4-cm length (Mansfield S-21-88). In cases where balloon alignment is impossible during inflation, the balloon catheter can be introduced through a 14 Fr long, preshaped

sheath (the same sheath as used for PBMV [18]). This will provide the required support to maintain the position of the inflated balloons across the stenotic tricuspid valve.

Balloon inflations up to five atmospheres are then performed under fluoroscopic control. Multiple inflations are required, not because of difficulty in splitting the commissures, but to ensure optimal alignment. Since splitting of only one or two of the fused commissures is required to produce an adequate result [62], slightly undersized balloon combinations, i.e., 20+18-mm or 18+18-mm diameter, should first be utilized. The waist around the inflated balloons caused by the stenotic tricuspid valve is less marked than that observed during balloon valvotomy of the stenotic mitral valve. Disappearance of the indentation of the inflated balloon indicates splitting of the fused commissures, thereby increasing the TVA. This will be corroborated by demonstrating that the transvalvular gradient, measured by simultaneous right atrial and right ventricular pressure recordings, has been eliminated or at least significantly reduced. Finally, a right ventricular angiogram is performed to assess any increase in tricuspid incompetence.

Results

In the eight reported cases of PBTV, all with the double-balloon technique [56–60], the overall mean TVA increased from 0.8 to 1.8 cm^2. There was an increase of more than 100% in valve area calculation after PBTV, apart from one case report [59]. Contrary to the belief that PBTV will most likely result in severe TR, no patient developed a significant increase in TR after PBTV, except for one in whom no increase in TVA occurred [59]. Short-term follow-up studies [55,57,60] at 6–12 weeks after PBTV showed clinical improvement. Three years follow-up study after PBTV has shown no evidence of restenosis, as defined by loss of 50% of the TVA acheived after PBTV. This achievement was associated with the persisting relief of symptoms [63].

Although symptoms of low cardiac output due to TS are usually vague and therefore difficult to assess, cardiac output calculation has shown obvious increase after PBTV [61]: resting cardiac output after PBTV increased from 2.5 to 3.6 l/min (p<0.02). Similarly, at peak treadmill exercise, cardiac output measurement also showed a marked increase from 5.6 to 7.4 l/min (p<0.01) at equivalent heart rate [61].

Complications. There has been no mortality in these reports of a small number of procedures. Serious complications, namely mortality, thromboembolic event, or cardiac tamponade, are unlikely to occur in those centers experienced in balloon valvotomy, since PBTV is relatively simple to perform compared to other balloon valvular dilatation.

Rupture of the papillary muscle of the tricuspid valve occurred during balloon inflation in a patient where the balloon catheter across the valve was directed towards the right ventricular outflow tract/pulmonary artery [64]. To avoid this possibility, we preferred to position the balloon across the tricuspid valve in the natural direction of the right ventricular inflow, i.e., toward the right ventricular apex. Transient and persistent conduction block has also occurred where this precaution has not been followed [57,59].

Future of PBTV

Despite the relatively few cases of PBTV reported, there is no practical or theoretical evidence that this procedure should not be attempted for TS, except when combined with severe TR.

ACKNOWLEDGMENT

We thank Dr. W. Sawyer for assistance with the manuscript.

REFERENCES

1. Inoue K, Owaki T, Nakamura T, Katamura F, Miyamota N (1984): Clinical application of transvenous mitral commissurotomy by a new balloon catheter. J Thorac Cardiovasc Surg 87 (3):394–402.
2. Al-Zaibag MA, Ribeiro PA, Al-Kasab SA, Al-Fagih MR (1986): Percutaneous double balloon mitral valvotomy for rheumatic mitral stenosis. Lancet 1:757–761.
3. Vahanian A, Michel PL, Cormier B, Vitoux B, Michel X, Slama M, Enriquez-Sarano L, Trabelsi S, Ismail MB, Acar J (1989): Results of percutaneous mitral commissurotomy in 200 patients. Am J Cardiol 63:847–852.
4. Ruiz CE, Allen JW, Lau F (1990) Percutaneous double balloon valvotomy for severe rheumatic mitral stenosis. Am J Cardiol 65:473–477.
5. Block PC, Palacios IF (1990): Aortic and mitral balloon valvuloplasty: The United States experience. In Topol EJ, (ed): "Textbook of Interventional Cardiology." Philadelphia: W.B. Saunders, pp 831–848.
6. Inoue K, Hung JS (1990): Percutaneous transvenous mitral commissurotomy: The Far East experience. In Topol EJ (ed): "Textbook of Interventional Cardiology." Philadelphia: W.B. Saunders, pp 887–899.
7. Al-Zaibag M, Ribeiro PA (1990): The future of balloon valvotomy. In Topol EJ (ed): "Textbook of Interventional Cardiology." Philadelphia: WB Saunders, pp 912–926.
8. Rediker DE, Block PC, Abascal VM, Palacios IF (1988): Balloon mitral valvuloplasty for mitral restenosis after surgical commissurotomy. J Am Coll Cardiol 11:252–256.
9. McKay RG, Lock JE, Keane JF, Safian RD, Aroesty JM, Grossman W (1986): Percutaneous mitral valvuloplasty in adult patients with calcific rheumatic stenosis (1986): J Am Coll Cardiol 7:1410–1415.
10. Palacios IF, Lock JE, Keane JF, Block P (1986): Percutaneous transvenous balloon valvotomy in a patient with severe calcific mitral stenosis. J Am Coll Cardiol 7:1416–1419.
11. Palacios IF, Block P, Wilkins G, Rediker D, Daggett W (1988): Percutaneous mitral balloon valvotomy during pregnancy in a patient with severe mitral stenosis. Cathet Cardiovasc Diagn 15:109–111.
12. Armando JM, Zuliani MF, Castillo JM, Noguera EA, Arie S (1989): Percutaneous double balloon mitral valvuloplasty in pregnant women Am J Cardiol 64:99–102.
13. Kaplan JD, Isner JM, Karas RH, Halaburka KR, Konstam MA, Hougen JJ, Cleveland RJ, Salem DN (1987): In vitro analysis of mechanisms of balloon valvuloplasty of stenotic mitral valves. Am J Cardiol 59:318–323.
14. Ribeiro PA, Al-Zaibag MA, Rajendran V, Ashmeg A (1988): Mechanism of mitral valve area increase by in vitro single and double-balloon mitral valvotomy. Am J Cardiol 62:264–270.

15. McKay RC, Lock JE, Safian RD, Come PC, Diver DJ, Baim DS, Berman AD, Warren SE, Mandel VE, Royal HD, Grossman W (1987): Balloon dilatation of mitral stenosis in adult patients: Post-mortem and percutaneous mitral valvuloplasty studies. J Am Coll Cardiol 9:723-731.

16. Lock JE, Khalilullah M, Shrivastava S, Bahl V, Keane JF (1985): Percutaneous catheter commissurotomy in rheumatic mitral stenosis. N Engl J Med 313:1515-1518.

17. Herrmann HC, Kussmaul WG, Hirshfeld JW Jr (1989): Single large balloon percutaneous mitral valvuloplasty. Cathet Cardiovasc Diagn 17:59-61.

18. Al-Zaibag M (1988): Percutaneous mitral valvotomy: The double balloon technique. In Vogel JHK, King SB III (eds): "Interventional Cardiology: Future Directions. St. Louis: C.V. Mosby, pp 194-209.

19. McKay RC, Kawanishi DT, Rahimtoola SH (1987): Catheter balloon valvuloplasty of the mitral valve in adults using a double-balloon technique—Early haemodynamic results. JAMA 257:1753-1761.

20. Palacios IF, Block PC, Brandi-Pifano S, Blanco P, Casal H, Pulido JI, Munoz S, D'empaire G, Ortega MA, Jacobs M, Vlahakes G (1987): Percutaneous balloon valvotomy for patients with severe mitral stenosis. Circulation 75:778-784.

21. Babic UU, Pejcic P, Djurisic Z, Vucinic M, Grujicic SM (1986): Percutaneous transarterial balloon valvotomy for mitral stenosis. Am J Cardiol 57:1101-1104.

22. Al-Kasab S, Ribeiro P, Al-Zaibag M, Bitar I, Idris M, Shahed M, Sawyer W (1989): Comparison of results of percutaneous balloon mitral valvotomy using single and double balloon technique. Am J Cardiol 63:135-136.

23. Palacios IF, Block P, Wilkin GT, Weyman AE (1989): Follow-up of patients undergoing percutaneous mitral' balloon valvotomy. Analysis of factors determining restenosis. Circulation 79:573-579.

24. Yoshida K, Yoshikawa J, Akasaka T, Yamura Y, Shakudo M, Hozumi T, Fukaya T (1989): Assessment of left to right atrial shunting after percutaneous mitral valvuloplasty by transoesophageal colour Doppler flow-mapping. Circulation 80: 1521-1526.

25. Chen CR, Huang ZD, Lo ZX, Cheng TO (1990): Comparison of single rubber nylon balloon and double polyethylene balloon valvuloplasty in 94 patients with rheumatic mitral stenosis. Am Heart J 119:102-111.

26. Mullins CE, Nihill MR, Vick GW (1987): Double-balloon technique for dilatation of valvular or vessel stenosis in congenital and acquired heart disease. J Am Coll Cardiol 10:107-114.

27. Labadidi Z, Wu JR, Wallis JT (1984): Percutaneous balloon aortic valvuloplasty results in 23 patients. Am J Cardiol 53:1194-1197.

28. Al-Zaibag MA, Ribeiro PA, Al-Kasab SA, Halim M: Percutaneous double balloon mitral valvotomy: Results using different sized balloon catheters, abstracted. J Am Coll Cardiol 9(suppl A):83A.

29. Brandi-Pifano S, Palacios IF, Block P, Blanco P, Pulido JI, Casal H, Bellera-Celli V (1989): Echocardiography in patients undergoing mitral balloon valvotomy (PMV): The learning curve. Am Heart J 117:25-31.

30. Herrmann HC, Kleaveland P, Hill JA, Cowley M, Goldberg S, Heilbrunn S, Hirshfeld JW, Lambert CR, Margolis JR, Martin JC, Nocero MA, Vetrovec G, Whitworth HB, Zalewski A, Pepine CJ (1990): Effects of balloon size on immediate haemodynamic results of percutaneous mitral valvuloplasty (PMV) in the M-Heart Registry, abstracted. J Am Coll Cardiol 15(suppl A):42A.

31. Chen C, Wang X, Wang Y, Lan Y (1989): Value of two-dimensional echocardiography in selecting patients and balloon sizes for percutaneous balloon mitral valvuloplasty. J Am Coll Cardiol 4:1651-1658.

32. Smith MD, Handshoe R, Handshoe S, Kwan OL, Demana AN (1986): Comparative accuracy of 2-D echocardiography and Doppler pressure half-time methods in assessing severity of MS in patients with and without prior commissurotomy. Circulation 73:100-107.

33. Wilkins GT, Weyman AB, Abascal VM, Block PC, Palacios IF (1988): Percutaneous mitral valvotomy: An analysis of echocardiographic variables relate to outcome and the mechanism of dilatation. Br Heart J 60:299-308.

34. Reid CL, Chandraratna PAN, Kawanishi DT, Kotlewski A, Rahimtoola SH (1989): Influence of mitral valve morphology on double-balloon catheter balloon valvuloplasty in patients with mitral stenosis. Circulation 80:515-524.

35. Abascal VM, Wilkins GT, Choong CY, Block P, Palacios IF, Weyman A (1988): Mitral regurgitation after percutaneous balloon mitral valvuloplasty in adults: Evaluation by Doppler echocardiography. J Am Coll Cardiol 11:257-263.

36. Smith WM, Neutze JM, Barratt-Boyes BG, Lowe JB (1981): Open mitral valvotomy: Effect of preoperative factors on result. J Thorac Cardiovasc Surg 82:738-751.

37. Vega JL, Fleitas M, Martinez R, Gallo JI, Gutierrez JA, Colman T, Duran CMG (1981): Open mitral commissurotomy. Ann Thorac Surg 31:266-270.

38. John S, Bashi VV, Jairaj PS, Muralidharan S, Ravikumar E, Rajarajeswari J, Krishnaswami S, Sukumar IP, Sundar PS (1983): Closed mitral valvotomy: Early results and long-term follow-up of 3274 consecutive patients. Circulation 68:891-896.

39. Shrestha NA, Morena FL, Nariciso FU, Torres L,

Calleja HB (1983): Two dimensional echocardiographic diagnosis of left atrial thrombus in rheumatic heart disease. A clinico-pathological study. Circulation 67:341–347.

40. Aschenberg W, Schluter M, Kremer P, Schroder E, Siglow V, Bleifeld W (1986): Transesophageal two-dimensional echocardiography for the detection of left atrial appendage thrombus. J Am Coll Cardiol 7:163–166.

41. Helmcke F, Nanda NC, Hsiung MC (1987): Color Doppler assessment of mitral regurgitation with orthogonal planes. Circulation 75:175–183.

42. Thomas JD, Wilkins GT, Choong CY, Abascal VM, Palacios IF, Block PC, Weyman AE (1988): Inaccuracy of mitral pressure half-time immediately after percutaneous mitral valvotomy . Dependence on transmitral gradient and left atrial and ventricular compliance. Circulation 78:980–993.

43. Chen C, Wang Y, Guo B, Lin Y (1989): Reliability of the Doppler pressure half-time method for assessing effects of percutaneous mitral balloon valvuloplasty. J Am Coll Cardiol 13:1309–1313.

44. Pandian N, Isner J, Hougen T, Desnoyers M, McInerney K, Salem D (1987): Percutaneous balloon valvuloplasty of mitral stenosis aided by cardiac ultrasound. Am J Cardiol 59:380–381.

45. Al-Zaibag M, Ribeiro P, Al-Kasab S, Halim M, Idris M, Habbab M, Shahed M, Sawyer W (1989): One year follow-up after percutaneous double balloon mitral valvotomy. Am J Cardiol 63:126–127.

46. Palacios IF, Block PC (1988): Percutaneous mitral balloon valvotomy: Update of immediate results and follow-up, abstracted. Circulation 78(suppl II):II–489.

47. Glover RP, Davila LD, O'Neill JJ, Jamon OH (1955): Does mitral stenosis recur after commissurotomy? Circulation 11:14–28.

48. Cequier A, Bonan R, Serra A, Dyrda I, Crepaeau J, Dethy M, Water D (1990): Left to right shunting after percutaneous mitral valvuloplasty: Incidence and long-term haemodynamic follow-up. Circulation 81:1190–1197.

49. Reyes VP, Raju BS, Raju ARG,Turi ZG; for the WSU–Nizam's Institute Valvuloplasty Study Group (1988): Percutaneous balloon mitral valvuloplasty vs surgery—Results of randomised clinical trial, abstracted. Circulation 78(suppl II):II–489.

50. Patel JJ, Shama D, Mitha AS, Blythe D, Le Roux BT, Chetty S (1990): Balloon mitral valvuloplasty vs closed commissurotomy: Randomised study, abstracted. J Am Coll Cardiol 15(suppl A):5A.

51. Shahed MS, Al-Zaibag M, Al-Kasab S, Al-Fagih MR, Ribeiro PA (1989): Comparson of results of percutaneous double-balloon mitral valvotomy with open surgical valvotomy, abstracted. Eur Heart J 10(suppl):373.

52. Kan JS, White RI, Mitchell SE, Gardner TJ (1982): Percutaneous balloon valvuloplasty: A new method for treating congenital pulmonary valve stenosis. N Engl J Med 307:540–542.

53. Cribier A, Savin T, Berland J, Saoudi N, Rocha P, Letac B (1986): Percutaneous transluminal valvuloplasty of acquired aortic stenosis in elderly patients: An alternative to valve replacement. Lancet 1:63–67.

54. Al-Zaibag MA, Ribeiro PA, Al-Kasab S (1987): Percutaneous balloon valvotomy in tricuspid stenosis. Br Heart J 57:51–53.

55. Al-Zaibag MA, Ribeiro PA, Al-Kasab S, Halim M, Idris M, Abdulla M, Shahed MS (1989): Percutaneous double balloon valvotomy in rheumatic tricuspid stenosis: Immediate and short term follow-up, abstracted. J Am Coll Cardiol 11(suppl A):220A.

56. Ribeiro PA, Al-Zaibag MA, Al-Kasab SA, Idris MT, Halim M, Abdullah M, Shahed M (1988): Percutaneous double balloon valvotomy for rheumatic tricuspid stenosis. Am J Cardiol 61:660–662.

57. Khalilullah M, Tyagi S, Yadav BS, Jain P, Choudhry A, Lochan R (1987): Double balloon valvuloplasty of tricuspid stenosis. Am Heart J 114:1232–1233.

58. Shrivastava S, Radhakrishnan S, Dev V (1988): Concurrent balloon dilatation of tricuspid and calcific mitral valve in a patient of rheumatic heart disease. Int J Cardiol 20.133–137.

59. Bourdillon PDV, Hookman LD, Morris SN, Waller BF (1989): Percutaneous balloon valvuloplasty for tricuspid stenosis: Haemodynamic and pathological findings. Am Heart J 117:492 195.

60. Goldenberg IFF, Pedersen W, Olson J, Madison JD, Mooney MR, Gobel FL (1989): Percuaneous double balloon valvuloplasty for severe tricuspid stenosis. Am Heart J 118:417–419.

61. Ribeiro PA, Al-Zaibag MA, Al-Kasab S, Hinchcliffe M, Halim M, Idris M, Abdullah M, Shahed M (1988): Provocation and amplication of the trans-valvular pressure grading for rheumatic tricuspid stenosis. Am J Cardiol 61:1307–1311.

62. Revuelta JM, Garcia-Rinaldi R, Duran CMG (1985): Tricuspid commissurotomy. Ann Thorac Surg 39:489–491.

63. Ribeiro PA, Al-Zaibag M, Idris M (1990): Percutaneous double balloon valvotomy for tricuspid stenosis—3 year follow-up study. Eur Heart J (Oct/Nov).

64. Attia I, Weinhaus L, Walls JT, Lababidi Z (1987): Rupture of tricuspid valve papillary muscle during balloon pulmonary valvuloplasty. Am Heart J 114:1233–1235.

9

Balloon Dilatation of Fixed Subaortic Stenosis

Zuhdi Lababidi, M.D.

Department of Pediatrics, Division of Pediatric Cardiology,
University of Missouri School of Medicine, Columbia, Missouri 65212

INTRODUCTION

Fixed discrete subaortic stenosis (DSAS) was first described by Chevers [1] in 1842. It accounts for approximately 8%–20% of all cases of congenital left ventricular outflow tract (LVOT) obstructions, and it occurs more frequently in males than in females by a ratio of 2:1. [2] Successful transluminal balloon dilatations have recently been widely used for obstructive left-sided cardiac lesions such as coarctation of the aorta and valvar aortic stenosis. This chapter deals with a less frequent left-sided obstructive lesion that is also less frequently treated with balloon dilatation. Although DSAS, *fixed subaortic stenosis, subaortic shelf, subaortic ridge,* and *diaphragmatic subaortic stenosis* are used as synonyms, they may represent a spectrum of lesions obstructing the LVOT. To understand why balloon dilatation works only in certain types of fixed subaortic obstructions one must understand the pathogenesis, pathology, and clinical features of these fixed subaortic obstructions.

PATHOGENESIS

The etiology of DSAS is still incompletely understood. In 1842, Chevers [1] believed that the lesion was caused by repeated infections and inflammatory proliferation of the endocardium of the LVOT. In 1924, Keith [3] speculated that it was due to failure of resorption of a portion of the bulbus cordis. In 1964, Seller and associates [4] suggested that it may be due to accessory mitral valve tissue or abnormal insertion of a normal or cleft mitral valve leaflet to the interventricular septum. Van Praag and associates [5] then (in 1970) speculated that it may be due to maldevelopment of the endocardial cushion tissue of the atrioventricular canal that usually forms the anterior leaflet of the mitral valve. In the same year Van Mierop [6] also noted that it may be associated with malformation of the proximal extremity of the truncus septum where it joins the conus septum. In 1971, Roberts [7] postulated that fibrous plaques in the LVOT can be attributed to trauma associated with the impact of septal hypertrophy and the mitral valve during systole, and in 1976 Pyle and associates [8] pointed out that in Newfoundland dogs the DSAS is caused by polygenic influences that manifest after birth due to proliferation of persistent embryonic tissue in the LVOT.

The acquired nature of the obstruction in humans has been documented by serial cardiac catheterizations. [2,9–11]. Important genetic inheritance has not been demonstrated in humans, and Ferrens and colleagues [12] demonstrated significant histological differences between the Newfoundland dog's and the human's DSAS. Congenital hemodynamic disturbances due to a variety of cardiac lesions have been described in association with DSAS, including coarctation of the aorta, ventricular septal defect, double outlet right ventricle, corrected transposition, and persistent ductus arteriosus. These associated anomalies have been reported in 27%–62% of patients with

LVOT obstructions [2] and may be responsible for subaortic proliferations. Other reports [13,14] indicate that isolated DSAS occurs in 75%-80% of the patients and therefore may not be secondary to associated hymodynamic disturbances. Acquired hemodynamic changes that occur after surgical repair or palliation of associated cardiac defects have also been incriminated. Acquired DSAS has been reported after ventricular septal defect repair [15], pulmonary artery banding [16], and atrioventricular septal defect repair [11,17,18]. On the other hand, Leichter and associates [11] reported 12/17 patients with ventricular septal defects who developed DSAS without previous repair or palliation, and there are other reports [19,20] of atrioventricular septal defects associated with DSAS even before surgical repair.

PATHOLOGY

Although the spectrum of presentation is broad, there are three types of fixed DSAS with a substantial overlap between them [2,11,13, 14,21-23]. It is not known whether the three types share the same pathogenesis.

Type I

Type I is a thin, discrete, fibrous membrane situated immediately subjacent to the aortic valve. It is 1-2 mm thick and is located 1-20 mm below the aortic valve annulus (i.e., anywhere at the level of the aortic-mitral annulus). It usually forms a crescent or complete ring of fibroelastic tissue. It is attached to the interventricular septum and extends to the superior part of the anterior leaflet of the mitral valve with a structurally normal mitral valve movement. It may or may not have continuity with the aortic cusps. The excised diaphragm or ring is described as a thin, pliable white fibrous membrane just below the aortic valve. There is no narrowing of the LVOT caused by excessive fibrous and muscular tissue. When attached to the septum and mitral valve annulus, it forms the floor of a small subaortic chamber and,

when severe, it is associated with concentric left ventricular hypertrophy.

Type II

Type II is a fibromuscular ridge with a muscular base that forms a collar-like LVOT obstruction. Compared with type I, it is thicker, situated lower, and is often attached to the anterior leaflet of the mitral valve. It is associated with a septal myocardial bulging with considerable muscular hypertrophy and narrowing of the LVOT. Usually the ridge is 2-3 mm thick and is more prominent anteriorly and laterally than posteriorly on the mitral-aortic annulus. It may be present as a complete fibrous diaphragm, and the stenotic orifice may be central, eccentric, or slit-like. Severe left ventricular hypertrophy is usually present. The aortic valve cusps are thickened and regurgitant, particularly after age 5 years, and mitral valve abnormalities occur in about 10% of the patients. Both type I and type II have been reported to occur in the same patient [24].

Type III

Type III is a diffuse subaortic tunnel obstruction. It is the extreme form of fibromuscular stenosis. It is a circumferential irregular stenosis commencing close to the aortic valve annulus and extending downward for 10-30 mm. The mitral-aortic annulus is longer than normal and the diameter of the aortic valve annulus, on the average, is smaller than normal. The LVOT appears hypoplastic, with fibrous thickened endocardium and muscular narrowing. It occurs less commonly than type I and type II obstructions.

Others

Other uncommon forms of fixed LVOT obstruction are caused by accessory endocardial cushion tissue in the LVOT, aberrant papillary muscle, aberrant mitral cusp tissue, herniation of the tricuspid valve through a closed ventricular septal defect in the presence of right ventricular hypertension, malalignment of the conal ventricular septum resulting in inferior ventricular septal defect, single ventricle with a narrow bulboventricular foramen, and Shone's syndrome (parachute mitral valve, supravalvar mitral stenosis, and coarctation of the aorta).

CLINICAL FEATURES

Infants with DSAS are asymptomatic. Symptoms are uncommon in children even when stenosis is severe, and they may present as effort syncope. Middle-aged adults may present with angina, dyspnea, endocarditis, or occasionally congestive heart failure [9]. Exertional dyspnea occurs in 17% of children [2] compared with 80% of adults [21]. The obstruction is usually severe. An outflow gradient of more than 60 mmHg is common [25]. Although the systolic murmur in DSAS is similar to that in valvar aortic stenosis, the absence of a systolic ejection click and the presence of an aortic regurgitant murmur are suggestive of DSAS. Trivial or mild aortic regurgitant murmur is found in 30%–55% of children [2,13] with DSAS and in 66% of adults [21]. Aortic regurgitation murmur is rare in infants and is reported to increase with age. There are several possible reasons for the aortic regurgitation in DSAS. In 1971, Roberts [7] emphasized aortic valve problems due to jet lesions from the stenotic subvalvar orifice, causing thickening and fibrosis of the valve leaflets [7,14]. It is also possible that it may be caused by intrinsic involvement of the valve cusps in the fibroelastic membranous process, with impaired mobility resulting in turbulence of blood flow that causes damage to the aortic cusps [14]. The aortic valve may be damaged by endocarditis, a not uncommon complication of DSAS [21]. The incidence increases with age to 13%–25% of untreated adults [21]. Fontana and Edwards [26] reported a 45% incidence of endocarditis in 29 postmortem patients with DSAS. Resection of the DSAS minimizes but does not completely prevent the occurrence of endocarditis [21]. The aortic valve is usually tricuspid and either entirely normal or with some diffuse thickening. Rosenquist and colleagues [27] found no commissural fusion in 22 postmortem heart specimens, although the leaflets were thickened.

Echocardiography [28] may be useful in distinguishing valvar and subvalvar stenoses. The subaortic lesion is best appreciated through the left parasternal long-axis view of the LVOT by two-dimensional echocardiography. The subaortic thin membrane domes toward the aortic valve with systole. Most patients exhibit systolic flutter and brisk partial closure of the aortic leaflets with subsequent reopening and gradual closure of the aortic valve. Unlike idiopathic hypertrophic subaortic stenosis, there is usually concentric left ventricular hypertrophy in DSAS. During cardiac catheterization the subvalvar obstruction is best evaluated by recording the pressure during a slow withdrawal of the catheter across the LVOT. Selective left ventricular angiogram in the tilted axial left anterior oblique view provides a good visualization of the DSAS, since this view overcomes the foreshortening of the LVOT present in the conventional left anterior oblique projection. A multipurpose catheter with end and side holes, with the end hole tip passing through the stenotic orifice and the sideholes just below the aortic leaflets, will demonstrate angiographically the thickness of the obstruction and the size of the subaortic chamber [29]. An aortic root angiogram may or may not show some degree of aortic regurgitation.

DSAS is not a static lesion. It is progressive in nature [9]. It may be absent at birth and then appears rapidly as an isolated lesion or may become manifest after surgical palliation or repair of associated anomalies. It is a rare cause of important obstruction in infancy. The obstruction begins to be evident after the first year of life. There is a striking absence of operations for DSAS in the first year of life. Isolated fixed subaortic stenosis becomes severe after age 10 years. Pyle and associates [8] demonstrated the absence of DSAS in Newfoundland dogs at birth, yet it became significant by age 12 weeks.

The fact that it recurs after surgical resection also indicates it is acquired and progressive in nature. The progression may be caused by proliferation of the fibrous tissue, or, with growth of the patient, the fixed narrowing may become significant [25].

SURGICAL TREATMENT

In 1959, Brock [30] reported transventricular dilatation as treatment for DSAS. Spencer and colleagues [31] published the first substantial set of results of cardiopulmonary bypass as treatment in 1960. With type I, the membrane is easily excised *in toto*, and resection of the adjacent tissue in the outflow may not be necessary. With type II, the fibromuscular ring is resected with some muscle tissue. Without the myectomy, significant residual obstruction may remain. Because of the likelihood of developing progressive obstruction and aortic regurgitation, the presence of mild to moderate

subaortic stenosis has warranted elective surgery. Most authors [2,23] agree that a gradient of 40–50 mmHg or more is a reasonable indication for surgery, especially if there is a thin membrane below the valve. It is still debatable whether early surgery prevents progressive aortic valve disease, including aortic regurgitation [21]. The early and late deaths are virtually all related to residual LVOT obstruction or subsequent efforts to relieve it. There is a tendency for the stenosis to recur or to progress postoperatively, especially in the fibromuscular and tunnel obstructions. Newfeld and colleagues [2] reported that 17/40 patients had surgical resection and had cardiac catheterization 1–8 years postoperatively. In nine patients the residual gradient was 50 mmHg or greater, and three had repeat surgical resection. Somerville et al. [9] found that the patients who had a good long-term result without restenosis were those operated on at less than 8 years of age, with less than 20 mmHg resid-

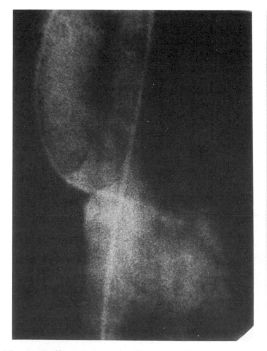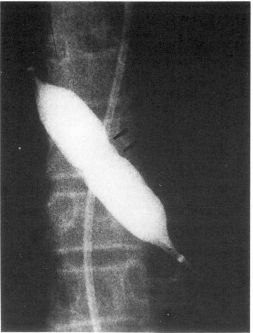

Fig. 1. Balloon subaortic dilatation. The balloon indentation from the subaortic stenosis is just below the aortic valve annulus indentation.

TABLE I. Transluminal Balloon Dilatation of DSAS

	Age (years)	Peak systolic gradient (mmHg)		
		Before	After	Follow-up
Type I (28 patients)				
Range	0.2 – 18	20 – 164	5 – 40	4 –30
Mean ± SD	9 ± 5	73 ± 34	18 ± 10	13 ±8
Type II (4 patients)				
Range	6 – 15	132 – 177	60 – 150	59
Mean ± SD	9 ± 3	155 ± 15	84 ± 37	±0

ual gradient after excision, and with normal aortic root size.

BALLOON DILATATION

Transluminal balloon dilatation is slowly being accepted as a nonsurgical technique to dilate thin subaortic fixed obstructions [32–37]. From 1982 to 1990, 32 patients with clinical, echocardiographic, and hemodynamic diagnoses of DSAS underwent percutaneous balloon dilatation at the University of Missouri Hospital and Clinics. They were 10 weeks to 18 years old. Before 1984, balloon dilatation was attempted on both type I and type II subaortic obstructions. Because all four patients with type II obstruction subsequently required open surgical resection and myotomy, only patients with type I obstruction have been dilated since then.

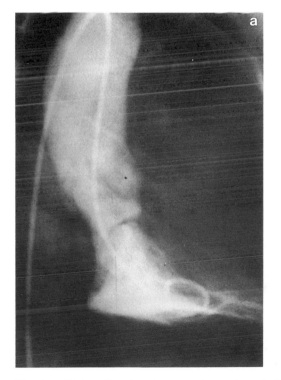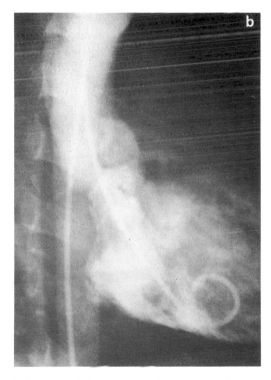

Fig. 2. a: Before dilatation the subaortic membrane bulges slightly toward the aortic valve during systole. **b:** After dilatation the subaortic membrane opens widely, extending toward the aortic annulus.

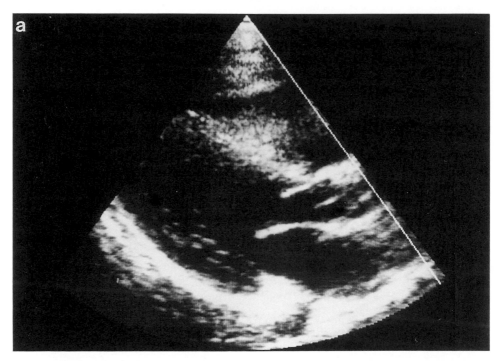

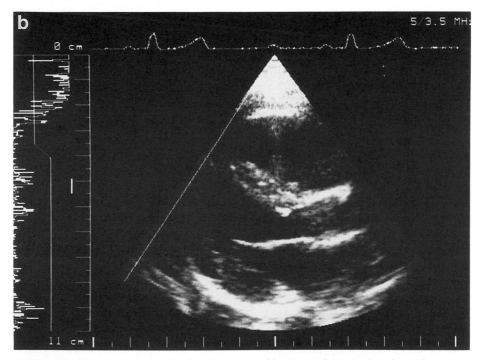

Fig. 3. a: The torn subaortic membrane the day after balloon dilatation is shown in the echocardiogram extending toward the apex in diastole. **b:** The subaortic membrane becomes a small globular ridge on the interventricular septum 1 year after the dilatation.

We now believe that both echocardiography and cineangiography must show a subaortic membrane less than 2 mm in thickness before balloon dilatation is attempted.

The technique of dilatation is similar to that of balloon aortic valvuloplasty (Fig. 1) and has been described earlier in detail [33]. Originally the balloon was chosen to be equal to or 1 mm less than the aortic valve annulus. If there is no associated valvar aortic stenosis we now use balloons equal to or 2 mm larger than the diameter of the aortic valve annulus. Such balloons seem to lower the gradients adequately without causing an increase in aortic regurgitation. The original balloons used were also 40 mm long, but now we use the 55 mm long and low-profile Mansfield balloons. They have a lesser chance of being ejected from the left ventricle and cause less femoral complications. Our results of DSAS dilatations are given in Table I. There were 28 patients with type I stenosis. Their mean age was 8.7 ± 4.7 years. The youngest was 10 weeks and the oldest 18 years. The mean predilatation gradient was 73 ± 34 mmHg, which was reduced to 17 ± 10 mmHg after dilatation. Follow-up gradients were obtained by repeat cardiac catheterization in 4 patients and continuous wave Doppler in 15 patients. The mean follow-up gradient was 13 ± 7 mmHg over a follow-up period of 4.5 years. There were four patients with type II stenosis who had a mean gradient of 155 ± 15 mmHg, which was reduced to 84 ± 37 mmHg. Because of their high residual gradients, they all had subsequent surgical myotomy.

The mechanism of gradient reduction is by tearing of the subaortic membrane. This was documented by cineangiography and echocardiography. When the membrane is intact, it bulges slightly toward the aortic valve during systole (Fig. 2a). After balloon dilatation, the torn membrane's edges open widely, flutter, and extend toward and sometimes protrude through the aortic valve during systole (Fig. 2b). On follow-up echocardiography, the obstruction changes to a small globular ridge on the interventricular septal surface (Fig. 3).

The complications of DSAS balloon dilatation are similar to previously reported complications of balloon aortic valvuloplasty. Femoral arterial complications are now less due to the use of low profile balloons, and aortic regurgitation is less frequently seen when there is no associated valvar aortic stenosis.[1]

---

[1]Editor's note: The author has presented an excellent review of pathogenesis, pathology, clinical features, and surgical treatment of fixed discrete subaortic stenosis. He also presented results of balloon angioplasty of subaortic stenosis performed at his institution. Though referenced, the results of other workers have not been adequately reviewed. Therefore, I believe it is worthwhile to summarize these data: The immediate results appear excellent (Table II), as are the follow-up results when the subaortic membrane is discrete and thin. When there is a fibromuscular obstruction, both the immediate results and the follow-up results are poor. Based on the data, Lababidi concluded that balloon angioplasty should not be attempted if the subaortic membrane is thick. I agree with this assessment.

The initial recommendation was to use balloons no larger than the aortic valve annulus for fear of producing aortic insufficiency. More recently, Lababidi (this chapter), Rao et al. [37], and others [32,34] used balloons larger than the aortic valve annulus for balloon dilatation of subaortic stenosis and have not observed any increase in aortic insufficiency. It may be surmised that nonstenotic aortic valve leaflets are simply compressed against the aortic wall without any damage to the valve mechanism, in contradistinction to valvar aortic stenosis, in which the valve mechanism may be distorted when balloons larger than the aortic valve annulus are used. However, when both valvar and subvalvar stenoses coexist, at least based on anecdotal experience [36], balloons larger than aortic valve annulus should not be used.

Several excellent hemodynamic studies documenting the natural history of discrete subaortic membranous stenosis suggested a progressive increase in the degree of obstruction with increasing age. These studies also suggested worsening of aortic insufficiency, presumably related to the damage to the aortic valve cusps by the jet flow through the subaortic obstruction. For this reason, the recommended gradient for surgical intervention is 30 or 40 mmHg [2,42], in contrast to valvar aortic stenosis, in which a much higher gradient is required prior to intervention. In line with this thinking, balloon angioplasty of subaortic membranous stenosis should be undertaken when the gradient is ≥ 40 mmHg. Based on our own experience and on that reviewed in this chapter, balloon angioplasty may be a preferable initial procedure in the treatment of membranous subaortic obstruction.

TABLE II. Results of Balloon Angioplasty of Subaortic Stenosis[a]

Investigators	No. of patients undergoing BA	Subvalvar gradient (mean ± SD), mm Hg[b]			Follow-up (No./duration)	Poor results (No. [%])	Comments
		Before	After	FU			
Suarez de Lezo et al. [32], 1986	7	65 ± 18	12 ± 9	15 ± 4	4/7 mo	0 (0)	AI remained mild
Lababidi et al. [33], 1987	6	82 ± 49	22 ± 15	27, 24	2/12 mo	0 (0)	Thin discrete membrane. No change in AI
	4	155 ± 18	85 ± 44	59	1/12 mo	4 (100)	Thick fibromuscular ring. No change in AI. Three patients underwent surgical resection
Arora et al. [34], 1988	3	112 ± 54	18 ± 10	22 ± 11	3/1 mo	0 (0)	No worsening of AI
Al Yousef et al. [35], 1988	6	115 ± 50	19 ± 16	14 ± 13[c]	6/9 mo	0 (0)	AI increased in one patient
Rao et al. [37], 1990	6	56 ± 19	12 ± 7	21 ± 5[c]	6/11 mo	1 (17)	AI remained mild. One infant with fibromuscular obstruction required surgery
Shrivastava et al. [39], 1991	7	87 ± 17	24 ± 13	29 ± 16[c]	7/3-24 mo	1 (14)	Thin membrane. No change in AI
	4	73 ± 32	27 ± 21	58 ± 19[c]	4/3 mo	3 (75)	Thick ridge. No change in AI
Suarez de Lezo et al. [40], 1991[d]	27	71 ± 32	21 ± 13	23 ± 9[c]	25/24 mo	7 (28)	AI has not increased
Lababidi and Walls [41], 1992[e]	28	73 ± 34	18 ± 10	13 ± 8[c]	19/4.5 yr	0 (0)	Thin discrete membrane

[a]AI, aortic insufficiency; BA, balloon angioplasty; FU, follow-up.
[b]Peak-to-peak gradients across the subaortic stenosis measured at cardiac catheterization in all but those qualified in footnote.
[c]Combined peak-to-peak catheterization gradient and peak instantaneous gradient by Doppler echocardiography.
[d]Includes seven cases previously reported in 1986 by the same authors.
[e]Includes six cases previously reported in 1987 by the same authors.

REFERENCES

1. Chevers N (1842): Observations on the diseases of the orifice and valves of the aorta. Guys Hosp Rep 7:387.

2. Newfeld EA, Muster AJ, Paul MM, Idriss FS, Richie WL (1976): Discrete subvalvar aortic stenosis in childhood. Am J Cardiol 38:53.

3. Keith A (1924): Schorstein Lecture on the Fate of the Bulbus Cordis in the Human Heart. Lancet 2:1267.

4. Sellers RD, Lillehie CW, Edwards JE (1964): Subaortic stenosis caused by anomalies of the atrioventricular valves. J Thorac Cardiovasc Surg 48:289.

5. Van Praagh R, Corwin RD, Dahlquist EH Jr, Freedom RM, Mattioli L, Nebesar RA (1970): Tetralogy of Fallot with severe left ventricular outflow tract obstruction due to anomalous attachment of the mitral valve to the ventricular septum. Am J Cardiol 26:93.

6. Van Mierop LHS (1970): Pathology and pathogenesis of the common cardiac malformations. Cardiovasc Clin 2:27.

7. Roberts WC In Kidd BSL, Keith JD (eds)· (1971): Pathologic aspects of valvular and subvalvular (discrete and diffuse) aortic stenosis. "Natural History and Progress in Treatment of Congenital Heart Defects." Springfield, IL: Charles C Thomas, pp 221.

8. Pyle RL, Patterson DF, Chacko S (1976): The genetics and pathology of discrete subaortic stenosis in the Newfoundland dog. Am Heart J 92:324.

9. Somerville J, Stone S, Ross D (1980): Fate of patients with fixed subaortic stenosis after surgical removal. Br Heart J 43:629.

10. Freedom RM, Pelech A, Brand A, Vogel M, Olley PM, Smallhorn J, Rowe RD (1985): The progressive nature of subaortic stenosis in congenital heart disease. Intra J Cardiol 8:137.

11. Leichter DA, Sullivan I, Gersony WM (1989): Acquired discrete subvalvular aortic stenosis: Natural history and hemodyamics. J Am Coll Cardiol 14:1539.

12. Ferrens VJ, Muna W FT, Jones M, Roberts WC (1978): Ultrastructure of the fibrous ring in patients with discrete subaortic stenosis. Lab Invest 39:30.

13. Kelly, DT, Wulfsberg E, Row RD (1972): Discrete Subaortic Stenosis. Circulation 46:309.

14. Champsaur G, Trusler GA, Mustard WT (1973): Congential discrete subvalvular aortic stenosis: Surgical experience and long-term follow-up in 20 Patients. Br Heart J 35:443.

15. Fisher DJ, Snider AR, Silverman NH, Stanger P (1982): Ventricular septal defect with silent subaortic stenosis. Pediatr Cardiol 2:265.

16. Freed, MD, Rosenthal A, Plauth WH, Nadas AS (1973): Development of subaortic stenosis after pulmonary artery banding. Circulation 48(Suppl III):3.

17. Lappen RS, Muster AJ, Idriss FS, Riggs TV, Iblawi M, Paul M, Bharati S, Lev M (1983): Masked subaortic stenosis in ostium primum atrial septal defect: Recognition and treatment. Am J Cardiol 52:336.

18. Ben-Shachar G, Moller JH, Castaneda-Zuniga W, Edwards JE (1981): Signs of membranous subaortic stenosis appearing after correction of persistent common atrioventricular canal. Am J Cardiol 48:340.

19. Heydarian M, Griffith BP, Zuberbuhler JR (1985): Partial atrioventricular canal associated with discrete subaortic stenosis. Am Heart J 109:915.

20. Spanos PK, Fiddler GI, Mair DD, McGoon DC (1977): Repair of atrioventricular canal associated with membranous subaortic stenosis. Mayo Clin Proc 52:121.

21. Sung C, Price EC, Cooley DA (1978): Discrete subaortic stenosis in adults. Am J Cardiol 42:283.

22. Chaikhouni A, Crawford FA, Sade RM, Taylor AB, Riopel DA, Hohn AR (1984): Discrete subaortic stenosis. Clin Cardiol 7:289.

23. Reis RL, Peterson LM, Mason DT, Simon AL, Morrow AG (1971): Congenital fixed subvalvular aortic stenosis: An anatomical classification and correlation with operative results. Circulation 43(Suppl I): 11.

24. Lemole GM, Tesler UF, Colombi M, Eldridge J (1976): Subaortic stenosis caused by two discrete membranes. Chest 69:104.

25. Khan MM, Varma MPS, Cleland J, O'Kane HO, Webb SW, Mulholland Hc, Adgey AAJ (1981): Discrete subaortic stenosis. Br Heart J 46:421.

26. Fontana RS, Edwards JE (1962): "Congenital Cardiac Disease. A Review of 357 Cases Studied Pathologically". Philadelphia; W.B. Saunders p 214.

27. Rosenquist GC, Clark EB, McAllister HA, Bharati S, Edwards JE (1979): Increased mitral–aortic separation in discrete subaortic stenosis. Circulation 60:70.

28. Wilcox WD, Seward JB, Hagler DJ, Mair DD, Tajik AJ (1980): Discrete subaortic stenosis: Two-dimensional echocardiographic features with angiographic and surgical correlation. Mayo Clin Proc 55:425.

29. Schaffer AI, Kania H, Cucci CE, DePasquale NP (1972): New technique for angiographic visualization of membraneous subaortic stenosis. Br Heart J 34:742.

30. Brock R: Aortic subvalvular stenosis: Surgical treatment. Guys Hosp Rep 108:144, 1959.

31. Spencer FC, Neill CA, Sank L, Bahnson HT (1960): Anatomical variations in 46 patients with congenital aortic stenosis. Am Surg 26.204, 1960.

32. Suarez de Lezo J, Pan M, Sancho M, Herrera N, Arizen J, Franko M, Concha M, Valles F, Romanos A (1986): Percutaneous transluminal balloon dilata-

tion for discrete subaortic stenosis. Am J Cardiol 58:619.

33. Lababidi Z, Weinhaus L, Stoeckle H, Jr., Walls JT: (1987): Transluminal balloon dilatation for discrete subaortic stenosis. Am J Cardiol 58:423.

34. Arora R. Goel PK, Lochan R, Mohan JC, Khalilullah M (1988): Percutaneous transluminal balloon dilatation in discrete subaortic stenosis. Am Heart J 116:1041.

35. Al Yousef S, Khan A, Lababidi Z, Mullins C (1988): Percutaneous balloon dilatation of discrete subvalvular aortic stenosis. Herz 13:32.

36. Biancaniello TM (1989): Balloon dilatation in discrete subaortic stenosis. Am Heart J 117:1397.

37. Rao PS, Wilson AD, Chapra PS (1990): Balloon angioplasty for discrete subaortic stenosis: Immediate and intermediate term results. J Invasive Cardiol 2:65.

38. Hellenbrand WE (1990): Balloon dilatation of six patients with discrete subaortic stenosis. In Symposium on Advances in Interventional Catheterization. ACC Annual Meeting, New Orleans, 1990.

39. Shrivastava S, Dev V, Bahl VK, Saxena A (1991): Echocardiographic determinants of outcome after percutaneous transluminal balloon dilatation of discrete subaortic stenosis. Am Heart J 122:1323.

40. Suarez de Lezo J, Medina A, Pan M, Hernandez E, Romero M, Melian F, Jimenez F, Sepura J, Pavlovic D, Coello I, Hidalgo R (1990): Long-term results after balloon dilatation for discrete subaortic stenosis, abstracted. Circulation 82(suppl III):583.

41. Lababidi ZA, Walls JE (1990): Balloon dilatation of thin fixed subaortic stenosis, abstracted. Circulation 82(suppl III): 583.

42. Wright GB, Keane JF, Nadar AS, Bernhard WF, Castaneda AR (1983): Fixed subaortic stenosis in the young: Medical and surgical course in 83 patients. Am J Cardiol 52:830.

10

Balloon Angioplasty of Native Aortic Coarctation

P. Syamasundar Rao, M.D.

Department of Pediatrics, Division of Pediatric Cardiology,
University of Wisconsin Medical School, University of Wisconsin
Children's Hospital, Madison, Wisconsin 53792-4108

INTRODUCTION

The prevalence of coarctation of the aorta (CoA) was found to vary between 5.1% and 8.1% of congenital heart defects [1,2]; however, coarctation may be found more frequently in infants presenting with symptoms prior to 1 year of age [3]. In the past, the CoA was designated as preductal (or infantile) or postductal (or adult), depending on whether the coarctation segment was proximal or distal to the ductus arteriosus, respectively. However, a closer examination of the anatomy suggests that all coarctations are juxtaductal. The presence of associated defects and aortic arch anomalies, the extent of patency of the ductus arteriosus, the rapidity of the process of closure of the ductus arteriosus, and the level of pulmonary vascular resistance determine the timing of clinical presentation and severity of symptoms. The coarctation may be discrete, or a long segment of aorta may be narrowed; the former is more common. Classic CoA is located in the thoracic aorta distal to the origin of the left subclavian artery, at about the level of the ductal structure. However, rarely, a coarcted segment may be present in the abdominal aorta. Varying degrees of hypoplasia of the isthmus of the aorta (that portion of the aorta between the origin of the left subclavian artery and the ductus arteriosus) are present in the majority of patients with thoracic CoA; this hypoplasia may be significant in symptomatic

CoA of the neonate and infant, whereas in older children there may be only a mild degree of narrowing. The transverse aortic arch (the arch between the origin of the innominate artery and the left subclavian artery) is also hypoplastic in symptomatic neonates and infants.

The most commonly associated defects are patent ductus arteriosus, ventricular septal defects, and aortic stenosis. The younger the infant presents, the more likely that there is a significant associated defect. Bicuspid aortic valve and abnormal mitral valves are also seen. Sometimes CoA is a complicating feature of more complex, cyanotic heart defects, such as transposition of the great arteries, Taussig-Bing anomaly, double-inlet left ventricle, tricuspid atresia with transposition of the great arteries, and hypoplastic left heart syndrome.

Pathologically, the constricted aortic segment consists of localized medial thickening with some infolding of the media and superimposed neointimal tissue. The localized constriction may form a shelf-like structure with an eccentric opening or it may be a membranous, curtain-like structure with a central or eccentric opening. There is dilatation of the aorta distal to coarctation (poststenotic dilatation). There is usually a jet lesion on the wall of the aorta distal to the coarctation site. Collateral vessels that connect arteries from the upper part of the body to the vessels below the level of coarctation may be seen; these can be present as early as a few weeks to a few months of life. Systemic hypertension is a feature of CoA; there is controversy with regard to its origin: mechanical, humoral, or a combination of both.

Infants with significant associated defects and occasionally those without associated cardiac defects may present in the neonatal period or in early infancy with signs of heart failure and/or failure to thrive. Rapid deterioration of the infant with symptoms of low output can be seen and may be associated with rapid closure of the ductus arteriosus. Children beyond infancy usually are asymptomatic; an occasional child will complain of pain or weakness in the legs. Most often, the coarctation is detected because of a murmur, or hypertension that are detected on routine examination. Physical findings depend on the type of associated defects. The classic findings in the absence of severe heart failure are absent or diminished and delayed femoral pulses and a systolic blood pressure difference between the arms and legs. The peak systolic pressure gradient may vary between a few to >100 mmHg, depending on the status of the ductus and the degree of systemic hypertension.

Chest roentgenograms may reveal cardiomegaly and increased pulmonary vascular markings in the infant coarctation, whereas in older children minimal cardiomegaly and rib-notching (secondary to collateral vessels) may be seen. The characteristic indentation of the barium-filled esophagus, the reversed E sign, may be seen on frontal view. Electrocardiograms in the neonate and infant usually show right ventricular hypertrophy. In older children, the electrocardiogram is normal or may show left ventricular hypertrophy. Echocardiographic studies usually reveal the coarctation in a suprasternal notch, two-dimensional echocardiographic view of the aortic arch. Increased Doppler flow velocity in the descending aorta by continuous-wave Doppler and a demonstrable jump in velocity at the coarcted segment by pulsed-Doppler technique are usually present.

In infants with congestive heart failure, the initial treatment consists of anticongestive medications, followed by relief of aortic obstruction by surgical intervention. Neonates benefit from prostaglandin E_1 (0.05–0.1 mcg/kg/min) intravenously because of its ductal-dilating effect. In children beyond the neonatal period, surgical resection is recommended to relieve hypertension, if present, or to prevent development of hypertension if no blood pressure elevation is present. With the availability of balloon angioplasty for aortic coarctation, many workers consider this treatment option an alternative mode to surgical therapy.

Sos and colleagues [4] demonstrated that the coarcted aortic segment could be dilated by balloon angioplasty; they performed this in a neonate postmortem. Lock, Castaneda-Zuniga, and their associates [5–7] extended these observations and showed that surgically excised coarcted aortic segments and experimentally created coarctation in lambs and dogs could be dilated by balloon angioplasty. Following these observations, several short-term and a few intermediate-term results of balloon angioplasty of previously unoperated ("native") aortic coarctations as well as postoperative recoarctations have been reported in the literature. However, there is considerable controversy among cardiologists and surgeons with regard to whether the aortic coarctations should be balloon dilated or surgically treated and, if balloon angioplasty is chosen, which coarctations should be dilated. I support the view that balloon angioplasty is an effective therapeutic alternative to surgical treatment of aortic coarctation.

Data from our own experience with balloon angioplasty in 58 consecutive patients performed during the last 7 years for relief of native aortic coarctations in infants and children between the ages of 3 days and 13 years, including that previously reported [8–25], and the experience reported in the literature will be used as supportive material. For the purpose of discussion, the coarctations are divided into two groups: 1) native coarctation in the neonate and small infant (<1 year old), usually associated with other defects, and 2) native coarctations in children (>1 year old).

INDICATIONS

The indications for balloon coarctation angioplasty is hypertension and/or congestive heart failure [9-11,18,24], very similar to the indications for surgery. Although there is some concern with regard to development of aneurysms [26-28] following balloon angioplasty of native coarctations, a general consensus is emerging that these coarctations should be balloon-dilated [9-11,24,29-31]. This is particularly true in the neonate and small infant because of high morbidity and mortality rates as well as a high recurrence rate with surgery. Balloon dilatation of coarctation of the aorta appears to offer a relatively safe and effective alternative to surgical repair in the neonates and young infants. With angioplasty, operative intervention may be avoided entirely or at least be postponed until the child is older and the body larger, when surgical results are much better with regard to operative mortality and recoarctation. Should recurrence follow the angioplasty, or should an aneurysm form at the site of dilatation, the infant could undergo surgical resection at a later date when not as acutely ill.

With regard to an older child with native coarctation, because of concern for developing aneurysm, the general recommendation has been that this procedure should probably be performed at selected medical centers with personnel who have expertise with this lesion, and its general use by others should be delayed until follow-up results and reports of follow-up on a larger number of patients are available. It is worthwhile noting differences in the evolution of recommendation for balloon angioplasty for native versus recoarctation. Balloon dilatation of postoperative recoarctations has been recommended [32,33] as the therapy of choice; such a recommendation was made

prior to the availability of data on immediate results in a significant number of patients and prior to the availability of any follow-up results. In contradistinction, balloon angioplasty for native coarctation was not recommended [34] despite the availability of convincing data (29). This type of recommendation is based in part on the speculation that the scar tissue in recoarctation may prevent progression of aneurysms, once they develop. Now that more data are available [32,35-43], the immediate results of balloon angioplasty in recoarctation appear good, with significant reduction in gradient across the coarctation. However, the follow-up data are scanty. Those available with regard to recurrence and aneurysmal formation in postoperative recoarctations are tabulated elsewhere [15,17] and compared with those associated with native aortic coarctations. Although the number of patients with follow-up catheterization after balloon angioplasty of postoperative recoarctation is not large, it can be seen that neither the recurrence rate nor the rate of aneurysmal formation following balloon angioplasty of postoperative recoarctation is significantly different ($P > 0.1$) from that seen with native coarctations. In addition, when mortality and complication rates of balloon angioplasty in both groups were compared [20], they were very similar. Therefore, it is hard to justify balloon angioplasty for postoperative recoarctation while not recommending it for native coarctations [15,17,24].

Symptomatic neonates and infants should undergo balloon angioplasty on an urgent basis soon after the infant is stabilized. Asymptomatic infants and children should undergo the procedure electively. If neither hypertension nor heart failure is present, elective balloon dilatation between ages 2 and 5 years is suggested. Waiting beyond 5 years of age is not advisable because of evidence for residual hypertension if the aortic obstruction is relieved after age 5 years [44].

It is generally recommended that only discrete, short-segment coarctations be dilated. Although such a recommendation appears reasonable, diffuse and long-segment coarctation can also be balloon-dilated effectively (Fig. 1).

TECHNIQUE

The diagnosis and assessment of CoA are made by the usual clinical and echo-Doppler studies. Once it is diagnosed and the criteria alluded to in the preceding section are met, cardiac catheterization and selective cineangiography are performed to confirm the clinical diagnosis and to indicate the need for balloon angioplasty. Once balloon dilatation is decided upon, 1) a 5-6 Fr multi-A-2 (Cordis) catheter is introduced into the femoral artery percutaneously and is positioned across the aortic coarctation; 2) a 0.032-0.035 inch J-shaped guidewire is passed through the catheter into the ascending aorta, and the tip of the wire is positioned in the ascending aorta; 3) a 4-9 French balloon angioplasty catheter is advanced over the guidewire, and the balloon

is positioned across the aortic coarctation; 4) the balloon is inflated with diluted contrast material (Fig. 2) to approximately 3-5 atm of pressure or higher, depending on the manufacturer's recommendations. Monitoring pressure of inflation via any of the commercially available pressure gauges is recommended. The balloon is inflated for a duration of 5 seconds. A total of two to four balloon inflations are performed, 5 minutes apart. While a double-balloon technique with two balloons simultaneously inflated across the stenotic region is required in a significant proportion of patients with pulmonic and aortic valve stenosis [45–48], such is not the case with aortic coarctation [24]; however, the double-balloon technique can be successfully used with CoA [49]; and 5) aortography and measurement of pressure gradients across the CoA are performed. Recording of heart rate, systemic pressure, and cardiac index prior to and after balloon dilatation are made to ensure that the change in pressure gradient is not

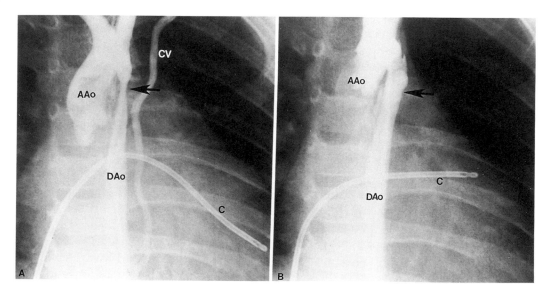

Fig. 1. A selected frame from a posteroanterior view of a cineaortogram **(A)** showing a long segment (arrow) of coarctation. Following balloon angioplasty, there is an excellent angiographic result **(B)**. The gradient across the coarctation was 105 mmHg prior to angioplasty, which was decreased to 15 mmHg after balloon dilatation. An intimal tear (arrow) is also shown in B. A collateral vessel (CV) that is seen prior to angioplasty (A) is no longer seen after angioplasty (B). AAo, ascending aorta; C, catheter in the left ventricle; DAo, descending aorta.

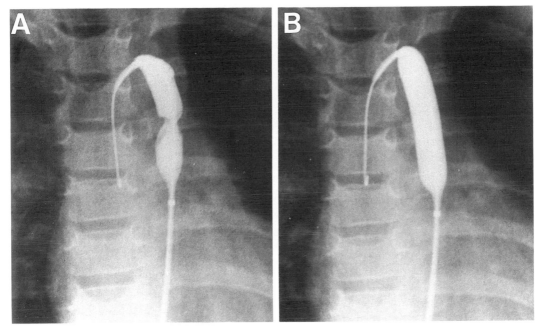

Fig. 2. A balloon catheter positioned across the aortic coarctation, showing waisting of the balloon during the initial phases of balloon inflation. (**A**) Note complete disappearance of the waisting after complete balloon inflation (**B**).

related to changes in patient status but is indeed related to the procedure.

We generally perform this procedure with the patient sedated with an intramuscular injection of a mixture of meperidine, promethazine, and chlorprazone supplemented with intermittent doses of midazolam, while others [50] advocate general anesthesia. The size of the balloon chosen for angioplasty is two or more times the size of the coarcted aortic segment, but no larger than the size of the descending aorta at the level of the diaphragm, as measured from a frozen frame of the video recording. I usually choose a balloon that is midway between the size of the aortic isthmus (or transverse aortic arch) and the size of the descending aorta at the level of the diaphragm. If there is not an adequate pressure gradient relief and angiographic improvement, a balloon as large as the descending aorta (at the level of the diaphragm) is selected for additional dilatation.

It is highly important that a catheter or a guidewire not be manipulated over the area of freshly dilated CoA. A guidewire should always be left in place across the coarctation segment, and all angiographic and balloon dilatation catheters should be exchanged over the guidewire.

Heparinization of the patient with 100 units/kg (maximum, 2,500 units) is recommended; I usually give heparin prior to introducing balloon angioplasty catheter. The heparin effect is neither reversed nor continued after the procedure. It is important to administer adequate doses of heparin to prevent thromboembolism [51,52].

When additional left ventricular outflow tract obstructions such as subvalvar or valvar stenosis are present in addition to aortic coarctation, both the stenotic lesions can be dilated [53] at the same sitting. Following initial dilatation of CoA, the other obstructive lesion (aortic valve or subaortic membranous stenosis) is dilated. It is important to keep a guidewire across the aortic coarctation to prevent inadvertent injury to the freshly dilated coarctation.

Most authors use a percutaneous femoral artery approach for cardiac catheterization and balloon angioplasty. Occasionally, femoral artery cut-down [54,55] or left axillary artery cut-down may have to be used [54] if percutaneous femoral artery entry is unsuccessful. We have utilized a transumbilical artery approach [56] in a manner similar to that described for balloon aortic valvuloplasty in the neonate [57]. In patients in whom the aorta can be entered from the right ventricle (either directly in patients with transposition of the great arteries or double-outlet right ventricle or indirectly through a ventricular septal defect), it may be possible to position the balloon catheter across the coarctation, antegrade [58]. Al Yousef et al. [58] used this technique successfully in five neonates. When feasible, this method should be employed, because the antegrade route has the advantage of sparing the femoral artery.

Relief of aortic obstruction can also be accomplished by dilating the ductus arteriosus via balloon [13]. This would allow flow from the proximal to the distal aorta (Fig. 3) with resultant improvement in pressure gradient

(Fig. 4) and angiographic appearance (Fig. 5). A balloon catheter is positioned within the ductus after having passed from the main pulmonary artery into the descending aorta, and then the ductus is dilated. This technique may be utilized if the femoral or transumbilical approaches are not successful. This is our last choice.

ACUTE RESULTS
Neonates and Infants Less Than 1 Year Old

Despite an initial report of poor results [36], subsequent experience with dilating the neonatal and infant coarctation [10,14,18,24,29, 30,36,58–64] appears encouraging. In our own case material, including that previously reported [10,18,24], 25 infants, aged 3 days to 12 months (median, 3.0 months), underwent balloon angioplasty with resultant reduction in peak systolic pressure gradient across the coarctation from 41 ± 12 to 11 ± 7 mmHg, $P < 0.001$ (Fig. 6) and increase in the size of the coarcted segment from 2.4 ± 0.8 to 4.9 ± 1.1 mm ($P < 0.001$). Examples of improvement in pressure gradient and angiographic appearance are shown in Figures 7 and 8, respectively. Sixteen of the 25 (64%) infants had associated significant cardiac defects. One infant died 2 days after balloon angioplasty, related to associated complex cyanotic heart defect. All other infants improved symptomatically and were discharged home within days of the procedure. Several infants who had been ventilator dependent prior to the procedure were extubated on the day following balloon angioplasty. The infants who were in heart failure improved, as did their systemic hypertension. One infant with severe heart failure and "hypertensive cardiomyopathy" improved clinically immediately following balloon angioplasty with normalization of cardiac size (Fig. 9) and function (Fig. 10) at follow-up [25]. The femoral pulses, which had been either absent or markedly reduced and delayed compared with brachial pulses, became palpable

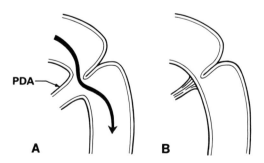

Fig. 3. Diagrammatic portrayal of the flow from the aortic isthmus to the descending aorta in coarctation of the aorta. **A:** With open ductus. **B:** With closed ductus. PDA, patent ductus arteriosus. (Reproduced from Rao and Solymar [13], with permission of the publisher.)

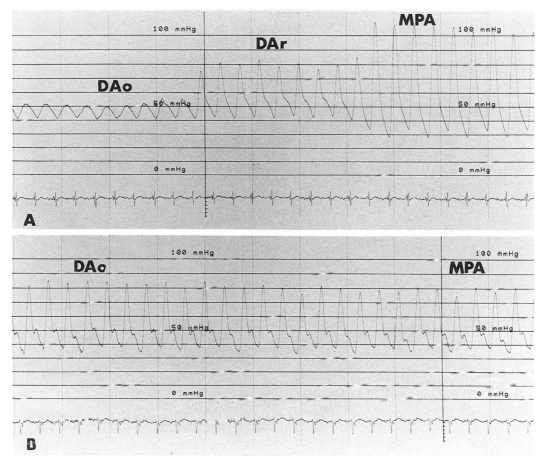

Fig. 4. Pressure pullback tracing across the segment of coarctation and ductus arteriosus before **(A)** and after **(B)** transductal balloon angioplasty. Note the marked improvement of the gradient. DAo, descending aorta; DAr, ductus arteriosus; MPA, main pulmonary artery. (Reproduced from Rao and Solymar [13], with permission of the publisher.)

with increased pulse intensity following angioplasty.

Review of the literature (excluding our reports and the Valvuloplasty and Angioplasty of Congenital Anomalies [VACA] Registry [65] patients) revealed that 47 neonates and infants underwent balloon coarctation angioplasty; these were derived from among nine reports [29,30,36,55,58,60–63]. Twenty-seven of the 36 (75%) infants for whom data on associated anomalies were available had severe associated defects, and these include moderate to large ventricular septal defect, mitral valve

atresia, Shone's syndrome, subvalvar aortic stenosis, transposition of the great arteries, and double-outlet right ventricle. Discrete and not so discrete coarctations were dilated by these workers, but long-segment coarctations were excluded by most. Adequate pressure data were available in 27 infants; these infants' ages ranged from 3 days to 12 months with a median of 3 weeks. Balloon angioplasty in these infants reduced peak systolic pressure gradients across the coarctation from 54 ± 32 (mean $\pm$ SD) to 18 ± 23 mmHg, $P < 0.001$ (Fig. 11). Three of these 47 infants required

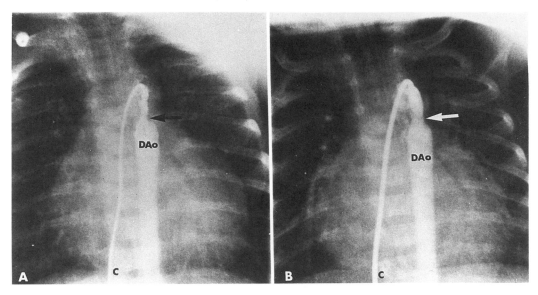

Fig. 5. Cineangiographic frame of the posteroanterior view of the area of coarctation before (A) and after (B) balloon angioplasty. Note marked improvement (arrows). DAo, descending aorta. (Reproduced from Rao and Solymar [13], with permission of the publisher.)

immediate surgical intervention [36,55,63]. There were four deaths [36,55,58,61], which are discussed in "Complications." The remaining infants improved clinically and were discharged home. Other workers [31,54,64] also

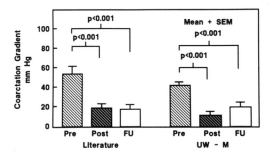

Fig. 6. Bar graph of peak systolic pressure gradients across the aortic coarctation and size of the coarcted segment before (pre) and immediately after (post) balloon angioplasty and at follow-up (FU) in neonates and young infants (≤1 year), showing significant (P < 0.001) improvement in both. Data from the literature [29,30,36,55,58,60–63] and from the University of Wisconsin (UW–M) are shown. SEM, standard error of mean.

reported good results, but their papers did not separately list neonatal and infant data. The pressure gradient reduction data in 27 neonates and infants from the VACA Registry (Fig. 11) are equally impressive [65].

Children Older Than 1 Year

From our study group, 33 children, aged 14 months to 13 years (median, 7.0 years), underwent balloon angioplasty of unoperated coarctation with resultant reduction in peak systolic pressure of gradient across the aortic coarctation from 48 ± 20 to 10 ± 10 mmHg, P < 0.001 (Fig. 12). The coarcted aortic segment increased from 4.4 ± 2.0 to 9.4 ± 2.9 mm (P < 0.001) after angioplasty. Examples of angiographic (Figs. 13, 14) and pressure gradient (Fig. 15) improvement after balloon dilatation are shown. Collateral vessels diminished promptly after balloon angioplasty (Fig. 16). No patient required immediate surgical intervention. The femoral pulses became palpable with increased pulse intensity following an-

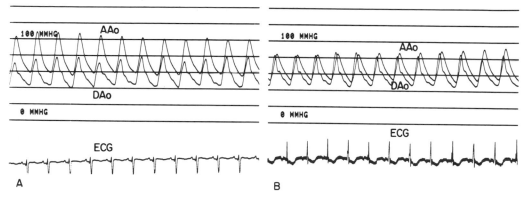

Fig. 7. Simultaneous ascending aortic (AAo) and descending aortic (DAo) pressures prior to **(A)** and following **(B)** balloon dilatation of coarctation of the aorta. Note equalization of pressures following balloon dilatation. ECG, electrocardiogram. (Reproduced from Rao *et al.* [8], with permission of the publisher.)

gioplasty, and the hypertension improved. All patients were discharged home within 24 hours following the procedure.

Review of the literature apart from our and the VACA Registry material revealed that 88 children underwent balloon coarctation angioplasty; these were derived from nine studies

[26,28–30,35,50,64,66,67]. There were other papers [31,54,64] that reported the results of balloon angioplasty in 33, 33, and 130 patients, respectively, but the descriptions did not indicate the numbers of neonates, children, and adults in the study populations. Of these 88 children, adequate pre- and postdilatation

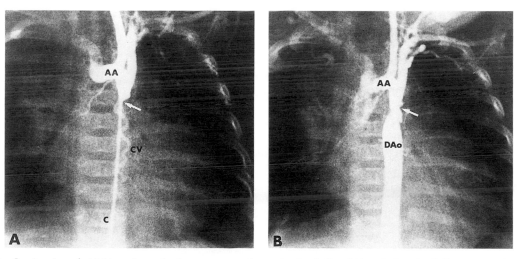

Fig. 8. Aortic arch (AA) angiography in posteroanterior projection before **(A)** and after **(B)** balloon angioplasty in an infant weighing 3.6 kg. Before balloon angioplasty, there was no opacification of the descending aorta (DAo); this is presumably because there was almost complete obstruction of the coarcted segment by the catheter (C). A collateral vessel (CV) was seen. Note clear-cut opacification of DAo after balloon angioplasty. The site of coarctation is marked with an arrow. Note the uneven opacification in the region of dilated coarctation; this probably represents intimal tears. (Reproduced from Rao [9], with permission of the publisher.)

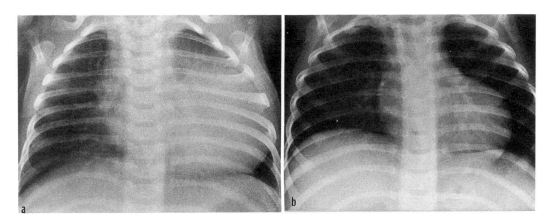

Fig. 9. Posteroanterior view of a chest x-ray film at presentation (**a**), showing marked cardiomegaly and pulmonary venous congestion. Note dramatic improvement in the cardiac size and pulmonary venous congestion on a chest x-ray film (**b**) taken 12 months following balloon angioplasty. (Reproduced from Salahuddin *et al.* [25], with permission of the publisher.)

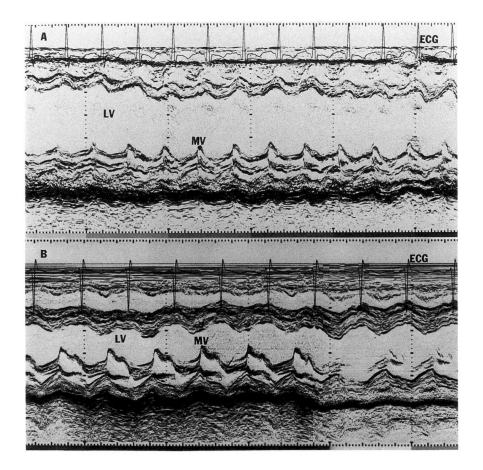

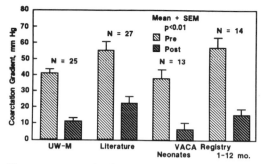

Fig. 11. Bar graphs showing peak-to-peak systolic pressure gradients across the aortic coarctation prior to (Pre) and following (Post) balloon angioplasty of aortic coarctation. There is a significant fall in the gradients in all three groups: UW–M, University of Wisconsin–Madison; literature, pooled data from nine papers [29,30,36,55,58,60–63] in the literature in which neonatal and infant (≤1 year) data are separately reported; VACA, Valvuloplasty and Angioplasty of Congenital Anomalies Registry. The N, number of subjects in each group, is marked at the top of the bar graph. SEM, standard error of mean.

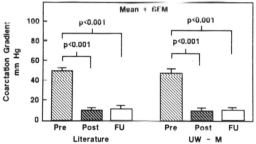

Fig. 12. Peak systolic pressure gradients across the aortic coarctation before balloon angioplasty (pre), immediately after angioplasty (post), and at follow-up (FU) in children >1 year of age from the literature group [26,28–30,35,50,62,66,67] and from our group (UW–M). Note significant (P < 0.001) fall in the peak-to-peak gradient immediately after angioplasty in both groups. The gradients at FU remained low and are significantly lower (P < 0.001) compared with preangioplasty values. SEM, standard error of mean.

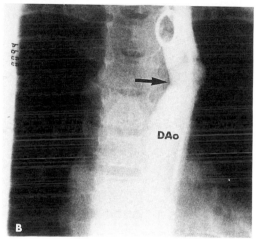

Fig. 13. Selected cine frame from a posteroanterior view of left ventricular (LV) angiogram prior to balloon angioplasty (A), showing discrete aortic coarctation (arrow) in a child aged 6 years. Following balloon angioplasty (B), aortic cineangiogram shows no evidence for a significant residua (arrow). Ao, aorta; DAo, descending aorta.

Fig. 10. M-mode tracing of two-dimensional directed echo images of the left ventricle (LV) at the time of initial presentation (A). Note marked LV enlargement and poor shortening fraction. The mitral valve (MV) is located in the posterior part of the LV, and its excursions are small. A similar echocardiographic view of the LV 12 months following balloon angioplasty (B) shows marked improvement in the LV size and function. ECG, electrocardiogram. (Reproduced from Salahuddin et al. [25], with permission of the publisher.)

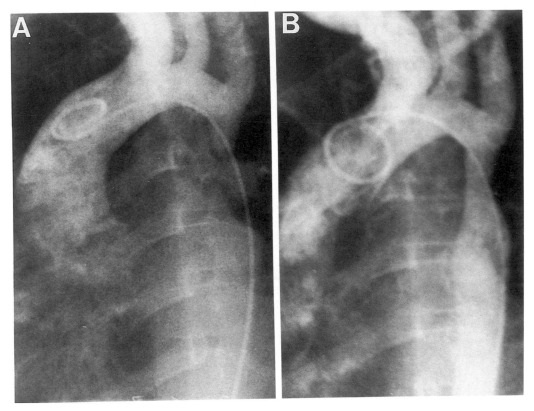

Fig. 14. Selected cineangiographic frames of aortograms in left anterior oblique projection, showing severe coarctation prior to balloon angioplasty **(A)**, which improved markedly following the procedure **(B)** in a 10-year-old child.

coarctation gradients were available from 43 children. These children ranged in age from 1 to 18 years (median, 5.8 years). The gradients across the coarctation were reduced from 52 ± 16 to 12 ± 11 mmHg, $P < 0.001$ (Fig. 12) following angioplasty. In three papers [28,50,62], pressure data from individual patients were not given, but group data were; in each of these studies, there was an impressive decrease in peak systolic pressure gradient from means of 51, 46, and 26 mmHg to means of 22, 8 and 6 mmHg, respectively. Of the 88 children from the literature review group who underwent balloon angioplasty, one child required surgical resection on the day following balloon dilatation [35]. Another patient from among 33 infants, children, and adults also

needed surgical resection 1 month after angioplasty [31]. The remaining patients did well with reduction in hypertension and improvement in symptoms when present [26,28,30, 35,50,62,66,67].

From the VACA Registry pressure gradient data were available for 97 children [65]. The gradient for the entire group (including neonates and infants) fell from 48 ± 19 to 12 ± 11 mmHg following balloon angioplasty.

FOLLOW-UP RESULTS
Neonates and Infants Less Than 1 Year Old

From our group of 25 neonates and infants who underwent balloon angioplasty, follow-up

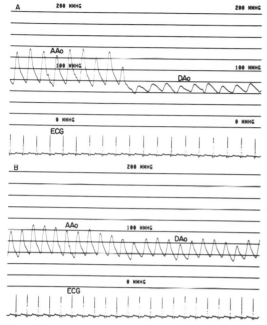

catheterization and angiography were performed in 16 patients 12 ± 4 months after angioplasty [18]. The residual gradient was 18 ± 16 mmHg (Fig. 6), significantly improved compared with the preangioplasty gradient of 45 ± 12 mmHg (P < 0.01). Angiographic improvement was observed in the majority of infants. Angiographic frames in one infant prior to, immediately following, and 1 year after balloon dilatation illustrate excellent result (Fig. 17). However, five (31%) of these patients developed recoarctation with gradients >20 mmHg [18]; two of these patients underwent surgical repair of residual coarctation early in our experience, and the remaining three infants underwent repeat balloon angioplasty with reduction of gradients from 30, 39 and 46 mm Hg, respectively to 0, 10, and 8 mmHg, respectively. Angiographic improvement in one infant following repeat angioplasty is documented in Figure 18.

Follow-up catheterization and angiographic data were available from 11 neonates and infants [29,30,57,59] of the 47 who underwent

Fig. 15. Pressure pullback tracings across the site of aortic coarctation prior to **(A)** and immediately after **(B)** balloon angioplasty. Note significant improvement in the pressure gradient across the coarctation and the pulse pressure in the descending aorta (DAo). AAo, ascending aorta; ECG, electrocardiogram.

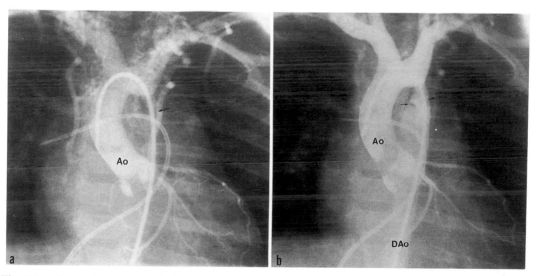

Fig. 16. Selected cineangiographic frame from posteroanterior view of an aortogram prior to balloon angioplasty, showing aortic coarctation (arrow) with a large number of collateral vessels **(a)**. Immediately following angioplasty **(b)**, the aortogram shows marked decrease in the collateral vessels. Both a and b were obtained at a similar phase of cineangiogram. In b, the area of dilated coarcted segment (longer arrow) and an intimal tear (shorter arrow) are shown. Also, note a greater opacification of the descending aorta (DAo) in b than in a. Ao, aorta.

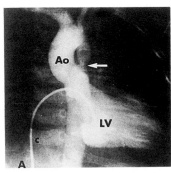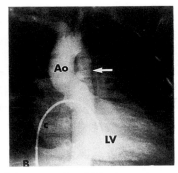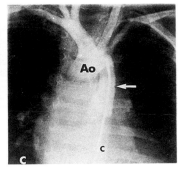

Fig. 17. Selected cine frames from left ventricular (LV) cineangiograms in posteroanterior view show aortic coarctation (arrows) prior to **(A)** and immediately following **(B)** balloon angioplasty. Note significant improvement. An aortogram performed 12 months following balloon angioplasty **(C)** showed no evidence for previous coarctation. Ao, aorta; C, catheter.

balloon angioplasty in the literature group. These data were obtained 10 ± 4 months after the procedure. The residual gradient at restudy was 17 ± 11 (Fig. 6), significantly improved compared with a preangioplasty gradient of 49 $\pm$ 26 mmHg ($P < 0.01$) in these infants. All surviving infants had clinical follow-up, and surgical resection of coarctation (in six) and repeat balloon (in one) were performed because of significant recoarctation [56,61,63]; five of these reinterventions were in neonates from a single institution [63]. The remaining infants seem to have done well clinically. No follow-up data were reported from VACA Registry [65] infants.

The high recurrence rate in the young infants is not too dissimilar to that seen following surgical intervention. In a previous study [14], we identified four factors for recurrence of aortic coarctation following balloon angioplasty: 1) age <12 months, 2) aortic isthmus less than two-thirds the size of the ascending aorta, 3) coarcted aortic segment <3.5 mm before angioplasty, and 4) coarcted aortic segment <6 mm after dilatation. We also observed that the larger the number of risk factors, the higher the chance for recurrence. The majority of the infants in this series had several of the risk factors, and therefore it is not surprising that the recoarctation rate is high. Despite this high recurrence, we believe balloon angioplasty is a worthwhile procedure, because repeat intervention, either by surgery [67a] or repeat balloon angioplasty [67b], to relieve residual or recurrent obstruction can be safely undertaken when the infant is large and not acutely ill.

Children Older Than 1 Year

From our study subjects, 29 children underwent repeat catheterization 14 ± 9 months following angioplasty, with a residual gradient of 10 ± 10 mmHg (Fig. 12). The preangioplasty gradient in these 29 patients was 47 ± 19 mmHg ($P < 0.001$). An example of pressure pullback at follow-up is shown in Figure 19. Repeat balloon angioplasty was required in one child, with good result. Two additional children had gradients of 30 mmHg; no intervention was recommended because of residual diffuse narrowing of the aorta and no significant systemic hypertension. The remaining children were asymptomatic with relief of hypertension (138 ± 27 vs. 110 ± 15 mmHg, $P < 0.01$) on follow-up.

Follow-up catheterization and angiographic data with pressure gradient information on individual patients were available for 26 of 88 patients [26,29,30,35] from the literature review group. The follow-up data were obtained 13 ± 4 months following angioplasty. The residual gradient at the time of follow-up study was $13 \pm$

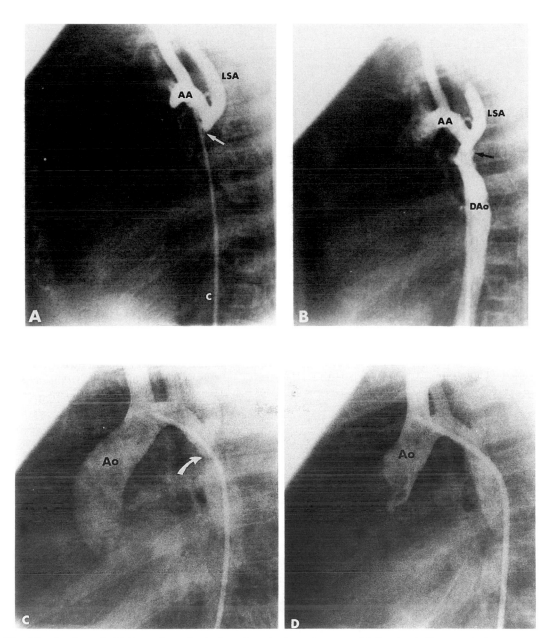

Fig. 18. Aortic arch (AA) angiography in lateral projection prior to and following balloon angioplasty in an infant weighing 3.6 kg. Prior to balloon angioplasty (**A**), there was no opacification of the descending aorta (DAo); this is presumably related to almost complete occlusion of the coarcted aortic segment by the catheter (C). Note clear-cut opacification of DAo following balloon angioplasty (**B**). The site of coarctation is marked with an arrow in each. Eleven months following angioplasty, significant recoarctation (arrow) developed (**C**), which was again balloon dilated with improvement (**D**). Ao, aorta; LSA, left subclavian artery. (Reproduced from Rao *et al.* [11], with permission of the publisher.)

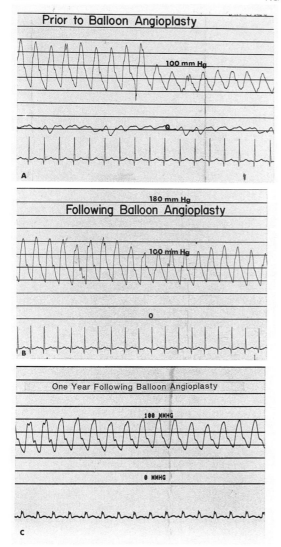

Fig. 19. Pressure pullback tracings across the site of aortic coarctation prior to **(A)**, immediately after **(B)**, and 1 year following **(C)** balloon angioplasty. Note immediate improvement in the gradient that persisted on follow-up. (Reproduced from Rao *et al.* [11], with permission.)

11 mmHg (Fig. 12), significantly lower (*P* < 0.001) than the preangioplasty value of 47 ± 15 mmHg in these 26 patients. In three studies comprising 45 patients (28,50,62) in whom only group data were given, the residual gradients were low; mean values were 7.6, 11.0, and

5.6 mmHg, which had been 51, 46, and 29 mm Hg prior to angioplasty. In another study [54], residual gradients were <20 mmHg in all 13 patients recatheterized. Adequate clinical follow-up information was available in 115 patients [26,28–31,35,50,54,62]; of these repeat intervention for recoarctation was required in six children. Elective surgery was performed in four children [28,30] to excise the recoarctation. In two children repeat balloon angioplasty was performed to relieve the residual coarctation [50]. The remaining children were asymptomatic with reduced hypertension at follow-up. No follow-up data are available from the VACA Registry [65].

APPLICABILITY TO ADULT PATIENTS

Although balloon angioplasty of aortic coarctation has most frequently been used in neonates, infants, and children, it can be used in adult patients as well. Lababidi *et al.* [68] were the first to apply this technique; they did so in a 27-year-old man, and it resulted in reduction of peak systolic pressure gradient across the coarctation from 70 to 15 mmHg, angiographic improvement, and reduced hypertension (190/124 *vs.* 130/80 mmHg). They subsequently reported [69] their experience with balloon dilatation of native coarctation in eight consecutive adults, aged 19–30 years (25 ± 5 years). The systolic pressure gradient across the coarctation was reduced from 48 ± 19 to 7 ± 5 mm Hg. The size of the coarcted segment increased from 6.8 ± 2.2 to 15.1 ± 5.0 mm. No complications were encountered. Clinical and echo-Doppler follow-up 1 year after the procedure revealed a good result with no more than a 15 mmHg peak systolic blood pressure difference, measured by cuff between arms and legs. They concluded that results in young adults are similar to those in children; balloon angioplasty should be considered as an option to surgical intervention; and follow-up studies (longer than 1 year) are required. Suarez de Lezo and associates [62] used balloon dilatation of aortic coarctation in nine young adults (22 ± 5 years), but the data were combined with those in children. Immediate postdilatation gradients (11 ± 9 mmHg) and follow-up gradients (17 ± 10 mmHg) suggest good results. Other reports [70–72] followed, which are described in Table I. Based on this review, it appears that aortic perforation during the procedure [71, 72a] and aneurysmal formation at follow-up [71, 72] are also seen in adults. In addition, intimal dissection that persisted at 6 month follow-up was seen in one patient [70]. Therefore, it is prudent to 1) avoid manipulation of tips of the catheters and guidewires in the region of freshly dilated coarctation; 2) choose an appropriate-sized balloon (no larger than the diameter of the descending aorta at the level of the diaphragm); and 3) monitor for development of aneurysms, and, if found, closely follow the progression of aneurysms by repeated angiography or magnetic resonance imaging.

APPLICABILITY TO OTHER STENOTIC LESIONS OF THE AORTA

Recoarctation following previous operation for native coarctation is discussed in Chapter 11. Congenital and acquired (atherosclerotic and Takayasu's disease) lesions of the descending aorta can be balloon dilated [73–81], with reduction in pressure gradient, increased distal perfusion, and decreased proximal hypertension. The principles of dilatation, selection of balloon size, and other technical issues are similar to those described for children. Follow-up studies for these lesions are also few and are needed.

COMPARISON WITH SURGERY

Neonates and Infants Less Than 1 Year Old

Forty-nine papers published since 1980[1] were scrutinized to assess the results of co-arctation surgery in neonates and infants less than 1 year old in a manner similar to our previous report [18]. These authors operated on 3 to 191 infants over a period of time from 1953 to 1990. Associated significant cardiac defects were present in 2,106 of 3,075 (68%) infants in whom such data were available. Operative mortality varied between 0% and 50%, with an overall mortality rate of 19% (617 of 3,292) (Table II). These investigators followed 3–152 infants and observed 3%–59% late mortality. The average mortality rate was 18% (483 of 2,648 infants) during a follow-up of 1 month to 25 years. Recurrence of coarctation ranged from 0% to 100%, with an average recurrence rate of 17% (421 of 2,540 infants, Table II). In an attempt to have comparable time periods during which both surgical and balloon interventions have been performed, we examined the results of infants who underwent coarctation surgery between 1979 and 1990.[2] The prevalence of associated significant heart defects was 70% (360 of 516 infants), similar ($P > 0.1$) to the balloon angioplasty group, with 70% (43 of 61) prevalence. The mortality and recoarctation rates in these two surgical groups (the 49 papers published since 1980 and the 11 papers reporting surgeries between 1979 and 1990) were compared with pooled data from our study plus nine balloon angioplasty reports dealing with infants less than 1 year [29,30,36,55,58,60–63] in Table II. As shown, the mortality rates are higher with surgery than with balloon angioplasty, while recoarctation rates are similar (Table II).

In conclusion, our data and those reported in the literature indicate that balloon angioplasty is effective in relieving aortic obstruction in the neonate and young infant with an acceptable complication rate, although the recoarctation rate is high. The latter can be relieved by repeat balloon angioplasty or surgery when the infant is stable and less acutely ill. Because of

---

[1]References are listed in Appendix I.

[2]References 13, 29, 32, 34, 35, 37, 38, 41, 42, 47, and 48 in Appendix I.

TABLE I. Results of Balloon Angioplasty of Aortic Coarctation in Adults Reported in the Literature[a]

Authors, year	No. undergoing BA	Age (Years) Mean ± SD	range	Gradient across coarctation (mean ± SD; mmHg)[b]			Follow-up (No.)/mean duration (months)	Comments
				Pre	Post	FU		
Attia & Lababidi, 1988 [69]	8	25 ± 5	19-30	48 ± 19	7 ± 5	<15[c]	8/12	No complications
Suarez de Lezo et al., 1989 [62]	9	22 ± 5	18-31	–	11 ± 9	13 ± 10	–/–	Pre-BA gradient for the group combined with 19 children was 49 ± 16 mmHg
Erbel et al., 1990 [70]	7	28 ± 14	14-49	59 ± 22	13 ± 7	6 ± 9	7/6	Intimal dissection in one patient at 6-month follow-up
Tyagi et al., 1992 [72]	35	23 ± 7	14-37	81 ± 23	15 ± 13	16 ± 13	26/13	Three aneurysms
Fawzy et al., 1992 [71]	23	23 ± 9	15-55	67 ± 20	9 ± 11	6 ± 7	22/15	One aortic perforation, two developed restenosis requiring reballooning, three developed small aneurysm

[a]BA, balloon angioplasty; FU, follow-up; pre, prior to angioplasty; post, immediately after angioplasty.
[b]Peak-to-peak systolic pressure gradient measured at cardiac catheterization except for that indicated in footnote c.
[c]Systolic pressure difference between arms and legs.

TABLE II. Comparison of Mortality and Recoarctation Rates Between Surgical and Balloon Angioplasty Groups in Neonates and Infants <1 Year Old

	49 Coarctation surgery papers 1953–1991[a]	P value	Balloon angioplasty 1982–1991[b]	P value	11 Coarctation surgery papers 1979–1991[c]
Initial mortality	617 of 3,292 (19%)	<0.01	5 of 72 (7%)	>0.1	82 of 607 (13.5%)
Late mortality	483 of 2,648 (18%)	<0.005	1 of 67 (1.5%)	<0.001	66 of 517 (12.8%)
Recoarctation rate	421 of 2,540 (17%)	>0.1	11 of 67 (16%)	>0.05	59 of 517 (11.4%)

[a]Pooled data from 49 papers published since 1980.
[b]Pooled data from the literature plus the author's case material.
[c]Pooled data from 11 papers reporting results of coarctation surgery performed between 1979 and 1990.

these results and the reported high mortality and morbidity rates after surgical repair in neonates and young infants, we recommend balloon angioplasty as the procedure of choice for relief of symptomatic native coarctation in neonates and infants less than 1 year old.

Children Older Than 1 Year

Sixteen papers published since 1980[3] were scrutinized to examine the results of surgery for aortic coarctation in children older than 1 year. There were a total of 1,998 children operated on over a period from 1953 to 1989; the number of children in each report varied between 9 to 263. The average operative mortality rate was 1.3% (22 of 1,706), although this varied from 0% to 5% from one study to the other. These authors followed 9 to 255 children for a period of 1 month to 30 years and observed 0%–27% late mortality; the mean was 5.6% (61 of 1,086 children). The recoarctation rate also varied between 0%–18%, with an average of 5.8% (104 of 1,806). The mortality and recoarctation rates between balloon and surgical groups are compared in Figure 20. As can be seen, the recoarctation rates are similar, while mortality rates are slightly higher in the surgical series.

[3]References are listed in Appendix II.

Other Complications

Aneurysms are discussed in a later section of this chapter. Other complications such as paraplegia and paradoxical hypertension occur with significant frequency following surgical repair while such complications are either rare or, if present, very mild and inconsequential following balloon angioplasty. The femoral artery occlusion rate may be higher with balloon than with surgical therapy. Vascular func-

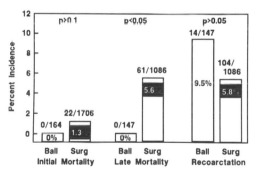

Fig. 20. Comparison of initial (operative) mortality, late mortality, and recoarctation rates after balloon angioplasty (Ball) and surgical correction (Surg) in children >1 year of age. The data for balloon angioplasty group were derived from both published literature [22,28–30,35,50,62,66,67] and our studies. The data for surgical correction were derived from 16 reports published after 1980 (see Appendix II). Note that the initial and late mortality rates are better with balloon angioplasty than with surgical intervention, although the recurrence rates are comparable.

tion and growth of the left upper limb following subclavian flap aortoplasty repair of coarctation [82–84] have been studied. Definitive reduction in the length and muscle mass of the upper arm [82,84] and forearm [83,84] have been observed. Shenberger and associates [82] detected no significant differences in forearm blood flow and vascular resistance between the right (normal) and left (disconnected subclavian artery) arms. However, Van Son et al. [84] observed compromised hemodynamics (as quantitated by Doppler spectrum analysis of blood flow velocities of left brachial artery at rest and during postocclusive reactive hyperemia) of the left arm with potential for symptoms of ischemia with exercise. Although not common, gangrene of the left arm can develop following subclavian flap repair of coarctation (85,86) in a manner similar to that seen following Blalock-Taussig shunts [85,86].

Conclusion

This review of comparison of surgical versus balloon therapy of aortic coarctation would suggest that balloon angioplasty is no more harmful than surgical intervention when mortality and major complication rates are compared. The longer hospital stay and the attendant increased costs, need for intubation and general anesthesia, and residual scar are additional disadvantages with surgery.

MECHANISM OF ANGIOPLASTY

Lock and associates [5] created aortic coarctations in animal models and balloon dilated the stenotic lesions in order to determine the mechanism of balloon angioplasty. Linear intimal tears were observed; they were located in the nonoperated aortic wall in experimentally produced aortic coarctations. The intimal tears were noted to extend into the media with intramedial hemorrhage. No evidence for adventitial rupture was observed [5]. These mechanisms of relief may be similar in postoperative recoarctations but may not be completely applicable to previously unoperated ("native")

coarctations. Intimal and medial tears following dilatation of human aortic coarctation were also observed by several workers [31,35,54,55,62,87], as well as by our group. As a matter of fact, the data from Suarez de Lezo et al. [62] suggest that there is less gradient at follow-up in patients with intimal tears immediately after angioplasty than those without intimal tears. Thus the mechanism of relief of aortic obstructions is by tearing of intima and media.

COMPLICATIONS

Acute

Complications during and immediately after balloon angioplasty have been remarkably minimal. Blood loss requiring transfusion has been reported in many studies. Cerebrovascular accident [30,51,62], transmural tears with or without vessel wall perforation [31,55, 65,88,89], balloon rupture at high inflation pressures [8,61], and hypertension with a *forme fruste* postcoarctectomy syndrome [9,35,68], though rare, have been reported. Although the reason why postcoarctectomy syndrome is not problematic following balloon coarctation angioplasty (in contradistinction to surgery) is not known, recent studies [90,91] suggest that there is either minimal or no stimulation of neurosympathetic activity and renin–angiotensin system after balloon dilatation.

Reopening of the ductal structure (Fig. 21) may occur following balloon angioplasty. Others [92] reported similar instances; however, these are infrequent. If there is a significant shunt across it, surgical ligation or transcatheter closure [93] may be performed.

Femoral artery thrombosis requiring heparin, streptokinase, or thrombectomy occurred in 39% (12 of 31) of patients undergoing balloon dilatation of aortic coarctation or stenosis, while such a complication occurred in only 2.2% of arterial catheterization not involving balloon dilatation [94]. In another study [95],

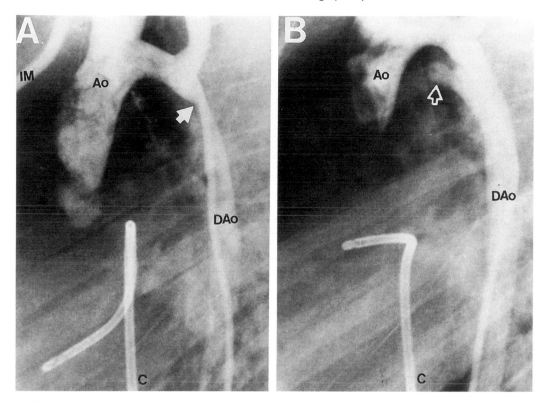

Fig. 21. Selected frames from lateral views of aortic angiograms prior to balloon angioplasty **(A)**. Note coarctation (solid arrow) without evidence of ductus arteriosus. Following balloon angioplasty **(B)**, opening of the ductal structure (open arrow) is seen. On review of the cineangiogram, there was no opacification of the pulmonary artery. Ao, aorta; C, venous catheter in the left ventricle; DAo, descending aorta; IM, internal mammary artery.

arterial complications were noted in 39 of 64 (45%) patients undergoing balloon dilatation procedure for systemic outflow obstruction; many of these children required heparin, thrombolytic therapy, and/or surgery. Understandably, these complications were found more often in patients with lower weight. A higher incidence of arterial complications documented in the series reported by Burrows et al. [95] than that observed in the VACA Registry [42,65,96] and other series tabulated by Rothman [97] may in part be related to systematic examination to detect arterial compromise used in this study. Furthermore, Burrows et al. [95] used large (8 and 9) French size catheters. The

availability of smaller catheters with low-profile balloons may reduce the arterial complication rate. If arterial compromise is noted, starting heparin infusion within hours of the procedure, changing to thrombolytic agents the next morning if no improvement is observed, and surgical intervention if threat of loss of tissue and/or no improvement on thrombolytic therapy are recommended [94,95].

Deaths associated with balloon dilatation have been reported after angioplasty of aortic coarctation [24,36,55,61]; these were related to vessel wall rupture [55], ventricular fibrillation [61], additional surgery [36], or severity of associated heart defect [24]. All the deaths were in the infant group, and to my knowledge no deaths have been reported in children.

Transient prolongation of the QTc interval following balloon valvuloplasty and angioplasty [98] has been reported. The Holter findings [99] of premature beats following valvuloplasty may have a significance in the light of prolongation of QTc interval [98], although to my knowledge ventricular ectopy has not been reported after balloon coarctation angioplasty. No patients from our series or from many other studies have been known to develop ventricular arrhythmias, although one case of sudden death from ventricular fibrillation shortly after balloon angioplasty of aortic coarctation [61] was reported. Whether these arrhythmias are related to QTc prolongation is not known. However, patient monitoring following balloon angioplasty is warranted [99].

Fellows et al. [100] carefully analyzed complications of catheter therapy over a 3 year period and reported 12% acute complications (6% were major and 6% were minor). The mortality rate was 0.7%. The complication rate appears to be related to age of the patients and type of lesion dilated. Patients younger than 6 months had a higher rate of complication than did the older children. Dilatation of recurrent coarctations appeared to have the lowest incidence of complications (4%), while aortic valvuloplasty had highest complication rate (40%). Booth's experience [89] with complications is similar. Some of these complications may be unavoidable. However, meticulous attention to the details of the technique, use of appropriate balloon diameter and length, low-profile balloon catheter, avoidance of extremely high inflation pressures, and use of short inflation/deflation cycles may prevent or reduce the complications.

Complications at Follow-Up

There was one late death from our infant study group, related to severe mitral and aortic stenoses and moderate hypoplasia of the left atrium and left ventricle, a forme fruste hypo-plastic left heart syndrome. There was one late death in the infants [58] from the literature group, and no late deaths were reported in the VACA Registry patients. No late deaths have been reported in children following balloon angioplasty from any of the above three groups.

With regard to other complications at follow-up, femoral artery occlusion, restenosis, and aneurysms at the site of coarctation dilatation have been noted. Data with regard to the incidence of femoral artery occlusion at follow-up are not readily available from the literature. In our study, we systematically looked at femoral artery complications at follow-up [11]. At the time of follow-up catheterization, arterial catheterization was performed on the side opposite to that used for angioplasty in two-thirds of the patients, and the same side was used in the remaining. In the former, iliac arteriography was done with visualization of the femoral artery previously used for angioplasty. Arterial entry in the latter group is considered evidence for arterial patency. Complete occlusion of the femoral artery previously used for balloon angioplasty was observed in 2 of 16 (13%) patients who had angioplasty during their infancy (≤ 1 year of age). Of the 29 children (>1 year) who underwent follow-up study, one femoral artery was completely occluded (14 months old at the time of balloon angioplasty), and two femoral arteries were found to be partially obstructed, but there was good collateral flow in all three children.

Residual or recoarctation in the infant group was discussed in the preceding section; 7 of the 47 infants from the literature group and 5 of 16 infants from our study required reintervention because of restenosis (12 of 63, 19%). The reasons for such a high recurrence are discussed in the next section.

The data with regard to recoarctation in children from the literature and from our study patients are listed in Table III. As indicated, significant recoarctation occurred in only 6 of 130 patients giving a recurrence rate of approximately 5%, although the recurrence rate is

TABLE III. Prevalence of Recoarctation and Aneurysm Formation at Follow-Up After Balloon Angioplasty of Native Coarctations in Children

Authors	No. of patients with follow-up[a]	Recoarctation gradients (mmHg)			Aneurysms No. (%)
		20–30	>30	Total (%)	
Lababidi et al., 1984 [29]	5	1	1	2 (40)	0 (0)
Allen et al., 1986 [35]	1	0	0	0 (0)	0 (0)
Cooper et al., 1987 [26]	7	0	1	1 (14)	3 (43)
Wren et al., 1987 [50]	15	2	0	2 (13)	1 (7)
Beekman et al., 1987 [30]	13	2	0	2 (15)	1 (8)
Brandt et al., 1987 [28]	11	1	2	3 (27)	4 (36)
Morrow et al., 1988 [31]	17	0	0	0 (0)	2 (12)
Suarez de Lezo et al., 1989 [62]	19	0	1	1 (5)	1 (5)
Fontes et al., 1990 [54]	13	0	0	0 (0)	1 (8)
Current series	29	2	1	3 (10)	1 (3)
Total	130	8	6	14 (11)	14 (11)

[a]Only patients in whom follow-up catheterization and/or NMR studies were available are included.

much higher (11%) if the gradient cut-off is lowered to 20 mmHg. The issues related to development of aneurysms are discussed in a later section of this chapter.

CAUSES OF RESTENOSIS

Recoarctation following balloon angioplasty has been reported [26,28–31,35,50,62], but the reasons for recurrence at intermediate-term follow-up have been studied only to a limited degree [30]. We have investigated causes of recoarctation following balloon angioplasty of aortic coarctation [14,19]. On the basis of results of 6–30 month follow-up catheterization data in 20 children, these were divided into: group A with good results (peak gradients ≤20 mmHg and no recoarctation of angiograms), 13 patients; group B with fair and poor results (peak gradients >20 mmHg with or without recoarctation on angiography), 7 patients. None developed aneurysms. Thirty demographic, anatomic, physiologic, and technical variables were examined by multivariate logistic regression analysis and four factors were identified as risk factors for developing recoarctation: 1) age less than 12 months, 2)

aortic isthmus less than half the size of ascending aorta, 3) coarcted aortic segment smaller than 3.5 mm prior to dilatation, and 4) coarcted aortic segment <6 mm after angioplasty. The larger the number of risk factors, the greater the chance of recoarctation (Fig. 22). Predilatation peak systolic pressure gradient across the aortic coarctation in excess of 50 mmHg previously implicated as a cause of recurrence [30] and ratio of balloon to coarcted aortic segment or descending aortic diameter were carefully scrutinized [30] but did not seem

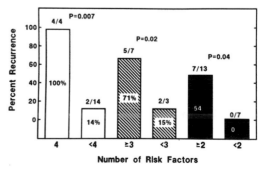

Fig. 22. Bar graph showing relationship of chance of recoarctation with the number of risk factors present in a given patient; the larger the number of risk factors, the higher the chance for recoarctation.

to influence the recoarctation. The identification of risk factors may help in selection of patients for balloon angioplasty. Avoiding or minimizing the number of risk factors may help to reduce the chance for recoarctation following angioplasty.

INFLUENCE OF TECHNICAL FACTORS ON ANGIOPLASTY

Use of very small balloons may not produce adequate relief of obstruction, and use of large balloons may produce aneurysms. These impressions are based on anecdotal experiences. Wren and associates [50] commented that the single patient in their series who had developed aneurysm follow-up was the patient in whom a balloon with the highest balloon-to-coarctation ratio was utilized for balloon angioplasty. In other series, no specific factor(s) were identified to cause either restenosis or aneurysmal formation. We have investigated the role of several technical factors (Table IV) in causing restenosis [14]. The good (group A) and poor (group B) results groups were identified, as detailed under "Causes of Restenosis." Although the ratio of balloon size to size of coarcted segment and the ratio of balloon size to size of the descending aorta at the level of the diaphragm are smaller in the poor results group, these differences did not attain statistical significance (Table IV). Other technical factors, such as maximum pressure achieved in the balloon, number of balloon inflations, and the total duration of balloon inflation, are similar in both groups.

As a rule of thumb, a balloon that is two times or more the diameter of the coarcted segment is necessary to produce any significant reduction of the obstruction. We initially start balloon dilatation using a balloon diameter midway between aortic isthmus and descending aorta at the level of the diaphragm. This type of approach can result in inadequate relief of obstruction (Table V). Then a larger balloon is used with effective relief of obstruction (Table V). We try not to use a balloon that is larger than the descending aorta. In our opinion, there is no reason to increase the size of the coarcted segment beyond the descending aortic diameter, because the latter is the limiting size of how much blood could be carried into the descending aorta. With this approach, the incidence of aneurysm formation is likely to be low.

Another technical factor of extreme importance is not to manipulate the tips of a guidewire or a catheter in the region of freshly dilated co-

TABLE IV. Technical Factors During Balloon Angioplasty[a]

	Group A (mean ± SD)	Group B (mean ± SD)	P value t	P value Logistic
Balloon size/size of coarcted segment	3.29 ± 1.19	2.85 ± 0.84	0.40	0.36
Balloon size/size of Isthmus	1.01 ± 0.22	1.09 ± 0.41	0.66	0.56
Balloon size/size of DAo immediately distal to coarction	0.74 ± 0.18	0.73 ± 0.42	0.92	0.90
Balloon size/size of DAo at diaphragm	0.95 ± 0.27	0.78 ± 0.24	0.18	0.14
Maximal pressure achieved in the balloon (atm)	5.6 ± 1.7	6.6 ± 1.4	0.22	0.20
Number of balloon inflations	3.92 ± 0.76	5.0 ± 1.8	0.18	0.07
Total duration of balloon inflation, (seconds)	33.0 ± 8.6	40.0 ± 21.0	0.43	0.28

[a]DAo, descending aorta. (Reproduced from Rao et al. [14], with permission of the publisher.)

TABLE V. Effect of Balloon Size on the Immediate Response of the Pressure Gradient Across the Coarctation After Balloon Angioplasty

Case No.	Age (Years)/Sex	Status	AAo (mmHg)	DAo (mmHg)	Gradient (mmHg)
1	5/F	Pre	118	87	31
		10 mm	111	87	24
		12 mm	109	99	10
2	10/F	Pre	137	79	58
		10 mm	125	90	35
		12 mm	130	113	17
3	2/F	Pre	133	103	30
		8 mm	96	76	20
		10 mm	90	76	14
4	1.5/M	Pre	103	72	31
		8 mm	106	71	35
		10 mm	96	79	17

AAo, ascending aorta; DAo, descending aorta; Pre, prior to balloon angioplasty.

arctation. Inadvertent manipulation may result in acutely perforating the aorta [55] or in aneurysms [11]. A guidewire should always be left in place across the area of coarctation and catheters exchanged over the guidewire.

NONINVASIVE EVALUATION OF FOLLOW-UP RESULTS OF ANGIOPLASTY
Echo-Doppler Studies

Intermediate-term follow-up results of balloon angioplasty of aortic coarctation were reported by several groups. In most of these studies cardiac catheterization was used for evaluation of long-term results. Allen et al. [35], Cooper et al. [26], and we [9–11] have used echo-Doppler (in addition to catheterization) for evaluation of follow-up results of balloon angioplasty of coarctation. These studies involved only small groups of patients. Cooper and associates [26] studied five patients with pulsed Doppler prior to and immediately after balloon angioplasty and found that the descending aortic flow pattern returned to normal in four of the five patients studied.

From our initial study cohort, echo-Doppler studies preceding and immediately following angioplasty were available for 19 patients, while intermediate-term follow-up studies were available for 18 patients [12]. Left ventricular end-diastolic dimension did not significantly change (30.0 ± 8.7 vs. 30.5 ± 7.4 mm; ($P >$ 0.1) immediately following balloon angioplasty. Left ventricular posterior wall thickness in diastole also did not change (6.8 ± 1.6 vs. 7.0 ± 1.7 mm; $P > 0.1$). Left ventricular shortening fraction (38 ± 10 vs. 35 ± 8 mm) remained unchanged ($P > 0.1$). Echographic improvement in the coarcted aortic segment (Fig. 23) and decreased Doppler flow velocity (Fig. 24) are seen. On follow-up, 3–22 months (mean, 12 months) after balloon angioplasty, the left ventricular dimension, though increased slightly (30.0 ± 8.7 vs. 35.2 ± 7.9 mm), did not attain statistical significance ($P > 0.05$). Left ventricular posterior wall thickness appears decreased (6.8 ± 1.6 vs. 5.9 ± 1.6 mm) but was not statistically significant ($P > 0.05$). Left ventricular shortening fraction (38.0 ± 10.1 vs. 42.7 ± 6.9) did not change ($P > 0.1$).

In a subsequent study, we examined the Doppler data from 27 patients who had undergone balloon angioplasty of native coarctation [101]. The mean Doppler flow velocity decreased from 3.62 ± 0.45 to 2.65 ± 0.53 m/s ($P > 0.001$) immediately following balloon

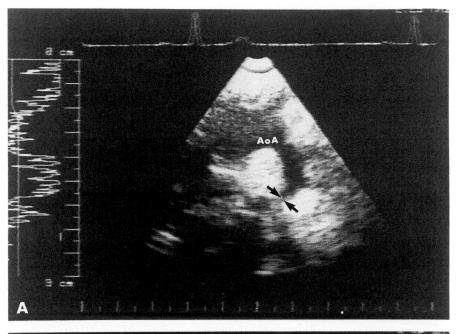

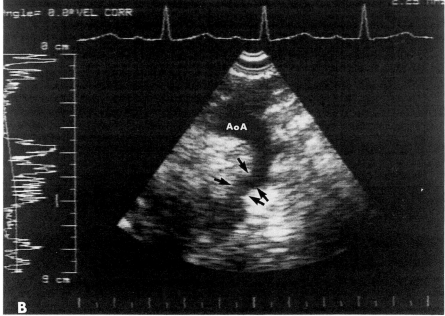

Fig. 23. Selected video frames from two-dimensional echographic suprasternal notch views of the aortic arch (AoA) prior to **(A)** and immediately **(B)** after balloon angioplasty. Note severe coarctation, arrows in A, which improved (arrows) following angioplasty.

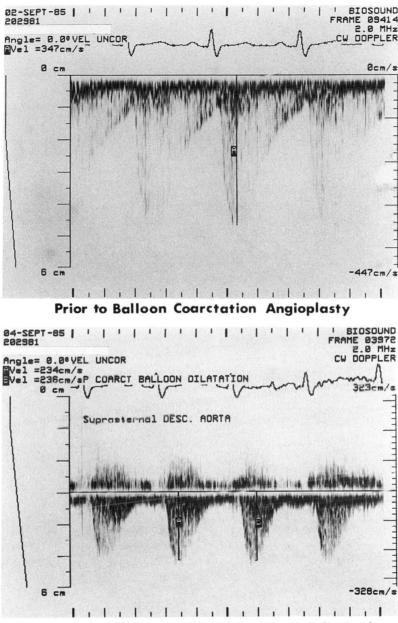

Prior to Balloon Coarctation Angioplasty

Twelve Hours Following Balloon Coarctation Angioplasty

Fig. 24. Continuous-wave Doppler flow velocity in the descending aorta recorded from suprasternal notch view prior to **(top)** and 12 hours following **(bottom)** balloon angioplasty. Note that Doppler flow velocity decreased from 3.47 to 2.35 m/s, corresponding to a drop in pressure gradient from 48 to 22 mm Hg across the coarctation of the aorta. Also, note that the flow was pandiastolic prior to angioplasty, while the diastolic flow, for the most part, disappeared after angioplasty. (Reproduced from Rao *et al.* [8], with permission of the publisher.)

angioplasty. A corresponding decrease in catheterization-measured peak-to-peak pressure gradient was from 53.0 ± 18 to 9 ± 8 mmHg (P < 0.001). On follow-up (6–30 months), the Doppler flow velocity remained unchanged (2.66 ± 0.5 m/s, P < 0.001) from that obtained immediately after angioplasty, but continued to remain improved (P < 0.001) compared with preangioplasty values. An example of such improvement is shown in Figure 25.

While there is improvement in Doppler flow velocity measures following balloon an-

gioplasty and a statistically significant (P < 0.001) relationship exists between catheterization-measured peak-to-peak systolic pressure gradients across the coarctation and Doppler-derived (using modified Bernouli equation) peak instantaneous gradients, the correlation coefficients are sufficiently low (r = 0.76) and Doppler-derived gradients may not accurately estimate the catheter gradient.

Duration-related measures of the Doppler flow curve were also examined [101]. Pandiastolic flow in the descending aortic flow

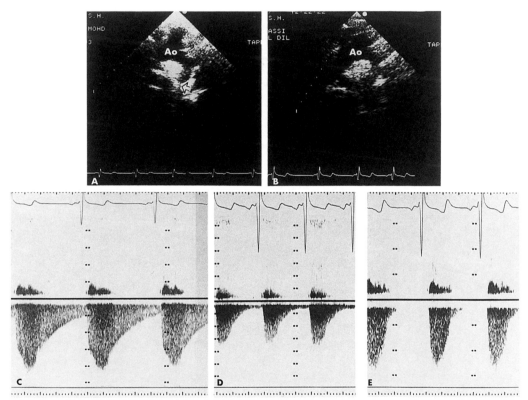

Fig. 25. Selected frames from two-dimensional echocardiograms from the suprasternal notch prior to (**A**) and immediately after (**B**) balloon angioplasty of aortic coarctation. The aorta (Ao) is shown with severe coarctation (arrow) in A, which improved markedly in the postangioplasty echocardiogram (B). Continuous-wave Doppler flow velocity recordings from the suprasternal notch while directing the ultrasound beam toward the descending aorta prior to (**C**), immediately after (**D**), and 6 months after (**E**) balloon angioplasty of aortic coarctation are shown. Note the immediate fall in the peak Doppler flow velocity (D), which decreased further on follow-up (E). Also note that the Doppler flow velocity was pandiastolic prior to balloon angioplasty (C), which was present only in early diastole (D) immediately after angioplasty. On further follow-up (E), there appears to be only systolic Doppler flow in the descending aorta. (Reproduced from Rao [12], with permission of the publisher.)

velocity curve, which was present in 16 of the 19 native coarctations, disappeared immediately after angioplasty. At follow-up, only 4 of 17 patients had pandiastolic flow. All four patients with pandiastolic flow had angiographic evidence for recoarctation with gradients in excess of 25 mmHg.

Other duration-related measures, namely, acceleration time (time from the onset of antegrade flow to peak systolic flow), antegrade flow time (time from the onset of antegrade flow to the point where the flow velocity curve became parallel to the base line), antegrade flow time (AFT) in excess of left ventricular ejection time (LVET) expressed as percentage of LVET,

$$(\frac{AFT - LVET}{LVET} \times 100),$$

and AFT fraction (AFT expressed as a fraction of R–R interval [RRI],

$$(\frac{AFT}{RRI} \times 100),$$

were examined [101]; all of them improved (Table VI) immediately following angioplasty ($P < 0.001$), and all but the uncorrected acceleration time remain improved ($P < 0.01-0.001$) at follow-up (Table VI). These results suggest that the magnitude and duration-related measures of descending aortic Doppler flow velocity curve immediately after and several months following balloon angioplasty are helpful in indicating the effectiveness of relief of aortic coarctation.

Nuclear Magnetic Resonance Imaging

As implied in the previous section, Doppler flow velocity in the descending aorta can be obtained easily. However, two-dimensional imaging of the area of the dilated coarctation may be difficult to obtain in some patients. Even the best imaging quality may not be able to identify or exclude aneurysms at the site of coarctation dilatation. Boxer et al. [102], Morrow et al. [31], and Bank et al. [103], have studied a limited number of patients with nuclear magnetic resonance (NMR) imaging techniques. Sagittal and 60° left anterior oblique views appear to demonstrate the anatomy best [102]. Residual coarctation and aneurysms can be detected by NMR imaging studies, and these data are comparable to those obtained at angiography. Our own limited experience confirms these observations. NMR imaging appears to be a useful adjunct in the evaluation of anatomic residua following balloon coarctation angioplasty.

OTHER ISSUES

Remodeling of the Aorta After Angioplasty

We have examined the data to see if remodeling of aorta takes place following successful balloon angioplasty of aortic coarctation [16]. The data from the same group of children in whom we examined the causes of recoarctation [14] were utilized for this purpose; group A with good results (peak gradient ≤20 mmHg and no recoarctation on angiography), 13 patients; and group B with fair and poor results (peak gradient >20 mmHg with or without recoarctation on angiography), 7 patients. Measurements of the aorta at five sites, namely, ascending aorta (immediately proximal to right innominate artery), isthmus, coarctation segment, and descending aorta distal to coarctation and at the level of diaphragm, were made (Fig. 26) in two angiographic views, corrected for magnification, and averaged. A standardized diameter of the aorta at the five locations measured was calculated (Fig. 27) for each case preangioplasty and at follow-up. The variance (variance is the sum of the squared differences of each measure divided by the degrees of freedom) from norm or unity was determined for each patient before angioplasty and at follow-up. The variance of standardized aortic measures (0.233 vs. 0.287) was similar ($P > 0.05$) in both groups prior to angioplasty (Table VII), whereas at follow-up (0.057 vs.

TABLE VI. Summary of Selected Variables Measured From Descending Aortic Flow Velocity Curve[a]

	AT (msec; mean ± SD)	CAT (msec; mean ± SD)	AFT (msec; mean ± SD)	CAFT (msec; mean ± SD)	Percent excess AFT (mean ± SD)	AFT fraction (mean ± SD)
All coarctations (N = 56)	105.5 ± 36.3	134 ± 33.4	418.2 ± 201.4	510.4 ± 207.6	61.0 ± 58.2	67.0 ± 25.1
Native aortic coarctations (N = 19)	123.0 ± 37.3	160.7 ± 29.2	592.6 ± 197.1	733.6 ± 138.6	118.3 ± 45.2	92.4 ± 15.5
Immediately following BA (N = 20)	83.7 ± 29.6*	112.6 ± 24.9*	269.8 ± 114.3*	360.0 ± 90.2*	21.5 ± 28.0*	50.8 ± 8.6*
6–30 Months following BA (N = 17)	104.9 ± 25.8***	131.3 ± 26.6**	347.2 ± 93.6*	444.0 ± 146.5*	34.1 ± 39.2*	57.6 ± 25.0*

[a]AFT, antegrade flow time; AT, acceleration time; BA, balloon angioplasty; CAFT, corrected antegrade flow time; CAT, corrected acceleration time. (Reproduced from Rao and Carey [101], with permission of the publisher.)
*$P < 0.001$ compared with native coarctations prior to balloon angioplasty.
**$P < 0.01$ compared with native coarctations prior to balloon angioplasty.
***$P < 0.005$ compared with native coarctations prior to balloon angioplasty.

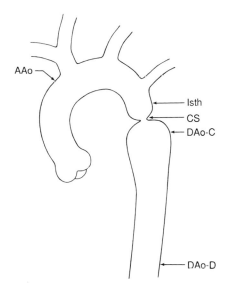

Fig. 26. Line drawing of the aorta to show the five locations from where the aortic measurements were obtained. AAo, ascending aorta immediately proximal to the origin of the right innominate artery; CS, coarcted segment; DAo-C, descending aorta distal to coarctation; DAo-D, descending aorta at diaphragm; Isth, aortic isthmus. (Reproduced from Rao and Carey [16], with permission of the publisher.)

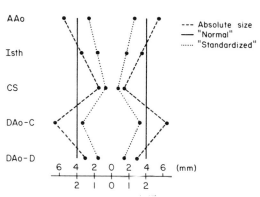

Fig. 27. A line drawing to demonstrate the method of obtaining standardized aortic measures. Absolute measurements (dashed lines) at all five locations (as detailed in Fig. 26) were averaged (represented by solid lines). The standardized aortic measure of each site was then calculated by dividing the absolute size by the average (mean) of all five measurements. The dotted lines represent the aortic shape, and the latter can be compared with those from other patients or those measured after an intervention. Abbreviations are as in Figure 26. (Reproduced from Rao and Carey [16], with permission of the publisher.)

0.129) they were different ($P = 0.01$). There was a greater percent improvement at follow-up (0.233 vs. 0.057) in group A with good results ($P = 0.002$) than in group B (0.287 vs. 0.129, $P = 0.04$) with fair and poor results (Table VII). Cluster analysis (Table VIII) and visual inspection of aortic shapes (Fig. 28) were also indicative of remodeling of the aorta in the group with good results. These data indicate a greater remodeling and normalization of the aorta following successful balloon angioplasty of aortic coarctation, suggesting that normalized flow across the dilated coarctation allows optimal growth of the aortic segments [16].

A quantitative analysis of angiographic data by Suarez de Lezo et al., [62] suggested a tendency to realignment as determined by a change in configuration angle between proximal and distal aortic segments following balloon angioplasty, and these data are supportive

of the remodeling of the aorta that we observed [16]. The data from Beekman et al. [30] showing improvement toward unity of the ratio of diameter of coarcted segment to isthmus diameter are also indicative of anatomic remodeling after balloon angioplasty.

Aneurysm Formation

The recommendations for use of balloon angioplasty as a treatment procedure of choice are clouded by the reports of development of aneurysms at the site of coarctation [26,27]. In this section, I will discuss issues related to development of aneurysms following balloon angioplasty and surgery for aortic coarctation.

To the best of my knowledge, aneurysms have not been reported after balloon angioplasty of native coarctation in the neonatal and infant (≤ 1 year) group. Detailed review of

TABLE VII. Nonparametric Comparison of Standardized Variance of Aortic Measures Between Groups[a]

Group	Preangioplasty median	Follow-up median	P value (Wilcoxan)
Group A	0.233	0.057	0.002
Group B	0.287	0.129	0.04
P value (Mann-Whitney)	0.08	0.01	

[a] Reproduced from Rao and Carey P [16], with permission of the publisher.

cases reported to have developed aneurysms [26–28,30,31,50,54,62] revealed that none of them were infants <1 year of age at the time of angioplasty. Also, the VACA Registry [65] did not have nay children <4 years of age in whom aneurysms developed. Although these data are encouraging in regard to lack of aneurysms in the infant group, longer term follow-up results than are currently available must be scrutinized before declaring this age group free from aneurysm development.

However, aneurysms at the site of balloon angioplasty have been reported with native coarctations in children >1 year of age [26–28,30,31,50,34,62]; a 6%–43% incidence has been reported by these workers. The reason for these differences in incidence are not clear. We postulated previously that development of aneurysms may reflect use of large balloons, inadvertent manipulation of catheters/guidewires in the region of freshly dilated aortic coarctation, and misinterpretation(Fig. 29) or overinterpretation of angiograms as possible causes. Other workers [31,62] also pointed out the potential problem of over- or misinterpre-

tation. Specific morphology of aortic coarctation (asymmetric in contrast to central) was also postulated [54] as a possible cause. The observation of Isner et al. [105] of severe depletion and disarray of elastic tissues (so-called cystic medial necrosis) in two-thirds of the resected aortic coarctation segments may give a pathologic basis for development of aneurysms, although such findings have not been supported as a cause of aneurysmal formation by others [106].

The aneurysms reported in the literature and that were observed by us (Fig. 30) are listed in Table III; there were 14 aneurysms out of a total of 130 patients, giving a 10.8% incidence. None of the patients with aneurysm required therapy, nor did any aneurysm rupture, although elective resection and repair were advocated by some workers [26,28]. The data available to date are limited with regard to the natural history of these aneurysms.

Both false aneurysms and true aneurysms have also been seen following surgical correction of aortic coarctation. Development of early false aneurysms appears to be unrelated to the

TABLE VIII. 2 × 2 Tables of Cluster Analysis (Anderberg) of Standardized Variance of Aortic Measures in Both Groups[a]

	Preangioplasty		Follow-up	
	Group A	Group B	Group A	Group B
Cluster 1	7	3	9	2
Cluster 2	6	4	4	4
P value[b]		0.4		0.025

[a]Reproduced from Rao et al. [16], with permission of the publisher.
[b]Chi square.

Schematic diagram of the aorta before and after treatment. Group A

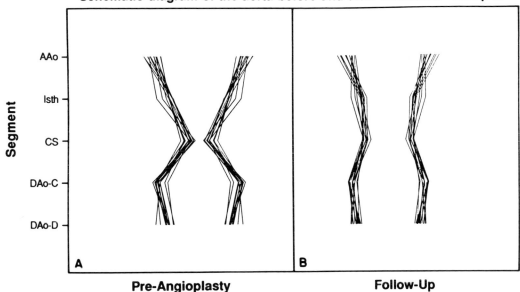

Pre-Angioplasty   **Follow-Up**

Schematic diagram of the aorta before and after treatment. Group B

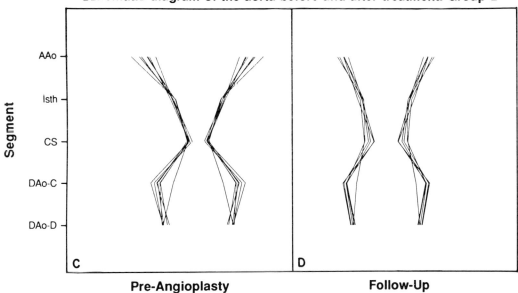

Pre-Angioplasty   **Follow-Up**

Fig. 28. Line drawings of the standardized aortic measurements in group A (**A,B**) and group B (**C,D**). Each pair of lines represents a single patient. Note that aortic shapes appear similar in both groups (A and C) before angioplasty. The shape of the aorta improved markedly in group A with good results (B), whereas in group B, the shape looked similar (D) to that before angioplasty (C). Abbreviations are as in Figure 26. (Reproduced from Rao and Carey [16], with permission of the publisher.)

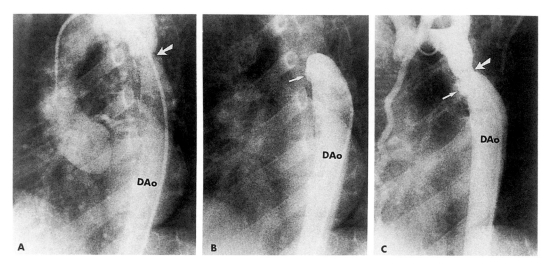

Fig. 29. A selected cine frame of an aortic root cineangiogram prior to **(A)** balloon angioplasty, showing coarctation (arrow). Repeat angiogram with the catheter tip close to the coarctation site revealed a better opacification of the area of coarctation **(B)**. Note the small area of bulging "aneurysm," marked by a small arrow. The same aneurysm was seen immediately after balloon angioplasty (not shown) and 8 months after angioplasty **(C)**. The small arrow points to the aneurysm, and the large arrow shows the site of coarctation. Had a better visualization of the area of coarctation (B) not been obtained, the aneurysm in C may have been interpreted to be the result of balloon angioplasty. DAo, descending aorta. (Reproduced from Rao *et al.* [11], with permission of the publisher.)

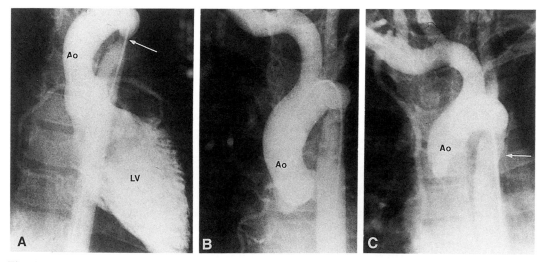

Fig. 30. A selected frame from a left ventricular (LV) cineangiogram prior to angioplasty showing prompt opacification of the aorta **(A)**. The site of the coarctation is marked with an arrow. An aortogram immediately following angioplasty **(B)** shows an excellent relief of the aortic coarctation. A repeat aortogram **(C)** 1 year following angioplasty shows a small bulge (arrow), interpreted as a small aneurysm. Ao, aorta.

type of coarctation repair [107,108] but appears to be related to the surgical technique or infection [109-111]. Late aneurysms have been well-documented following Dacron tube grafts and synthetic onlay patch grafts [112-122]. Although the exact etiology of these aneurysms is not known, compliance mismatch between the normal aortic wall and the synthetic patch [114-118], intimal resection [123], and translocated ductal tissue onto aortic wall [114,119,124] have been postulated as possible causes. A review of 10 studies [113-122] published since 1980 revealed an incidence of 5%-100% aneurysmal formation, with a mean of 13% (74 of 556 patients) following synthetic patch angioplasty of aortic coarctation. The true incidence is probably on the order of 24%, as observed by Bromberg et al. [119], who determined the prevalence rate prospectively and with objective, measurable criteria. Rapid progression of these aneurysms has been observed [125]. Sudden deaths secondary to rupture of the aneurysm have been reported [113,117,118]. Elective surgical repair of these aneurysms has been carried out with good success [113,115,117,118].

The prevalences of aneurysm following balloon angioplasty and Dacron patch angioplasty are similar, at 11% and 13% (Table III), respectively. Occurrence of aneurysms following resection with end-to-end anastomosis and subclavian flap angioplasty is also well documented [126,127], although the prevalence rate is not yet determined. Pinzon and associates [127] analyzed 215 angiograms of the aorta, performed 4.2 ± 4.1 years (range, 0.002-15.6 years) after surgical repair. These 215 patients represent 27% of the total population (796) undergoing coarctation repair at the Hospital for Sick Children in Toronto during a 13 year (1976-1988) period of their review. The indications for the study were associated cardiovascular malformations and clinical signs of residual or recoarctation. None were studied because of suspected aneurysms. Sixty-four of 215 patients (30%) were found to have aneurysms, defined as the ratio of the

repair site to the descending aorta at the level of diaphragm >1.5 [127]. The aneurysms consisted of diffuse enlargement in 20 patients, a focal anterior bulge in 24, and a focal posterior bulge in 20. The incidences of these aneurysms are similar in all three types of repair: 26 out of 97 (27%) with resection and end-to-end repair, 29 out of 92 (32%) with subclavian flap repair, and 9 out of 26 (35%) with synthetic patch repair. These data [127] clearly demonstrated that aneurysms do occur following all types of repair and that their prevalence is significant. However, the exact incidence remains to be determined, since only 27% of the total group undergoing coarctation repair were studied by the authors.

Irregularities of the region of the coarctation are frequently present [122], and these should be carefully scrutinized before ascribing "aneurysmal formation" to an interventional technique, whether it be surgical or balloon angioplasty. Furthermore, coarctation may not be an isolated arterial abnormality [128], but it may be a feature of a more generalized disease.

Intravascular Ultrasound

Cross-sectional images of the vessel wall can be obtained with an intravascular ultrasound catheter system (InterTherapy, Inc. Costa Mesa, CA). Luminal diameters and the architecture of the aortic wall proximal to, at, and distal to the coarctation segment prior to and after angioplasty can be obtained [129,130]. Intimal and medial disruption and intimal flaps can be identified. Limited experience in intravascular ultrasound imaging before and after balloon angioplasty of aortic recoarctation following previous surgery suggests that a more accurate assessment of arterial morphologic changes, not detected by conventional angiographic techniques, can be made with this technique [129,130]. Although intravascular ultrasound imaging has not to date been reported in native coarctation, there is every reason to believe that similar information as derived in recoarctation can be obtained in native aortic coarctations. However, the potential risk of injuring the freshly dilated site with multiple catheter exchanges that are required to record intravascular imaging should be kept in mind. Furthermore, controlled injury is what is intended by balloon angioplasty, and the value of documenting the same by intravascular ultrasound imaging should be determined. Further clinical trials on the utility and safety of this technique may be necessary prior to adapting it to general use.

SUMMARY AND CONCLUSIONS

The technique of balloon angioplasty of aortic coarctation has been available since 1983, and several workers have used this technique in native coarctations. Immediate- and intermediate-term follow-up results are generally good, with a small chance for recoarctation and aneurysmal formation at the site of coarctation. Echo-Doppler and NMR imaging techniques are useful adjuncts to cardiac catheterization and selective cineangiography in the evaluation of follow-up results.

The causes of recoarctation have been identified and include age <1 year, isthmus hypoplasia, and very small coarcted segment prior to and immediately after angioplasty. The aorta appears to remodel itself to approach a near-normal aortic shape following successful balloon angioplasty. Complications of the procedure are modest in degree, although arterial complications in the neonate and young infant may be significant.

Although good immediate and intermediate-term follow-up results of balloon angioplasty of aortic coarctation have been reported, recommendations for the use of this technique as a choice of treatment have been clouded by the reports of development of aneurysms at the site of coarctation dilatation. We feel that balloon coarctation angioplasty is the treatment of choice in the neonates and small infants, whereas general use of this technique in native coarctation in older children should await follow-up results in larger numbers of children at selected medical centers.

A substantial miniaturization of balloon catheter systems has taken place. Further miniaturization and improving rapidity of inflation–deflation of balloons are necessary for increasing the safety and effectiveness of this technique in infants and children. Meticulous attention to the details of the technique and to further refinements of the procedure are likely to reduce the complication rate further.

Despite the problems enumerated above, I consider balloon angioplasty to be an effective and safe alternative to surgical intervention for native aortic coarctation. Periodic reassessment of this recommendation is in order as more data are accumulated. In my opinion, the following data should be gathered in order to arrive at a final conclusion: First, longer term (5–10 years) follow-up data than are currently available should be collected after balloon coarctation angioplasty in a larger number of patients; second, such data should be compartmentalized into three separate groups, namely, neonates, infants aged 1–12 months, and children >1 year of age; third, the above subgroups, particularly the neonatal and infant groups, should be separated into those with isolated lesions and those with coarctations associated with cardiac defects; fourth, the causes and natural history of aneurysms occurring following balloon angioplasty should be investigated; fifth, actuarial evaluation of surgical versus balloon angioplasty is needed, including actuarial calculations of survival, time free of reintervention, and time free of complications; and, finally, multiinstitutional, preferably randomized, clinical trials should be attempted.

REFERENCES

1. Nadas AS, Fyler DC (1972): "Pediatric Cardiology," 3rd ed. Philadelphia: W.B. Saunders, p 683.
2. Keith JD, Rowe RD, Vlad P (1978): "Heart Disease in Infancy and Childhood," 3rd ed. New York: Macmillan Co, pp 4–6.
3. Gersony WM (1989): Coarctation of the aorta. In Adams FH, Emmanouilides GC, Riemenschneider TA (eds): "Moss' Heart Disease in Infants,

Children, and Adolescents," 4th ed. Baltimore: William & Wilkins, pp 243–255.

4. Sos T, Sniderman KW, Rettek-Sos B, Strupp A, Alonso DR (1979): Percutaneous transluminal dilatation of coarctation of thoracic aorta post mortem. Lancet 2:970–971.

5. Lock JE, Niemi T, Burke BA, Einzig S, Castaneda-Zuniga WR (1982): Transcutaneous angioplasty of experimental aortic coarctation. Circulation 66:1280–1286.

6. Lock JE, Castaneda-Zuniga WR, Bass JL, Foker JE, Amplatz K, Anderson RW (1982): Balloon dilatation of excised aortic coarctations. Radiology 143:689–692.

7. Castaneda-Zuniga WR, Lock JE, Vlodaver Z, Rusnak B, Rysavy JP, Herrera M, Amplatz K (1982): Transluminal dilatation of coarctation of the abdominal aorta: An experimental study in dogs. Radiology 143:693–697.

8. Rao PS, Mardini MK, Najjar HN (1986): Relief of coarctation of the aorta without thoracotomy: The experience with percutaneous balloon angioplasty. Ann Saudi Med 6:193–203.

9. Rao PS (1986): Transcatheter treatment of pulmonary stenosis and coarctation of the aorta: Experience with percutaneous balloon dilatation. Br Heart J 56:250–258.

10. Rao PS (1987): Balloon angioplasty for coarctation of the aorta in infancy. J Pediatr 110:713–718.

11. Rao PS, Najjar HN, Mardini MK, Solymar L, Thapar MK (1988): Balloon angioplasty for coarctation of the aorta: Immediate and long-term results. Am Heart J 115:657–664.

12. Rao PS (1988): Value of echo-Doppler studies in the evaluation of the results of balloon angioplasty of aortic coarctation. J Cardiovasc Ultrasonogr 7:215–220.

13. Rao PS, Solymar L (1988): Transductal balloon angioplasty for coarctation of the aorta in the neonate: Preliminary observations. Am Heart J 116:1558–1562.

14. Rao PS, Thapar MK, Kutayli F, Carey P (1989): Causes of recoarctation after balloon angioplasty of unoperated aortic coarctation. J Am Coll Cardiol 13:109–115.

15. Rao PS (1989): Balloon angioplasty of aortic coarctation: A review. Clin Cardiol 12:618–628.

16. Rao PS, Carey P (1989): Remodeling of the aorta following successful balloon coarctation angioplasty. J Am Coll Cardiol 14:1312–1317.

17. Rao PS (1989): Which aortic coarctations should we balloon-dilate? Am Heart J 117:787–789.

18. Rao PS, Thapar MK, Galal O, Wilson AD (1990): Follow-up results of balloon angioplasty of native coarctation in neonates and infants. Am Heart J 120:1310–1314.

19. Rao PS (1990): Causes of restenosis following balloon angioplasty/valvuloplasty: A review. Pediatr Rev Commun 4:157–172.

20. Rao PS (1990): Balloon angioplasty of native coarctations. Am J Cardiol 66:1401.

21. Rao PS (1991): Pseudoaneurysm following balloon angioplasty. Cathet Cardiovasc Diagn 23:150–153.

22. Rao PS (1991): Fatal aortic rupture following balloon angioplasty of aortic coarctation. Br Heart J 66:406–407.

23. Rao PS (1991): Balloon angioplasty of native aortic coarctation. Int J Cardiol 31:363–367.

24. Rao PS, Chopra PS (1991): Role of balloon angioplasty in the treatment of aortic coarctation. Ann Thorac Surg 52:621–631.

25. Salahuddin N, Wilson AD, Rao PS (1991): An unusual presentation of coarctation of the aorta in infancy: Role of balloon angioplasty in the critically ill infant. Am Heart J 122:1772–1775.

26. Cooper RS, Ritter SB, Rothe WB, Chen CK, Griepp R, Golinko RJ (1987): Angioplasty for coarctation of the aorta: Long-term results. Circulation 75:600–604.

27. Marvin WJ, Mahoney LT, Rose EF (1986): Pathologic sequelae of balloon dilation angioplasty for unoperated coarctation of the aorta in children, abstracted. J Am Coll Cardiol 7:117A.

28. Brandt B III, Marvin WJ Jr, Rose EF, Mahoney LT (1987): Surgical treatment of coarctation of the aorta after balloon angioplasty. J Thorac Cardiovasc Surg 94:715–719.

29. Lababidi ZA, Daskalopoulos DA, Stoeckle H Jr (1984): Transluminal balloon coarctation angioplasty: Experience with 27 patients. Am J Cardiol 54:1288–1291.

30. Beekman RH, Rocchini AP, Dick M II, Snider AR, Crowley DC, Serwer GA, Spicer RL, Rosenthal A (1987): Percutaneous balloon angioplasty for native coarctation of the aorta. J Am Coll Cardiol 10:1078–1084.

31. Morrow WR, Vick GW III, Nihill MR, Rokey R, Johnston DL, Hedrick TD, Mullins CE (1988): Balloon dilatation of unoperated coarctation of the aorta: Short- and intermediate-term results. J Am Coll Cardiol 11:133–138.

32. Kan JS, White RI Jr, Mitchell SE, Farmiett EJ, Donahoo JS, Gardner TJ (1983): Treatment of restenosis of coarctation by percutaneous transluminal angioplasty. Circulation 68:1087–1094.

33. Lock JE, Keane JF, Fellows KE (1986): The use of catheter intervention procedures for congenital heart disease. J Am Coll Cardiol 7:1420–1423.

34. Lock JE (1984): Now that we can dilate, should we? Am J Cardiol 54:1360.

35. Allen HD, Marx GR, Ovitt TW, Goldberg SJ

(1986): Balloon dilatation angioplasty for coarctation of the aorta. Am J Cardiol 57:828–832.

36. Lock JE, Bass JL, Amplatz K, Fuhrman BP,
Castaneda-Zuniga W (1983): Balloon dilation angioplasty of aortic coarctations in infants and children. Circulation 68:109–116.

37. Hess J, Mooyaart EL, Busch HJ, Bergstra A, Landsman MI (1986): Percutaneous transluminal balloon angioplasty in restenosis of coarctation of the
aorta. Br Heart J 55:459–461.

38. Lorber A, Ettedgui JA, Baker EJ, Jones ODH,
Reidy J, Tynan M (1986): Balloon aortoplasty for
recoarctation following the subclavian flap operation. Int J Cardiol 10:57–63.

39. Saul JP, Keane JF, Fellows KE, Lock JE (1987):
Balloon dilation angioplasty of postoperative aortic obstructions. Am J Cardiol 59:943–948.

40. Cooper SG, Sullivan ID, Wren C (1989): Treatment of recoarctation: Balloon dilation angioplasty. J Am Coll Cardiol 14:413–419.

41. Lo RNS, Leung MP, Yau KK, Cheung DLC
(1989): Transvenous antegrade balloon angioplasty for recoarctation of the aorta in an infant. Am
Heart J 117:1157–1158.

42. Hellenbrand WE, Allen HD, Golinko RJ, Hagler
DJ, Lutin W, Kan J (1990): Balloon angioplasty
for aortic recoarctation: Results of Valvuloplasty
and Angioplasty of Congenital Anomalies Registry. Am J Cardiol 65:793–797.

43. Rao PS, Wilson, AD, Chopra PS (1990): Immediate and follow-up results of balloon angioplasty of
postoperative recoarctation in infants and children. Am Heart J 120:1315–1320.

44. Liberthson RR, Pennington DG, Jacobs ML,
Daggett WM (1979): Coarctation of the aorta:
Review of 243 patients and clarification of man-
agement problems. Am J Cardiol 43:835–845.

45. Rao PS, Fawzy ME (1988): Double balloon technique for percutaneous balloon pulmonary
valvuloplasty: Comparison with single balloon
technique. J Interventional Cardiol 1:257–262.

46. Mullins CE, Nihill MR, Vick GW III, Ludomirsky
A, O'Laughlin MP, Bricker JT, Judd VE (1987):
Double balloon technique for dilation of valvular
or vessel stenosis in congenital and acquired heart
disease. J Am Coll Cardiol 10:107–114.

47. Beekman RH, Rocchini AP, Crowley DC, Snider
AR, Serwer GA, Dick M II, Rosenthal A (1988):
Comparison of single and double balloon
valvuloplasty in children with aortic stenosis. J Am
Coll Cardiol 12:480–485.

48. Rao PS, Thapar MK, Wilson AD, Levy JM,
Chopra PS (1989): Intermediate-term follow-up
results of balloon aortic valvuloplasty in infants
and children with special reference to causes of
restenosis. Am J Cardiol 64:1356–1360.

49. D'Souza VJ, Velasquez G, Weesner KM, Prabhu
S (1984): Transluminal angioplasty of aortic coarctation with a two-balloon technique. Am J Cardiol
54:457–458.

50. Wren C, Peart I, Bain H, Hunter S (1987): Bal-
loon dilatation of unoperated aortic coarctation:
Immediate results and one year follow-up. Br
Heart J 58:369–373.

51. Treacy EP, Duncan WJ, Tyrrell MJ, Lowry NJ
(1991): Neurological complications of balloon angioplasty in children. Pediatr Cardiol 12:98–101.

52. Rao PS: Neurologic complications following balloon angioplasty. Pediatr Cardiol (in press).

53. Pan M, Suarez de Lezo J, Herrera N, Sancho M,
Arizon J, Romero M, Franco M, Concha M,
Valles F, Romanos A (1987): Two-level left ventricular outflow balloon dilatation: Sequential therapeutic approach. Am Heart J 114:162–165.

54. Fontes VF, Esteves CA, Brago SLM, da Silva
MVD, e Silva MAP, Sousa EMR, de Souza
JAM (1990): It is valid to dilate native aortic
coarctation with a balloon catheter. Int J Cardiol
27:311–316.

55. Finley JP, Beaulieu RG, Nanton MA, Roy DL
(1983): Balloon catheter dilatation of coarctation
of the aorta in young infants. Br Heart J 50:411–
415.

56. Rao PS, Wilson AD, Brazy J (1992): Transumbilical balloon angioplasty for the neonate with aortic
coarctation. Am Heart J 124:1622–1624.

57. Beekman RH, Rocchini AP, Andes A (1991):
Balloon valvuloplasty for critical aortic stenosis in
the newborn: Influence of new catheter technology. J Am Coll Cardiol 17:1172–1176.

58. Al Yousef S, Khan A, Nihill M, Lababidi Z,
Mullins C (1988): Perkutane transvenose ange-
grade Ballonangioplastie bei Aortenisthmusstenose. Herz 13:36–40.

59. Lababidi Z (1983): Neonatal transluminal balloon
coarctation angioplasty. Am Heart J 106:752–753.

60. Sperling DR, Dorsey TJ, Rowen M, Gazzaniga AB
(1983): Percutaneous transluminal angioplasty of
congenital coarctation of the aorta. Am J Cardiol
51:562–564.

61. Suarez de Lezo J, Fernandez R, Sancho M, et al.
(1984): Percutaneous transluminal angioplasty for
aortic isthmic coarctation in infancy. Am J Cardiol
54:1147–1149.

62. Suarez de Lezo J, Sancho M, Pan M, Romero M,
Olivera C, Luque M (1989): Angiographic follow-
up after balloon angioplasty for coarctation of the
aorta. J Am Coll Cardiol 13:689–695.

63. Redington AN, Booth P, Shore DF, Rigby ML
(1990): Primary balloon dilatation of coarctation
of the aorta in neonates. Br Heart J 64:277–281.

64. Osman K (1990): Percutaneous balloon angioplas-

ty for the coarctation of the aorta in neonates and children. Radiogr Today 56:14-17.

65. Tynan M, Finley JP, Fontes V, Hess J, Kan J (1990): Balloon angioplasty for the treatment of native coarctation: Results of valvuloplasty and angioplasty of congenital anomalies registry. Am J Cardiol 65:790-792.

66. Cooper RS, Ritter SB, Golinko RJ (1984): Balloon dilation angioplasty: Nonsurgical management of coarctation of the aorta. Circulation 70:903-907.

67. Brodsky SJ (1984): Percutaneous balloon angioplasty: Treatment for congenital coarctation of the aorta and congenital valval pulmonic stenosis. Am J Dis Child 138:851-854.

67a. Minich LL, Beekman RH, Rocchini AP, Heidelberger K, Bove EL (1992): Surgical repair is safe and effective after unsuccessful balloon angioplasty of native coarctation of the aorta. J Am Coll Cardiol 19:389-393.

67b. Rao PS (1992): Balloon Angioplasty of Native aortic coarctation. J Am Coll Cardiol 20:749-752.

68. Lababidi Z, Madigan N, Wu J, Murphy TJ (1984): Balloon coarctation angioplasty in an adult. Am J Cardiol 53:350-351.

69. Attia IM, Lababidi ZA (1988): Early results of balloon angioplasty of native aortic coarctations in young adults. Am J Cardiol 61:930-931.

70. Erbel R, Bednarezyk I, Pop T, Todt M, Henrichs KJ, Brunier A, Thelen M, Meyer J (1990): Detection of dissection of the aortic intima and media after angioplasty of coarctation of the aorta. Circulation 81:805-814.

71. Fawzy MF, Dunn B, Gulal O, Wilson N, Shaikh A, Sriram R, Duran CMG (1992): Balloon coarctation angioplasty in adolescents and adults: Early and intermediate results. Am Heart J 124:167-171.

72. Tyagi S, Arora R, Kaul UA, Sethi KK, Gambhir DS, Khalilullah M (1992): Balloon angioplasty of native coarctation of the aorta in adolescents and young adults. Am Heart J 123:674-680.

72a. Kulick DL, Kotlewski A, Hurvitz RJ, Jamison M, Rahimtoola SH (1990): Aortic rupture following percutaneous catheter balloon coarctoplasty in an adult. Am Heart J 119:190-193.

73. Velasquez G, Castaneda-Zuniga W, Formaneck A, Zollikofer C, Barrelo A, Nicoloff D, Amplatz K, Sullivan A (1980): Nonsurgical aortoplasty in Leriche syndrome. Radiology 134:359-360.

74. Grollman JH, Del Vicario M, Mittak AK (1980): Percutaneous transluminal abdominal aortic angioplasty. Am J Radiol 134:1053-1054.

75. Tegtmeyer CJ, Wellons HA, Thompson RN (1980): Balloon dilatation of the abdominal aorta. J Am Med Assoc 244:2636-2637.

76. Khalilullah M, Tyagi S, Lochan R, Yadav BS, Nair M, Gambhir DS, Khanna SK (1987): Percutaneous transluminal balloon angioplasty of the aorta in patients with aortitis. Circulation 76:597-600.

77. Yakes WF, Kumpe DA, Brown SB, Parker SH, Lattes RG, Cook PS, Haas DK, Gibson MD, Hopper KD, Reed MD, Cox HE, Bourne EE, Griffin DJ. (1989): Percutaneous transluminal aortic angioplasty: Techniques and results. Radiology 172:965-970.

78. Yagura M, Sano I, Akioka H, Hayashi M, Uchida H (1984): Usefulness of percutaneous transluminal angioplasty for aortitis syndrome. Arch Intern Med 144:1465-1468.

79. Park JH, Han MC, Kim SH, Oh BH, Park YB, Seo JD (1989): Takayasu arteritis: Angiographic findings and results of angioplasty. Am J Radiology 153:1069-1074.

80. Kumar S, Mandalam KR, Rao VRK, Subramanyan R, Gupta AK, Joseph S, Unni M, Rao AS (1989): Percutaneous transluminal angioplasty in nonspecific aortoarteritis (Takayasu's disease): Experience of 16 cases. Cardiovasc Intervent Radiol 12:321-325.

81. Dev V, Shrivastava S, Rajani M (1990): Percutaneous transluminal balloon angioplasty in Takayasu's aortitis: Persistent benefit over two years. Am Heart J 120:222-224.

82. Todd PJ, Dangerfield PH, Hamilton DI, Wilkinson JL (1983): Late effects on the left upper limb of subclavian flap aortoplasty. J Thorac Cardiovasc Surg 85:678-681.

83. Shenberger JS, Prophet SA, Waldhausen JA, Davidson WR Jr, Sinoway LI (1989): Left subclavian flap aortoplasty for coarctation of the aorta: Effects on forearm vascular function and growth. J Am Coll Cardiol 14:953-959.

84. Van Son JAM, Van Asten WNJC, Van Lier HJJ, Daniels O, Vincent JG, Skotnicki SH, Lacquet LK (1990): Detrimental sequelae on the hemodynamics of upper left limb after subclavian flap angioplasty in infancy. Circulation 81:996-1004.

85. Kittle CF, Schafer PW (1953): Gangrene of the forearm after subclavian arterio-aortostomy for coarctation of the aorta. Thorax 8:319-322.

86. Geiss D, Williams WG, Lindsay WK, Rowe RD (1980): Upper extremity gangrene: A complication of subclavian artery division. Ann Thorac Surg 30:487-489.

87. Hagemo PS, Birnstad PG, Smevik B, Foerster A (1988): Aortic wall lesion in balloon dilatation of coarctation of the aorta. Eur Heart J 9:1271-1273.

88. Krabill KA, Bass JL, Lucas RV Jr, Edwards JE (1987): Dissecting transverse aortic arch aneurysm after percutaneous transluminal balloon dilatation angioplasty of an aortic coarctation. Pediatr Cardiol 8:39-42.

89. Booth P, Redington AN, Shinebourne EA, Rigby ML (1991): Early complications of interventional balloon catheterization in infants and children. Br Heart J 65:109–112.

90. Choy M, Rocchini AP, Beekman RH, Rosenthal A, Dick M, Crowley D, Behrendt D, Snider AR (1987): Paradoxical hypertension after repair of coarctation of the aorta in children: balloon angioplasty versus surgical repair. Circulation 75:1186–1191.

91. Lewis AB, Takahashi M (1988): Plasma catecholamine responses to balloon angioplasty in children with coarctation of the aorta. Am J Cardiol 62:649–650.

92. Galal O, Qureshi SA, Al Halees Z (1990): Reopening of the arterial duct after balloon dilatation of native coarctation. Int J Cardiol 27:133–135.

93. Pavlovic D, Suarez de Lezo J, Medina A, Romero M, Hernandez E, Pan M, Tejero I, Melian F (1992): Sequential transcatheter treatment of combined coarctation of aorta and persistent ductus arteriosus. Am Heart J 123:249–250.

94. Wessel DL, Keane JF, Fellows KE, Robichaud H, Lock JE (1986): Fibrinolytic therapy for femoral arterial thrombosis after cardiac catheterization in infants and children. Am J Cardiol 58:347–351.

95. Burrows PE, Benson LN, Williams WG, Trusler GA, Coles J, Smallhorn JF, Freedom RM (1990): Iliofemoral arterial complication of balloon angioplasty for systemic obstructions in infants and children. Circulation 82:1697–1704.

96. Rocchini AP, Beekman RH, Ben Shachar G, Benson L, Schwartz D, Kan JS (1990): Balloon aortic valvuloplasty: Results of the Valvuloplasty and Angioplasty of Congenital Anomalies Registry. Am J Cardiol 65:784–789.

97. Rothman A (1990): Arterial complications of interventional cardiac catheterization in patients with congenital heart disease. Circulation 82:1868–1871.

98. Martin GR, Stanger P (1986): Transient prolongation of the QTc interval after balloon valvuloplasty and angioplasty in children. Am J Cardiol 58:1232–1235.

99. Kveselis DA, Rocchini AP, Snider AP, Rosenthal A, Crowley DC, Dick M (1985): Results of balloon valvuloplasty in the treatment of congenital valvar pulmonary stenosis in children. Am J Cardiol 56:527–532.

100. Fellows KE, Radtke W, Keane JF, Lock JE (1987): Acute complications of catheter therapy for congenital heart disease. Am J Cardiol 60:679–683.

101. Rao PS, Carey P (1989): Doppler ultrasound in the prediction of pressure gradients across aortic coarctation. Am Heart J 118:299–307.

102. Boxer RA, LaCorte MA, Singh S, Cooper R, Fishman MC, Goldman M, Stein HL (1986): Nuclear magnetic resonance imaging in evaluation and follow-up of children treated for coarctation of the aorta. J Am Coll Cardiol 7:1095–1098.

103. Bank ER, Aisen AM, Rocchini AP, Hernandez RJ (1987): Coarctation of the aorta in children undergoing angioplasty: Pretreatment and posttreatment MR imaging. Radiology 162:235–240.

104. Anderberg MR (1973): "Cluster Analysis for Applications." New York: Academic Press.

105. Isner JM, Donaldson RF, Fulton D, Bhan I, Payne DD, Cleveland RJ (1987): Cystic medial necrosis in coarctation of the aorta: A potential factor contributing to adverse consequences observed after percutaneous balloon angioplasty of coarctation sites. Circulation 75:689–695.

106. Ho SY, Somerville J, Yip WCL, Anderson RH (1988): Transluminal balloon dilatation of resected coarcted segments of thoracic aorta: Histologic study and clinical implications. Int J Cardiol 19:99–105.

107. Crafoord C, Elrup B, Gladnikoff H (1947): Coarctation of the aorta. Thorax 2:121–147.

108. Olsson P, Soderland S, Dabiel WT, Ovenfors CO (1976): Patch grafts or tabular grafts in repair of coarctation of the aorta. Scand J Thorac Cardiovasc Surg 10:139–143.

109. Davis DB, Fell EH, Taylor CB (1965): Postoperative aneurysm following surgery for coarctation of the aorta. Surg Gynecol Obstet 121:1043–1048.

110. Callard GM, Wright CB, Wray RC, Minor GER (1971): False aneurysm due to macromycosis following repair of coarctation with Dacron prosthesis. J Thorac Cardiovasc Surg 61:181–185.

111. Kirsh MM, Perry B, Spooner E (1977): Management of pseudoaneurysm following patch grafting for coarctation of the aorta. J Thorac Cardiovasc Surg 74:636–639.

112. McGoldrick JP, Brown IW, Ross DN (1988): Coarctation of the aorta: Late aneurysm formation with Dacron only patch grafting. Ann Thorac Surg 45:89–90.

113. Bergdahl L, Ljunqvist A (1980): Long-term results after repair of coarctation of the aorta by patch grafting. J Thorac Cardiovasc Surg 80:177–181.

114. Clarkson PM, Brandt PWT, Barratt-Boyers BG, Rutherford JD, Kerr AR, Neutze JM (1985): Prosthetic repair of coarctation of the aorta with particular reference to Dacron onlay patch grafts and late aneurysm formation. Am J Cardiol 56:342–346.

115. del Nido PJ, Williams WG, Wilson GJ, Coles JG, Moes CAF, Hosokawa Y, McLaughlin PR, Fowler RS, Izukawa T, Rowe RD, Trusler GA (1986): Synthetic patch angioplasty for repair of coarctation of the aorta: Experience with aneurysm formation. Circulation 74:132–136.

116. Rheuban K, Gutgesell HP, Carpenter MA, Jedeikin R, Damman JF, Kron IL, Wellons J, Nolan SP (1986): Aortic aneurysms after patch angioplasty for aortic isthmic coarctation in childhood. Am J Cardiol 58:178-180.

117. Hehrlein FW, Mulch J, Rautenburg HW, Schlepper M, Scheld HH (1986): Incidence and pathogenesis of late aneurysms after patch graft aortoplasty for coarctation. J Thorac Cardiovasc Surg 92:226-230.

118. Ala-Kalju K, Heikkinen L (1989): Aneurysms after patch graft aortoplasty for coarctation of the aorta: long-term results of surgical management. Ann Thorac Surg 47:853-856.

119. Bromberg BI, Beekman RH, Rocchini AP, Snider AR, Bank ER, Heidelberger K, Rosenthal A (1989): Aortic aneurysm after patch aortoplasty repair of coarctation: A prospective analysis of prevalence, screening tests and risks. J Am Coll Cardiol 14:734-741.

120. Kron IL, Flanagan TL, Rheuban KS, Carpenter MA, Gutgesell HP Jr, Blackbourne LH, Nolan SP (1990): Incidence and risk of reintervention after coarctation repair. Ann Thorac Surg 49:920-926.

121. Malan JE, Benatar A, Levin SE (1991): Long-term follow-up of coarctation of the aorta repaired by patch angioplasty. Int J Cardiol 30:23-32.

122. Parik SR, Hurwitz RA, Hubbard JE, Brown JW, King H, Girod DA (1991): Preoperative and postoperative "aneurysm" associated with coarctation of the aorta. J Am Coll Cardiol 17:1367-1372.

123. DeSanto A, Bills RG, King H, Waller B, Brown JW (1987): Pathogenesis of aneurysm formation opposite prosthetic patches used for coarctation repair: An experimental study. J Thorac Cardiovasc Surg 94:721-723.

124. Ho SY, Anderson RH (1979): Coarctation, tabular hypoplasia, and ductus arteriosus: Histologic study of 35 patients. Br Heart J 41:268-274.

125. Mendelsohn AM, Crowley DC, Lindauer A, Beekman RH (1992): Rapid progression of aortic aneurysms after patch aortoplasty repair of coarctation of the aorta. J Am Coll Cardiol 20:381-385.

126. Martin MM, Beekman RH, Rocchini AP, Crowley DC, Rosenthal A (1988): Aortic aneurysms after subclavian angioplasty repair of coarctation of the aorta. Am J Cardiol 61:951-953.

127. Pinzon JL, Burrows PE, Benson LN, Moës CAF, Lightfoot NE, Williams WG, Freedom RM (1991): Repair of coarctation of the aorta in children: Postoperative morphology. Radiology 180:199-203.

128. Mitchell IM, Pollock JCS (1990): Coarctation of the aorta and post-stenotic aneurysmal formation. Br Heart J 64:332-333.

129. Harrison JK, Sheikh KH, Davidson CJ, Kisslo KB, Leithe ME, Himmelstein SI, Kantor RJ, Bashore TM (1990): Balloon angioplasty of coarctation of the aorta evaluated with intravascular ultrasound imaging. J Am Coll Cardiol 15:906-909.

130. Jain A, Ramee SR, Culpeper WR, Mesa JE, Murgo JP, White CJ (1992): Intravascular ultrasound-assisted percutaneous angioplasty of aortic coarctation. Am Heart J 123:514-515.

APPENDIX I

Results of surgery for native aortic coarctation in neonates and infants: 49 papers published since 1980.

1. Beerman LB, Neches WH, Patnode RE, Fricker FJ, Mathews RA, Park SC (1980): Coarctation of the aorta in children: Late results after surgery. Am J Dis Child 134:464-466.

2. Fyler DC, Buckley LP, Hellenbrand WE, Cohn HE (1980): Report of the New England Regional Infant Cardiac Program. Pediatrics 65(Suppl):375-461.

3. Williams WG, Shindo G, Trusler GA, Dische MR, Olley PM (1980): Results of repair of coarctation of the aorta during infancy. J Thorac Cardiovasc Surg 79:603-608.

4. Campbell J, Delorenzi R, Brown J, Girod D, Hurwitz R, Caldwell R, King H (1980): Improved results in newborns undergoing coarctation repair. Ann Thorac Surg 30:273-280.

5. Kamau P, Miles V, Toews W, Kelminson L, Friesen R, Lockhart C, Butterfield J, Hernandez J, Hawes CR, Pappas G (1981): Surgical repair of coarctation of the aorta in infants less than six months of age including the question of pulmonary artery banding. J Thorac Cardiovasc Surg 81:171-179.

6. Hesslein PS, McNamara DG, Morris MJH, Hallman GL, Cooley DA (1981): Comparison of resection versus patch aortoplasty for repair of coarctation in infants and children. Circulation 64:164-168.

7. Leanage R, Taylor JFN, de Leval MR, Stark J, Macartney FJ (1981): Surgical management of coarctation of the aorta with ventricular septal defect: Multivariate analysis. Br Heart J 46:269-277.

8. Lerberg DB, Hardesty RL, Siewers RD, Zuberbuhler JR, Bahnson HT (1982): Coarctation of the aorta in infants and children: 25 years of experience. Ann Thorac Surg 33:159-170.

9. Bergdahl LAL, Blackstone EH, Kirklin JW, Pacifico AD, Bargeron LM Jr (1982): Determinants of early success in repair of aortic coarctation in infants. J Thorac Cardiovasc Surg 83:736-742.

10. Waldman JD, Lamberti JJ, Goodman AH, Mathewson JW, Kirkpatrick SE, George L, Turner SW, Pappelbaum SJ (1983): Coarctation of the aorta in

the first year of life: Patterns of postoperative effect. J Thorac Cardiovasc Surg 86:9-17.

11. Nair VK, Jones O, Walker DR (1983): Surgical management of severe coarctation of the aorta in the first month of life: Review of 48 consecutive cases. J Thorac Cardiovasc Surg 86:587-590.

12. Harlan JL, Doty DB, Brandt B III, Ehrenhaft JL (1984): Coarctation of the aorta in infants. J Thorac Cardiovasc Surg 88:1012-1019.

13. Moulton AL, Brenner JL, Roberts G, Tavares S, Ali S, Nordenberg A, Burns JE, Ringel R, Berman MA, McLaughlin JS (1984): Subclavian flap repair of coarctation of the aorta in neonates: Realization of growth potential. J Thorac Cardiovasc Surg 87:220-235.

14. Penkoske PA, Williams WG, Olley PM, LeBlanc J, Trusler GA, Moes CAF, Judakin R, Rowe RD (1984): Subclavian anterioplasty: Repair of coarctation of the aorta in the first year of life. J Thorac Cardiovasc Surg 87:894-900.

15. Schumacher G, Peters DR, Schreiber R, Meisner H, Heimisch W, Sebening F, Bühlmeyer K (1984): Isolated coarctation of the aorta: Indication for surgery and results. Herz 9:362-370.

16. Campbell DB, Waldhausen JA, Pierce WS, Fripp R, Whitman V (1984): Should elective repair of coarctation of the aorta be done in infancy? J Thorac Cardiovasc Surg 88:929-938.

17. Cobanoglu A, Teply JF, Grunkemeier GL, Sunderland CO, Starr A (1985): Coarctation of the aorta in patients younger than three months: A critique of the subclavian flap operation. J Thorac Cardiovasc Surg 89:128-135.

18. Körfer R, Meyer H, Kleikamp G, Bricks W (1985): Early and late results after resection and end-to-end anastomosis of coarctation of the thoracic aorta in early infancy. J Thorac Cardiovasc Surg 89:616-622.

19. Pennington DG, Dennis HM, Swartz MT, Nouri S, Chen S, Azzam F, Schweiss JF (1985): Repair of aortic coarctation in infants: Experience with intraluminal shunt. Ann Thorac Surg 40:35-40.

20. Palatianos GM, Kaiser GA, Thurer RJ, Garcia O (1985): Changing trends in the surgical treatment of coarctation of the aorta. Ann Thorac Surg 40:41-45.

21. Kopf GS, Hellenbrand W, Kleinman C, Lister G, Talner N, Laks H (1986): Repair of aortic coarctation in the first three months of life: Immediate and long-term results. Ann Thorac Surg 41:425-430.

22. Beekman RH, Rocchini AP, Behrendt DM, Bove EL, Dick M, II, Crowley DC, Snider AR, Rosenthal A (1986): Long-term outcome after repair of coarctation in infancy: Subclavian angioplasty does not reduce the need for reoperation. J Am Coll Cardiol 8:1406-1411.

23. Ziemer G, Jonas RA, Perry SB, Freed MD,

Castaneda AR (186): Surgery for coarctation of the aorta in the neonate. Circulation 74:1-25-1-31.

24. Sanchez GR, Balsara RK, Dunn JM, Mehta AV, O'Riordan AC (1986): Recurrent obstruction after subclavian flap repair of coarctation of the aorta in infants: Can it be predicted or prevented? J Thorac Cardiovasc Surg 91:738-746.

25. Goldman S, Hernandez J, Pappas G (1986): Results of surgical treatment of coarctation of the aorta in the critically ill neonate: Including the influence of pulmonary artery banding. J Thorac Cardiovasc Surg 91:732-737.

26. Hehrlein FW, Mulch J, Rautenburg HW, Schlepper M, Scheld HH (1986): Incidence and pathogenesis of late aneurysms after patch graft aortoplasty for coarctation. J Thorac Cardiovasc Surg 92:226-230.

27. Yee ES, Soifer SJ, Turley K, Verrier ED, Fishman NH, Ebert PA (1986): Infant coarctation: A spectrum in clinical presentation and treatment. Ann Thorac Surg 42:488-493.

28. Kirklin JW, Barratt-Boyes BG (1986): "Cardiac Surgery." New York: John Wiley & Sons, pp 1036-1080.

29. Lansman S, Shapiro AJ, Schiller MS, Ritter S, Cooper R, Galla JD, Lowery RC, Golinko R, Ergin A, Griepp RB (1986): Extended aortic arch anastomosis for repair of coarctation in infancy. Circulation 74(Suppl I):37-41.

30. Palatianos GM, Thurer RJ, Kaiser GA (1987): Comparison of operations for coarctation of the aorta in infants. J Cardiovasc Surg 28:128-131.

31. Koller M, Rothlin M, Senning A (1987): Coarctation of the aorta: Review of 362 operated patients. Long-term follow-up and assessment of prognostic variables. Eur Heart J 8:670-679.

32. Mellgran G, Friberg LG, Eriksson BO, Sabel K, Mellander M (1987): Neonatal surgery for coarctation of the aorta: The Gothenburg experience. Scand J Thorac Cardiovasc Surg 21:193-197.

33. Fenchel G, Steil E, Seybold-Epting W, Seboldt H, Apitz J, Hoffmeister H (1988): Repair of symptomatic aortic coarctation in the first three months of life: Early and late results after resection and end-to-end anastomosis and subclavian flap angioplasty. J Cardiovasc Surg 29:257-263.

34. Vouhe PR, Trinquet F, Lecompte Y, Vemant F, Roux P, Touati G, Pome G, Leca F, Neveux J (1988): Aortic coarctation with hypoplastic aortic arch: Results of extended end-to-end aortic arch anastomosis. J Thorac Cardiovasc Surg 96:557-563.

35. Trinquet F, Vouhe PR, Vernant F, Touati G, Roux P, Rome G, Leca F, Neveux J (1988): Coarctation of the aorta in infants: Which operation? Ann Thorac Surg 45:186-191.

36. Hopkins RA, Kostic I, Klages U, Armiru U, de Leval M, Sullivan I, Wyse R, McCartney F, Stark J (1988):

Correction of coarctation of the aorta in the neonates and young infants: An individualized surgical approach. Eur J Cardio-Thorac Surg 2:296-304.

37. Yamaguchi M, Tachibana H, Hosokawa Y, Ohashi H, Oshima Y (1989): Early and late results of surgical treatment of coarctation of the aorta in the first three months of life. J Cardiovasc Surg 30:169-172.

38. Ladusans EJ, Campalani G, Parsons JM, Qureshi SA, Opie J, Baker EJ, Tynan M, Deverall PB (1989): Recurrence of aortic coarctation following repair by reimplantation of the subclavian artery. Int J Cardiol 2:321-325.

39. Rostad H, Abdelnoor M, Sørland S, Tjønneland S (1989): Coarctation of the aorta, early and late results of various surgical techniques. J Cardiovasc Surg 30:885-890.

40. Ehrhard EP, Walker DR (1989): Coarctation of the aorta corrected during the first month of life. Arch Dis Child 64:330-332.

41. Baudet E, Al-Qudah A (1989): Late results of the subclavian flap repair of coarctation in infancy. J Cardiovasc Surg 30:445-449.

42. Lacour-Gayet F, Bruniaux J, Serraf A, Chambran P, Blaysat G, Lossy J, Petit J, Kachaner J, Planché C (1990): Hypoplastic transverse arch and coarctation in neonates. J Thorac Cardiovasc Surg 100:808-816.

43. Kron IL, Flanagan TL, Rheuban KS, Carpenter MA, Gutgesell HP, Blackbourne LH, Nolan SP (1990): Incidence and risk of reintervention after coarctation repair. Ann Thorac Surg 49:920-926.

44. Sciolaro C, Copeland J, Cork R, Barkenbush M, Donnerstein R, Goldberg S (1991): Long-term follow-up comparing subclavian flap angioplasty to resection with modified oblique end-to-end anastomosis. J Thorac Cardiovasc Surg 101:1-13.

45. Malan JE, Benatar A, Levin SE (1991): Long-term follow-up of coarctation of the aorta repaired by patch angioplasty. Int J Cardiol 30:23-32.

46. Shrivastava CP, Monro JL, Shore DF, Lamb RK, Sutherland GR, Fong LV, Keeton BR (1991): The early and long-term results of surgery for coarctation of the aorta in the 1st year of life. Eur J Cardio-Thorac Surg 5:61-66.

47. Amato JJ, Galdieri RJ, Cotroneo JV (1991): Role of extended aortoplasty related to the definition of coarctation of the aorta. Ann Thorac Surg 52:615-620.

48. Messmer BJ, Minale C, Mühler E, Bernuth GV (1991): Surgical correction of coarctation in early infancy: Does surgical technique influence the results? Ann Thorac Surg 52:594-603.

49. Siewers RD, Ettedgui J, Pahl E, Tallman T, del Nido PJ (1991): Coarctation and hypoplasia of the aortic arch: Will the arch grow? Ann Thorac Surg 52:608-614.

APPENDIX II

Results of surgery for native aortic coarctation in children: 16 papers published since 1980.

1. Beerman LB, Neches WH, Patnode RE, Fricker FJ, Mathews RA, Park SC (1980): Coarctation of the aorta in children: Late results after surgery. Am J Dis Child 134:464-466.

2. Hesslein PS, McNamara DG, Morris MJH, Hallman GL, Cooley DA (1981): Comparison of resection versus patch aortoplasty for repair of coarctation in infants and children. Circulation 64:164-168.

3. Hamilton DI, Medici D, Dickinson DF (1981): Aortoplasty with the left subclavian flap in older children. J Thorac Cardiovasc Surg 82:103-106.

4. Lerberg DB, Hardesty RL, Siewers RD, Zuberbuhler JR, Bahnson HT (1982): Coarctation of the aorta in infants and children: 25 years of experience. Ann Thorac Surg 33:159-170.

5. Bergdahl L, Bjork VO, Jonasson R (1983): Surgical correction of coarctation of the aorta: Influence of age on late results. J Thorac Cardiovasc Surg 85:532-536.

6. Clarkson PM, Nicholson MR, Barratt-Boyes BG, Neutze JM, Whitlock RM (1983): Results after repair of coarctation of the aorta beyond infancy: A 10 to 28 year follow-up with particular reference to late systemic hypertension. Am J Cardiol 51:1481-1488.

7. Schumacher G, Peters DR, Schreiber R, Meisner H, Heimisch W, Sebening F, Bühlmeyer (1984): Isolated coarctation of the aorta: Indication for surgery and results. Herz 9:362-370.

8. Palatinos GM, Kaiser GA, Thurer RJ, Garcia O (1985): Changing trends in the surgical treatment of coarctation of the aorta. Ann Thorac Surg 40:41-45.

9. Hehrlein FW, Mulch J, Rautenburg HW, Schlepper M, Scheld HH (1986): Incidence and pathogenesis of late aneurysms after patch graft aortoplasty for coarctation. J Thorac Cardiovasc Surg 92:226-230.

10. Kirklin JW, Barratt-Boyes BG (1986): "Cardiac Surgery." New York: John Wiley & Sons, pp 1036-1080.

11. Koller M, Rothlin M, Senning A (1987): Coarctation of the aorta: Review of 362 operated patients. Long-term follow-up and assessment of prognostic variables. Eur Heart J 8:670-679.

12. Presbitero P, Demarie D, Villani M, Perinetto EA, Riva G, Orzan F, Bobbio M, Morea M, Brusca A (1987): Long term results (15-30 years) of surgical repair of aortic coarctation. Br Heart J 57:462-467.

13. Behl PR, Sante P, Blesovsky A (1987): Surgical treatment of isolated coarctation of the aorta: 18 years' experience. Thorax 42:309–314.

14. Rostad H, Abdelnoor M, Sørland S, Tjønneland S (1989): Coarctation of the aorta, early and late results of various surgical techniques. J Cardiovasc Surg 30:885–890.

15. Kron IL, Flanagan TL, Rheuban KS, Carpenter MA, Gutgesell HP, Blackbourne LH, Nolan SP (1990): Incidence and risk of reintervention after coarctation repair. Ann Thorac Surg 49:920–926.

16. Malan JE, Benatar A, Levin SE (1991): Long-term follow-up of coarctation of the aorta repaired by patch angioplasty. Int J Cardiol 30:23–32.

11

Balloon Angioplasty for Aortic Recoarctation Following Previous Surgery

P. Syamasundar Rao, M.D.

Department of Pediatrics, Division of Pediatric Cardiology,
University of Wisconsin Medical School, University of Wisconsin
Children's Hospital, Madison, Wisconsin 53792-4108

INTRODUCTION

Aortic recoarctation following previous surgery may be due to either significant residua or development of restenosis. Since a distinction between these two types cannot always be made, the term *recoarctation* encompasses both of these types and will be so used in this chapter. Recoarctation occurs irrespective of age at surgical repair. However, the younger the child at surgery, the higher is the chance for recurrence. In the previous chapter on balloon angioplasty of native aortic coarctation, surgical experience with aortic coarctation was reviewed [1]. In neonates and infants <1 year of age, the average recoarctation rate was 17% when 49 papers published after 1980 were reviewed (see Appendix I, Chapter 10, this volume). When 11 papers reporting on surgery performed between 1979 and 1991 were analyzed, the average recurrence rate was 11.4%. In children >1 year of age, the recurrence rate varied from 0%–18%, with an average of 5.6% (see Appendix II, Chapter 10, this volume). Since a substantial proportion of these patients were not catheterized, it is likely that the recoarctation rate is much higher.

When Pinzon and associates [2] restudied 215 children a mean of 4.2 years after coarctation surgery, there were 150 children who had significant obstruction; two-thirds were thought to be secondary to hypoplasia of the arch of the aorta and isthmus, and the remaining one-third, constituting 23% of the total group, had recoarctation. Development of recoarctation is independent of the type of surgical repair used [3–9]; it has been reported following resection with end-to-end anastomosis, subclavian flap repair, prosthetic patch repair, subclavian turn-down procedures, and interposition tube grafts. The causes of recoarctation are not clearly understood, and many hypotheses have been advanced, including technically inadequate repair (including failure to resect obstructive intimal ridge); hypoplasia of the aortic segment proximal to the repair site; presence of left ventricular outflow tract obstruction; lack of growth of suture line; presence of abnormal mesodermal or ductal tissue that may proliferate and cause marked intimal and medial hypertrophy; relative increase in the chondroitin sulfate fraction; and fibrous reaction secondary to exposure of suture line to turbulent flow [3,7,10–12]. Variations in the technique of anastomosis, such as interrupted versus continuous sutures and absorbable (polydioxanone [13]) *versus* nonabsorbable monofilament suture material, did not seem to have significantly affected the problem of recoarctation.

Pathologically, fibrous reactions in the vessel wall at the sites of anastomosis and significant periaortic fibrosis have been noted. These changes are in addition to histologic changes seen with native coarctation [1] if the coarcted segment had not been resected.

In general, the symptoms are dependent on associated heart defects. Despite significant obstruction, the symptoms are less dramatic than prior to surgery, presumably related to the gradual process of renarrowing. Hypertension and signs of heart failure may be present. Absent or diminished and delayed femoral pulses and systolic blood pressure differences between arms and legs may be found. Chest roentgenograms, electrocardiograms, and echo-Doppler studies are useful adjuncts in the evaluation of residual coarctation and associated cardiac defects. Increased Doppler flow velocity in the descending aorta, especially in the presence of pandiastolic flow [14], is indicative of significant aortic recoarctation. An arm to leg pressure difference >20 mmHg or a peak-to-peak systolic pressure difference of >20 mmHg at cardiac catheterization are generally considered to indicate recoarctation. Angiography usually reveals localized obstruction.

Castaneda-Zuniga et al. [15] and Lock et al. [16] created experimental aortic recoarctations in dogs and lambs and attempted balloon angioplasty to relieve the obstruction. Their initial experience in the dog model [15] was disappointing and prompted them to conclude that balloon dilatation of recoarctation after end-to-end anastomosis is difficult or impossible. However, they were able to dilate and relieve recoarctations successfully [16] in their newborn lamb model. A 65% increase in the size of the coarcted segment and a 60% drop in peak systolic pressure gradient were observed, but high dilating pressures of 6–8 atm were required. To the best of my knowledge, Singer et al. [17] were the first to report clinical (human) application of balloon angioplasty to treat aortic recoarctation following previous surgery. They reported a 7-week-old infant who developed recoarctation after a Teflon patch graft repair of severe coarctation on the first day of life. A 5 mm diameter balloon was used for transluminal angioplasty with reduction of peak-to-peak systolic pressure gradient from 65 to 15 mmHg and angiographic improvement of recoarctation site [17]. They suggested that

relief of recoarctation by balloon angioplasty offers an alternative method of treatment without the risks of thoracotomy in an acutely ill infant [17]. Subsequently, several investigators [18–28], including our group [30–32], applied this technique to aortic recoarctations following previous surgery. The purpose of this chapter is to present the current state of knowledge of balloon angioplasty of recoarctation following previous surgery for aortic coarctation; our experience, including that reported previously [30–32] and that in the literature, is used as supportive material.

INDICATIONS

Balloon angioplasty of postoperative recoarctations has been recommended as the therapy of choice [20,33], although it was not recommended for native coarctations [33,34]. A positive recommendation for recoarctations was made before the availability of data on the immediate results in a significant number of patients and before the availability of any follow-up data. This type of recommendation was based in part on the speculation that circumferential scar tissue at the recoarctation site may prevent formation of aneurysms and, if formed, prevent their rupture [11,23,28,34]. Such a hypothesis may not be tenable in some patients; in the Valvuloplasty and Angioplasty of Congenital Anomalies (VACA) Registry [28], it was observed that there was little scar tissue surrounding the previous repair site in a patient with aortic rupture after balloon angioplasty. Comparison of results and complications of balloon angioplasty in native versus postsurgical aortic coarctations (Table I) reveals that these are essentially similar in both groups. Based on this type of analysis, we have argued [36,37] against different types of recommendation for these two lesions. Now that more data are available, immediate and follow-up results appear good; complications are modest; and the risks of repeat surgical repair are high [31,32]. Therefore, balloon angioplasty of recoarctations following previous surgery

TABLE I. Comparison of Results of Balloon Angioplasty From VACA Registry[a]

	Native coarctation [35]	Recoarctation [28]	P value
Pressure gradient relief			
Before angioplasty	48 ± 9^b	42 ± 20^b	>0.1
After angioplasty	12 ± 11^b	9 ± 3^b	
Arterial complications	14 ± 114 (9.9%)	17/200 (8.5%)	>0.1
Deaths	1/141 (0.7%)	5/200 (2.5%)	0.05-0.1

[a]Reproduced from Rao [37], with permission of the publisher.
[b]mmHg: mean ± standard deviation.

has emerged as a therapeutic procedure of choice.

The indications for catheterization and angiographic study in patients with suspected recoarctation are systemic hypertension, defined as an arm systolic pressure above the 95th percentile for age, and/or congestive heart failure. The indications for balloon angioplasty are a peak-to-peak systolic pressure gradient >20 mmHg across the previous surgical repair site and angiographically demonstrable narrowing [31].

TECHNIQUE

The technique of balloon angioplasty [31] of recoarctations is very similar to that used for native aortic coarctations [38–41]. It is described in detail in Chapter 10 (this volume), which deals with native coarctations [1] and therefore will not be detailed here. A few important features will be mentioned. The importance of heparinization [42] and avoidance of manipulation of tips of catheters and guidewires in the vicinity of a freshly dilated site cannot be overemphasized. It is generally believed that a higher pressure of inflation is required to dilate recoarctations successfully, presumably related to circumferential scar tissue. Balloon size is important in not only providing adequate relief of obstruction but also in preventing acute rupture [28,43,44] and immediate or late formation of aneurysms [25,45,46]. The diameter of the balloon used for dilatation should be two or more times the

size of the coarcted segment [19], but no larger than the descending aorta at the level of the diaphragm [32,39,40]. In practice, I select a balloon size that is midway between the diameter of the aortic isthmus or arch (segment proximal to recoarctation site) and the diameter of the descending aorta at the level of the diaphragm. If there is no adequate improvement (see Fig. 1, Chapter 4, this volume), a balloon as large as the descending aorta at the level of the diaphragm is chosen for additional dilatation. The objective is to apply "controlled" injury. Meticulous attention to the technique and balloon size is necessary to prevent complications and to produce good results. Finally, it is important to prevent balloon rupture, especially in view of the requirement for high inflation pressures to dilate recoarctations. Selecting a balloon that can tolerate high inflation pressures (Chapter 5, this volume) knowledge of the manufacturers' recommendations with regard to pressure of inflation tolerated by the balloon and monitoring pressure of inflation via a commercially available pressure gauge to avoid balloon rupture [43,44] are important.

ACUTE RESULTS

Our own experience with balloon angioplasty of recurrent coarctation, including that reported previously [30–32], is in 11 patients. These procedures were performed during a 70 month period preceding July 1991. These children developed recoarctation 6 months to 7.5

years (31 ± 30 [mean ± SD] months; median, 20 months) following surgical repair of aortic coarctation (N = 10) and interruption of the aortic arch (N = 1). Previous surgery included end-to-end anastomosis after resection of coarctation in five; patch angioplasty in five (Dacron, two; subclavian flap, three); and repair of interrupted aortic arch in one. Surgical repair was performed in the neonatal period in seven children and at 2, 8, 10, and 18 months of age, respectively, in the remaining four children (mean, 3.8 ± 5.8 months; median, 1.0 month). At the time of balloon angioplasty, they were 6 months to 9 years of age (median, 20 months). There were eight boys and three girls. Their weights ranged between 5.1 and 30 kg (median, 10.9 kg). Preangioplasty peak-to-peak systolic pressure gradients ranged from 30 to 94 mmHg, with a median of 48 mmHg. The peak gradient across the recoarcted area decreased from 48 ± 25 to 14 ± 8 mmHg ($P < 0.001$) following angioplasty. The residual gradients after angioplasty varied from 2 to 25 mmHg (median,

12 mmHg). As a result of angioplasty, the recoarcted aortic segment increased from 3.1 ± 1.3 to 6.2 ± 1.6 mm ($P < 0.01$). Examples of improvement are shown in Figures 1 through 5.

There are several reports in the literature of balloon angioplasty for recoarctation [17–29,47,48]. Immediate results (excluding single case reports) are given in Table II and are comparable with our results. Thus a review of the data from the literature and from our own experience indicates that balloon angioplasty can be successfully performed and that the aortic obstruction is relieved in the vast majority of patients. Balloon angioplasty produces significant pressure gradient relief irrespective of the type of the previous coarctation surgery (Figs. 1 through 3). Data from the VACA Registry [28] suggest that the pressure gradient relief is inversely proportional to the age at angioplasty, although there was considerable overlap between the groups. Other investigators [29] were unable to show such an age-dependent result.

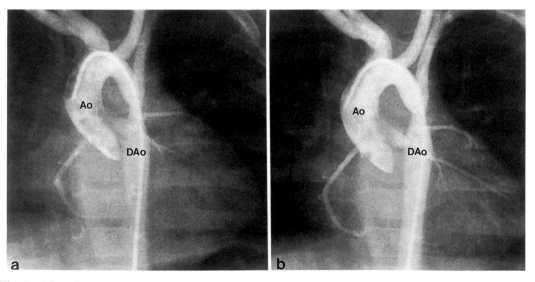

Fig. 1. Selected cineangiographic frames from aortic (Ao) root cineangiograms in posteroanterior view prior to (**a**) and immediately following (**b**) balloon angioplasty aortic recoarctation that developed after resection and end-to-end anastomosis. Note significant improvement in the size of the coarcted aortic segment. DAo, descending aorta.

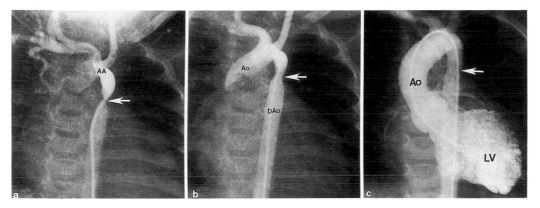

Fig. 2. Aortic arch (AA) cineangiographic frames in posteroanterior view prior to (**a**) and immediately after (**b**) balloon angioplasty of aortic recoarctation that developed (arrow) following surgical repair of aortic coarctation by a subclavian flap angioplasty. Note significant improvement after angioplasty (**b**). Left ventricular (LV) angiography 1 year following balloon dilatation (**c**) revealed excellent results. Also note marked improvement in collateral vessels both immediately after (**b**) and 12 months following (**c**) balloon angioplasty. Ao, aorta; DAo, descending aorta.

FOLLOW-UP RESULTS

From our study group, follow-up catheterization and angiography were performed in eight children aged 8–42 months (18 ± 11 months; median, 18 months) after balloon angioplasty. All 11 patients were studied for clinical and echo-Doppler follow-up data 6–54 months (30± 16 months; median, 36 months) after angioplasty. Residual gradient across the dilated postsurgical recoarctation was calculated by combining the peak-to-peak catheterization-derived pressure gradient in ten children, with arm and leg cuff peak systolic pressure differences in the remaining children. The residual gradients in these 11 children were 6 ± 6 mmHg, with a range of 0–21 mmHg (median, 4 mmHg). The gradients were 48 ± 25 mmHg prior to angioplasty and 14 ± 8 mmHg immediately after angioplasty in these children and indicate a further fall ($P<0.01$) in gradient at follow-up. The follow-up pressure gradients reported herein suggest further improvement in gradient across the dilated recoarctation in a manner similar to that observed by Allen and Cooper and their associates [22,26]. The

coarcted aortic segment was 8.7 ± 1.3 mm, which was 6.2 ± 1.6 mm immediately after angioplasty. Examples of improvement at follow-up are shown in Figures 2, 4, and 5. No aneurysms were seen in the area of the previously dilated recoarctation.

In the literature, there are few studies reporting a limited number of patients for whom follow-up data are recorded. The available studies are listed in Table III. Of the 76 patients for whom follow-up data are available, 19 (25%) had significant residua or restenosis at follow-up. Aneurysms were found in 7 of 76 (9%) at follow-up. Follow-up information on a larger number of patients for a longer duration of follow-up may be necessary before one can be certain of the long-term favorable effects of balloon angioplasty of postoperative recoarctation.

COMPARISON WITH SURGERY

The operative mortality rate for the second operation for recoarctation following the initial surgical repair of aortic coarctation is high and varied from 0% to 33% [5,7,8,10,26,49–57].

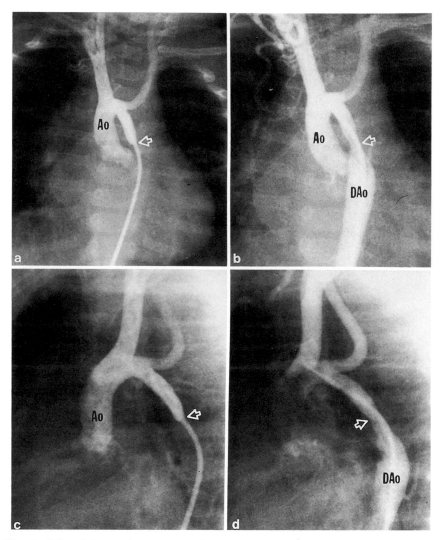

Fig. 3. Selected frames from aortic arch cineangiography in posteroanterior (**a,b**) and lateral (**c,d**) views prior to (a,c) and immediately following (b,d) balloon angioplasty in a child who developed recoarctation after repair of interrupted aortic arch with subclavian artery turn-down procedure. Note complete obstruction to blood flow (a,c) prior to angioplasty (arrows) with improvement in flow to the descending aorta (DAo) and an increase in coarcted segment size (b,d) following angioplasty (arrows). Ao, aorta.

The mortality rate following balloon angioplasty of aortic coarctations varied from 0% to 2.5% [19,28] and compares favorably with the operative mortality rate following the second surgery quoted above. Recoarctation rates following the second operation for postsurgical recoarctation were also high and varied from 6% to 30%, and these recoarctation rates appear comparable with those reported (25%, 19 of 76; Table III) for balloon angioplasty for postoperative recoarctation [18–32]. However, there are limitations to comparing the surgical

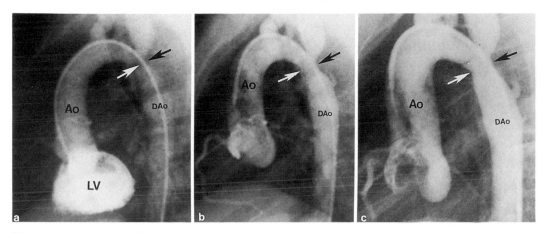

Fig. 4. Left ventricular (LV) cineangiogram in lateral view showing severe aortic recoarctation **(a)** (arrow) in a child who previously underwent resection and end-to-end anastomosis. Note improvement immediately following **(b)** and 1 year after **(c)** balloon angioplasty demonstrated by aortic (Ao) root angiography (arrows). DAo, descending aorta.

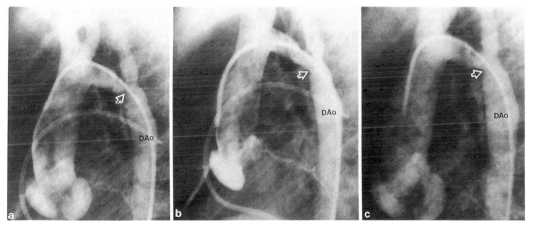

Fig. 5. Aortograms in the lateral view showing severe recoarctation **(a)** (arrow), which improved immediately following balloon angioplasty **(b)** and at follow-up 14 months later **(c)** (arrows). DAo, descending aorta.

data with balloon angioplasty data because of the small number of balloon angioplasty patients available for follow-up, the shorter duration of follow-up, and the possible inaccuracy of comparing "older" surgical studies with "current" balloon angioplasty. Nonetheless, there are advantages to balloon therapy, namely, avoidance of intubation, anesthesia, repeat thoracotomy, possible bleeding while isolating the recoarcted segment, risk of spinal cord injury, and stay in the intensive care unit. In addition, shorter duration of hospitalization and less expense are advantages of balloon angioplasty.

TABLE II. Acute Results of Balloon Angioplasty of Postsurgical Recoarctation [a]

Authors	Year	No. of patients undergoing BA	Age (mo, mean ± SD; range)	Types of previous surgery	Interval between surgery and BA (mo)	Pre-BA and post-BA gradients, (mmHg)	Patients with residual coarctation [b] No. (%)	Complications
Lock et al.	1983	5	90 ± 107 (1.5–264)	EE-3 SF-2	–	51 ± 19 22 ± 19	2 (40)	Surgery in two patients within 1 week of BA
Kan et al.	1983	7	113 ± 64 (10–204)	EE-3 TG-2 PA-1 IA-1	95 ± 59 (10-198)	58 ± 12 13 ± 9	1 (14)	One patient died 2° to ventricular fibrillation
Lababidi	1984	7	121 ± 53 (36–192)	EE-3 PA-4	74 ± 36 (36-132)	39 ± 21 8 ± 6	1 (14)	None reported
Allen et al.	1986	8	97 ± 102 (7–240)	EE-5 SF-2 TG-1	15 ± 10	51 ± 18	2 (25)	Severe post-BA hypertension in one patient
Hess et al.	1986	5	8.2 (mean) (1.5–14.3)	EE-3 SF-1 ST-1	–	27 (mean) 12 (mean)	–	Balloon rupture in three patients
Lorber et al.	1986	5	4 ± 2 (3–9)	SF-5	4 ± 2 (3–9)	59 ± 16 22 ± 16	2 (40)	Femoral artery thrombosis, 1; hypotension, 1
Saul et al.	1987	27	67 ± 75 (3–264)	EE-14 SF-7 PA-3 NP-3	24 (median) (3–180)	42 ± 14 14 ± 15	5 (19)	Blood loss, 6; femoral artery occlusion, 5; and 3 procedures failed

Author	Year	N		Procedure				Complications
Cooper et al.	1989	44	288 ± 64 (2–240)	EE-21 SF-13 PA-5 MO-5	49 = 54 (1.5–180)	37 ± 16 14 ± 11	—	Femoral artery occlusion, 4; aneurysm, 1; deaths, 2
Hellenbrand (VACA Registry)[c]	1990	190	84 (mean) (1–312)	EE-84 SF-48 PA-40 NP-12 TG-4 UK-12	65 (mean) (1.5–420)	42 ± 20 13 ± 12	41 (22)	Deaths, 5; femoral artery occlusion, 17; hypertension, 4; neurologic event, 3; fair to poor result, 41; balloon rupture, 19
Anjos et al.	1992	26	8[d] (2.6–220)	EE-4 SF-17 PA-5	7.5[d] (2–2.5)	49 ± 17 20 ± 17	9 (35)	Femoral artery occlusion, 1; spontaneous ophthalmoplegia, 1; balloon rupture, 2; aneurysm, 1
Current series	1992	11	33 ± 32 (6–108)	EE-5 SF-3 PA-2 IA-1	31 ± 30 (6–90)	48 ± 25 14 ± 8	2 (18)	Blood loss, 2

[a]Papers reporting single cases were not included BA, balloon angioplasty; EE, end-to-end anastomosis; IA, interrupted aortic arch repair; MO, multiple operations; PA, patch angioplasty (Dacron, Goretex, or pericardial patch); NP, Norwood procedure; SD, standard deviation; SF, subclavian flap; ST, subclavian artery to thoracic aorta anastomosis—end-to-side; TG, tube graft; UK, type of surgical procedure is unknown. (Reproduced in part from Rao et al. [31], with permission of the publisher.)

[b]Residual coarctation, defined as peak-to-peak gradient >20 mmHg.

[c]Only means values without SD were available.

[d]This is median; mean and SD were not given.

TABLE III. Follow-Up Results of Balloon Angioplasty of Postoperative Recoarctations[a]

Authors	Year	No. of patients followed	Duration of follow-up (mo; mean ± SD range)	Follow-up gradients (mm Hg; range)	Aneurysm (%)	Restenosis (%)[b]	Comments
Lock et al.	1983	3	3.4 ± 2.9 (0.25–6.0)	15 ± 13 (5–30)	0	1 (33)	
Lababidi et al.	1984	4	–	10 ± 6 (5–18)	0	0	Duration of follow-up not given
Allen et al.	1986	6	7 ± 2 (4–11)	7 ± 8 (0–20)	0	1 (17)	Femoral artery occlusion at follow-up
Lorber et al.	1986	5	12 ± 12 (2–30)	24 ± 17 (0–45)	0	4 (80)	Repeat BA in two
Saul et al.	1987	5	–	24 ± 22 (3–50)	2 (40)	2 (40)	Repeat BA in two
Cooper et al.	1989	21	12 ± 8 (2–24)	12 ± 9	3 (14)[c]	3 (14)	Repeat BA in three
Anjos et al.[d]	1992	26	22 ± 22 (2–80)	–	2 (8)	11 (42)	Follow-up mean gradients for the entire group were not given; repeat BA in three; surgery in five
Current series	1991	11	30 ± 16 (8–42)	6 ± 6 (0–21)	0	1 (9)[e]	Femoral artery occlusion in one
Totals		76		–	7 (9)	19 (25)	

[a]Modified from Rao PS et al., [31], with permission of the publisher.
[b]Restenosis is defined as peak-to-peak gradient >20 mmHg.
[c]Includes one aneurysm that developed immediately after BA.
[d]Includes Lorber's cases previously reported, and therefore, the latter are excluded from totals.
[e]The gradient was across the hypoplastic aortic arch and not across the dilated aortic coarctation.

MECHANISM OF ANGIOPLASTY

Castaneda-Zuniga et al. [15] and Lock et al. [16] investigated the feasibility and mechanism of balloon angioplasty in surgically created aortic coarctations in animal models. They detected intimal tears extending into media to varying degrees in the nonoperated aortic wall. The tears were found to be healed within 2 months without formation of aneurysms or atheroma. Although these surgically created coarctations are not perfect models of human aortic recoarctations, based on these data and on the data regarding native coarctations re-viewed elsewhere (see Chapter 5, this volume), it is likely that intimal and medial tears are the most possible mechanisms for relief of obstruction following balloon angioplasty.

COMPLICATIONS

In the present small series, the complications are modest. In the VACA Registry involving 200 patients, five (2.5%) deaths were reported following balloon angioplasty [28], and this death rate is higher than that seen with native coarctations (0.7%, 1 of

141), also reported by the VACA Registry [35], although this difference did not attain statistical significance ($P = 0.056$–0.1). Other significant complications reported by the Registry [28] included balloon rupture (9.5%), femoral artery complications (8.5%), postcoarctectomy syndrome (2%), and neurologic event (1.5%).

Other workers reported acute complications of balloon angioplasty of recoarctation; these include fatal aortic rupture [43], pseudoaneurysm formation [45], and cerebrovascular accidents [58,59]. A review of acute complications following balloon dilatation by Fellows et al. [60] revealed a lower complication rate (4%) for recoarctation than for any other lesion undergoing balloon dilatation.

Development of aneurysms at follow-up is another complication that needs to be addressed. The incidence of this complication appears to be 9% (Table III), similar to that seen following balloon angioplasty of native coarctation [30]. It has previously been thought that circumferential scar tissue at the recoarctation site following previous surgical repair may prevent formation of aneurysms and, if formed, prevent their rupture [11,23,28,34]. Such a hypothesis may not be tenable, at least in some patients. In the VACA Registry [28], it was observed that there was little scar tissue surrounding a previous surgical repair site in a patient with aortic rupture following balloon angioplasty.

CAUSES OF RESTENOSIS

As stated in the previous section (Table III), a 9%–80% restenosis rate has been reported; the average for the entire group of 76 patients with follow-up data was 25% (19 of 76). Anjos et al. [29] found a 42% recurrence rate at a mean follow-up of 1.8 years. They examined several factors and found that aortic arch diameter and the ratio of balloon:aortic diameter at the level of the diaphragm were significantly smaller in the poor result group. The high prevalence of smaller aortic arches in the poor result group is similar to that found with recoarctation after balloon dilatation of native coarctation [61].

INFLUENCE OF TECHNICAL FACTORS ON ANGIOPLASTY

In the VACA Registry [28], a good to excellent immediate result, defined as a peak-to-peak systolic pressure gradient ≤ 20 mmHg, was observed in 79% of 190 patients for whom such data were available. Examination of ratios of balloon diameter to coarcted segment size and aortic diameter proximal and distal to the coarctation site did not reveal significant correlation between the ratios and favorable results. Similarly, pressure of balloon inflation had no effect. However, age at angioplasty is inversely related to adequacy of angioplasty, while age at initial surgery and the time interval between surgery and angioplasty had no effect.

While the VACA Registry data, despite the large numbers, were unable to show any relationship between the balloon diameter and success of angioplasty (reduction of peak gradient and angiography improvement), our personal experience in both native and postsurgical coarctation is contrary to this. Perhaps this is related to the method of how we choose balloon size for balloon angioplasty. We initially use a balloon whose diameter is midway between the diameters of the aortic isthmus (or aortic segment proximal to coarcted site) and descending aorta at the level of the diaphragm. If there is not adequate relief of obstruction, we go to a larger balloon size. We limit maximum size used to the diameter of the descending aorta at the level of the diaphragm (see Table V, Chapter 10, and Fig. 1, Chapter 4, this volume). With this approach there is likely to be adequate relief of obstruction and hopefully no aneurysms.

With regard to influence of technical factors on follow-up results, there are very few data. However, it should be recognized that residual, immediate, postdilatation gradients do improve at follow-up [22,26,31]. Of the 11 patients in our study group, the gradient further decreased at follow-up in eight children and remained the same in three patients. Confirmation of this phenomenon in a larger series may give credence to this observation. As mentioned in the previous section, Anjos et al. [29] found that larger balloon:descending aortic (at the level of the diaphragm) ratios are associated with better follow-up results than when smaller balloons are used.

NONINVASIVE EVALUATION OF FOLLOW-UP RESULTS

A review of papers reporting follow-up results of balloon angioplasty for aortic recoarctations [19,21,22,24–26] suggested that most workers used cardiac catheterization for evaluation of short-term results. Few have reported use of echo-Doppler studies [29]. We have reported echo-Doppler findings from our initial study cohort [31]. I will now review the findings in all 11 children studied.

Left ventricular end diastolic dimension did not significantly change (29 ± 5.5 vs. 28 ± 5.1 mm, $P > 0.1$) immediately following balloon angioplasty. Left ventricular posterior wall thickness (5.9 ± 1.0 vs. 5.8 ± 1.0 mm, $P > 0.1$) also did not change. Left ventricular shortening fraction (42% ± 5% vs. 38% ± 7%), though diminished (more toward normal), was not statistically significant ($P > 0.1$). Left atrial size to aortic root ratio diminished (1.6 ± 0.4 vs. 1.4 ± 0.4), but not to a statistically significant degree ($P > 0.1$). Peak Doppler flow velocity in the descending aorta decreased significantly ($P < 0.01$) from 3.7 ± 0.9 m/s prior to angioplasty to 2.6 ± 0.4 m/s immediately after balloon dilatation. This corresponded to a decrease in peak instantaneous gradient across the aortic coarctation (calculated by using the formula $\Delta P = 4(V_2^2 - V_1^2)$, where ΔP is the pressure gradient, V_1 and V_2 are velocities distal (V_2) and proximal (V_1) to aortic coarctation) [14] from 51 ± 25 to 22 ± 7 mmHg ($P < 0.01$).

At follow-up 6 months to 4.5 years (30 ± 16 months) after balloon angioplasty, the left ventricular dimension (33 ± 5.3 mm) increased lightly ($P < 0.05$), which probably could be explained by the increase in mean body surface area from 0.49 ± 0.13 to 0.62 ± 0.09 m². The left ventricular posterior wall thickness (6.3 ± 0.9 mm), left ventricular shortening fraction (38% ± 6%), and left atrial to aortic root ratio (1.4 ± 0.4) remain unchanged ($P > 0.1$) compared with immediate postangioplasty values. The peak Doppler flow velocity in the descending aorta (2.6 ± 0.4 m/s) and the calculated peak instantaneous gradient across the area of dilated recoarctation (23 ± 6 mmHg) remain unchanged from postangioplasty ($P > 0.1$) values, but continue to remain improved ($P < 0.01$) compared with preangioplasty Doppler velocity measures. The echo-Doppler data indicate that left ventricular and left atrial chamber size, left ventricular wall thickness, and function do not significantly change following angioplasty, while peak Doppler flow velocity and calculated gradient improve following angioplasty.

Measurement of peak systolic blood pressure differences between the arm and leg can also be used to assess the adequacy of relief of obstruction. In addition, the degree of hypertension, as measured by cuff blood pressure, is also indicative of the success of angioplasty. Kan et al. [20] measured arm to leg pressure differences 4–14 months following angioplasty in five of the seven recoarctation patients undergoing balloon dilatation. The peak gradient was reduced from 57 ± 14 to 13 ± 10 mmHg immediately after balloon angioplasty, which was reduced further to 4 ± 6 mmHg 4–14 months later. Lorber and associates [24] documented blood pressure-measured gradients in three of five children undergoing balloon angioplasty, and they were 35, 45, and 20 mmHg, respectively, at 4, 10, and 2 months after angioplasty. These had been 80, 45, and 65 mmHg prior to balloon angioplasty. Saul and colleagues [25] mentioned noninvasive gradients, presumably measured by cuff blood pressure differences between the arm and leg, in 20 of 27 patients undergoing balloon angioplasty. These follow-up data were obtained 1 day to 1 year after angioplasty and reveal gradients ≤20 mmHg in all patients. From our group of 11 patients, evaluation of arm blood pressures and arm to leg blood pressure differences were performed prior to and immediately following balloon dilatation and 6 months to 4.5 years (30 ± 16 months) after angioplasty. The systolic arm blood pressure prior to angioplasty was 143 ± 27 mmHg (range, 110 to 200 mmHg; median, 134 mmHg), which decreased ($P = 0.05$ to 0.1) to 121 ± 26 mmHg (range, 90–186; median, 117 after angioplasty. At follow-up 30 months (mean) later, the blood pressure was 104 ± 11 mmHg (range, 90–127 mmHg; median, 101 mmHg), representing a significant ($P<0.001$) reduction compared with preangioplasty blood pressures. At follow-up, the arm to leg pressure gradients were 6 ± 7 mmHg (range, 0–20 mmHg; median, 2 mmHg), which were 48 ± 28 mmHg prior to angioplasty and 14 ± 8 mmHg immediately following angioplasty. Thus our series, though small, does suggest that blood pressure differences can be utilized at follow-up for evaluation of residual gradients after balloon dilatation of recoarctation.

Nuclear magnetic resonance (NMR) imaging may be useful in the evaluation of postoperative recoarctation [62]. Both the area of narrowing and the aneurysmal bulges can be identified in a manner similar to angiography [62]. NMR studies following balloon angioplasty for recoarctation may also be useful in a manner described for native aortic coarctations [62,63].

OTHER ISSUES

Aneurysms

Formation of aneurysms appears to be a significant complication at follow-up. As indicated in Complications and in Table III, 7 of 76 (9%) of children studied angiographically were found to have aneurysms. Since the number of patients studied is small, the true incidence of aneurysms after balloon dilatation of recoarctation is not known. In addition, reports of "aneurysms" without any intervention [64] and following surgery without balloon intervention [2] makes the evaluation of aneurysms and the establishing of a causal relationship between the aneurysmal bulge and a procedure (surgery or balloon angioplasty) difficult. Careful review of angiograms (in multiple projection) performed prior to surgery and/or balloon angioplasty and their comparison with postdilatation studies is necessary to detect "new aneurysms" presumably related to the procedure. Once detected, careful follow-up studies with NMR or angiography are highly recommended to document the natural history of such aneurysms. For further discussion on aneurysms, the reader is referred to Chapter 10 (this volume) dealing with native aortic coarctations.

Intravascular Ultrasound

Intravascular ultrasound [65,66] has been used to document intimal and medial disruption and formation of intimal flaps following balloon angioplasty of aortic coarctation. The value of morphologic documentation of the intended, controlled injury of balloon angioplasty, in addition to hemodynamic and angiographic relief of obstruction, should be scrutinized in future studies prior to adoption of this technique for routine use.

SUMMARY AND CONCLUSIONS

Since the first human application of balloon angioplasty of the postoperative aortic recoarctation in 1982 by Singer and his associates, the technique has been used extensively by many other workers. Balloon dilatation of aortic recoarctation is next only to valvar pulmonic stenosis with regard to the acceptability by cardiologists. Immediate results seem excellent, with an acceptable complication rate. The results and risks appear comparable with those seen with repeat surgical intervention. Follow-up results are available in only a limited number of patients, with recurrence and aneurysm formation rates of 25% and 9%, respectively. These and arterial complication rates are likely to diminish because of progressive improvement of the balloon catheter technology and a greater understanding by cardiologists of the angioplasty technique.

Most cardiologists agree that balloon angioplasty is the treatment of choice for management of aortic recoarctations. A peak-to-peak systolic pressure gradient across the operative site in excess of 20 mmHg with angiographic demonstration of discrete narrowing is an indication for balloon dilatation. Use of heparin, appropriate choice of balloon diameter, and avoidance of manipulation of the tips of the catheters/guidewires in the vicinity of freshly dilated coarctation are important technical features of balloon angioplasty. Periodic evaluation for evidence of renarrowing after angioplasty and for development of aneurysms is necessary; these may be performed by clinical, echo-Doppler, NMR, and angiographic studies.

The mechanism for effectiveness of angioplasty appears to be the intimal and medial disruption produced by controlled injury through radial forces of balloon inflation. Further miniaturization of balloon/catheter systems, a better understanding of the technique of balloon angioplasty, longer duration of follow-up in a larger number of patients than is currently available, and causes and natural history of aneurysm formation following angioplasty are all important in further advancing balloon angioplasty as a successful therapeutic option for the management of postoperative aortic recoarctations.

REFERENCES

1. Rao PS (1993): Balloon angioplasty of native aortic coarctation. In Rao PS (ed): "Transcatheter Therapy in Pediatric Cardiology." New York: Wiley-Liss, pp. 153–196.

2. Pinzon JL, Burrows PE, Benson LN, Moës CAF, Lightfoot NE, Williams WG, Freedom RM (1991): Repair of coarctation of the aorta in children: Postoperative morphology. Radiology 180:199–203.

3. Moulton AL (1991): Introduction to the symposium. Ann Thorac Surg 52:592–593.

4. Hesslein PS, McNamara DG, Morris MJH, Hallman GL, Cooley DA (1981): Comparison of resection versus patch aortoplasty for repair of coarctation in infants and children. Circulation 64:164–168.

5. Kron IL, Flanagan TL, Rheuban KS, Carpenter MA, Gutgesell HP, Jr, Blackbourne LH, Nolan SP (1990): Incidence and risk of reintervention after coarctation repair. Ann Thorac Surg 49:920–926.

6. Messmer BJ, Minale C, Mühler E, Bernuth GV (1991): Surgical correction of coarctation in early infancy: Does surgical technique influence the result? Ann Thorac Surg 52:594–603.

7. Kirklin JW, Barratt-Boyes BG (1986): "Cardiac Surgery." New York: John Wiley & Sons, pp 1036–1080.

8. Beekman RH, Rocchini AP, Behrendt DM, Bove EL, Dick M II, Crowley DC, Snider AR, Rosenthal A (1985): Long-term outcome after repair of coarctation in infancy: Subclavian angioplasty does not reduce the need for reoperation. J Am Coll Cardiol 8:1406–1411.

9. Trinquet F, Vouhé PR, Vernant F, Touati G, Roux P, Pome G, Leca F, Neveux J (1988): Coarctation of the aorta in infants: Which operation? Ann Thorac Surg 4:186–191.

10. Foster ED (1984): Reoperation for aortic coarctation. Ann Thorac Surg 38:81–89.

11. Huhta JC (1989): Angioplasty for recoarctation. J Am Coll Cardiol 14:420–421.

12. Jonas RA (1991): Coarctation: Do we need to resect ductal tissue? Ann Thorac Surg 52:604–607.

13. Myers JL, Waldhausen JA, Pae WE Jr, Abt AB, Prophet GA, Pierce WS (1982): Vascular anastomoses in growing vessels: The use of absorbable sutures. Ann Thorac Surg 34:529–537.

14. Rao PS, Carey P (1989): Doppler ultrasound in the prediction of pressure gradients across aortic coarctation. Am Heart J 118:299–307.

15. Castaneda-Zuniga WR, Lock JE, Vlodaver Z, Rusnak B, Rysavy JP, Herrera M, Amplatz K (1982): Transluminal dilatation of coarctation of the abdominal aorta: An experimental study in dogs. Radiology 143:693–697.

16. Lock JE, Niemi T, Burke BA, Einzig S, Castaneda-Zuniga WR (1982): Transcutaneous angioplasty of experimental aortic coarctation. Circulation 66:1280–1286.

17. Singer MI, Rowen M, Dorsey TJ (1982): Transluminal aortic balloon angioplasty for coarctation of the aorta in the newborn. Am Heart J 103:131–132.

18. Finley JP, Beaulieu RG, Nanton MA, Roy DL (1983): Balloon catheter dilatation of coarctation of the aorta in young infants. Br Heart J 50:411–415.

19. Lock JE, Bass JL, Amplatz K, Fuhrman BP, Castaneda-Zuniga W (1983): Balloon dilation angioplasty of aortic coarctations in infants and children. Circulation 68:109–116.

20. Kan JS, White RI, Mitchell SE, Farmlett EJ, Donahoo JS, Gardner TJ (1983): Treatment of restenosis of coarctation by percutaneous transluminal angioplasty. Circulation 68:1087–1094.

21. Lababidi ZA, Daskalopoulos DA, Stoeckle H Jr (1984): Transluminal balloon coarctation angioplasty: Experience with 27 patients. Am J Cardiol 54:1288–1291.

22. Allen HD, Marx GR, Ovitt TW, Goldberg SJ (1986): Balloon dilatation angioplasty for coarctation of the aorta. Am J Cardiol 57:828–832.

23. Hess J, Mooyaart EL, Busch HJ, Bergstra A, Landsman MLJ (1986): Percutaneous transluminal balloon angioplasty in restenosis of coarctation of the aorta. Br Heart J 55:459–461.

24. Lorber A, Ettedgui JA, Baker EJ, Jones ODH, Reidy J, Tynan M (1986): Balloon aortoplasty for recoarctation following the subclavian flap operation. Int J Cardiol 10:57–63.

25. Saul JP, Keane JF, Fellows KE, Lock JE (1987): Balloon dilation angioplasty of postoperative aortic obstructions. Am J Cardiol 59:943–948.

26. Cooper SG, Sullivan ID, Wren C (1989): Treatment of recoarctation: Balloon dilation angioplasty. J Am Coll Cardiol 14:413–419.

27. Lo RNS, Leung MP, Yau KK, Cheung DLC (1989): Transvenous antegrade balloon angioplasty for recoarctation of the aorta in an infant. Am Heart J 117:1157–1158.

28. Hellenbrand WE, Allen HD, Golinko RJ, Hagler DJ, Lutin W, Kan J (1990): Balloon angioplasty for aortic recoarctation: Results of Valvuloplasty and Angioplasty of Congenital Anomalies Registry. Am J Cardiol 65:793–797.

29. Anjos R, Qureshi SA, Rosenthal E, Murdoch I, Hayes A, Parsons J, Baker EJ, Tynan M (1992): Determinants of hemodynamic results of balloon dilation of aortic recoarctation. Am J Cardiol 69:665–671.

30. Rao PS (1989): Balloon angioplasty of aortic coarctation: A review. Clin Cardiol 12:618–628.

31. Rao PS, Wilson AD, Chopra PS (1990): Immediate and follow-up results of balloon angioplasty of postoperative recoarctation in infants and children. Am Heart J 120:1315–1320.

32. Rao PS, Chopra PS (1991): Role of balloon angioplasty in the treatment of aortic coarctation. Ann Thorac Surg 52:621–631.

33. Lock JE, Keane JF, Fellows KE (1986): The use of catheter intervention procedures for congenital heart disease. J Am Coll Cardiol 7:1420–1423.

34. Lock JE (1984): Now that we can dilate, should we? Am J Cardiol 54:1360.

35. Tynan M, Finley JP, Fontes V, Hess J, Kan J (1990): Balloon angioplasty for the treatment of native coarctation: Results of Valvuloplasty and Angioplasty of Congenital Anomalies Registry. Am J Cardiol 65:790–792.

36. Rao PS (1989): Which aortic coarctations should we balloon-dilate? Am Heart J 117:987–989.

37. Rao PS (1990): Balloon angioplasty of native coarctations. Am J Cardiol 66:1401.

38. Rao PS (1986): Transcatheter treatment of pulmonary stenosis and coarctation of the aorta: Experience with percutaneous balloon dilatation. Br Heart J 56:250–258.

39. Rao PS (1987): Balloon angioplasty for coarctation of the aorta in infancy. J Pediatr 110:713–718.

40. Rao PS, Najjar HN, Mardini MK, Solymar L, Thapar MK (1988): Balloon angioplasty for coarctation of the aorta: Immediate and long-term results. Am Heart J 115:657–664.

41. Rao PS, Thapar MK, Galal O, Wilson AD (1990): Follow-up results of balloon angioplasty of native coarctation in neonates and infants. Am Heart J 120:1310–1314.

42. Rao PS (1992): Neurologic complications following balloon angioplasty. Pediatr Cardiol (in press).

43. Balaji S, Oommen R, Rees PG (1991): Fatal aortic rupture during balloon dilatation of recoarctation. Br Heart J 65:100–101.

44. Rao PS (1991): Fatal aortic rupture during balloon dilatation of recoarctation. Br Heart J 66:406–407.

45. Joyce DH, McGrath LB (1990): Pseudo-aneurysm formation following balloon angioplasty for recurrent coarctation of the aorta. Cathet Cardiovasc Diagn 20:133–135.

46. Rao PS (1991): Pseudoaneurysm following balloon angioplasty? Cathet Cardiovasc Diagn 23:150–153.

47. Da Costa AG, Iwahashi ER, Atik E, Rati MAN, Ebaid M (1992): Persistence of hypoplastic and recoarcted fifth aortic arch associated with type A aortic arch interruption: Surgical and balloon angioplasty results in an infant. Pediatr Cardiol 13:104–106.

48. Nawa S, Nakayama Y, Teramoto S, Mori K, Dohi T (1989): Coarctation restenosis after isthmosubclavioplasty: A consideration on operative procedure and intraluminal balloon angioplasty. Chest 9:247–250.

49. Cerilli J, Lauridsen P (1965): Reoperation for coarctation of the aorta. Acta Chir Scand 129:391–394.

50. Ibarra-Perez C, Castaneda AR, Varco RL, Lillehei CW (1969): Recoarctation of the aorta: Nineteen year clinical experience. Am J Cardiol 23:778–784.

51. Castaneda AR, Norwood WI (1979): Residual co-arctation of the aorta: Surgical experience. In Tucker BI, Lindesmith GC (eds): "First Clinical Conference on Congenital Heart Disease." New York: Grune & Stratton, pp 167–178.

52. Williams WG, Shindo G, Trusler GA, Dische MR, Olley PM (1980): Results of repair of coarctation of the aorta during infancy. J Thorac Cardiovasc Surg 79:603–608.

53. Beekman RH, Rocchini AP, Behrendt DM, Rosenthal A (1981): Reoperation for coarctation of the aorta. Am J Cardiol 48:1108–1114.

54. Pollack P, Freed MD, Castaneda AR, Norwood WI (1983): Reoperation for isthmic coarctation of the aorta: Follow-up of 26 patients. Am J Cardiol 51:1690–1694.

55. Sweeney MS, Walker WE, Duncan M, Hallman GL, Livesay JJ, Cooley DA (1985): Reoperation for aortic coarctation: Techniques, results, and indications for various approaches. Ann Thorac Surg 40:48–49.

56. Campbell DB, Bartholomew M, Waldhausen JA (1986): The case for subclavian flap repair. J Am Coll Cardiol 8:1412.

57. Hopkins RA, Kostic I, Armiru U, de Leval M, Sullivan I, Wyse R, Macartney F, Stark J (1988): Correction of coarctation of the aorta in neonates and young infants: An individualized surgical approach. Eur J Cardiovasc Surg 2:296–304.

58. Benson LN, Freedom RM, Wilson GJ, Halliday WC (1986): Cerebral complications following balloon angioplasty of coarctation of the aorta. Cardiovasc Intervent Radiol 9:184–186.

59. Booth P, Redington AN, Shinebourne EA, Rigby ML (1991): Early complications of interventional balloon catheterization in infants and children. Br Heart J 65:109–112.

60. Fellows KE, Radtke W, Keane JF, Lock JE (1987): Acute complications of catheter therapy for congenital heart disease. Am J Cardiol 60:679–683.

61. Rao PS, Thapar MK, Kutayli F, Carey P (1989): Causes of recoarctation after balloon angioplasty of unoperated aortic coarctation. J Am Coll Cardiol 13:109–115.

62. Bank ER, Aisen AM, Rocchini AP, Hernandez RJ (1987): Coarctation of the aorta in children undergoing angioplasty: Pretreatment and posttreatment MR imaging. Radiology 162:235–240.

63. Boxer RA, La Corte MA, Singh S, Cooper R, Fishman MC, Goldman M, Stein HL (1986): Nuclear magnetic resonance imaging in evaluation and follow-up of children treated for coarctation of the aorta. J Am Coll Cardiol 7:1095–1098.

64. Parik SR, Hurwitz RA, Hubbard JE, Brown JW, King H, Girol DA (1991): Preoperative and postoperative "aneurysm" associated with coarctation of the aorta. J Am Coll Cardiol 17:1367–1372.

65. Harrison JK, Sheikh KH Davidson CJ, Kisslo KB, Leithe ME, Himmelstein SI, Kantor RJ, Bashore TM (1990): Balloon angioplasty of coarctation of the aorta evaluated with intravascular ultrasound imaging. J Am Coll Cardiol 15:906–909.

66. Jain A, Ramee SR, Culpeper WR, Mesa JE, Murgo JP, White CJ (1992): Intravascular ultrasound-assisted percutaneous angioplasty of aortic coarctation. Am Heart J 123:514–515.

12

Balloon Angioplasty for Peripheral Pulmonary Artery Stenosis

Albert P. Rocchini, M.D.

Division of Pediatric Cardiology, University of Minnesota, Minneapolis, Minnesota 55455; Division of Pediatric Cardiology, University of Michigan, Ann Arbor, Michigan

INTRODUCTION

Schwalbe [1] and Mangars [2] described the first cases of isolated peripheral pulmonary artery stenosis. In addition to peripheral pulmonary arterial stenosis, or hypoplasia occurring as an isolated lesion [3], it can also occur in association with tetralogy of Fallot [4,5], post-rubella syndrome [6], William's syndrome [7], and Alagille's syndrome [8]. The reported frequency of peripheral pulmonary artery stenosis has been estimated to range from 2% to 3% of all patients with congenital heart disease [9,10].

PATHOLOGY

The pathogenesis of peripheral pulmonary artery stenosis is unknown. The high frequency of associated intracardiac anomalies suggests that the pathogenesis may be developmental in origin. Any teratogenic insult that affects components of the developing pulmonary arteries may arrest their development, leading to atresia, hypoplasia, or stenosis. At least one teratogenic agent, the rubella virus, has been implicated [11–14]. It appears that the virus interferes with the normal formation of elastic tissue, and this is believed to be the principle mechanism for the development of the stenoses [11].

Peripheral pulmonary artery stenosis can also occur in association with a number of syndromes. The association of peripheral pulmonary artery stenosis, supravalvar aortic stenosis, mental retardation, and elfin facies is know as *William's syndrome* [15]. In several families peripheral pulmonary artery stenosis has been observed in siblings or in a mother and child [13,16,17]. Recently, a hereditary syndrome consisting of intrahepatic cholestasis, varying degrees of peripheral pulmonary artery stenosis, or diffuse hypoplasia of the pulmonary arteries and its branches, have been reported (Alagille's syndrome) [18–22].

In addition to the congenital forms of peripheral pulmonary artery stenosis the lesion can also result as a squella of congenital heart disease surgery. Thus, because of the marked heterogencity of peripheral pulmonary stenosis, no one form of therapy has been successfully used in its treatment.

TREATMENT

The prognosis of children with severe congenital or acquired peripheral pulmonary artery stenosis is poor [23,24]. Surgical correction of these stenotic arteries remains difficult and is at times impossible [23,24]. Because of poor surgical results for treatment of peripheral pulmonary artery stenosis, balloon dilatation angioplasty has been attempted. In 1980, Martin et al. [25] described the first trial of percutaneous transluminal angioplasty for periph-

Transcatheter Therapy in Pediatric Cardiology, pages 213–228

eral pulmonary arterial stenosis. Following that report, Lock and coworkers [26] described the use of transvenous angioplasty in newborn lambs with experimentally produced branch pulmonary arterial stenosis. These investigators were able to dilate the experimentally induced peripheral stenoses with a modified Gruntzig balloon catheter. In the lamb, the balloon dilatation was associated with a significant reduction in the systolic gradient across the narrowed site and an increase in both the diameter of the site and the amount of blood flow across the stenosis. These investigators demonstrated histologically that the dilatation resulted from both intimal tearing and medial stretching of the pulmonary artery [27]. As a result of these experiments, clinical trials of balloon dilatation angioplasty of peripheral pulmonary artery stenosis have been initiated [28–32].

METHOD FOR BALLOON ANGIOPLASTY OF PERIPHERAL PULMONARY ARTERIAL STENOSIS

The protocol for angioplasty of peripheral pulmonary arteries is similar to that of pulmonary valve stenosis. After a selective pulmonary artery angiogram, an end hole catheter is positioned across the stenotic peripheral pulmonary artery. Since it is frequently very difficult to enter stenotic, hypoplastic branch pulmonary arteries, no one type of end hole catheter will always work. Initially, we use a 7 Fr end hole balloon wedge catheter, and if we fail to cross the stenotic site with this catheter we will try any one of the following other catheters: a right Judkins coronary catheter, an Amplatz coronary catheter, a cobra-curved catheter, or a sidewinder-curved catheter. Once the stenosis is traversed a balloon dilatation catheter is positioned across the stenotic peripheral pulmonary artery over a 0.038 inch Teflon-coated Amplatz heavy-duty exchange guidewire.

We and others recommend that the diameter of the dilatation balloon be three to four and one-half times the diameter of the most

narrow segment of pulmonary artery. The balloon should be inflated to a low pressure (1 or 2 atm) with diluted contrast material and positioned such that the stenotic pulmonary artery segment, indicated by a "waist," is centered in the balloon. Under continuous fluoroscopic monitoring the balloon should be further inflated either until the "waist" deformity disappears or until a dilatation pressure of 4–7 atm is achieved. The pressure in the balloon should be maintained for 10–60 seconds. During the dilatation we strongly recommend that systemic arterial pressure, systemic oxygen saturation, and heart rate be continuously monitored. After dilatation, the balloon catheter is removed, an angiographic catheter is carefully exchanged over a guidewire, and pressure pullback and a repeat angiogram are performed. As with angioplasty of coarctation of the aorta, if the exchange guidewire becomes dislodged, the angioplasty site should not be recrossed, but rather a repeat angiogram should be performed in the main pulmonary artery. For safety (in case the pulmonary artery perforates or thromboses) we usually recommend that only one major branch pulmonary artery be dilated at a time.

RESULTS

Acute Results

Results of balloon angioplasty for peripheral pulmonary arterial stenosis have been less impressive than those for valvar pulmonary stenosis. To date, we have attempted balloon dilatation of 53 pulmonary arteries in 42 patients at the University of Michigan. Since successful relief of vascular obstruction should increase the diameter of the obstructing segment, decrease the pressure gradient, and increase blood flow across the site, we consider an angioplasty of a peripheral pulmonary artery successful if two or more of the following criteria are met: an increase in pulmonary artery size by more than 75% of predilatation size; a greater than 50% reduction in the distal pulmonary artery to main pulmonary artery systolic pressure gradient; a 50% reduction in either peak systolic right ventricular pressure and/or the ratio of right to left ventricular systolic pressures; or a 25% increase in total pulmonary blood flow.[1]

Using these criteria, we have successfully dilated 27 of 53 vessels (51%). We have found that, regardless of the location or type of stenosis (discrete, proximal, or diffuse stenosis) balloon angioplasty can successfully treat peripheral pulmonary artery stenosis (Fig. 1–3). Figure 4 depicts the changes in pulmonary artery size and pulmonary artery gradients that we have observed in our patients. Our results are in agreement with those of Ring and coworkers [31], who reported successful angioplasty on 26 of 52 (50%) dilatations in 24 children. Both our study and the Ring et al. study are very representative of the results recently reported from the Valvuloplasty and Angioplasty of Congenital Anomalies (VACA) Registry [32]. One hundred eighty-two peripheral pulmonary artery dilatations in 156 patients were reported by the VACA registry, and the acute hemodynamic and angiographic results are depicted in Figure 5.

Reasons why angioplasty is unsuccessful in children with peripheral pulmonary artery stenosis include inadequate technique (balloon too small, inability to position balloon or wire across the stenotic site), the refractory nature of the lesion itself, and the age of the subject.

1. Balloon size is an important determinate of angioplasty success. In our own experience, we observed a significant linear relationship between balloon size/stenosis size and both percent increase in pulmonary artery size (r = 0.515, P < 0.0004) and percent decrease in systolic gradient across the stenosis (r = 0.374, P < 0.02). The data from the VACA registry [32] also document a significantly greater increase in pulmonary artery dimension at the site of stenosis if the angioplasty balloon diameter was more than three times the original dimension of the stenosis.

2. In our initial 13 patients, we could not advance the angioplasty catheter across the stenotic segment in three (23%); however, with increased experience and with the development of small angioplasty catheters and stiff guidewires the inability to cross stenotic arteries has been nearly eliminated. In those patients in whom the pulmonary arteries could not be entered at the time of cardiac catheterization, balloon angioplasty has been utilized successfully in the operating room [33].

3. With regard to the refractory nature of the stenosis, we have found that the following factors are associated with stenoses that are unlikely to be dilatable: stenosis at the site of a previous Blalock-Taussig, Waterston-Cooley, or Potts shunt; stenosis of the origin of the left pulmonary artery associated with the placement of a right ventricle to pulmonary artery conduit; stenosis associated with the arterial switch repair of d-transposition of the great arteries[2]; and the presence of either William's syndrome or Alagille's syndrome. Of the nine peripheral pulmonary artery stenoses due to a previous systemic-to-pulmonary artery shunt (Blalock-Taussig shunt in 6, a Waterston-Cooley shunt in two and a Potts shunt in one), only 3 of 9 (33%) were successfully dilated.

---

[1]Editor's note: Quantitative radionudide pulmonary blood flow scans prior to and after dilatation showing an increase in relative distribution to the lung ipsilateral to the dilated pulmonary artery (Ring JR et al. J Thorac Cardiovasc Surg 90:35, 1985) is another indicator of successful balloon angioplasty.

[2]Editor's note: The results of balloon dilatation of pulmonary artery stenoses that develop following arterial switch procedure depend on whether the narrowing is diffuse or discrete. Balloon angioplasty is successful in discrete obstructions (Zeevi B et al. J Am Coll Cardiol 14:401, 1989; Rao PS: Curr Prob Cardiol 14(8): 417, 1989) while it is not beneficial in diffuse obstructions (Zeevi B et al. J Am Coll Cardiol 14:401, 1989; Saxena A, et al. Br Heart J 4:151, 1990).

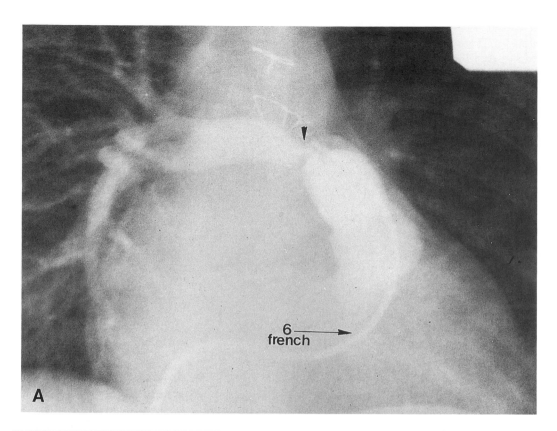

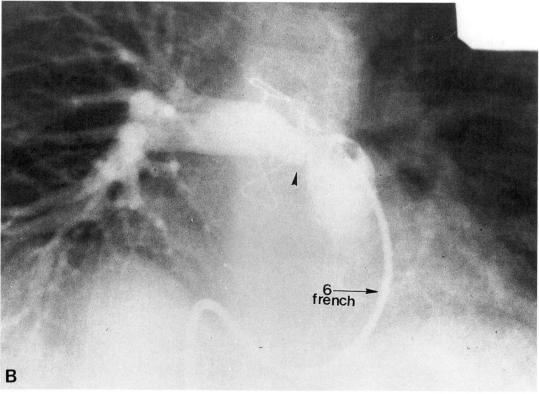

Since despite the use of large balloons and inflation pressures of up to 6 atm the "waist" of the balloon could not be eliminated, we believe that the failure to dilate the peripheral pulmonary artery stenosis may be related to the fact that, at the site of an old systemic-to-pulmonary artery shunt, the stenosis is caused by external fibrosis rather than an anatomic defect of the pulmonary artery wall itself. A similar explanation may also address why we were unable to dilate both patients in whom proximal left pulmonary artery stenoses were caused by the placement of a right ventricle-to-pulmonary conduit and patients in whom main pulmonary artery stenoses were associated with the arterial switch repair of d-transposition of the great arteries. Despite our findings that previous surgical intervention may make angioplasty less likely to improve the branch pulmonary artery narrowing, the results of the entire VACA registry were unable to document a relationship between previous surgery and angioplasty success.

4. We have found that branch pulmonary artery stenosis that is associated with various syndromes such as Alagille's or William's is unlikely to be improved by angioplasty. Of the seven patients with either Alagille's syndrome ($N = 3$) or William's syndrome ($N = 4$) in only one patient (a boy with Alagille's syndrome who developed an aneurysm at the angioplasty site) was angioplasty successful in relieving the peripheral pulmonary artery stenosis (Fig. 6). In most cases a large angioplasty balloon (four to five times the size of the stenosis) was inflated until the "waist" in the balloon was nearly eliminated, yet with deflation of the balloon the stenosis returned. Because of this experience we feel that balloon angioplasty is unlikely to be successful in children with either William's or Alagille's syndrome.[3]

5. We and the VACA Registry have observed no relationship between angioplasty success and patient age. However, Ring and coworkers [31] have reported that nondilatable lesions appear to be more common in children over age 2 years.

Complications

Significant complications have been reported to occur following percutaneous balloon dilatation of peripheral pulmonary arterial stenosis. In the 53 angioplasties performed at the University of Michigan, seven (13%) major complications have occurred. 1) One child had the right pulmonary artery perforated by the guidewire. The patient required multiple transfusions and was taken to the operating room, where a small circular perforation of a distal branch pulmonary artery was sutured [29]. 2) One patient who had balloon angioplasty performed at the time of surgical placement of a right ventricle-to-pul-

---

[3]Editor's note: Although the success rate is low with William's syndrome, there are some reports (e.g., D'Orsogna L et al: Am Heart J 116:647, 1987) that suggest that successful dilatation of branch pulmonary artery stenosis can be accomplished. I therefore suggest that balloon angioplasty be commended as a viable treatment option in these patients also.

Fig. 1. A: Predilatation pulmonary angiogram from a 6-year-old who had previously undergone repair of tetralogy of Fallot. The arrowhead indicates the severe proximal right pulmonary arterial stenosis. The smallest diameter measured was 3.5 mm. The angiogram was performed in the right pulmonary artery using a 6 Fr Berman angiographic catheter. **B:** The postdilatation pulmonary artery angiogram in the same patient is depicted. The arrow localizes the area of the proximal right pulmonary artery that was dilated. After angioplasty the narrowest diameter of the right pulmonary artery was 10 mm. Again the angiogram was performed in the right pulmonary artery using a 6 Fr Berman angiographic catheter. (Adapted from Rocchini et al. [29], with permission of the publisher.)

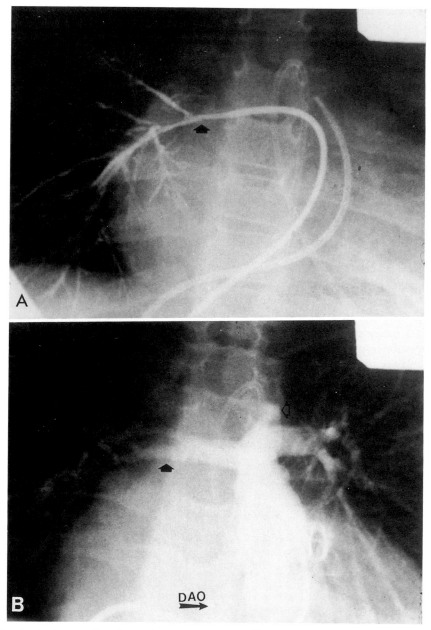

Fig. 2. A: The predilatation pulmonary angiogram of a patient with congenital diffuse branch pulmonary artery stenosis. There is marked, diffuse hypoplasia of the distal right pulmonary artery. The narrowest diameter of the pulmonary artery is indicated by the arrow and was 2.8 mm. The angiogram was performed using a 7 Fr Berman angiographic catheter. **B:** The postdilatation pulmonary angiogram from the same patient is depicted. The arrow indicates the area of the right pulmonary artery that was dilated. After angioplasty the narrowest diameter of the right pulmonary artery 5.4 mm. The angiogram was performed using an 8 Fr Berman catheter. The ductus and descending aorta (DAO) fill are shown. (Adapted from Rocchini et al. [29], with permission of the publisher.)

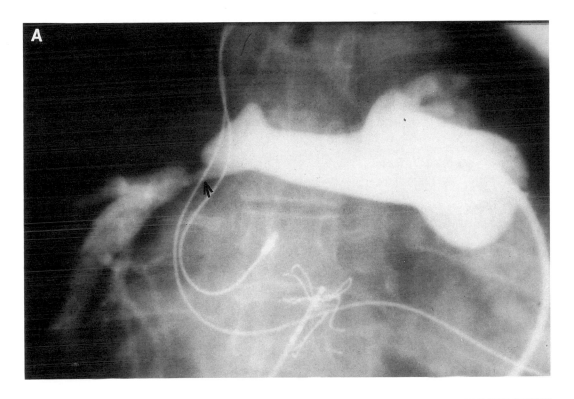

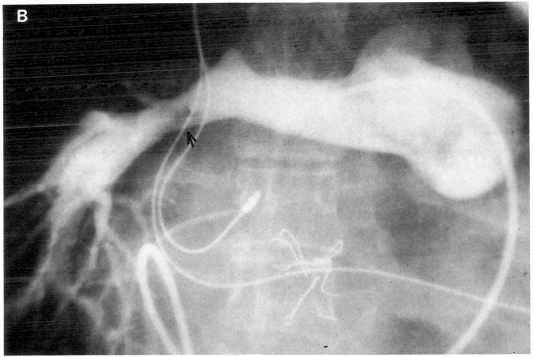

Fig. 3. A: Predilatation right pulmonary artery angiogram from a 45-year-old woman with postoperative tetralogy of Fallot is depicted. A discrete stenosis of the distal right pulmonary artery is well visualized. The systolic pressure gradient across the stenosis measured 40 mmHg. **B:** The postdilatation right pulmonary artery angiogram from the same patient is depicted. The distal stenosis has been almost completely eliminated. Postangioplasty the systolic pressure gradient across the stenosis was only 5 mmHg.

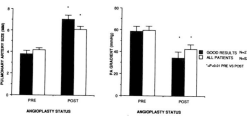

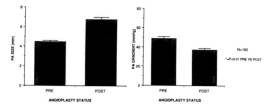

Fig. 4. The results of angioplasty to treat branch pulmonary artery stenosis from the University of Michigan are depicted. It can be seen that for the group of 53 angioplasties as a whole, angioplasty (open bars) resulted in a significant increase in pulmonary artery size and a significant decrease in pressure gradient. The improvement in pulmonary artery size and reduction in gradient is even more dramatic when the 27 angioplasties that were thought to have a good result (closed bars) were looked at separately. We defined an angioplasty of a peripheral pulmonary artery to have a good result if two or more of the following criteria were met: an increase in pulmonary artery size by more than 75% of predilation size; a >50% reduction in the distal pulmonary artery to main pulmonary artery systolic pressure gradient; a 50% reduction in either peak systolic right ventricular pressure and/or in the ratio of right to left ventricular systolic pressures; or a 25% increase in total pulmonary blood flow.

Fig. 5. Combined findings from 182 angioplasties in the VACA Registry showing the ability of angioplasty to treat branch pulmonary artery stenosis. Angioplasty resulted in a significant decrease in branch pulmonary artery systolic gradient and a significant increase in pulmonary artery size.

monary conduit developed hemoptysis and severe hypoxemia and died 20 hours after surgery. At postmortem examination, the lungs were congested with blood, but no discrete site of pulmonary artery perforation was visualized [29]. 3) Four patients have developed asymptomatic pulmonary edema 2–4 hours after a successful peripheral pulmonary angioplasty. The x-ray evidence of edema resolved in all within a period of 1 month (Fig. 7). 4) One child developed an aneurysm of the left pulmonary artery after a successful angioplasty (Fig. 6). The child was recatheterized

10 months later, and no change in the aneurysm was noted. Others have reported complications, including exanguination from a pulmonary artery rupture during the dilatation; clotted iliac veins; and transient arrhythmias, cyanosis, and hypotension [28,29,31,34]. The complications reported by the VACA Resistry are outlined in Table I.

Follow-Up

We have followed our successful angioplasties for up to 6 years. Each child has remained well and without signs of subsequent deterioration. Seven of the subjects have undergone repeat cardiac catheterization. In all but one patient, both the diameter of the stenosis and the systolic gradient across the stenosis remained similar to their postdilatation values. Others have also demonstrated that angioplasty of peripheral pulmonary stenosis when effective appears to be long-lasting [28–31]; however, there are no large prospective studies to document the long-term results of balloon angioplasty for branch pulmonary artery stenosis.

Fig. 6. A: Preangioplasty angiogram from a 9-year-old boy with Alagille's syndrome. Diffuse bilateral peripheral pulmonary stenosis is present. The most severe stenosis was thought to exist in the left pulmonary artery, and angioplasty was performed on that side. **B:** The 1 year postangioplasty angiogram from the same patient is depicted. Although the left pulmonary artery was enlarged by the angioplasty, an aneurysm of the left pulmonary artery developed (arrow). This aneurysm was not present on the immediate postangioplasty angiogram. There has been no progression of the aneurysm over a 3 year period of follow-up.

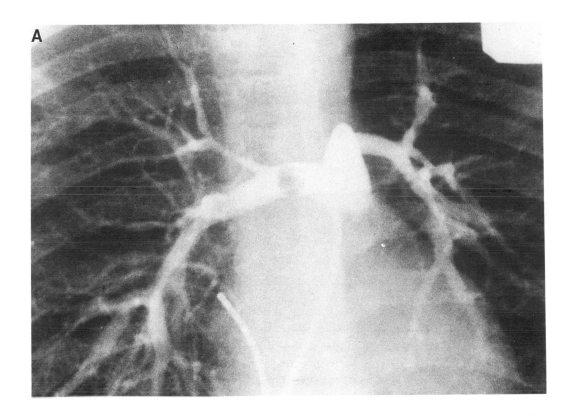

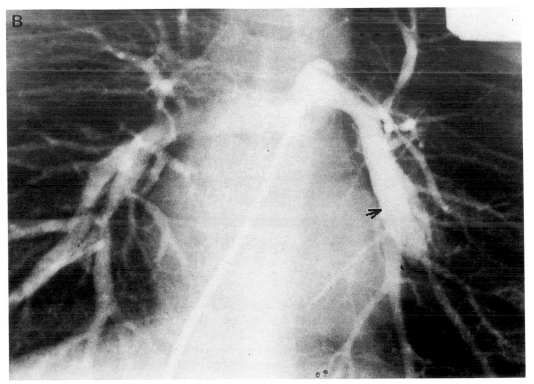

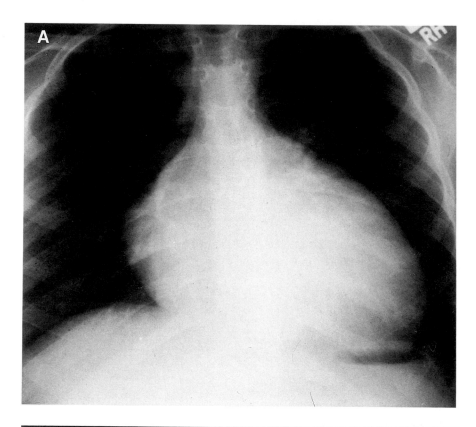

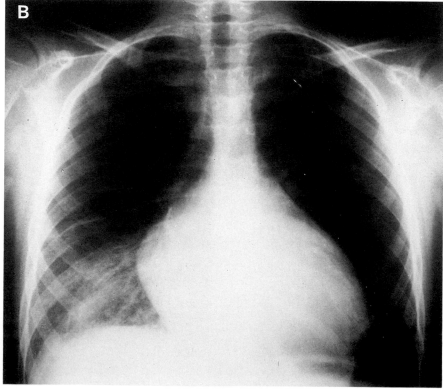

TABLE I. Complications Reported During the Balloon Angioplasty Procedure: Occurrence With Possible Risk Factors [a]

Complication	Age	Balloon diameter more than three times the stenosis diameter	Balloon rupture	Total No. reported
Tear or perforation of pulmonary artery	1	2	1	9
Death	2	1	0	5
Technical failure	1	–	–	4
Bleeding requiring transfusion	1	0	0	3
Arrhythmia	1	0	0	2
Acute aneurysm formation	1	0	0	2
Interstitial lung edema	0	0	0	1
Paradoxical embolus	1	1	0	1
Cerebral accident	1	1	0	1
Loss of arterial pulse	0	0	1	1

[a]Adapted from Kan J et al. [32], with permission of the publisher.

USE OF BALLOON-EXPANDABLE INTRAVASCULAR STAINLESS STEEL STENTS TO TREAT BRANCH PULMONARY ARTERY STENOSIS

A stainless steel balloon-expandable graft (stent) was recently developed by Palmaz and coworkers [35,36]. Both Mullins and coworkers [37] and Benson and coworkers [38] recently demonstrated the feasibility of placing such stents into the normal pulmonary arteries of dogs and pigs. Mullins et al. successfully implanted 11 of 13 stents in normal pulmonary arteries, and 11 of 14 were implanted in normal nonstenotic tributaries of precava or postcava. Some of their dogs were recatheterized at intervals ranging from 56 to 270 days. Twelve stents were patent and nonobstructive, two were malpositioned, and one was obstructive. When the animals were sacrificed the stents were evaluated pathologically and were found to be completely covered with neointima and patent without any evidence of thrombus formation.

There is only limited experience with the use of these stents to treat experimentally created stenoses. Mullins and coworkers [37] described dilating one experimentally created peripheral pulmonary artery narrowing, and Benson et al. [38] described in an abstract the successful use of stents to dilate surgically created stenoses in the pulmonary arteries of pigs. We recently developed a dog model of the peripheral pulmonary artery and have been able to establish the efficacy of relieving the experimentally created stenosis with a balloon-expandable stainless steel stent.

Peripheral pulmonary artery stenosis was created in 12 adult mongrel dogs [39] by placing two pieces of 2-O vicryl suture (three loops each) around the pulmonary artery 1–2 cm from its origin. Two to 3 months after creation of the stenosis all dogs underwent cardiac catheterization stent placement. The technique used for stent placement was as follows: A 7 Fr end-hole catheter was passed into the distal pulmonary artery, and a 0.038 inch Teflon-coated 250 cm exchange guidewire

Fig. 7. A: Preangioplasty chest x-ray from a 7-year-old girl with severe distal right pulmonary artery stenosis. **B:** Postangioplasty chest x-ray from the same patient demonstrates the new finding of pulmonary edema in the right lower lobe. The child was asymptomatic from this edema, and it resolved within 1 month postangioplasty.

was advanced into the distal vessel. The end hole catheter was removed, leaving the wire fixed in the vessel, and a 12 Fr long sheath and dilator was introduced over the guidewire into the vessel beyond the stenosis. A stainless steel stent 0.076 mm in thickness, 3 cm in length, and 3.7 mm in diameter before expansion (provided by Johnson and Johnson, Inc.) was placed on an 8 mm diameter balloon angioplasty catheter (Fig. 8). The size of the angioplasty catheter was chosen to be~1 mm larger than the normal vessel diameter. The long dilator was removed from the sheath, and the stent-mounted balloon angioplasty catheter was advanced through the long sheath into the distal pulmonary artery or vena cava. After the angioplasty catheter was positioned across the stenosis, the sheath was withdrawn off the proximal end of the catheter into the main pulmonary artery or right ventricle. The balloon was then expanded to 4–6 atm of pressure and after deflation was exchanged for an end hole catheter, leaving the expanded stent across the area of stenosis.

Successful stent placement was accomplished in all nine dogs in which the stenotic site could be crossed with the 7 Fr wedge catheter (Fig. 9). In all cases the stent abolished the gradient across the stenosis. In all but the first dog, there were no significant complications associated with stent placement. In the first dog in which stent placement was attempted two of the stents inadvertently embolized from the angioplasty catheter. In this animal the stent dislodgements occurred while we were trying to advance the angioplasty catheter and stent across the tricuspid valve without the use of a long sheath. When a long sheath was use to deliver the stent in this and the remaining dogs, no inadvertent embolization occurred. At follow-up catheterization 3 and 6 months after stent placement, all stents were patent without evidence of thrombosis. In the five dogs with distal pulmonary artery stent placement, multiple branch pulmonary arteries were crossed by the stent, and, at follow-up catheterization, angiography demonstrated that these branch pulmonary vessels

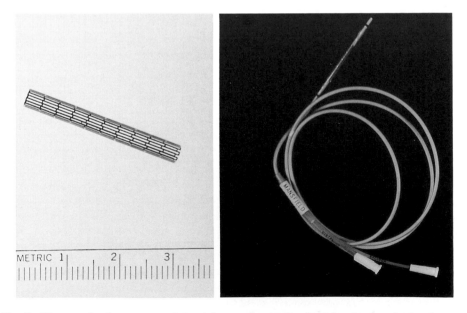

Fig. 8. Photograph of an unexpanded stainless steel stent. On the right, the stent is placed on a 8 mm balloon angioplasty catheter.

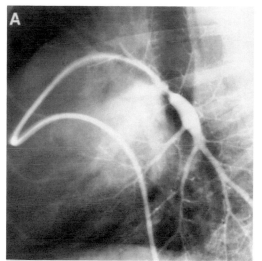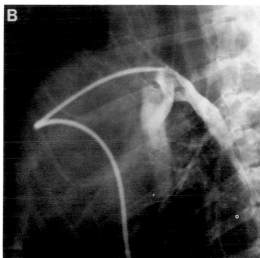

Fig. 9. A series of angiograms before (A) and 6 months after (B) placement of a stent in a branch pulmonary artery. **A:** The discrete stenosis of the proximal left pulmonary artery is visualized. **B:** Angiographic demonstration that the stent and pulmonary artery are widely patent 6 months after initial placement.

remained patent (Fig. 10). Finally, there was no evidence for either late stent migration to a more distal position in the pulmonary artery or for the development of aneurysms.

Our results, along with the work of Mullins and coworkers [37] and Benson et al. [38], suggest that stainless steel balloon-expandable stents should be ideal for treating subjects with refractory branch pulmonary artery stenosis.

O'Laughlin et al. [41] has recently reported the preliminary results of using a 45 balloon-expandable stent in 30 patients to treat refractory stenosis. Branch pulmonary artery stenosis was present in 23 patients and was treated with the placement of 36 stents. Stent placement resulted in a reduction of pulmonary artery branch pressure gradient (50 ± 24 to 15.9 ± 13.4 mmHg). Five patients had stents placed after atrial surgery—three for Fontans and one for an obstructed superior vena cava after repair of sinus venous defect. One patient each had stent placement for pulmonary venous stenosis and coarctation of the aorta. Follow-up catheterization in nine patients documented patency of the stents and sustained

hemodynamic improvement in all but the patient with pulmonary venous stenosis.

However, before these stents can be widely recommended for children and infants, a number of other questions need to be addressed. Children frequently will require placement of a stent at a young age prior to achieving full growth. Since these stents are made of stainless steel, they will not grow with the patient, and stenosis may therefore recur. Thus the question of whether these stents can be progressively expanded months or years after initial placement needs to be addressed before they can be clinically used in young children and infants. Vick et al. [40] have shown that stents placed in the descending aorta of normal juvenile minipigs could be redilated 6 months after initial placement without damage to the aortic wall or stent. Further animal studies will be necessary to establish that balloon-dilatable stents can also be redilated when positioned in a branch pulmonary artery.

A second question that needs to be addressed relates to the ideal length of the stent. In our dogs with proximally placed stenoses,

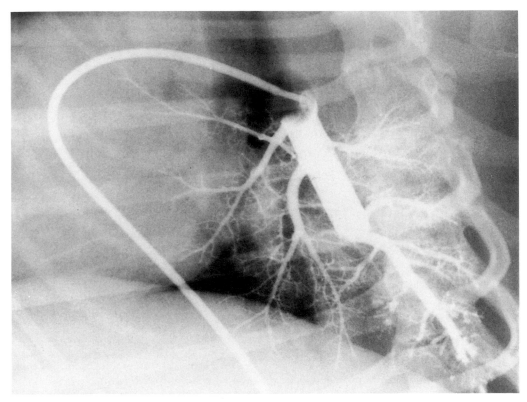

Fig. 10. An angiogram of a distally placed stent 6 months after initial placement demonstrates that the branch pulmonary arteries that were crossed by the stent are widely patent. Although there appears to be a narrowing of the distal pulmonary artery, no hemodynamic gradient was present.

the use of a 3 cm stent resulted in a portion of the stent extending into the main pulmonary artery. For these proximal discrete stenoses the use of a shorter stent length would appear to be more appropriate. In many cases of pulmonary artery branch stenosis, long segment stenosis or multiple stenoses are present. In these situations two or more stents could be implanted in series, as has been done in systemic peripheral arterial disease. Experimental studies will need to document that implantation of stents in series in the pulmonary artery will preserve the curvature of the pulmonary vessel without damaging the vessel.

Finally, although we and others [35,36] have documented that these stents remain patent without local or distal thrombosis formation for up to 6 months, we do not known if thrombi will not develop after longer periods of implantation. Despite the many unknowns still associated with the use of intravascular stents, we believe that they will become the therapy of choice for treating patients with branch pulmonary artery stenosis.

RECOMMENDATIONS

In summary, balloon angioplasty for peripheral pulmonary artery stenosis can provide significant hemodynamic relief to a group of patients in whom traditional operative management is usually not successful. It also appears that, if the peripheral stenosis is the result of a previous systemic-to-pulmonary artery shunt or related to either William's or Alagille's syndrome, angioplasty is unlikely to be beneficial. Based on our animal experience with intravascular balloon-expandable stents, we believe that these stents will make it possible to treat many if not most of the patients with branch pulmonary artery stenosis in whom angioplasty is not currently effective.

REFERENCES

1. Schwalbe E: "Morphologie der Missbidungen." Pt 3, p 426.
2. Mangars (1802): Rec Period Soc Med (Paris) p 74.
3. Orell SR, Kaineil J, Wahlgren F (1960): Malformation and multiple stenoses of the pulmonary arteries with pulmonary hypertension. Acta Radiol 54:449–520.
4. Blackstone EH, Kirklin JW, Bertranou EG, Labrosse CJ, Soto B, Bergeron LM (1979): Preoperative prediction from cineangiograms of post repair right ventricular pressure in tetralogy of Fallot. J Thorac Cardiovasc Surg 73:542–553.
5. Wilson JM, Mack JW, Turley K, Ebert PA (1981): Persistent stenosis and deformity of the right pulmonary artery after correction of the Waterston anastomosis. J Thorac Cardiovasc Surg 82:169–175.
6. Hastreeiter AR, Joorabchi B, Pujatti G, Van der Horst RL, Patersil G, Sever JL (1967): Cardiovascular lesions associated with congenital rubella. J Pediatr 71:59.
7. Beuren AJ, Schulze C, Eberle P, Harmjanz D, Apitz J (1964): The syndrome of supravalvular aortic stenosis, peripheral pulmonary stenosis, mental retardation and similar facial appearance. Am J Cardiol 13:471.
8. Greenwood RD, Rosenthal A, Crocker AAC (1976): Syndrome of intra-hepatic biliary dysgenesis and cardiovascular malformations. Pediatrics 58:243.
9. Mudd CM, Walter KF, Wilman VL (1965): Pulmonary artery stenosis: Diagnosis and therapeutic consideration. Am J Med Sci 249:125.
10. Fouron JC, Favreau-Ethier M, Marion P, Davignon A (1967): Les stenoses pulmonaires peripheriques congenitales: Presentation de 16 observations et revue de la literature. Can Med Assoc J 96:1084.
11. Campbell PE (1965): Vascular abnormalities following maternal rubella. Br Heart J 27:134.
12. Emmanoulilides GC, Linde LM, Crittenden IH (1964): Pulmonary artery stenosis associated with ductus arteriosis following maternal rubella. Circulation 29:514.
13. McCue CM, Robertson LW, Lester RG, Mauck HP Jr (1965): Pulmonary artery coarctation: A report of 20 cases with review of 319 cases from the literature. J Pediatr 67:222.
14. Rowe RD (1973): Cardiovascular disease in the rubella syndrome. Cardiovasc Clin 4:5.
15. Jue KL, Noren GR, Anderson RC (1965): The syndrome of idiopathic hypercalcemia in infancy with associated heart disease. J Pediatr 47:1130.
16. Roberts N, Moes CAF (1973): Supravalvular pulmonary stenosis. J Pediatr 82:838.
17. Gay BB, Franch RH, Shuford WH, Rogers JV (1963): Roentgenologic features of simple and multiple coarctation of the pulmonary artery and branches. Am J Roentgenol 90:599.
18. Alagille D, Odievre M, Gautier M, Dommergues JP (1975): Hepatic ductular hypoplasia associated with characteristic facies, vertebral malformations, retarded physical, mental and sexual development, and cardiac murmur. J Pediatr 86:63.
19. Devloo-Blancquaaert A, Van Den Bosaert-Van Hegesvelde AM, Van Aken Crean R, Essermont-Wirtsen M, Kunnen M, Hooft C (1980): Supravalvular pulmonic and aortic stenoses and intrahepatic bile duct hypoplasia. Acta Paediatr Belg 33:95.
20. Greenwood RD, Rosenthal A, Crocker AC (1976): Syndrome of intrahepatic biliary dysgenesis and cardiovascular malformations. Pediatrics 58:243.
21. Rosenfield MS, Kelley MJ, Jensen PS (1980): Radiology of arteriohepatic dysplasia Am J Radiol 1980,135.1217.
22. Riely CA, Labrecque DR, Ghent C, Horwich A, Klatskin G (1978): A father and son with cholestasis and peripheral pulmonic stenosis. J Pediatr 92:406.
23. Gill CC, Moodie DS, McGoon DC (1977): Staged surgical management of pulmonary atresia with diminutive pulmonary arteries. J Thorac Cardiovasc Surg 73:436–448.
24. Haworth SG, Rees PG, Taylor JRN, MacCartney FJ, DeLeval M, Stark J (1981): Pulmonary atresia with ventricular septal defect and major aortopulmonary collateral arteries: Effect of systemic pulmonary anastomosis. Br Heart J 45:133–142.
25. Martin EC, Diamond NG, Casarella WJ (1980): Percutaneous transluminal angioplasty in non-atherosclerotic disease. Radiology 135:27–33.
26. Lock JE, Niemi T, Einzig S, Amplatz K, Burke B, Bass JL (1981): Transvenous angioplasty of hypoplastic and stenotic pulmonary arteries in newborn lambs. Circulation 64:886–893.
27. Edwards BS, Lucas RV Jr, Lock JE, Edwards JE (1986): Morphologic changes in the pulmonary arteries following percutaneous balloon angioplasty for pulmonary arterial stenosis. Circulation 74:135–143.

28. Lock JE, Castaneda-Zuniga WR, Fuhrman BP, Bass JL (1983): Balloon dilatation angioplasty of hypoplastic and stenotic pulmonary arteries. Circulation 67:962–967.

29. Rocchini AP, Kveselis D, Dick M, Crowley D, Snider AR, Rosenthal A (1984): Use of balloon angioplasty to treat peripheral pulmonary stenosis. Am J Cardiol 54:1069–1073.

30. Kveselis D, Rocchini AP (1984): Percutaneous transluminal angioplasty of peripheral pulmonary arterial stenosis, coarctation of the aorta, superior vena caval and pulmonary venous stenosis, and other great-artery stenosis. Semin Intervent Radiol 1:201–214.

31. Ring JC, Bass JL, Marvin W, Furhman BP, Kulek JJ, Foker JE, Lock JE (1985): Management of congenital stenosis of a branch pulmonary artery with balloon dilation angioplasty. Report of 52 procedures. J Thorac Cardiovasc Surg 90:35–44.

32. Kan JS, Marvin WJ, Bass JL, Muster AJ, Murphy J (1990): Balloon angioplasty–branch pulmonary artery stenosis: Results from the valvuloplasty and angioplasty of congenital anomalies registry. Am J Cardiol 65:798.

33. Foker JE, Turley K, Lock JE, Ring WS, Stanger P (1983): Intraoperative balloon dilation of stenotic and hypoplastic pulmonary arteries. Circulation 68(Suppl II):213.

34. Fellows K, Radtke W, Keane JF, et al. (1987): Acute complications of catheter therapy for congenital heart disease. Am J Cardiol 60:679.

35. Palmaz JC, Sibbitt RR, Tio F, et al. (1986): Expandable intraluminal vascular graft: A feasibility study. Surgery 99:199.

36. Palmaz JC, Windeler SA, Reuter SR, et al. (1987): Expandable intrahepatic portacaval shunt stents: Early experience in the dog. Am J Radiol 145:821.

37. Mullins CE, O'Laughlin MP, Vick GW III, et al. (1988): Implantation of balloon-expandable intravascular grafts by catheterization in pulmonary arteries and systemic veins. Circulation 77:188.

38. Benson LN, Hamilton F, Dasmahapatra HK, Coles JG (1988): Implantable stent dilation of the pulmonary artery: Early experience. Circulation 78(Suppl II): II-100.

39. Rocchini AP, Gundry SR, Beekman RH, et al. (1988): A reversible pulmonary artery band: Preliminary experience. J Am Coll Cardiol 11:172.

40. Vick GW III, O'Laughlin M, Myers T, Nakatani T, Palmaz J, Schatz R, Morrow WR, Mullins C (1989): Evaluation of aortic implantation and redilation of balloon expandable intravascular stents in juvenile minipigs. J Am Coll Cardiol 13:223A.

41. O'Laughlin MP, Perry SB, Lock JE, Mullins CE (1991): Use of endovascular stents in congenital heart disease. Circulation 83:1923.

13

Role of Balloon Dilatation and Other Transcatheter Methods in the Treatment of Cyanotic Congenital Heart Defects

P. Syamasundar Rao, M.D.

Department of Pediatrics, Division of Pediatric Cardiology,
University of Wisconsin Medical School, University of Wisconsin
Children's Hospital, Madison, Wisconsin 53792-4108

INTRODUCTION

Cyanotic congenital heart defects as a group constitute up to one-fifth to one-fourth of all congenital heart defects [1,2]. In cyanotic congenital heart defects, the arterial oxygen desaturation is secondary to right-to-left shunting at the atrial, ventricular, or great artery level or because of transposition of the great arteries in which deoxygenated blood recirculates through the body. In the latter group, balloon or blade atrial septostomy may be of use to augment admixture at the atrial level, and these procedures have been discussed in Chapters 2 and 3 (this volume) and thus are not dealt within here. In the former group, obstruction to pulmonary blood flow by stenotic or atretic pulmonary valve is an integral part of the cardiac malformation causing right-to-left shunt. These patients usually present with symptoms in the neonatal period or in early infancy. The degree of cyanosis and the level of hypoxemia determine the symptomatology. Physical findings and laboratory data (EGG, chest x-ray, and echo-Doppler) depend on the defect complex and are reasonably characteristic for each of them. Total surgical correction and, if that is not feasible, palliation with some type of systemic-to-pulmonary artery anastomosis to augment pulmonary blood flow are usually recommended. Since the

introduction of transluminal balloon dilatation technique in children by Kan and associates [3], we [4–7] and others have utilized this technique to augment pulmonary blood flow instead of employing an initial or a repeat systemic-to-pulmonary artery shunt. For the purpose of discussion in this chapter, the subject is divided into four distinct groups: 1) pulmonary stenosis with right-to-left shunt at the ventricular level; 2) Pulmonary stenosis with intact ventricular septum and right-to-left atrial shunt; 3) pulmonary atresia; and 4) narrowed systemic-to-pulmonary artery shunts.

PULMONARY STENOSIS WITH VENTRICULAR RIGHT-TO-LEFT SHUNT (VENTRICULAR SEPTAL DEFECT)

The patients considered in this section are those who have severe pulmonary stenosis in association with a (usually) large interventricular communication. The most common type of defect in this category is tetralogy of Fallot (TOF). Other defects include transposition of the great arteries, double-outlet right (or left) ventricle, and ventricular inversion (corrected transposition of the great arteries), all with a large ventricular septal defect and severe pulmonic stenosis. Other

Transcatheter Therapy in Pediatric Cardiology, pages 229–253
© 1993 Wiley-Liss, Inc.

defects such as single ventricle and tricuspid atresia fall into this category provided pulmonary stenosis is present.

Indications

The indications for balloon pulmonary valvuloplasty that we have used [4,7] were cardiac defects not amenable to surgical correction for the age and size at the time of presentation but at the same time requiring palliation for pulmonary oligemia. Symptoms related to hypoxemia and polycythemia are indications for intervention. Hypoplasia of the pulmonary valve ring and main and/or branch pulmonary arteries is another indication even if symptoms are not present. Two or more sites of obstruction to pulmonary blood flow (Fig. 1) were considered a prerequisite when employing balloon valvuloplasty because, if valvar stenosis is the sole obstruction, relief of such an obstruction may result in a marked increase in pulmonary blood flow and elevation of pulmonary artery pressure and resistance.

Technique

The technique of balloon pulmonary valvuloplasty in this group of patients is similar to that used in isolated valvar pulmonic stenosis described in Chapter 6 (this volume), although at times it may be more difficult to accomplish balloon valvuloplasty in this group than in a simple pulmonary valve stenosis group. A few examples of balloon catheters across the pulmonary valve are shown in Figures 2 through 4. We chose a balloon size that is 1.2–1.4 times the size of the pulmonary valve annulus [8,9].

Results

Immediate results. Balloon pulmonary valvuloplasty for infants with cyanotic congenital heart defects with pulmonary oligemia was

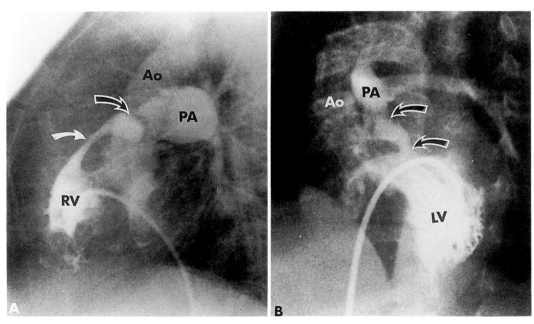

Fig. 1. Selected cineangiographic frames from patients with tetralogy of Fallot (**A**) and d-transposition of the great arteries (**B**), demonstrating two sites of pulmonary outflow obstruction (two arrows). When the pulmonary valve obstruction is relieved by balloon valvuloplasty, the subvalvar obstruction remains and prevents flooding of the lungs. Ao, aorta; LV, left ventricle; PA, pulmonary artery; RV, right ventricle.

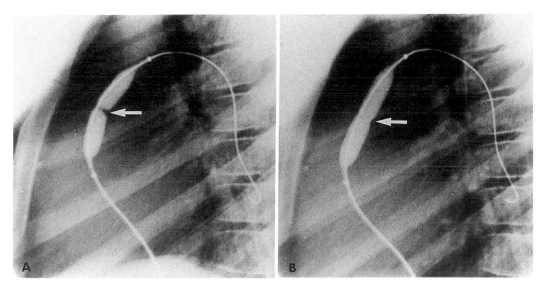

Fig. 2. Selected cineradiographic (lateral view) frames of a balloon dilatation catheter placed across the pulmonic valve in an infant with tetralogy of Fallot. Note "waisting" of the balloon during the initial phases of balloon inflation (**A**, arrow), which is almost completely abolished during the later phases of balloon inflation (**B**, arrow).

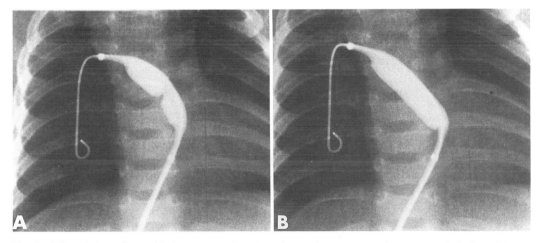

Fig. 3. Selected cineradiographic (posteroanterior view) frames demonstrating the position of a balloon dilatation catheter across the pulmonic valve in a patient with tetralogy of Fallot. Note the indentation (waist) of the balloon (**A**), which disappeared (**B**) following full inflation. Although we prefer to place the guidewire in the left pulmonary artery, balloon valvuloplasty can also be successfully performed with the guidewire positioned in the right pulmonary artery, as in the illustrated case.

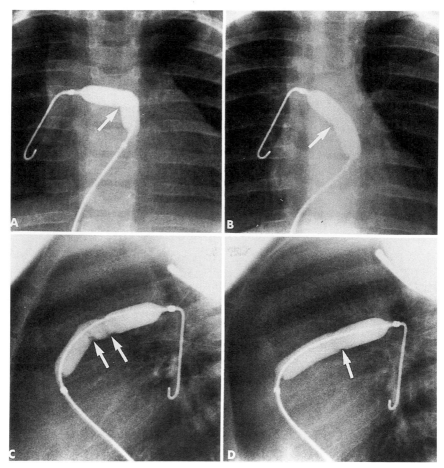

Fig. 4. Selected cineradiographic views in posteroanterior **(A,B)** and lateral **(C,D)** projections showing a balloon catheter during the initial **(A,C)** and final **(B,D)** phases of inflation. Note the initial prominent "waisting", which was subsequently almost completely abolished (arrows). In this patient with tetralogy of Fallot, a lower "waist" (C, left arrow) produced by infundibular constriction is also seen, which completely disappeared after balloon inflation (D).

used by us [5,7] and others [10–14] to augment pulmonary blood flow. McCredie and associates [10] balloon dilated a stenotic pulmonary valve in two patients, one with TOF and the other with tricuspid atresia, and reported improvement in exercise tolerance in both and improvement in oxygen saturation from 83% to 89% in one child. Boucek et al. [11] were successful in performing balloon pulmonary valvuloplasty in seven of the eight patients in whom they attempted the procedure. The diagnoses in these seven patients were TOF in five;

transposition of the great arteries, ventricular septal defect, and pulmonic stenosis in one; and ventricular inversion, ventricular septal defect, and pulmonic stenosis in the final patient. The systemic arterial oxygen saturations increased from 72% ± 5% to 83% ± 5% (P < 0.005). The pulmonary blood flow and pulmonary arterial pressure also increased. Qureshi et al. [12] reported their observations after balloon dilatation of the pulmonary valve in 15 patients with TOF; the systemic arterial oxygen saturation increased in the majority of patients.

In four of these children, either no significant change or a deterioration in oxygen saturation occurred, and they received systemic-to-pulmonary artery shunts an average of 1.6 months (0–3 months) after the procedure. Six children did not require further intervention. Qureshi et al. concluded that balloon dilatation may be useful in the management of infants with severe TOF and that it should be considered for the initial palliative treatment. Mehta and Perlman [13] reported a single patient with TOF in whom balloon pulmonary valvuloplasty increased oxygen saturation from 80% to 90%.

Our experience with this procedure, including that previously reported [4,5,7], was in 14 infants with cyanotic congenital heart defects aged 3 months to 27 years (median, 10 months), weighing 5.4–16 kg (median, 8.0 kg), who underwent balloon pulmonary valvuloplasty as a palliative procedure to improve pulmonary oligemia. All but one were < 3 years of age. The diagnoses in these cases were TOF in ten; transposition of the great arteries, with ventricular septal defect and valvar and subvalvar pulmonary stenoses in three; and dextrocardia, ventricular inversion with ventricular septal defect, and valvar and subvalvar

pulmonary stenosis in the final case. Following balloon pulmonary valvuloplasty, the arterial oxygen saturation increased from 69% ± 13% to 84% ± 12% (P < 0.01). The pulmonary blood flow index (2.2 ± 0.8 l/min/m² vs. 3.5 ± 1.2 l/min/m², P < 0.05), pulmonary-to-systemic flow ratio (Qp:Qs; 0.7 ± 0.4 vs. 1.2 ± 0.5, P < 0.02), and pulmonary artery pressure (16 ± 5 vs. 26 ± 9 mmHg, P < 0.02) increased following balloon dilatation (Table I). The pulmonary valvar gradients (56 ± 20 vs. 31 ± 21 mmHg) fell (P < 0.05), whereas infundibular gradients (33 ± 12 vs. 39 ± 17 mmHg) and total pulmonary ventricular outflow tract (valvar plus subvalvar) gradients (77 ± 14 vs. 66 ± 17 mmHg) remained unchanged (P > 0.1) after valvuloplasty. An example is shown in Figure 5. None required immediate surgical intervention. No complications were encountered during the procedure. All children were discharged home within 24 hours of the procedure.

Follow-up results. There are limited follow-up data available. Boucek et al. [11] reported 0.5–2.8 year follow-up results; four TOF patients underwent surgical correction, one patient underwent systemic-to-pulmonary

TABLE I. Results of Balloon Pulmonary Valvuloplasty—Group 1[a]

	Prior to BPV (N = 11)	Immediately after BPV (N = 11)	P value[b]	4–36 Months after BPV (N = 11)	P value[b]
Arterial O_2 sat (%)	67 ± 13	83 ± 13	<0.01	82 ± 9	<0.01
Qp:Qs	0.7 ± 0.4	1.2 ± 0.5	<0.02	1.3 ± 0.7	<0.05
Qp (liters/min/m²)	2.1 ± 0.8	3.2 ± 1.3	<0.05	4.0 ± 1.7	<0.01
PA pressure (mmHg)	16 + 5	26 ± 11	<0.02	22 ± 6	>0.05
Pulmonary valve gradient (mmHg)	52 ± 16	32 ± 22	<0.05	18 ± 7	<0.001
Infundibular gradient (mmHg)	33 ± 12	42 ± 16*	>0.1	53 ± 18*	<0.02
Total gradient across, PV outflow (mmHg)	77 ± 14	66 ± 12	>0.05	69 ± 13	>0.1
Hemoglobin (gm%)	16.5 ± 2.9	—	—	15.8 ± 2.7	>0.1

[a]PV, pulmonary ventricle; other abbreviations, as in Table II.
[b]Compares with value obtained prior to BPV.
*P > 0.1.

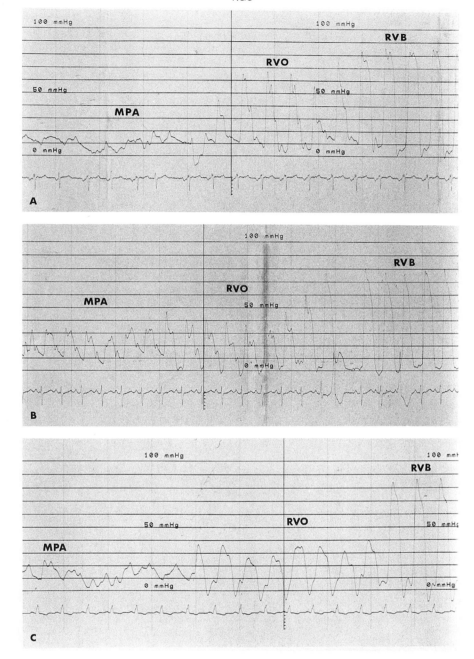

Fig. 5. Pressure pullback tracings across the pulmonic valve and right ventricular outflow tract before **(A)**, 15 minutes after **(B)**, and 12 months after **(C)** balloon pulmonary valvuloplasty in a patient with tetralogy of Fallot. Note that both valvar and infundibular gradients were present prior to valvuloplasty (A), whereas the valvar gradient almost completely disappeared and the infundibular gradient persisted immediately after (B) and 12 months after (C) valvuloplasty. MPA, main pulmonary artery; RVB, right ventricular body; RVO, right ventricular outflow tract. Reproduced from Rao *et al.* [7], with permission of the publisher.

artery anastomosis, and the other two did not require surgical correction. Qureshi and associates [12] reported follow-up observations after balloon angioplasty of 15 TOF patients. Seven children did not require further palliation during a mean follow-up period of 12.9 months (3.5–26 months). Four children required a systemic-to-pulmonary artery shunt operation 0–3 months (mean, 1.6 months) after angioplasty. The final four patients had a corrective operation 6–16 months (mean, 8 months) after balloon dilatation.

In our study [7], all 4 children have been followed for 3 to 48 months (15 ± 3 months) with pulse oximetry and hemoglobin determinations. Cardiac catheterization was also performed in 3 children 4–40 months (median, 11 months) following valvuloplasty. Arterial oxygen saturation (82% ± 9%), pulmonary blood flow (4 ± 1.7 l/min/m²), and the Qp:Qs ratio (1.3 ± 0.7) remain unchanged (P > 0.1) from the immediate postvalvuloplasty values, but remain im-

proved (P < 0.05–0.001) compared with prevalvuloplasty values (Table I). The hemoglobin level (16.2 ± 2.5 gm%) did not increase (P > 0.1) compared with a prevalvuloplasty value of 16.8 ± 3.0 gm%. The pulmonary valve gradient (18 ± 7 mmHg) remains improved compared with both that recorded prior to (P < 0.001) and that immediately after (P < 0.05) valvuloplasty (Table I). The subvalvar (53 ± 18 mmHg) and total pulmonary ventricular outflow tract (69 ± 13 mmHg) gradients remain unchanged (P > 0.1). An example is shown in Figure 5. None of the patients had significant elevation of peak systolic pulmonary artery pressure: 22 ± 6 mmHg (range, 12–30 mmHg).

Eight children with TOF underwent successful total surgical correction 4–24 months (12 ± 9 months) following valvuloplasty. Five of these children had very small pulmonary arteries prior to valvuloplasty and were initially considered unsuitable for total surgical correc-

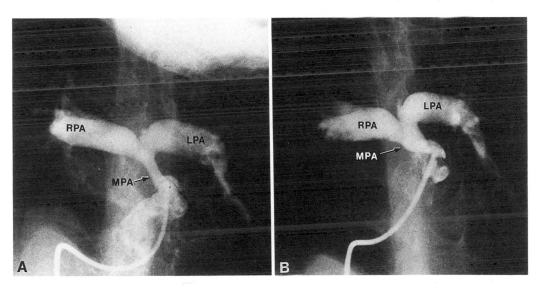

Fig. 6. Selected frames from pulmonary artery cineangiograms in a "sitting-up" view in a patient with tetralogy of Fallot prior to (**A**) and 12 months following (**B**) balloon pulmonary valvuloplasty. Note significant improvement in the size of the valve annulus and main and branch pulmonary arteries following valvuloplasty. LPA, left pulmonary artery; MPA, main pulmonary artery; RPA, right pulmonary artery. Reproduced from Rao et al. [7], with permission of the publisher.

tion. Approximately 12 months later, the pulmonary artery anatomy improved (Fig. 6) and total surgical correction was performed without incident. The other three children were operated on 4, 5 and seven months, respectively) after balloon valvuloplasty because they developed cyanotic spells. The remaining two patients with TOF are clinically doing well and awaiting surgery.

Two children in the transposition group showed evidence for significant hypoxemia on follow-up and Blalock-Taussig shunts were performed, 6 and 18 months, respectively, following initial balloon valvuloplasty. An increase in the size of the pulmonary artery (Fig. 7), as previously reported [4], was observed. The remaining transposition patient and the single patient with corrected transposition (ventricu-

lar inversion) are clinically well, and no further intervention is planned.

Complications

Complications have been remarkably minimal. A transient decrease in systemic arterial saturation occurs while the balloon is inflated but rapidly improves following balloon deflation. Surprisingly, cyanotic spells following balloon valvuloplasty have not been a problem, presumably because of improvement of pulmonary blood flow following the procedure. However, increasing cyanosis has been observed by some workers [12]. Hypotension during balloon inflation, which is common in balloon dilatation of pulmonic stenosis with intact ventricular septum [15], is usually not seen in this group of patients; presumably the

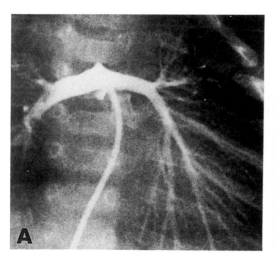
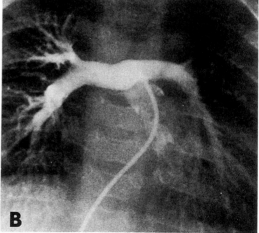

RPA — 5.0 mm
LPA — 3.3 mm

RPA — 9.4 mm
LPA — 7.8 mm

Fig. 7. Pulmonary arteriogram immediately before (**A**) and 6 months after (**B**) balloon pulmonary valvuloplasty in an infant with transposition of the great arteries, ventricular septal defect, and valvar and subvalvar pulmonic stenosis. Note increased size of the pulmonary arteries after pulmonary valvuloplasty. There were differences in the magnification between both cineangiographic frames; catheters in both frames were 5 Fr. After correcting for magnification, the right pulmonary artery (RPA) size increased from 5.0 to 9.4 mm, whereas the left pulmonary artery (LPA) increased from 3.3 to 7.8 mm. Part of the growth was attributed to an increase in forward flow following balloon valvuloplasty. (Reproduced from Rao and Brais [4], with permission of the publisher.)

flow through the ventricular septal defect provides systemic flow. Pulmonary arterial tear [16] has been reported in a 3-year-old child, which was noted at the time of total surgical correction 15 months following valvuloplasty. Femoral venous occlusion may be seen at follow-up [4,7], but without adverse effects.

Comments

To the best of my knowledge, Lababidi and colleagues [17,18] were the first to report balloon valvuloplasty in patients with tetralogy of Fallot. However, they did not advocate the procedure for patients with TOF. While evaluating the mechanism of balloon pulmonary valvuloplasty [17,18], they also examined its role in TOF and suggested that, in the presence of combined infundibular and valvar pulmonic stenosis, balloon fixation by infundibulum causes retraction of the balloon into the ventricle during systole, which may cause avulsion of the valve cusp. Therefore they did not recommend balloon valvuloplasty in these patients [18]. Subsequently, several groups of workers, including ours [4,5,7,10–14], reported successful balloon pulmonary valvuloplasty to improve pulmonary oligemia, which were just reviewed.

The immediate results of balloon pulmonary valvuloplasty in this group of patients appear good, and it attained the objective of improving pulmonary oligemia and systemic arterial hypoxemia. Immediate surgical intervention was avoided in most cases. Intermediate-term results are also good, the augmentation of pulmonary blood flow continuing to be present at follow-up in most children. The size of the pulmonary arteries improved in most patients, making them more suitable for further palliative or total surgical corrective procedure.

Battistessa et al. [19] reported their observations of surgery for TOF patients who had previously undergone balloon pulmonary valvuloplasty. Results in 27 patients (which included 15 patients previously reported by Qureshi et al. [12] and probably form a subgroup of their larger experience [14]) were scrutinized. They found anatomic alterations in the right ventricular outflow tract in 20 (74%) patients, whereas no change was seen in seven (26%). They also noted that there was no evidence for significant growth of the pulmonary valve annulus and that the need for transannular patch was not abolished at the time of intracardiac repair. In view of the damage to the pulmonary valve mechanism and no evidence for enough growth of the pulmonary valve to obviate the need for transannular patch at a later corrective surgery, they were not very supportive of balloon valvuloplasty as a palliative procedure. While these observations are important, we [4,7] and others [11,14,20] have documented an increase in the size of the pulmonary artery and/or annulus following balloon pulmonary valvuloplasty. The increased size was demonstrated in a larger group of patients [14], which included the patients of Battistessa et al. [19]. An increased ($P < 0.001$) pulmonary valve annulus was demonstrated in 24 patients who also had increased systemic arterial oxygen saturations following balloon valvuloplasty, and this increase in pulmonary annulus size was greater ($P < 0.005$) than expected from normal growth. This improvement in the size of the pulmonary arteries [4,7,11,14,20] is similar to that observed following the Brock [22] procedure [21], and systemic-to-pulmonary arterial shunts [23–26].

In view of the varied observations, it would seem prudent that balloon pulmonary valvuloplasty in TOF (or any other cyanotic defects) be performed only in selected patients. General criteria that I propose are the following: 1) the infant/child requires palliation of pulmonary oligemia but is not a candidate for total surgical correction because of the size of the patient, the type of the defect, or anatomic aberrations; 2) valvar obstruction is a significant component of the right ventricular outflow tract obstruction; and 3) multiple obstructions in series (Fig. 1) are present so that there is residual subvalvar obstruction after relief of pulmonary valvar obstruction and flooding of lungs is prevented. Once balloon valvuloplasty is decided upon, we would recommend balloons large enough to produce balloon/annulus ratios of 1.2–1.4 [4,7–9,27].

New Developments

Obstruction to pulmonary outflow tract is usually at multiple levels in TOF; the sites of obstruction are pulmonary arteries, pulmonary valve leaflets, pulmonary valve ring, and infundibulum. Relief of valvar obstruction can in some patients increase forward flow and encourage growth of the pulmonary valve ring and pulmonary arteries, as discussed above. If severe infundibular stenosis is present, relief of pulmonary valve stenosis alone may not accomplish the objectives of relieving systemic hypoxemia and encouraging growth of the pulmonary arteries. Qureshi and associates [28] used a Simpson coronary atherectomy catheter to perform an infundibular myectomy in a 14-month-old child with TOF. The systemic arterial saturation improved from 78% prior to the procedure to 85% 1 month later, and the right ventricular outflow tract became wider. They suggested that the type of transcatheter resection of the infundibulum may be important in the palliation of TOF. Further clinical trials of this method in selected patients are warranted because this method may serve as a useful adjunct to balloon pulmonary valvuloplasty in the management of TOF.

Conclusions

Balloon pulmonary valvuloplasty appears to offer excellent relief of pulmonary oligemia and systemic arterial hypoxemia in patients with a TOF type of hemodynamics. Based on the data presented, we recommend balloon pulmonary valvuloplasty to manage patients with cyanotic heart defects and pulmonary oligemia. We believe it is an effective alternative to surgical creation of a systemic-to-pulmonary arterial anastomosis, thus avoiding potential complications associated with surgical shunts [29–32]. The procedure is likely to be beneficial if the valvar obstruction is the dominant obstruction. The presence of two or more obstructions in series is desirable to prevent flooding the lungs when the procedure proves successful.

PULMONARY STENOSIS WITH ATRIAL RIGHT-TO-LEFT SHUNT (INTACT VENTRICULAR SEPTUM)

Some patients have very severe pulmonary stenosis with a resultant increase in right ventricular and atrial pressures and consequent right-to-left shunting across either a patent foramen ovale or an atrial septal defect.

Indications

Any patient with severe enough pulmonary valve obstruction to produce right-to-left atrial shunting and arterial desaturation is a candidate for relief of the pulmonary valve stenosis. No age or weight (size) are contraindications. It is important to relieve the pulmonary valve obstruction prior to deterioration of right ventricular function.

Technique

The procedure of balloon pulmonary valvuloplasty is exactly the same as that used for isolated valvar pulmonary stenosis, as described in Chapter 6. However, the procedure may be slightly more difficult to accomplish because of the greater severity of the pulmonary outflow obstruction and the more frequent association of right ventricular hypoplasia and infundibular obstruction. Sometimes, even introducing a 5 Fr catheter across the pulmonary valve may cause bradycardia and hypoxemia because of further obstruction to pulmonary blood flow by the catheter. On such occasions, we leave a 0.014 inch guidewire (wires used for coronary arterial lesions) across the pulmonic valve and then perform rapid dilatation with a 4 Fr coronary balloon dilatation catheter carrying a 4 mm low-profile balloon. Subsequent to that, a more appropriate-sized balloon dilatation catheter (1.2–1.4 times the size of the pulmonary annulus) can be used. Such progressive dilatation technique [33,34] should be employed when dealing with severe pulmonary valve stenosis patients with suprasystemic right ventricular peak systolic pressure and in neonates and small infants after spontaneous ductal closure. At times it may be difficult to advance a catheter across the severe infundibular obstruction secondary valvar stenosis; administration of propranolol (0.1 mg/kg) by slow intravenous route may help position the catheter across the right ventricular obstruction [35] and allow balloon valvuloplasty.

Hypotension during balloon inflation is minimal in these children because of maintenance of systemic perfusion by right-to-left shunting across the patent foramen ovale [36]. However, when monitored by pulse oximetry, the systemic arterial oxygen saturation falls, but returns to normal after balloon deflation.

Results

Immediate results. Although some of the investigators, as listed elsewhere [34], may have mentioned of patients with right-to-left shunt, none have grouped the patients in a manner similar to that in this chapter. From our study group, we had 12 patients, aged 3 days to 11.5 years (median, 8 months), who underwent balloon pulmonary valvuloplasty [7]. All had severe valvar pulmonic stenosis with intact ventricular septum and interatrial right-to-left shunting. The right ventricle was hypoplastic in three infants; severe infundibular stenosis was present either before or immediately after balloon angioplasty in five children, in a manner described elsewhere [37]; poor right ventricular function was evident in two children; and Ebstein's anomaly of the tricuspid valve was present in one infant. The right ventricular peak systolic pressure was above that in the left ventricle in nine children and was similar in both ventricles in the remaining three. There was a varying level of hypoxemia, with a mean arterial oxygen saturation of 83% ± 8% (mean ± SD; range = 64%–91%). The arterial desaturation was secondary to interatrial right-to-left shunting in all cases.

Following balloon pulmonary valvuloplasty, the arterial oxygen saturation increased from 83% ± 8% to 94% ± 5% ($P < 0.001$); in only one child was the oxygen saturation less than 91% after valvuloplasty. The pulmonary blood flow index (1.9 ± 0.5 vs. 2.8 ± 0.6 liters/min/m^2, $P < 0.001$), Qp:Qs ratio (0.7 ± 0.1 vs. 1.0 ± 0.2, $P < 0.001$), and pulmonary artery pressure (15 ± 6 vs. 27 ± 9 mmHg, $P < 0.01$) increased after valvuloplasty. Peak systolic pressure gradients across the pulmonary valve decreased ($P < 0.001$) from 105 ± 48 to 25 ± 18 mmHg. Infundibular pressure gradients were recorded prior to valvuloplasty in two children; these were 20 and 130 mmHg, respectively. They changed respectively, to 27 and 30 mmHg after balloon valvuloplasty. Infundibular gradients that were not present prior to valvuloplasty appeared in two children; these were 30 and 115 mmHg. Right ventricular cineangiography revealed a greater movement of the leaflets of the pulmonary valve and a larger jet of contrast material passing across the pulmonary valve than in prevalvuloplasty cineangiograms. A hyperactive infundibular region was observed before and/or after valvuloplasty in five children, including the four in whom pressure gradients were recorded. The size of the right ventricle increased dramatically in a 7-day-old infant with critical pulmonary stenosis and hypoplastic right ventricle (Fig. 8) [4]. The size of the right ventricle decreased markedly in one child with associated Ebstein's anomaly of the tricuspid valve (Fig. 9). All but the two neonates were discharged home on the morning following balloon pulmonary valvuloplasty. The two neonates aged (3 and 7 days) who were on ventilators at the time of valvuloplasty were discharged home within 1 week after valvuloplasty. No complications other than an episode of supraventricular tachycardia in one neonate (which resolved spontaneously) were encountered.

Follow-up results. Clinical and echo-Doppler follow-up data are available for 11 children, aged 1–31 months (mean, 12

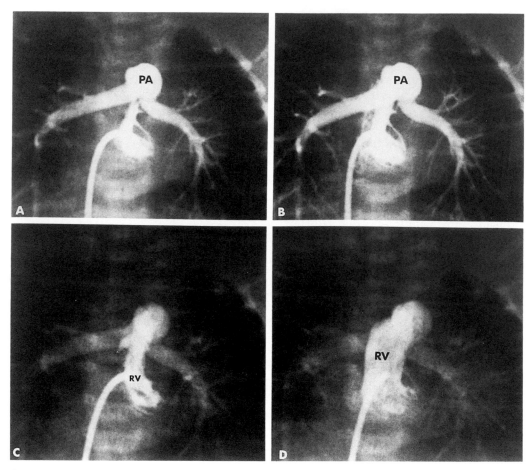

Fig. 8. Systolic **(A,B)** and diastolic **(C,D)** cine frames from right ventricular angiograms before **(A,C)** and after **(B,D)** balloon pulmonary valvuloplasty in a neonate with critical pulmonary stenosis with intact ventricular septum and hypoplastic right ventricle (RV). Note increased size of the right ventricle **(B,D)** after balloon valvuloplasty. PA, pulmonary artery. (Reproduced from Rao and Brais [4], with permission of the publisher.)

months) following balloon dilatation, and cardiac catheterization was performed in seven children aged 6–18 months (11 ± 4 months) after valvuloplasty. Arterial oxygen saturation (94% ± 6%), pulmonary blood flow (3.5 ± 0.9 liters/min/m^2), and the Qp:Qs ratio (1.0 ± 0.1) remain improved ($P < 0.01$–0.001) compared with prevalvuloplasty values but essentially unchanged ($P > 0.1$) compared with immediate postvalvuloplasty values (Table II). The pulmonary valvar gradient (33 ± 33 mmHg) continues to be lower ($P < 0.001$) than

that prior to valvuloplasty, but unchanged ($P > 0.1$) compared with the immediate postvalvuloplasty gradient. Infundibular gradients disappeared in two children and fell further in one child, and significant residual (50 mmHg) was present in the remaining child.

Despite improvement as a group, two children had significant residual pulmonary valvar gradients, and repeat balloon pulmonary valvuloplasty was performed at the follow-up catheterization with reduction of gradients from 94 and 61 mmHg to 26 and 18 mmHg,

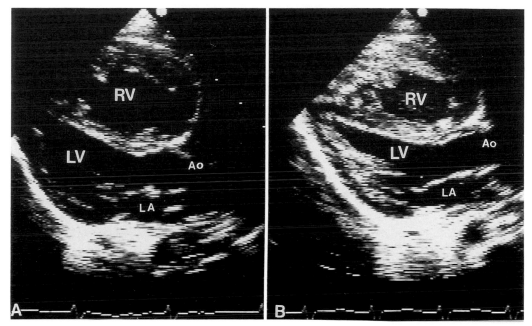

Fig. 9. Two-dimensional echographic views of the right ventricle (RV) demonstrating markedly enlarged right ventricle in a patient with severe valvar pulmonic stenosis and Ebstein's anomaly of the tricuspid valve prior to balloon pulmonary valvuloplasty (**A**), which markedly decreased after valvuloplasty (**B**). RV, right ventricle; LV, left ventricle; Ao, aorta; LA, left pulmonary artery.

respectively. None required surgical intervention, and two children remain on β-blocking agents.

Doppler studies (performed in a manner similar to that described elsewhere [38,39]) at the last follow-up examination revealed a mean Doppler flow velocity of 2.6 ± 0.7 m/s across the pulmonary valve, which had been 4.9 ± 0.9 m/s prior to valvuloplasty (Table II). Calculated instantaneous pressure gradients (26 ± 10 mmHg) were lower (P < 0.001) than those prior to valvuloplasty (100 ± 36 mmHg). No complications were observed at the follow-up catheter and clinical evaluations.

Comments.

Both the immediate and intermediate-term follow-up results were good, with relief of right ventricular hypertension and systemic arterial hypoxemia. The group with intact ventricular septum and interatrial right-to-left shunting behaved in a manner similar to that seen with isolated pulmonary valve stenosis [40–42]. Despite restenosis of the pulmonary valve in two children, requiring repeat balloon dilatation, the overall results are gratifying. Persistent hypoxemia was seen in only one child with hypoplastic right ventricle and severe residual infundibular obstruction. This child might need surgical resection of infundibular obstruction at a later date. Infundibular obstruction resolved in the remaining patients in a manner described by us [37] and others [43].

Conclusions

Balloon pulmonary valvuloplasty appears to offer excellent relief of pulmonary oligemia, systemic arterial hypoxemia, and right ventricular hypertension in patients with pulmonary stenosis with intact ventricular septum and

TABLE II. Results of Balloon Pulmonary Valvuloplasty—Group II[a]

	Prior to BPV (N = 12)	Immediately after BPV (N = 12)	P value[b]	1–31 Months after BPV[c]	P Value[b]
Arterial O$_s$ sat (%)	83 ± 8	94 ± 5	<0.001	94 ± 6	<0.01
Qp:Qs	0.7 ± 0.1	1.0 ± 0.16	<0.001	1.0 ± 0.1	<0.001
Qp (liters/min/m^2)	1.9 ± 0.5	2.8 ± 0.6	<0.001	3.5 ± 0.9	<0.001
PA pressure (mm Hg)	15 ± 6	27 ± 9	<0.01	17 ± 6	>0.1
Pulmonary valve gradient (mm Hg)	105 ± 48	25 ± 18	<0.001	33 ± 33	<0.001
Hemoglobin (gm%)	15.4 ± 2.8	–	–	12.1 ± 1.4	<0.01
PA Doppler flow velocities (m/s)	4.9 ± 0.9	2.7 ± 0.8	<0.001	2.6 ± 0.7	<0.001

[a]BPV, balloon pulmonary valvuloplasty; O$_2$ sat, oxygen saturation; PA, pulmonary artery; Qp, pulmonary blood flow; Qp:Qs, pulmonary-to-systemic blood flow ratio.
[b]Compares with values obtained prior to BPV.
[c]N = 11 for noninvasive and N = 7 for catheterization data.

right-to-left atrial shunting. Based on the data presented, we suggest that it is the procedure of choice for treatment of this group of patients.

PULMONARY ATRESIA

Pulmonary atresia may be present with or without a ventricular septal defect. Multiple palliative procedures are usually necessary [44,45] prior to any corrective surgery. Pulmonary atresia patients with ventricular septal defects usually have underdeveloped main pulmonary artery and/or infundibular atresia and may not be amenable to transcatheter treatment, to be discussed below, although an occasional patient may have isolated valvar atresia. Patients with pulmonary atresia with an intact ventricular septum usually have a well-developed main pulmonary artery with only valvar atresia, although some patients in this category may also have infundibular atresia. In this section, I discuss transcatheter approaches that have potential utility in the management of valvar pulmonary atresia with intact ventricular septum. These methods could also be employed in the ventricular

septal defect group, provided the infundibulum and main pulmonary artery are wide open.

The prognosis for patients who have pulmonary atresia with an intact ventricular septum is poor with or without conventional surgical intervention [44,46–48]. Therefore, we suggested [44,49] the adoption of a comprehensive medical and surgical treatment program leading to complete surgical correction of the lesion. The objectives of such a program were 1) to relieve hypoxemia and acidosis by a timely and appropriate procedure to increase pulmonary blood flow at initial presentation (usually in the newborn period); 2) to facilitate adequate egress of blood from the right atrium; and 3) to stimulate the growth of the right ventricle [44,49]. The objectives of the program can often be achieved by appropriately timed, multiple surgical procedures. These have been detailed elsewhere [44]. Two transcatheter treatment strategies have been suggested for the management of these difficult patients [50,51]: 1) primary perforation of the atretic pulmonary valve by transcatheter methods [50] and 2) limited opening of the pulmonary valve at surgery [51], both followed by balloon valvuloplasty [50, 51].

Transcatheter Perforation of Atretic Pulmonary Valve

Perforation of the atretic pulmonary valve with a blunt wire, though feasible [52], is not generally used. Lee et al. [53] and Riemenschneider et al. [54] applied laser irradiation to relieve obstructed valves and create atrial septal defects in animal models and human postmortem specimens. Arapov et al. used laser for pulmonary valvotomy introperatively [55]. Qureshi et al. [50] utilized laser via a catheter to perforate the atretic pulmonary valve and followed this with balloon enlargement of the pulmonary valve. They were successful in perforating the pulmonary valve with an Nd-YAG laser wire in four of the five patients in whom they tried this procedure. Perforation of the right ventricle and cardiac tamponade occurred in the fifth patient. An increase in the pulmonary artery pressure and a decrease in the right ventricular pressure occurred in all four patients. At 2–6 month follow-up examinations, forward flow across the laser-opened pulmonary valve was demonstrated; there was a 50–70 mmHg residual gradient across the pulmonic valve. The oxygen saturations ranged from 70% to 87%.

These preliminary observations are of interest, and, with further refinement of the technique and additional clinical trials, the laser techniques are likely to be useful in the management of these complex pulmonary atresia patients.

Surgical Pulmonary Valvotomy Followed by Balloon Valvuloplasty

Latson and associates [51] advocated a limited incision (4 mm) in the atretic pulmonary valve by direct vision via the main pulmonary artery in order to allow antegrade flow and future access for balloon dilatation. They performed this procedure either at the time of the initial shunt procedure or at a subsequent sitting. They performed balloon pulmonary valvuloplasty in patients aged 2–12 months and reduced the pulmonary valvar gradients to less than 20 mmHg. The right ventricular peak systolic pressure was less than 60% of systemic pressure. They applied this technique in four infants. Two patients had undergone complete repair, and the other two are acyanotic and have biventricular physiology.

Kan et al. [56] and Sullivan et al. [57] also attempted balloon dilatation following surgical pulmonary valvotomy for pulmonary atresia, but without success. Ballerini al. [58] also performed balloon valvuloplasty after surgical valvotomy for pulmonary atresia with intact ventricular septum; in six patients, they reduced peak pulmonary valve gradients from 50 ± 8 to 30 ± 6 mmHg. Our experience in two patients is similar to that reported by Ballerini et al. [58]. Both of the above approaches are innovative methods and may have clinical utility. Appropriate clinical trials are warranted to assess their effectiveness and safety.

NARROWED SYSTEMIC-TO-PULMONARY ARTERY SHUNTS

Cyanotic congenital heart defects with pulmonary oligemia secondary to severe pulmonary stenosis or pulmonary atresia usually require a systemic arterial-to-pulmonary arterial shunt operation to augment pulmonary blood flow and to improve arterial oxygen saturation. Narrowing of these shunts can occur postoperatively with resultant inadequate oxygenation. These narrowed shunts can be balloon dilated [6,59–63,63a]. Gibbs and associates [59] reported balloon dilatation of a narrowed Waterston (ascending aorta-to-right pulmonary artery) shunt in a 13-year-old child with pulmonary atresia and multiple shunts. The size of the stoma of the Waterston anastomosis was 3 mm. They initially used an 8 mm balloon catheter, did not observe "waisting" of the balloon and, therefore repeated the procedure with a 12 mm balloon. There was a dramatic increase in arterial oxygen saturation (from 76% to 96%) and pulmonary artery pressure (from 15/11 to 42/30 mmHg). However, the child died 12 hours later because of unilateral pulmonary edema. Autopsy findings were enlargement of the Waterston shunt to 10 mm and congested and edematous right lung. The other shunts were completely occluded without any blood supply to the left lung. The complication in this child may have been caused by the use of a very large balloon to dilate the Waterston shunt. More data and experience with this lesion are necessary prior to making any definitive recommendation. The experience in dilating narrowed classical and modified Blalock-Taussig (BT) shunts [6,60–63,63a] is more favorable and is discussed in detail.

Indications

The indication for dilating narrowed BT shunts is the presence of cyanotic heart defects not amenable to total surgical correction at the time of presentation either because of age and size of the patient or because of anatomic complexity, while requiring palliation of pulmonary oligemia [6]. The majority of these patients have associated pulmonary atresia or a pulmonary artery that cannot be catheterized directly because of either the severity of obstruction or an abnormal or atypical position. Measurement of pulmonary arterial pressure and demonstration of pulmonary arterial anatomy are of obvious value in the overall patient management. This is an additional indication for balloon angioplasty of narrowed BT shunts.

Technique

After clinical assessment and after the usual laboratory studies suggest hypoxemia and pulmonary oligemia in association with a complex cyanotic heart defect, cardiac catheterization is performed both to confirm the clinical diagnosis and to assess for possible balloon angioplasty. In each case, 100 units/kg of heparin (maximum 2,500 units) is administered immediately after introduction of an arterial catheter. After obtaining arterial oxygen saturation, right or left innominate artery (depending on the side of aortic arch) or subclavian artery cineangiogram is performed in order to determine the location and size of the BT anastomosis. Attempts to advance a 5 Fr multi-A2 and/or a right coronary artery catheter into BT shunt and pulmonary artery are made. Failing this, the tip of the catheter is positioned in the mouth of the subclavian artery or as close to it as possible, and a 0.014–0.035 inch flexible-tip guidewire is advanced into the BT shunt and from there into the pulmonary artery (In our previous experience with one child [6] with almost complete occlusion of the BT shunt [Fig. 10A], the tip of the catheter was wedged against the tip of the nipple-like blind end of the subclavian artery stump, and the stiff end of an 0.018 inch guidewire was gently threaded into the pulmonary artery; eventually balloon angioplasty was performed with a 4 mm balloon catheter.) Once the guidewire is positioned in the distal pulmonary artery, a low-profile balloon dilatation catheter is positioned across the narrowed BT shunt. The objective is to try to position a balloon with a diameter equivalent to the diameter of the subclavian artery. If a balloon angioplasty catheter cannot be passed across the BT shunt, a balloon-on-a-wire[1] (2 mm or 3 mm) should be advanced across the narrowed BT shunt (Fig. 11). Three successive inflations at 3–10 atm pressure, depending on the catheter manufacturer's recommendations of 5–10 seconds duration each is performed with a 5-minute interval between each dilatation. The procedure of dilatation with the balloon-on-a-wire and with a 4 Fr coronary dilatation catheter can be performed through a 5 Fr sheath placed into the femoral artery at the beginning of the procedure. Larger balloon catheters may be advanced via a 6 Fr sheath, or dilatation could be performed without the use of a sheath. Fifteen minutes following the

---

[1]The balloon-on-a-wire that we used in a USCA Probe balloon-on-a-wire [6]. Other alternatives are the ACS Hartzler Micro XR and Sci Med Dilating Guidewire.

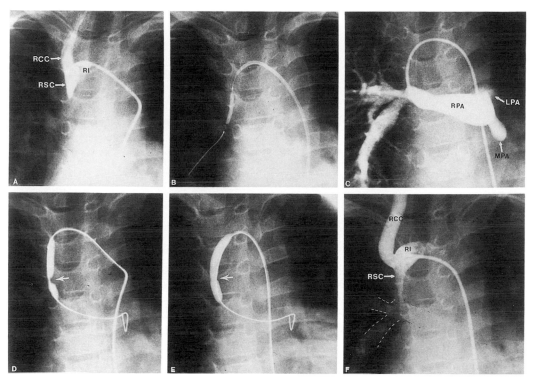

Fig. 10. Technique of catheterization of Blalock-Taussig shunt when it is completely or almost completely occluded. Right innominate (RI) artery cineangiographic frame **(A)** shows right common carotid (RCC) artery and right subclavian (RSC) artery; the latter is completely blocked. Having not been able to catheterize it in the usual manner, a 2 mm balloon-on-a-wire was advanced into the shunt, and the balloon was inflated **(B)**. Subsequently, a 5 Fr multi-A2 catheter was introduced into the pulmonary artery, and a cineangiogram **(C)** was performed. Note the main (MPA), right (RPA), and left (LPA) pulmonary arteries; the LPA was not completely opacified because of flow from the left Blalock-Taussig shunt. Then a 4 Fr coronary balloon angioplasty catheter carrying a 4 mm balloon was positioned across the narrowed BT shunt **(D,E)**; note "waisting" of the balloon (D) during the initial phases of balloon inflation. A right innominate artery cineangiogram **(F)** following balloon angioplasty shows the open Blalock-Taussig shunt and opacification of the pulmonary artery through the shunt, although the shunt is still narrow. (Reproduced Rao et al. [6], with permission of the publisher.)

last balloon dilatation, pulmonary artery to aorta pressure pullback across the BT shunt and aortic saturation are obtained and the innominate or subclavian artery cineangiogram repeated.

Results

Acute results. Balloon angioplasty of a narrowed BT shunt was initially reported by Fischer et al. [60] and subsequently by others [6,61–63,63a]. Fischer et al. [60] dilated a narrowed classic BT shunt in a 4-year-old child

and increased systemic arterial saturation from 68% to 80%. Marx and associates [61] successfully performed this procedure in five of six patients in whom they attempted the dilatation. Two of the five patients benefited markedly and one moderately. In the remaining two patients, no benefit could be seen. It is not clear whether these are classic or modified BT shunts that were dilated. Parsons and colleagues [62] balloon dilated a proximal stenosis of a modified right (Gore-Tex) BT shunt in a 17-month-old child with tricuspid atresia and

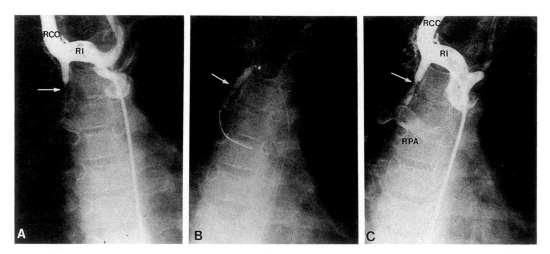

Fig. 11. Right innominate (RI) artery cineangiogram shows a markedly narrowed, thread-like right subclavian artery (**A**) which was initially entered with the help of a 0.014 inch guidewire. Then a 3 mm balloon-on-a-wire could be advanced across the shunt (**B**), and the shunt was dilated with angiographic improvement (**C**). Catheters carrying larger balloons could not be advanced into the shunt. The arrows show the narrowed shunt prior to (**A**), during (**B**) and after balloon dilation. RCC, right common carotid artery. Reproduced from Rao *et al.* [6], with permission of the publisher.

increased arterial oxygen saturation from 73% to 80%. There was angiographic improvement also. Rheuban and Carpenter [63], while discussing pediatric interventional procedures, presented angiograms of a patient who underwent balloon dilatation of a narrowed proximal anastomosis of what appears to be a modified (Gore-Tex) BT shunt. Significant angiographic improvement was noted, but no oxygen saturation data were provided. Marks *et al.* [63a] used balloon angioplasty to dilate discrete stenoses (at the pulmonary end) of classic BT shunts in 5 children, aged 11–67 months, and increased stenotic diameter from 2.8 ± 0.8 to 5.7 ± 1.1 mm and systemic arterial oxygen saturation from 73 ± 9% to 84 ± 3%.

Our experience with this procedure, including that previously reported [6], is in eight children. There were four boys and four girls, with a weight range of 6.2–19.6 kg (mean, 11.0 kg). The diagnoses in these children were pulmonary atresia in four (one with intact ventricular septum; two with large ventricular septal defects; and the final patient with mitral atresia, hypoplastic left ventricle, and double-outlet right ventricle); tricuspid atresia in three; and single ventricle, single atrium, and severe valvar and subvalvar pulmonic stenoses in the final patient. Each of these children underwent a BT shunt either in the neonatal period (five patients) or in early infancy (three patients). All children were cyanotic with increased hemoglobin values, 19.0 ± 2.7 gm% (mean ± SD), with a range of 14.8–22.1 gm%. Three children were severely symptomatic and were unable to attend school. Three toddlers were severely cyanotic with hyperpnea. The remaining two children were cyanotic and tolerated normal activity. There was moderate to severe hypoxemia with a mean oxygen saturation of 71% (SD ± 7%), with a range of 62%–82%. The pulmonary artery pressure was low normal in four children in whom the pulmonary artery pressure could be measured prior to angioplasty. In one child with long segmental narrowing of the left subclavian artery (in a patient with right aortic arch) proximal to its entry into the left pulmonary (Fig. 12), there was no significant improvement in the oxygen saturation or in the angiographic appearance of the BT shunt. The angioplasty was considered to be a failure, and the child underwent a right BT shunt within several weeks after balloon angioplasty. In the remaining children, there was significant improvement. The arterial oxygen saturation increased from 71% ± 7% to 81% ± 4% following balloon angioplasty. Pulmonary artery pressure was measured in each case following angioplasty, and the peak systolic pressure was 14 ± 5 mmHg, with a range of 9–23 mmHg; none had elevated pulmonary artery pressures. Angiographic improvement of the BT shunt with greater degree of opacification of the pulmonary circuit was observed in each of the seven children. Examples are shown in Figures 10, 11, and 13 through 15. No complications were encountered during the procedure.

Follow-up results. Follow-up data after balloon angioplasty of narrowed BT shunts is scanty. Fischer et al. [60] commented that the dilated shunt was patent 2 months after angioplasty. Marx et al. [61] stated that, on short-term follow-up, three patients (out of five) improved and two did not benefit. The patient of Parsons et al. [62] maintained clinical improvement for 4 months following angioplasty. At repeat catheterization, the arterial oxygen saturation was 76% (which was 73% prior to angioplasty and 80% immediately after angioplasty), and the dilated proximal anastomotic site was patent without restenosis or aneurysmal formation. Marks et al. [63a] followed five children after balloon angioplasty for 6 ± 2 months, and the oxygen saturations (86 ± 3%) remained high at follow-up.

From our series, the single child with failed balloon angioplasty (of left BT shunt) underwent successful right BT shunt and improved arterial oxygen saturation. The remaining seven children were followed for 3–24 months (mean, 12 months). The children with symptoms of exercise intolerance improved markedly, although all of them remained cyanotic. The hemoglobin level decreased from 19.0 ±

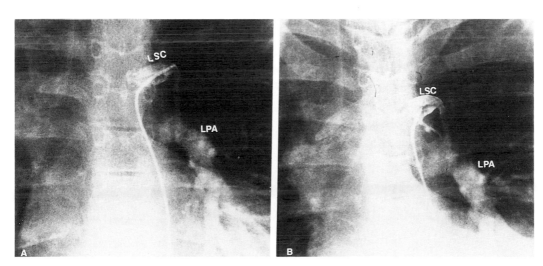

Fig. 12. Selected cineangiographic frames of the left subclavian artery (LSC) prior to (A) and immediately following (B) balloon angioplasty with a 4 mm coronary balloon angioplasty catheter. Catheters carrying larger balloons could not be advanced across the shunt. Note long segment narrowing of the left subclavian artery, which did not significantly change following angioplasty. LPA, left pulmonary artery. (Reproduced from Rao et al. [6], with permission of the publisher.)

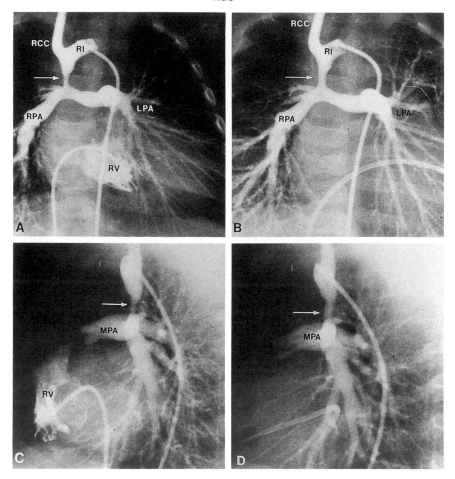

Fig. 13. Selected cineangiographic frames of Blalock-Taussig shunt prior to **(A,C)** and immediately after **(B,D)** balloon angioplasty. Anteroposterior (A,B) and lateral (C,D) views are shown; the arrows point to the narrow Blalock-Taussig shunt. Note angiographic improvement in both views. RI, right innominate artery; RCC, right common carotid artery; RPA, right pulmonary artery; LPA, left pulmonary artery; RV, right ventricle. (Reproduced from Rao *et al.* [6], with permission of the publisher.)

2.7 to 17.1 ± 1.9 gm%. Arterial oxygen saturation by pulse oximeter remains improved as a group (78% ± 10%). Auscultation revealed continuous murmur of the shunt in five patients, but on echo-Doppler study the shunt was patent in six children.

Repeat catheterization was undertaken in two children because of progressive hypoxemia. The O_2 saturations decreased. Although the shunts were patent, because of continued hypoxemia the BT shunts were successfully

performed on the contralateral side 8 and 10 months after the balloon angioplasty. The remaining children were doing well clinically with continued palliation of pulmonary oligemia.

Complications

No complications were detected either in our series or in the patients reported by other workers [60–62]. It is somewhat surprising that there was no significant hypoxemia during

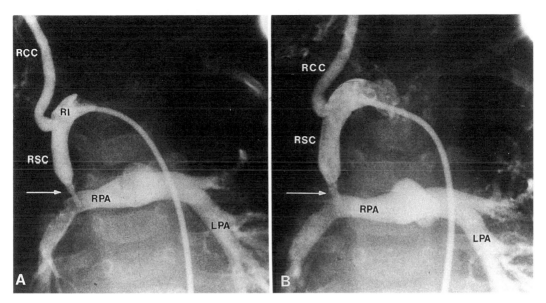

Fig. 14. Right innominate artery (RI) cineangiographic frames prior to (A) and immediately following (B) balloon angioplasty. Note slight, but significant, improvement in the narrowed segment of the right subclavian artery (RSC) and the anastomotic site (arrow). LPA, left pulmonary artery; RCC, right common carotid artery; RPA, right pulmonary artery.

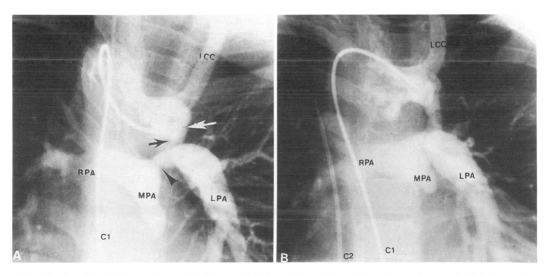

Fig. 15. Aortic arch cineangiographic frames with the catheter tip positioned very close to the left innominate artery. Note the two areas of narrowing (arrows) in the left subclavian artery (SCA) prior to balloon angioplasty (A), which completely disappeared after angioplasty (B). A was obtained with cranial angulation of the camera, and B is a straight posteroanterior view. Note constriction (arrowhead) of the left pulmonary artery (LPA) at its junction with the main pulmonary artery (MPA) in A. C1, arterial catheter in the aorta (right aortic arch); C2, venous catheter in superior vena cava; LCC, left common carotid artery; RPA, right pulmonary artery.

balloon inflation (and consequent complete occlusion of BT shunt); presumably this is because of an alternative pulmonary blood supply either through bronchial collateral vessels, contralateral BT shunt, or the stenotic pulmonary valve [6].

Because of reported instances of acute blockage of the BT shunts following catheter manipulation [64,65], such complications can occur following balloon angioplasty. Close monitoring to ensue patency of the BT shunt in the postdilatation period is highly recommended. If such blockage occurs, consideration for administration of intravenous streptokinase [65] or similar thrombolytic agents should be given.

Comments

The immediate results of balloon angioplasty of narrowed BT shunts are good; the procedure accomplished the objective of improved pulmonary blood flow and hypoxemia in most patients. It appears that balloon angioplasty can be performed in both classic and modified (Gore-Tex) BT shunts. These results are similar to those following balloon pulmonary valvuloplasty for cyanotic congenital heart defects [4,7,10–14]. During the short follow-up period, more than 50% of the patients maintained symptomatic relief, whereas the others required additional palliation or correction.

There are other benefits. In two children from our study group with either complete or almost complete blockage of the BT shunt, we were unable to advance any catheter into the BT shunt, but we were able to advance a balloon-on-a-wire, dilate the shunt, and introduce a catheter. This has resulted in obtaining pulmonary artery pressure measurements directly and in good quality pulmonary arteriograms (Fig. 10), information of obvious value in patient management, in addition to helping improve the arterial oxygen saturation.

Although there are many different ways of catheterizing the BT shunt and dilating it, the method that we used (first, positioning an end-hole type of catheter in the vicinity of subclavian artery, passing a flexible (0.014 inch) guidewire into the BT shunt and pulmonary artery, and dilating with low-profile coronary-dilating catheters; or second, failing above, passing a balloon-on-a-wire to dilate the shunt initially and then to redilate with a coronary-dilating catheter) have been successful in our hands. Others [61] have used Cook Cobra and Headhunter catheters with success.

It is not clear what the most appropriate-sized balloon is for balloon angioplasty; it should probably be 2.5–3.0 times the narrowest site. We have generally used balloons as large as the size of the subclavian artery feeding the shunt, and such large balloons may be necessary to achieve adequate dilatation [6]. As pointed out by Marx et al. [61], small balloons may not produce adequate improvement in oxygen saturation, and this may be the reason for the only modest success of this procedure in the Marx et al. patients [61]. Use of balloons as large as or only slightly smaller than the diameter of the unobstructed shunt were also suggested by Marks et al. [63a]. When there is difficulty in advancing a large balloon-dilating catheter, use of extra-stiff guidewire (e.g., extra-stiff Amplatz Cook guidewire) has been helpful in our hands and is recommended.

We generally use heparin (100 units/kg) during the procedure to prevent thrombosis. We suggest continuing heparinization for 24 hours following the procedure. Others [62] have used aspirin and dipyridamole in postdilatation period.

The type of BT shunt constriction that responds to balloon angioplasty is not clear. Our experience indicates that diffusely narrowed shunts (Fig. 12) do not favorably respond, while discrete obstructions are likely to improve.

Conclusions

Based on our experience and on that reported by others [60–63,63a], we recommend balloon angioplasty of narrowed BT shunt as the procedure of choice to augment pulmonary blood flow if the patient's size or the complexity of the cardiac defect will not permit total surgical correction. However, at the same time, the child requires palliation of systemic hypoxemia and pulmonary oligemia.

SUMMARY AND CONCLUSIONS

In this chapter, I discussed the role of transcatheter methods in the management of cyanotic congenital heart defects. Cyanotic children with interatrial right-to-left shunt secondary to severe valvar pulmonary stenosis respond in a manner similar to that seen with isolated pulmonary valve stenosis. In these patients, balloon valvuloplasty is the treatment of choice and may be corrective in most patients.

In a substantial proportion of patients with interventricular right-to-left shunting secondary to pulmonary outflow tract obstruction, and in patients with narrowed BT shunts, balloon dilatation may be an effective palliative procedure, obviating the need for an initial or second palliative shunt. I would recommend this if the patients' size or cardiac anatomy make them unsuitable for safe total surgical correction.

In patients with pulmonary atresia, either opening of the atretic pulmonary valve by laser or initial opening by surgery with subsequent balloon dilatation are potentially beneficial in reducing the total number of surgical procedures that these children are likely to require. However, further clinical trials are needed prior to their general use.

REFERENCES

1. Nadas AS, Fyler DC (1972): "Pediatric Cardiology," 3rd ed. Philadelphia: W.B. Saunders, Co, p 683.
2. Keith JD, Rowe RD, Vlad P (1978): "Heart Disease in Infancy and Childhood," 3rd ed. New York: Macmillan Co, pp 4-6.
3. Kan JS, White RI, Jr, Mitchell SE, et al. (1982): Percutaneous balloon valvuloplasty: A new method for treating congenital pulmonary valve stenosis. N Engl J Med 307:540-542.
4. Rao PS, Brais M (1988): Balloon pulmonary

valvuloplasty for congenital cyanotic heart defects. Am Heart J 115:1105-1110.
5. Rao PS (1989): Balloon angioplasty and valvuloplasty in infants, children, and adolescents. Curr Probl Cardiol 14:417-500.
6. Rao PS, Levy JM, Chopra PS (1990): Balloon angioplasty of stenosed Blalock-Taussig anastomosis: Role of balloon-on-a-wire in dilating occluded shunts. Am Heart J 120:1173-1178.
7. Rao PS, Wilson AD, Thapar MK, Brais M (1992): Balloon pulmonary valvuloplasty in the management of cyanotic congenital heart defects. Cathet Cardiovasc Diagn 25:16-24.
8. Rao PS (1987): Influence of balloon size on the short-term and long-term results of pulmonary valvuloplasty. Texas Heart Inst J 14:57-61.
9. Rao PS (1988): Further observations on the role of balloon size on the short-term and intermediate-term results of balloon pulmonary valvuloplasty. Br Heart J 60:507-511.
10. McCredie RM, Lee CL, Swinburn MJ, Warner G (1986): Balloon dilatation pulmonary valvuloplasty in pulmonary stenosis. Aust NZ J Med 16:20-23.
11. Boucek MM, Webster HE, Orsmond GS, Ruttenberg HD (1988): Balloon pulmonary valvotomy: Palliation for cyanotic heart disease. Am Heart J 115:318-322.
12. Qureshi SA, Kirk CR, Lamb RK, Arnold R, Wilkinson JL (1988): Balloon dilatation of the pulmonary valve in the first year of life in patients with tetralogy of Fallot: A preliminary study. Br Heart J 60:232-235.
13. Mehta AV, Perlman PE (1990): Palliative percutaneous balloon valvuloplasty in a cyanotic child with tetralogy of Fallot. South Med J 83:360-361.
14. Sreeram N, Saleem M, Jackson M, Peart I, McKay R, Arnold R, Walsh K (1991): Results of balloon pulmonary valvuloplasty as a palliative procedure in tetralogy of Fallot. J Am Coll Cardiol 8:159-165.
15. Rao PS (1991): Percutaneous balloon valvuloplasty/angioplasty in congenital heart disease. In Bashore TM, Davidson CJ (eds): "Percutaneous Balloon Valvuloplasty and Related Techniques." Baltimore: Williams & Wilkins, pp 251-277.
16. Lamb RK, Qureshi SA, Arnold R (1987): Pulmonary artery tear following balloon valvuloplasty in Fallot's tetralogy. Int J Cardiol 15:347-349.
17. Lababidi Z, Wu JR (1983): Percutaneous balloon pulmonary valvuloplasty. Am J Cardiol 52:560-562.
18. Walls JT, Lababidi Z, Curtis JJ, Silver D (1984): Assessment of percutaneous balloon pulmonary and aortic valvuloplasty. J Thorac Cardiovasc Surg 88:352-356.

19. Battistessa SA, Robles A, Jackson M, Miyamoto S, Arnold R, McKay R (1990): Operative findings after percutaneous pulmonary balloon dilatation of the right ventricular outflow tract in tetralogy of Fallot. Br Heart J 64:321-324.

20. Parsons JM, Ladusans EJ, Qureshi SA (1989): Growth of the pulmonary artery after neonatal balloon dilatation of the right ventricular outflow tract in an infant with tetralogy of Fallot and atrioventricular septal defect. Br Heart J 62:65-68.

21. Brock RC (1974): Late results of palliative operations for Fallot's tetralogy. J Thorac Cardiovasc Surg 67:511-518.

22. Matthews HR, Belsey RHR (1973): Indications for the Brock operation in the current treatment of tetralogy of Fallot. Thorax 28:1-9.

23. Kirklin JW, Bargeron LM, Pacifico AD (1977): The enlargement of small pulmonary arteries by preliminary palliative operations. Circulation 56:612-617.

24. Gale AW, Arciniegas E, Green EW, Blackstone EH, Kirklin JW (1979): Growth of the pulmonary annulus and pulmonary arteries after the Blalock-Taussig shunt. J Thorac Cardiovasc Surg 77:459-465.

25. Alfieri O, Blackstone EH, Parenzan L (1979): Growth of the pulmonary annulus and pulmonary arteries after the Waterston anastomosis. J Thorac Cardiovasc Surg 78:440-444.

26. Guyton RA, Owens JE, Waumett JD, Dooley KJ, Hatcher CR, Williams WH (1983): The Blalock-Taussig shunt: Low risk, effective palliation, and pulmonary artery growth. J Thorac Cardiovasc Surg 85:917-922.

27. Radtke W, Keane JF, Fellows KE, Lang P, Lock JE (1986): Percutaneous balloon valvotomy of congenital pulmonary stenosis using oversized balloons. J Am Coll Cardiol 8:909-915.

28. Qureshi SA, Parsons JM, Tynan M (1990): Percutaneous transcatheter myectomy of subvalvar pulmonary stenosis in tetralogy of Fallot: A new palliative technique with an atherectomy catheter. Br Heart J 64:163-165.

29. Rao PS, Covitz W, Moore HV (1982): Principles of palliative management of patients with tricuspid atresia. In Rao PS (ed): "Tricuspid Atresia." Mt. Kisco, NY: Futura Publishing Co, pp 233-253.

30. Rao PS, Ellison RG (1978): The causes of kinking of the right pulmonary artery in the Waterston anastomosis: a growth phenomenon. J Thorac Cardiovasc Surg 76:126-129.

31. Monarrez CN, Rao PS, Moore HV, Strong WB (1979): False aneurysm of the right pulmonary artery: A new complication of aorta-right pulmonary artery anastomosis. J Thorac Cardiovasc Surg 77:738-741.

32. Feteih W, Rao PS, Whisennand HW, Mardini MK, Lawrie GM (1983): Chylopericardium: A new complication of Blalock-Taussig anastomosis. J Thorac Cardiovasc Surg 85:791-794.

33. Qureshi SA, Ladusans EJ, Martin RP (1989): Dilatation with progressively larger balloons for severe stenosis of the pulmonary valve presenting in the late neonatal period and early infancy. Br Heart J 62:311-314.

34. Rao PS (1993): Balloon pulmonary valvuloplasty for isolated pulmonic stenosis. In Rao PS (ed): "Transcatheter Therapy in Pediatric Cardiology." New York: Wiley-Liss, pp. 59-104.

35. Thapar MK, Rao PS (1990): Use of propranolol for severe dynamic infundibular obstruction prior to balloon pulmonary valvuloplasty. Cathet Cardiovasc Diagn 19:240-241.

36. Shuck JW, McCormick DJ, Cohen IS, et al (1984): Percutaneous balloon valvuloplasty of the pulmonary valve: Role of right-to-left shunt through a patent foramen ovale. J Am Coll Cardiol 4:132-135.

37. Thapar MK, Rao PS (1989): Significance of infundibular obstruction following balloon valvuloplasty for valvar pulmonic stenosis. Am Heart J 118:99-103.

38. Rao PS (1986): Value of echo-Doppler studies in the evaluation of the results of balloon pulmonary valvuloplasty. J Cardiovasc Ultrasonogr 5:309-312.

39. Rao PS (1987): Doppler ultrasound in the prediction of transvalvar pressure gradients in patients with valvar pulmonic stenosis. Int J Cardiol 15:195-203.

40. Rao PS (1986): Transcatheter treatment of pulmonary stenosis and coarctation of the aorta: The experience with percutaneous balloon dilatation. Br Heart J 56:250-258.

41. Rao PS, Fawzy ME, Solymar L, Mardini MK (1988): Long-term results of balloon pulmonary valvuloplasty of valvar pulmonic stenosis. Am Heart J 115:1291-1296.

42. Rao PS (1989): Balloon pulmonary valvuloplasty: A review. Clin Cardiol 12:55-74.

43. Fontes VF, Esteves CA, Eduardo J, Sousa JEMR, Silva MVD, Bembom MCB (1988): Regression of infundibular hypertrophy after pulmonary valvuloplasty for pulmonic stenosis. Am J Cardiol 62:977-979.

44. Rao PS (1985): Comprehensive management of pulmonary atresia with intact ventricular septum. Ann Thorac Surg 40:409-413.

45. Puga FJ, Leoni FE, Julsrud PR, et al. (1989): Complete repair of pulmonary atresia, ventricular septal defect and severe peripheral arborization abnormalities of the central pulmonary arteries:

Experience with preliminary unifocalization procedures in 38 patients. J Thorac Cardiovasc Surg 98:1018-1028.

46. Cobanoglu A, Metzdorff MT, Pinson CE, et al. (1985): Valvotomy for pulmonary atresia with intact ventricular septum. J Thorac Cardiovasc Surg 89:482-490.

47. de Leval M, Bull C, Hopkins R, et al. (1985): Decision-making in the definitive repair of the heart with a small right ventricle. Circulation 72(Supp II):52-60.

48. Coles JG, Freedom RM, Lightfoot ME, et al. (1989): Long-term results in neonates with pulmonary atresia and intact ventricular septum. Ann Thorac Surg 47:213-217.

49. Rao PS, Liebman J, Borkat G (1976): Right ventricular growth in a case of pulmonic stenosis with intact ventricular septum and hypoplastic right ventricle. Circulation 53:389-394.

50. Qureshi SA, Rosenthal E, Tynan M, et al (1991): Transcatheter laser-assisted balloon pulmonary valve dilatation in pulmonic valve atresia. Am J Cardiol 67:428-431.

51. Latson LA, Flemming WH, Hofschire PJ, et al (1991): Balloon valvuloplasty in pulmonary valve atresia. Am Heart J 121:1567-1569.

52. Wexler L: Personal communication.

53. Lee G, Ikeda RM, Kozina J, et al. (1981): Laser-dissolution of coronary atherosclerotic obstruction. Am Heart J 102:1074-1076.

54. Riemenschneider TA, Lee G, Ikeda RM, et al. (1983): Laser irradiation of congenital heart disease: Potential for palliation and correction of intracardiac and intravascular defects. Am Heart J 106:1389-1393.

55. Arapov AD, Vishnerski AA, Jr, Abdullaev FZ, et al (1974): A preliminary report on laser application in cardiosurgery. Eksp Khiv Anesteziol 4:10-12.

56. Kan JS, White RI, Jr, Mitchell SE, Anderson JH, Gardner TJ (1984): Percutaneous transluminal balloon valvuloplasty for pulmonary valve stenosis. Circulation 69:554-560.

57. Sullivan ID, Robinson PJ, Macartney FJ, Taylor JFN, Rees PG, Bull C, Deanfield JE (1985): Percutaneous balloon valvuloplasty for pulmonary valve stenosis in infants and children. Br Heart J 54:435-441.

58. Ballerini L, Mullins CE, Cifarelli A, et al. (1990): Percutaneous balloon valvuloplasty of pulmonary valve stenosis, dysplasia, and residual stenosis after surgical valvotomy for pulmonary atresia with intact ventricular septum: Long-term results. Cathet Cardiovasc Diagn 19:165-169.

59. Gibbs JL, Wilson N, daCosta P (1988): Balloon dilatation of a Waterston aortopulmonary anastomosis. Br Heart J 59:596-597.

60. Fischer DR, Park SC, Neches WH, et al (1985): Successful dilatation of a stenotic Blalock-Taussig anastomosis by percutaneous transluminal balloon angioplasty. Am J Cardiol 55:861-862.

61. Marx GR, Allen HD, Ovitt TW, Hanson W, Keiter-Marek J (1988): Balloon dilatation angioplasty of Blalock-Taussig shunts. Am J Cardiol 62:824-827.

62. Parsons JM, Ladusans EJ, Qureshi SA (1989): Balloon dilation of a stenosed modified (polytetrafluoroethylene) Blalock-Taussig shunt. Br Heart J 62:228-229.

63. Rheuban KS, Carpenter MA (1988): Diagnostic cardiac catheterization, angiography, and interventional catheterization. In Lake CL (ed): "Pediatric Cardiac Anesthesia." Norwalk, CT: Appleton & Lange, p 8.

63a. Marks LA, Mehta AV, Marangi D (1991): Percutaneous transluminal balloon angioplasty of stenotic standard Blalock-Taussig shunts: Effect on choice of initial palliation in cyanotic congenital heart disease. J Am Coll Cardiol 546-551.

64. McKay R, de Leval MR, Rees P, Taylor JFN, Macartney FJ, Stark J (1980): Postoperative angiographic assessment of modified Blalock-Taussig shunts using expanded polytetrafluoroethylene (Gore-Tex). Ann Thorac Surg 30:137-145.

65. Rajani RM, Dalvi BV, Kulkarni HL, Kale PA (1990): Acutely blocked Blalock-Taussig shunt following cardiac catheterization: Successful recanalization with intravenous streptokinase. Am Heart J 120:1238-1239.

14

Balloon Dilatation of Stenotic Bioprosthetic Valves

P. Syamasundar Rao, M.D.

Department of Pediatrics, Division of Pediatric Cardiology,
University of Wisconsin Medical School, University of Wisconsin
Children's Hospital, Madison, Wisconsin 53792-4108

INTRODUCTION

When the porcine heterografts became available [1–3], they were rapidly adopted for use in children [4–7]. Despite initial enthusiasm [4–7], calcific degeneration and valve dysfunction, reviewed and referenced in detail elsewhere [8,9], occurred, with the resultant reduced use of the heterografts in children, particularly in left heart lesions. Calcific degeneration appears to occur more frequently and with greater rapidity in younger children than in older children. Data from our group [9] with regard to mitral heterografts and from others [10] with regard to the aortic heterografts suggest that heterografts in children ≤15 years calcify rapidly, whereas those in patients >15 years do so less frequently and less rapidly. It also appears that the calcific degeneration also occurs more frequently and more rapidly in left heart valve replacements than in right-sided valve replacements. However, significant valve dysfunction and a need for re-replacement in the right side of the heart is also documented [11–20].

Beginning in the early 1960s homografts have also been used to replace cardiac valves [21–24]. Unfortunately, calcification and obstruction of homografts are also observed [25–29].

The incidence of valve dysfunction requiring intervention varies with the age of the patient, the location of the bioprosthetic valve (right or left heart), and the type of bioprosthetic valve used. By and large, 20%–30% of the valves need replacement within 5 years of valve insertion, 40% within 7 years, and essentially in all patients by 10 years.

Pathologically, stiffening of the valve cusp, which causes valve stenosis or cusp degeneration that produces regurgitation across the valve, may also be found [30–40,40a–d]. Cusp tears secondary to calcification or collagen disruption may also be seen. Calcium deposits along the commissures have also been observed; sometimes these deposits may cause commissural fusion. Gross calcific lesions in the basal and central regions of the cusp have been seen. Microscopically, breakdown of the collagen fibers, which forms a nidus for intrinsic calcification, has been observed. Because a bioprosthetic valve does not have a reparative mechanism to replace the degenerated collagen fibers, calcification ensues. This intrinsic calcification usually appears years after valve implantation; the degree of calcification is dependent on the length of the time since valve implantation. This type of calcification occurs more frequently in children than in adults and perhaps more frequently in left-sided than in right-sided valves. Calcification from the surface either secondary to surface thrombi or vegetations of bacterial endocarditis, the so-called extrinsic calcification, can also occur; this is unrelated to the duration since valve implantation. Degenerative and calcific changes have been observed in gluteraldehyde-

Transcatheter Therapy in Pediatric Cardiology, pages 255–274
© 1993 Wiley-Liss, Inc.

preserved porcine valves, irrespective of the manufacturer (Hancock, Carpentier-Edwards, or Tascon); bovine pericardial xenografts (Ionescu-Shiley, Mitroflow®); and homografts. When bioprostheses are used in conduits, problems such as peel formation [41,42] can occur in addition to valve degeneration and calcification. Obstruction of anastomotic sites of the conduit (proximal and distal) have also been reported. In this chapter, I review the experience with balloon dilatation of stenotic bioprosthetic valves.

BIOPROSTHETIC VALVES IN PULMONARY POSITION

Several groups of workers [43–45] have independently and almost simultaneously applied balloon dilatation techniques to relieve stenotic lesions of porcine heterografts in pulmonary position. Soon after, several other workers [46–51] reported their observations.

Indications

The indications for balloon dilatation of stenotic bioprosthetic valves are not clearly defined. Symptoms of right heart failure [47], systemic (or near systemic) levels of peak systolic pressures in the right ventricle [43], right ventricular systolic pressure >60% of systemic pressure [47], and peak-to-peak gradient across the valve conduit =50 mmHg [44] have been suggested as indications for balloon therapy. Avoidance of surgical replacement of the valved conduit or at least postponement of the timing for surgery is the objective of balloon dilatation of stenotic bioprosthetic valves. I believe that the indications for balloon valvuloplasty of stenotic bioprosthetic valves in a pulmonary position should be similar to that used for native pulmonary valve [45,52]; a peak-to-peak systolic pressure gradient in excess of 50 mmHg with normal cardiac index (measured by a thermodilution [or indocyanine green dye dilution] technique or by the Fick method with measured oxygen consumption) is an indication for balloon dilatation.

Distal obstructions may become evident following relief of valvar obstruction [43]; these should be sought out and balloon dilated concurrently.

All types of bioprosthetic valves appear to be dilatable. Porcine heterografts of all varieties (Hancock, Carpentier-Edwards, Tascon), bovine heterografts (Ionescu-Shiley) [43–51], and homografts [44,47,53] are amenable for dilatation. When the conduit is between the right atrium and the pulmonary artery or right ventricle, as an integral part of the Fontan operation, the indication for dilatation is any significant pressure gradient across the tissue valve with or without evidence for systemic venous congestion.

Technique

The general technique of balloon valvuloplasty is similar to that used for pulmonary valve stenosis, as described in Chapter 6 (this volume). Therefore this technique will not be described in detail, but specific issues related to bioprosthetic valves will be mentioned.

Positioning the balloon catheter. Examples of position of the balloon dilatation catheter across porcine heterografts (Hancock) are shown in Figure 1. It is slightly more difficult to position a balloon catheter across the stenotic heterograft than across a natural pulmonary valve. Therefore an extra-stiff Amplatz (Cook) or a similar extra-stiff guidewire should be used in all such cases. Also, it is advisable to position the tip of the guidewire as far distally in the left or right pulmonary artery as possible so that the wire provides an "anchor" [43] and the balloon catheter can be advanced over the wire. Some workers [46,51] used additional maneuvers, such as application of silicone lubricant on the balloon, placement of a transseptal catheter in the right ventricular outflow tract to prevent buckling of the balloon catheter, and wedging a small balloon in one of the valve commissures in order to position an appropriate-sized balloon dilatation catheter across the stenosed conduit. While these methods may be helpful, use of an extra-stiff

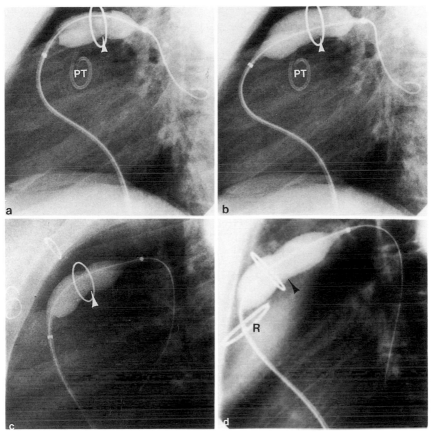

Fig. 1. Selected cineradiographic frames in lateral view of the balloon dilatation catheter(s) positioned across the porcine heterografts (Hancock). Partially inflated balloon (a), showing balloon "waisting" (arrowheads) that is almost completely abolished (b) with further balloon inflation. Fully inflated balloons are shown in two other patients (c,d). Note that the "waisting" (arrows) was not completely ablated in these two frames. Also, note that the "waisting" (arrows) is just distal to the opaque metallic ring of the Hancock prosthesis. In d, the connection of the conduit to the right ventricle is marked by another ring (R). PT, pigtail catheter in the ascending aorta.

Amplatz guidewire has been the most helpful in our hands. With the greater availability of lower profile balloons than in the past, the difficulties in positioning the catheter have decreased.

Balloon size. The method of balloon choice has varied among cardiologists using balloon dilatation in this lesion. Most workers [43,46] use a balloon size similar to the conduit or valve size. Lloyd et al. [44] start with a balloon size that is 60%–75% of the valve

diameter at the time of conduit insertion. If this is unsuccessful, they repeat balloon dilatation with an 18 mm balloon [44]. The final balloon size used was 2–3 mm smaller than the original valve diameter. Some other workers [47] choose a balloon that is twice the narrowest site. If a waist is not seen, the next larger sized balloon is chosen. In no case was a balloon larger than the diameter of the conduit used [47]. We prefer to use a balloon that is equal to the size of the conduit valve [54] specified by the manufacturer. Waldman et al. [43], after analyzing their clinical and in vitro studies, concluded that balloon sizes similar to the valve annulus should be chosen for porcine heterograft stenosis. The rigid metallic ring used in most bioprosthetic valves limits the possible benefit of oversized balloons such as those used for isolated valvar pulmonic stenosis [45]. In addition, such large balloons may cause transverse rupture of the balloon [54,55]. Circumferential constriction of the balloon is produced by the rigid, metallic, nonyielding ring of the heterografts. This shearing stress along the circumference of the balloon [54–57] may cause transverse balloon rupture [55]. In such cases, the double-balloon technique may have advantages in that the stress is not on the entire balloon circumference, and consequently there is a lesser chance for transverse balloon rupture [58].

Unmasking obstructive lesions. Waldman and associates [43] demonstrated unmasking of the distal (branch pulmonary artery) obstruction following relief of valvar obstruction by balloon dilatation. They suggested that it is imperative to seek out distal obstructions and to relieve them if feasible. After balloon dilatation of valve stenosis, main pulmonary artery pressure should be measured. If it is elevated, branch pulmonary artery stenosis may be present. Appropriate angiography to visualize the obstruction and balloon angioplasty to relieve the obstruction should then be carried out.

There may be additional problems of a similar nature. In the presence of multiple obstructions in series, when the distal obstruction is severe, the pressure gradient across the proximal obstruction may be diminished or abolished [59,60]. This atypical pressure gradient manifestation was thought to be due to "forced vibration" with greater energy transfer into the cardiovascular segment upstream from the distal obstruction [59,60]. Once the distal obstruction is relieved, proximal gradient manifests. For example, if there is severe supravalvar or branch pulmonary artery stenosis, a gradient across the stenotic bioprosthesis may not be recorded. After the branch or supravalvar pulmonary artery stenosis is relieved, the valvar gradient appears.

These principles of multiple obstructions in the cardiovascular system must be understood so that appropriate documentation of the obstructions and balloon dilatation, if needed, can be accomplished at the same time.

Oxygen administration during valvuloplasty. Some authors [43] advocated administration of oxygen via face mask during balloon dilatation. This was done with the belief that ventricular hypoxia should be avoided during balloon dilatation. While the concerns of these workers are understandable, we do not believe that face mask administration of oxygen serves any useful purpose. During the balloon dilatation procedure, there is no problem of oxygenation, but there is a problem of flow into the lungs. Brief periods of balloon inflation are all that are necessary. As a matter of fact, attempts to put on a face mask and to administer oxygen may disturb and awaken the child, which is not desirable during the procedure.

Acute Results

Balloon dilatation of stenotic bioprosthetic valves has been utilized to avoid or postpone reoperation. Waldman et al. [43] reported four children who developed stenosis of porcine heterografts 10–24 months after their insertion and who underwent balloon dilatation. The average peak-to-peak valvar gradient was reduced from 48 to 25 mmHg. There was only mild pulmonary insufficiency. Additional branch pulmonary artery stenosis became evident, requiring further balloon angioplasty. In a later review [49] by the same authors, 10 children were stated to have had balloon dilatation of stenosed pulmonary outflow conduits. No detailed data were given, however. A substantial reduction in the gradient occurred, and conduit replacement could be deferred in 8 of the 10 patients.

Lloyd and associates [44] presented results

of balloon dilatation in five children who developed stenosis of bioprosthetic valves inserted 4–14 years previously. The peak gradient was reduced from 78 ± 15 mmHg to 39 ± 18 mmHg. In three children, systolic pressure gradients were reduced significantly; no surgical intervention was required. The remaining two children did not have significant gradient reduction; one of these was secondary to peel formation and underwent successful conduit replacement, whereas the other patient had only a modest degree of stenosis and is being followed clinically.

We reported our experience [45] in dilating porcine heterografts in three children, and these, along with our up-to-date experience, are summarized in the latter part of this section. Ensing et al. [46] used balloon dilatation in nine patients with stenosis of a variety of heterografts (Hancock, Ionescu-Shiley, Carpentier-Edwards, and Tascon) that had been implanted 3–9.8 years earlier. Balloon valvuloplasty reduced the peak gradient from a mean of 51 mmHg to a mean of 21 mmHg. The right ventricular peak systolic pressure in all patients was >70% of the systemic pressure prior to valvuloplasty but <70% in seven of the nine children after balloon dilatation. In eight of these children, surgery was postponed or avoided [46]. In a later study [51], they report the results in 14 patients with essentially similar results. Zeevi et al. [47] utilized balloon dilatation in nine patients with stenosed bioprosthetic valves. In three children, the gradient decreased from 38, 52, and 70 mmHg to 16, 25, and 12 mmHg, respectively. In five other children, the gradient did not change, while in the final patient there was only a 37% decrease in gradient. Five of these nine children required conduit valve replacement in 0.5–12 months after balloon dilatation, and the sixth patient awaits replacement. Unwala et al. [48] balloon dilated a stenosed porcine heterograft (Carpentier-Edwards) in a 35-year-old male and reduced the peak-to-peak gradient from 56 to 15 mmHg. The Valvuloplasty and Angioplasty of Congenital Anomalies (VACA)

Registry [50] listed 23 patients with pulmonary conduits as having had balloon dilatation. In eight of them, the result was stratified as a success; in nine, as failure; and in eight, unknown. No details with regard to the ages of the patients, types of prosthetic valves dilated, sizes of balloon used, or pressure gradient data were given in the VACA Registry report. Murdoch et al. [53] reduced the peak gradient from 57 to 34 mmHg by balloon dilatation of a stenotic homograft valve in an 8-year-old boy. The results reported in the literature are summarized in Table I.

We have used balloon dilatation in five patients with stenotic porcine heterografts. These heterografts had been implanted 4.2–11 years (9.9 ± 3.5 years) prior to balloon dilatation as a part of total correction of severe tetralogy of Fallot (in two), truncus arteriosus (in two), or pulmonary atresia with a ventricular septal defect (in one). The patients were 5–21 years (14.9 ± 6.2 years) of age at the time of balloon dilatation (Table II). The right ventricular peak systolic peak systolic pressure (108 ± 33 vs. 88 ± 24 mmHg), gradient across the porcine heterograft (77 ± 25 vs. 46 ± 29 mmHg), and right ventricle/left ventricle peak systolic pressure ratio (0.94 ± 0.19 vs. 0.72 ± 0.22), though decreased after balloon dilatation, did not reach statistical significance (P > 0.1). The percent reduction of valve gradient varied from 0% to 84% (43% ± 31%). When individual values were examined (Table III), the heterograft gradients decreased significantly in some patients. Two patients underwent conduit replacement (one secondary to peel formation), and the other three were followed clinically. No procedure-related complications have been encountered.

Balloon dilatation of right-atrium-to-right-ventricle or right-atrium-to-pulmonary-artery conduit (Fontan) has also been attempted [46,51,61]. Ensing et al. [46], who attempted balloon dilatation of a stenosed Dacron graft (right-atrium-to-pulmonary-artery) in a 14-year-old, was unsuccessful. Pelikan et al. [61] dilated a stenotic right-atrium-to-pulmonary-artery ho-

TABLE I. Results of Balloon Dilatation of Bioprosthetic Valves in Pulmonary Position (Conduits) From the Literature[a]

Author	Year	N	Age at BD (years, mean ± SD; range)	Diagnosis	Type of bioprosthetic valve	Time since conduit placement (years, mean ± SD; range)	Gradient (mmHg, mean ±6 SD;range) Pre	Gradient (mmHg, mean ±6 SD;range) Post	Comments
Waldman et al. [43]	1987	4	2.0 ± 1.1 (1.1–3.5)	Truncus, 2; TGA, 2	Porcine, 4	1.2 ± 0.6 (0.8–2.0)	48[b]	25[b]	CR avoided in three patients
Lloyd et al. [44]	1987	5	15.2 ± 4.4 (8–20)	TGA, 2; TOF, 2; PA; VSD, 1	Porcine, 3; homograft, 2	10.4 ± 3.4 (5–14)	80 ± 15 (62–100)	39 ± 18 (20–60)	CR avoided in three patients
Rao [45]	1989	3	13.1 ± 7.3 (5–19)	TOF, 2; truncus, 1	Porcine, 3	9.7 ± 4.8 (4–13)	73 ± 6 (68–79)	43 ± 34 (11–79)	CR avoided in two patients
Ensing et al. [46]	1989	10	14.5 ± 5.3 (7–21)	PA; VSD, 5; TOF, 2; TGA, 3;	Porcine, 6; bovine, 3	6.4[c] (3–9.8)	57 ± 22 (–)	21[b] (–)	CR postponed or avoided in eight patients
Zeevi et al. [47]	1989	9	12.2 ± 6.9 (1.3–19.5)	PA; VSD, 6; TOF, 1; TGA, 1; truncus, 1	Porcine, 8; homograft, 1	5.3 ± 4.5 (0.6–11.5)	62 ± 21 (38–100)	47 ± 30 (12–95)	CR avoided in four patients

	Year			PI[d]					CR avoided
Unwala et al. [48]	1990	1	35		Porcine, 1	6	56	15	CR avoided
Waldman and Swenson [49]	1990[e]	10	–	–	–	–	–	–	CR deferred in eight patients
VACA Registry [50]	1990[f]	23	–	–	–	–	–	–	Success, eight; failure, seven; unknown, eight
Murdoch et al. [55]	1991	1	8	Truncus, 1	Homograft, 1	7.2	57	34	CR avoided
Hagler [51]	1992[g]	14	13.9 ± 5.1 (7–21)	PA; VSD, 7; TGA, 4; TOF, 2; truncus, 1	Porcine, 10; bovine, 4	–	46[b]	18[b]	CR postponed or avoided in 12 patients
Current series	1992[h]	5	14.9 ± 6.2 (5–21)	TOF, 2; truncus, 2; PA; VSD, 1	Porcine, 5	9.9 ± 3.5 (4.2–13.0)	77 ± 25 (50–117)	46 ± 29 (11–79)	CR postponed or avoided in three patients

[a]BD, balloon dilatation; CR, conduit replacement; PA, pulmonary atresia; PI, pulmonary insufficiency; TGA, transposition of the great arteries; TOF, tetralogy of Fallot; VACA, Valvuloplasty and Angioplasty of Congenital Anomalies; VSD, ventricular septal defect.

[b]Only mean values were given.

[c]This is a median; mean and standard deviation were not given.

[d]Severe pulmonary insufficiency secondary to a previous episode of bacterial endocarditis.

[e]Includes 4 cases previously published by Waldman et al. [43]. No other details were given.

[f]No other details were given. May include many of the previously reported patients.

[g]Includes 10 cases previously reported by Ensing et al. [46].

[h]Includes three cases previously reported by Rao [45].

TABLE II. Patient Characteristics[a]

Patient no.	Age at BD (years)	Gender	Diagnosis	Size of Hancock conduit valve (mm)	Age of the conduit (years)
1	5.0	F	Truncus	14	4.2
2	19.0	F	TOF	20	13.0
3	15.5	M	TOF	18	12.0
4	14.0	F	Truncus	18	9.5
5	21.0	M	PA, VSD	18	11.0

[a]BD, balloon dilatation; F, female; M, male; PA, pulmonary atresia; TOF, tetralogy of Fallot; VSD, ventricular septal defect.

mograft in a 28-year-old woman who had developed the obstruction 4 months after a Fontan operation. Balloon dilatation resulted in an increase in the stenotic diameter from 5 to 11 mm, complete disappearance of peak systolic gradient, and clinical improvement. Two months following balloon dilatation, symptoms recurred, necessitating repeat balloon dilatation. A double-balloon (10 + 15 mm) technique was used, which resulted in a fall in the peak gradient from 5 to 1 mmHg and in angiographic improvement. Continued clinical improvement was documented 11 months following a second balloon dilatation. Hagler [51] balloon dilated a stenotic porcine heterograft in a 20-year-old patient. The peak

gradient was reduced from 10 to 5 mmHg. Because of persistence of elevated right atrial pressure, surgical conduit replacement was performed.

Follow-Up Results

The follow-up results are scanty. The data from the published reports [43–49,51,52,61a] are listed in Table IV. Of the 42 patients who underwent balloon dilatation, nine required conduit replacement within 3 months of the balloon dilatation procedure [44–47]. In 3 patients, no follow-up information was available [43–47]. The remaining 18 patients were followed for a few months to 4 years. Ten of these children required replacement of the

TABLE III. Results of Balloon Dilatation of Heterografts[a]

Patient no.	Valve size (mm)	Balloon size (mm)	Peak-to-peak valve gradient			RV/LV peak systolic pressure ratio		Outcome
			Pre-BD (mmHg)	Post-BD, (mmHg)	Percent reduction	Pre-BD	Post-BD	
1	14	15	72	45	38	1.2	0.88	Conduit replaced
2	20	18	68	11	84	0.8	0.60	Clinical FU, 4 years
3	18	18	79	79[b]	0	1.0	1.00	Conduit replaced
4	18	18	50	24	52	0.7	0.45	Clinical FU, 4 years
5	18	18	117	69	41	1.0	0.66	Clinical FU, 1.25 years[c]

[a]BD, balloon dilatation; FU, follow-up; RV/LV, right-ventricle-to-left-ventricle.
[b]There was tubular narrowing of the conduit, secondary to neointimal formation.
[c]Recatheterization 15 months after BD revealed recurrence. Successful replacement of the conduit with a homograft was undertaken.

TABLE IV. Follow-Up Results After Balloon Dilatation of Bioprosthetic Conduits

Author	N	Comments
Waldman et al. [43]	4	Replacement of conduit in one patient 4 months after BD.[a] No follow-up in three patients
Lloyd et al. [44]	5	Elective replacement of conduits in two patients. No follow-up reported in three patients
Waldman et al. [61a]	7[b]	4 conduits were replaced 4 days, 7 mo, 19 mo, and 28 mo following balloon dilatation.
Ensing et al. [46]	10	Two patients underwent conduit replacement initially
Hagler [51]	14[c]	Two additional patients had the conduit replaced 1.5 and 4 years after BD. One patient died suddenly (presumably due to arrhythmia) 2 years following BD. No follow-up data given for the remaining 9 patients
Zeevi et al. [47]	9	Conduit replacement was performed in five patients 0.5–12 months (mean, 5.7 months) after BD. One patient with obstructed conduit is awaiting replacement. No follow-up data given for three patients
Unwala et al. [48]	1	Doppler study 14 months after BD showed no increase in gradient
Murdoch et al. [53]	1	Doppler-estimated gradient (38 mmHg) 6 months following BD remained similar to that (34 mmHg) immediately after BD
Current series	5	Two conduits were replaced immediately. One conduit was replaced 15 months after the procedure. Two children followed for 4 and 3.5 years, respectively, without need for replacement of the conduits

[a]BD, balloon dilatation.
[b]Includes 4 patients reported by Waldman et al. [43].
[c]Includes all 10 patients reported by Ensing et al. [46].

conduit 4 months to 4 years (median, 12 months) [43,45–47] later. The reasons for replacement were obstruction at additional sites (proximal or distal anastomosis of the conduit and peel formation) or significant residual or restenosis of the biological valve. One child is awaiting valve replacement [47]. One child, with a known history of ventricular ectopy, died suddenly 2 years after balloon dilatation [51]; this was presumably due to arrhythmia. The final four patients [48,53] (Table IV) are clinically well, with Doppler evidence of mild to moderate residual conduit obstruction.

Complications

Some workers [44,46,58] have reported significant complications, whereas others [43,45,47,48,53] have not. Balloon rupture appears to be a significant complication. For example, in one study, six balloon ruptures were reported in 10 patients undergoing balloon dilatation [46]. Some of these were circumferential balloon ruptures [44,46,58], causing avulsion and breakage of balloon/catheter fragments [11,16]. The cause of the high incidence of balloon ruptures is not known, but may be related to calcific deposits on the bioprosthetic valve, rigid metallic ring, and perhaps some balloon damage secondary to insertion of the balloon through scarred tissue in the groin. Use of high-strength balloons, perhaps insertion of the balloon catheter via a sheath instead of the Seldinger type of balloon catheter insertion, and use of a balloon no larger than the valve ring into which the prosthetic valve had been mounted may help to decrease balloon ruptures. Avoidance of balloons larger than the valve ring is particularly important. A larger one will produce a waist on the balloon, which will have a greater circumferential stress [55,58], thus predisposing it to transverse balloon rupture. Use of a double-balloon technique may reduce balloon ruptures, because this technique may allow redistribution of the stress.

Development of obstructive pannus, observed several months after balloon dilatation [43], is of concern, but this may not be causally related to balloon dilatation. Dislodgement of pseudointimal peel, causing further enhancement of obstruction, is another potential complication and should be kept in mind.

Comments

Based on our limited experience and on this review, it appears that all types of heterografts and homografts can be balloon dilated. It is important to realize that the site of obstruction in the valved conduits is variable; multiple sites may be involved [41,42], which include valve stenosis (46%), stenosis of anastomotic sites (24%), and neointimal peel formation (30%). It has been demonstrated that relief of one obstruction may unmask other obstructive lesions. These should be sought out following the initial balloon dilatation and balloon dilated as well. Obstruction caused by neointimal peel is not amenable to balloon dilatation. Appropriate precautions to prevent balloon rupture, as reviewed, should be taken. While the results reported by various groups are different, it seems logical to attempt balloon dilatation as an initial therapeutic option at the time of hemodynamic study for evaluation of conduit obstruction. The objective of balloon dilatation is to avoid or postpone replacement of these conduits. Some hitherto undilatable lesions may be relieved by placement of stents [62]. These stents may make the valve nonfunctional, causing pulmonary regurgitation, but this may be tolerated in a manner similar to replacing valved conduits with nonvalved conduits [19]. Studies in animal models [62] and preliminary clinical trials [62a] suggest that stent implantation is feasible and that significant relief of obstruction can be accomplished by this modality. Further experimental work, including clinical trials, is

necessary prior to general application of this technique.

BIOPROSTHETIC VALVES IN TRICUSPID POSITION

To the best of my knowledge, Feit and associates [63] were the first to report balloon valvuloplasty of stenosed tricuspid valve prosthesis. Subsequently, several other workers [64–68] reported their experience. Symptomatic patients with clinical and echo-Doppler evidence for tricuspid stenosis are candidates for balloon valvuloplasty. The technique of valvuloplasty is similar to that used for other valves. Introduction of a flow-directed balloon catheter across the tricuspid valve for positioning the guidewire is advisable [67] in order to prevent inadvertent dilatation through a perivalvar space or perforated valve cusp. Some workers use curved guidewires positioned in the right ventricular apex for positioning the balloon catheter(s), while others position the tips of the guidewires in the main or branch pulmonary arteries; our preference is the latter. An example is shown in Figure 2. The size of the single balloon or the effective size of the double balloon [69] should be similar to the prosthetic valve ring into which the biologic valve has been mounted. Recording of the mean diastolic pressure difference across the tricuspid valve, cardiac index, and calculation of tricuspid valve area prior to and following balloon dilatation is essential for the evaluation of the results of the procedure. Similarly, right ventricular angiography is needed to assess the degree of residual tricuspid insufficiency.

Immediate results reported in the literature are tabulated (Table V). Patient ages ranged from 19 to 67 years (Table V) at the time of balloon valvuloplasty, and their tricuspid valves had been replaced 7–13 years earlier. A decrease in the mean diastolic gradient across the tricuspid valve, improvement (though slight) in cardiac output, and increase in calculated tricuspid valve area have been

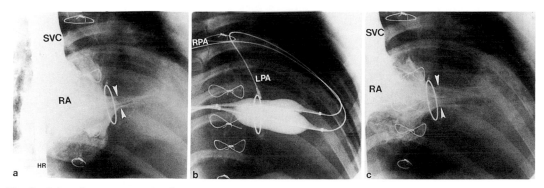

Fig. 2. Selected cineangiographic frame of a superior vena caval (SVC) angiogram in a 30° right anterior oblique projection, showing opacification of the right atrium (RA) and a small jet of contrast material (arrowheads) traversing the porcine heterograft (Hancock), suggesting severe prosthetic tricuspid stenosis (**a**). Balloon valvuloplasty was performed with two balloons positioned across the prosthetic valve (**b**). The guidewires were positioned in the left (LPA) and right (RPA) pulmonary arteries. Following balloon valvuloplasty (**c**), a much wider jet of contrast than in a is seen to pass the heterograft. There was a decrease in diastolic pressure gradient and a slight increase in cardiac index (Table V).

noted. An increase in width of the opening of the tricuspid valve leaflets can sometimes be demonstrated by angiography (Fig. 2). The degree of tricuspid insufficiency did not significantly increase. Symptomatic improvement was present in most. However, at least half of them required either repeat dilatation or valve replacement within months of the initial balloon procedure. Significant complications have not been reported. In the remaining patients, only short-term follow-up data are available.

Based on the limited experience available, it is difficult to assess the role of balloon dilatation in stenotic tricuspid bioprosthetic valves. Perhaps it has a role in temporary palliation of these patients as a bridge to surgery. Until more data are available, definitive recommendations cannot be made. Once balloon dilatation is decided on, the diameter of the balloon(s) used should be at least as large as the prosthetic valve ring.

BIOPROSTHETIC VALVES IN MITRAL POSITION

Calvo et al. [70] reported successful balloon dilatation of stenotic mitral valve heterografts

(both porcine, one Hancock and one Carpentier-Edwards) in two patients, aged 29 and 37 years, respectively, with improvement in transmitral valve gradient, cardiac index, and calculated mitral valve area. They suggested that this is an effective palliative method for some groups of patients with stenosed bioprosthetic mitral valves. This appears to be the first report of application of a balloon dilatation technique to relieve stenosed mitral heterograft valves. Subsequently, other investigators [71–74] have also applied this technique. The indications for and the technique of balloon valvuloplasty are similar to those for native mitral valve stenosis, as described in detail elsewhere in this volume (Ch. 8) and thus will not be listed here. The acute results are encouraging, and the data reported in the literature [70–74] are tabulated (Table VI). The follow-up data are scanty. Based on those available, the balloon dilatation techniques appear to be useful in acutely relieving mitral obstruction secondary to bioprosthetic valve stenosis and help with avoiding or postponing replacement of the bioprosthesis. Because of the lack of follow-up results, it is difficult to assess the role of this technique in the overall management of patients with stenotic mitral heterograft valves.

TABLE V. Balloon Dilatation of Stenosed Tricuspid Valve Bioprosthesis[a]

Author	Year	Age at BD and Gender	Basic cardiac defect	Type of bio-prosthesis	Age of bio-prosthetic valve (years)	Size of balloon(s) (mm)	Mean diastolic gradient across TV (mm Hg) Pre	Post	Cardiac index (liters/min/m²) Pre	Post	TV area (cm²/m²) Pre	Post	Tricuspid insufficiency Pre	Post	Comments
Feit et al. [63]	1987	46/M	TV endo-carditis	Porcine (No. 31 Hancock)	10	20	22	15	2.3	3.6	0.69	1.22	Mild	Mild	Continued improvement at 1 month FU
Rao [64]	1989	21/F	Ebstein's anomaly	Porcine (No. 31 Carpentier-Edwards)	13	20 + 18	6	2	2.0	2.7	—	—	Mild	Mild	Recurrence of symptoms 3 months later; pros-thetic valve replaced
Wren and Hunter [65]	1989	19/F	TV endo-carditis	Bovine (No. 29 Ionescu-Shiley)	6	20	8-12	4-6	3.4	3.2	0.52	0.65	Mild	Mild	Recurrence of symptoms 3 months later; repeat balloon with 23 mm balloon; eventual replacement of TV (9 months after initial BD)

Attrubato et al. [66]	1990	35/F	TV endo-carditis	Porcine (Carpentier-Edwards)	9	20 + 15	11	6	1.4	3.6	0.6	1.5	Mild	Mild	No follow-up data were given for either patient
		29/F	TV endo-carditis	Porcine (Carpentier-Edwards)	2	20 + 15	8	4	3.1	2.7	1.0	1.6	Mild	Mild	
Chow et al. [67]	1990	67/F	Rheumatic valvular disease	Porcine (No. 29 Carpentier-Edwards)	7	23	6	2.5	2.76[b]	2.86[b]	0.9	4.4	None	Mild	Continued improvement 6 months after BD
Benedick et al. [68]	1990	37/F	TV endo-carditis	Porcine (No. 27 Carpentier-Edwards)	0.33	15 + 15	21	7	2.7[b]	4.6[b]	0.3	1.3	Mild	Mild	Death 20 days later, probably unrelated to BD

[a]BD, balloon dilatation; F, female; FU, follow-up; M, male; TV, tricuspid valve.
[b]Cardiac output, not indexed.

TABLE VI. Balloon Dilatation of Stenosed Mitral Valve Bioprosthesis[a]

Author	Year	Age at BD & gender	Basic cardiac defect	Type of bioprosthesis	Age of Bioprosthetic valve (years)	Size of balloon(s), mm	Mean diastolic gradient across MV (mm Hg)		Cardiac index (L/min/m²)		MV area (cm²/m²)		Mitral insufficiency		Comments
							Pre	Post	Pre	Post	Pre	Post	Pre	Post	
Calvo et al. [70]	1987	29/M	–	Porcine (No. 31 Hancock)	10	25[b]	15	11	4.3[c]	3.5[c]	1.1	1.3	1+	2+	No atrial shunt
		37/F	–	Porcine (No. 29 Carpentier-Edwards)	3	25[b]	13	3	4.4[c]	4.0[c]	1.3	2.5	0	0	No atrial shunt; marked symptomatic improvement
Arie et al. [71]	1989	62/F		Dura matter bioprosthesis	30	20[d]	13	8	1.8	2.6	1.0	2.6	0	0	Symptomatic improvement; FU, 60 days
De Felice [72]	1989	67/F	–	Porcine (Carpentier-Edwards)	5	20	22	12	3.6[c]	3.6[c]	0.9	1.3	0	0	No atrial shunt; restenosis by 8 months

Fernandez et al. [73]	1990	62/F	—	Porcine (No. 25 Hancock)	10	20	22	6	4.25[c]	4.4[c]	0.77	1.53	Minimal	Minimal	No atrial shunt; symptomatic improvement; FU, 3 weeks
Babic et al. [74]	1991	39/M	—	Bovine pericardial (Ionescu-Shiley)	3	25[e]	29	9	1.9	2.4	0.7	1.7	Trace	Trace	Hemodynamic study 10 months after BD revealed MV area of 1.7 cm^2/m^2

[a] BD, balloon dilatation; F, female; FU, follow-up; L, liter; M, male; MV, mitral valve.
[b] Trefoil balloon.
[c] Cardiac output, not indexed.
[d] Dilatation with the 20 mm balloon followed sequential dilatation of the mitral valve with 15 and 18 mm balloons.
[e] Dilatation with the 25 mm balloons followed dilatation with a 20 mm balloon.

For discussion of the potential for embolization during and immediately after balloon dilatation, the reader is referred to the next section,
regarding bioprosthetic aortic valve dilatation.

BIOPROSTHETIC VALVES
IN AORTIC POSITION

I was able to find only two reports [75,76]
in which balloon valvuloplasty of a stenosed
bioprosthetic valve in the aortic position has
been utilized. McKay *et al.* [75] performed
balloon dilatation of stenotic bioprosthetic
(both porcine heterografts) aortic valves in two
adult patients, aged 28 and 31 years respectively. In one patient, there was good relief of
aortic valve peak gradient, whereas in the other
no significant gradient reduction occurred. In
the patient with gradient relief, severe aortic
insufficiency developed, related to torn-away
aortic valve cusps. Because of clinically unpredictable results, these authors recommended
that balloon valvuloplasty of aortic porcine
heterografts should be restricted to highly selected patients [75]. Ramondo *et al.* [76] presented a 60-year-old male who underwent balloon dilatation of a 27 mm Hancock porcine
heterograft that had been implanted 6.5 years
earlier. They used a 15–18 mm Schneider
balloon and reduced peak-to-peak gradient
across the aortic valve from 110 to 25 mmHg;
the aortic valve area increased from 0.59 to
1.07 cm^2m^2. The left ventricular end-diastolic
pressure decreased (14 *vs.* 4 mmHg), and there
was negligible aortic insufficiency. Short-term
follow-up was uneventful. Long-term follow-up
was not reported [76]. They concluded that
balloon valvuloplasty is a suitable and safe
procedure for relief of stenosis of all
bioprosthetic valves, including those in the
aortic position.

There appears to be a significant chance of
dislodgement of calcific nodules and debris
during balloon positioning and inflation
[40,75,77] when stenotic calcified
heterographs are balloon dilated. These fragments can embolize. Such an embolism is of

particular concern when mitral or aortic
bioprostheses are dilated because of the potential for systemic embolization. This is an additional consideration in favor of limiting application of balloon dilatation techniques to
left-sided bioprosthetic valves. However, Babic
and associates [74] employed a custom-made,
emboli-protecting device to capture embolic
materials, should they dislodge during left
heart prosthetic valve dilatation. This device is
made up of nylon netting connected to six
stainless steel wires, which can be positioned
in the aortic root and opened such that the
emboli can be caught in the net and removed.
In the single case in which they employed this
technique, they were able to filter several particulate clot materials measuring 3/2/1 to
4/3/3 mm [74]. This is an ingenious approach
and may resolve the issue of embolism, and it
may become useful in older adolescents and
adults. The device-carrying catheter may be too
bulky for the younger patients. Further experimental work on the utility of the emboli-protecting device and clinical trials are needed
prior to wide usage of this device.

MECHANISM OF BALLOON
DILATATION

The effects of balloon dilatation of the
heterografts were studied *in vitro* by several
workers [43,77]. *In vitro* balloon inflation of
the porcine valved conduits with oversized balloons did not produce cuspal tears or commissural dehiscence, and the valve patency or competence was not affected [43]. This is
irrespective of whether the balloon had ruptured. In a single specimen, there were longitudinal tears in the atrial muscle shelf that was incorporated into the valve by the manufacturer.
In contrast to the benign effects of balloon inflation in "normal" porcine heterografts, significant structural changes were observed in valve
structure when *in vitro* balloon dilatation was
performed in calcified, stenotic heterografts
[40,77]. Waller and associates [77] performed
in vitro balloon dilatation of 20 surgically ex-

cised porcine heterografts from patients aged 26–68 years (mean, 53 years). The valves had been implanted 1–10 years (mean, 6.6 years) prior to surgery. Fourteen of these valves were explanted from a mitral position and six from an aortic position. Balloon dilatation produced commissural splitting in all 18 valves in which primary degeneration was the cause of valve stenosis. In addition, half of these had cuspal fractures. Extensive cuspal fracture with fragmentation (and potential emboli) occurred in three valves (17%). Dislodgement of calcific debris was observed in 10 valves. Annular ruptures were not seen. In two valves with intracuspal thrombus formation as a cause of stenosis, balloon dilatation resulted in crumbling of the thrombus (with consequent dislodgement) in both valves and cuspal tearing in one valve.

Based on these observations, the mechanism of balloon dilatation appears to be related to commissural splitting and cusp fracture. The potential for dislodgement of calcific or thrombotic debris appears high. These *in vitro* observations of the mechanism of relief of prosthetic valve obstruction are indeed similar following *in vivo* balloon dilatation [75].

SUMMARY AND CONCLUSIONS

Calcific degeneration and obstruction of bioprosthetic valves have been well documented. Conventional treatment of choice is repeat valve replacement. Recently, balloon dilatation techniques have been applied to relieve obstruction of biological valves in an attempt to avoid or postpone surgery for repeat replacement of the valve. The largest experience is with bioprosthetic valve conduits in the pulmonary position. All varieties of heterografts and homografts can be balloon dilated. Although the results are not uniformly successful, repeat valve replacement could be avoided or at least postponed for several years in some patients. The indication for intervention is a peak systolic pressure gradient in excess of 50 mmHg across the pulmonary bioprosthetic valve. A balloon size equal to the size of the

bioprosthesis should be used. Relief of valvar obstruction may unmask additional obstructive lesions at the proximal or distal anastomosis. These should be searched for and, if feasible, balloon dilated concurrently. The high incidence of balloon rupture is of concern; appropriate precautions should be taken to prevent or reduce balloon ruptures. Follow-up results are few and are needed.

There are also reports of balloon dilatation of stenotic heterografts in the tricuspid position. Acute improvement in valve stenosis was observed in most, but nearly one-half of them required additional intervention within months after balloon valvuloplasty. Because of limited experience with this lesion, definitive recommendations with regard to the role of balloon dilatation of tricuspid heterograft stenosis cannot be made.

Balloon dilatation of mitral and aortic heterograft valve stenosis has also been performed. The results are unpredictable. This and the potential for dislodgement of calcific debris and fractured valve cusps and consequent systemic embolization indicate a limited role of balloon dilatation procedures in the management of left heart bioprosthetic valve stenosis. However, development of an embolic-protecting device may resolve the latter issue. Mechanisms of balloon dilatation have been studied and include commissural splitting and valve leaflet fracture.

Because of the limited experience with balloon valvuloplasty of prosthetic biologic valve stenosis, it is imperative that careful documentation of both immediate and follow-up results is made. Additional clinical trials are necessary prior to adoption of the balloon dilatation technique as a procedure of choice in the management of bioprosthetic valve stenosis.

REFERENCES

1. Binet JP, Duran CG, Carpentier A, Langlois J (1965): Heterologous aortic valve transplantation. Lancet 2:1275–1277.
2. Carpentier A, Lemaigre G, Robert L, Carpentier S (1969): Biologic factors affecting long-term re-

sults of valvular heterografts. J Thorac Cardiovasc Surg 58:467–482.

3. Zuhdi N, Hawley W, Voehl V, Hancock W, Carey J, Greer A (1974): Porcine aortic valves as replacement for human heart valves. Ann Thorac Surg 17:479–491.

4. Van der Horst RL, le Roux BT, Rogers NMA, Gotsman MS (1973): Mitral valve replacement in childhood: A report of 51 patients. Am Heart J 85:624–634.

5. Mathew RA, Neches WH, Lenox CC, Zuberbuhler JR, Fricker FJ (1977): Valve replacement in children and adolescents. J Thorac Cardiovasc Surg 73:872–876.

6. Sade RM, Ballenger JF, Hohn AR, Arrants JE, Riopel DA, Taylor AB (1979): Cardiac valve replacement in children: Comparison of tissue with mechanical prostheses. J Thorac Cardiovasc Surg 78:123–127.

7. Galioto FM, Jr, Midgley FM, Shapiro SR, Perry LW, Ciaravella JM, Scott LP III (1981): Mitral valve replacement in infants and children. Pediatrics 67:230–235.

8. Solymar L, Rao PS, Mardini MK, Fawzy ME, Guinn G (1991): Prosthetic valves in children and adolescents. Am Heart J 121:557–568.

9. Rao PS, Solymar L, Fawzy ME, Guinn G (1991): Reassessment of usefulness of porcine heterografts in mitral position in children. Pediatr Cardiol 12:164–169.

10. Dunn JM (1981): Porcine valve durability in children. Ann Thorac Surg 32:357–368.

11. Bailey WW, Kirklin JW, Bargeron LM, Jr, Pacifico AD, Kouchoukos NT (1977): Late results with synthetic valved external conduits from venous ventricles to pulmonary arteries. Circulation 56(Suppl II):73–79.

12. Heck HA, Schieken RM, Lauer RM, Dotty DB (1978): Conduit repair for complex congenital heart disease—Late follow-up. J Thorac Cardiovasc Surg 75:806–814.

13. Bisset GS, Schwartz DC, Benzig G, Helmsworth J, Schreiber JT, Kaplan S (1981): Late results of reconstruction of the right ventricular outflow tract with porcine xenografts in children. Ann Thorac Surg 31:437–444.

14. Miller DC, Stinson EB, Oyer PE, Billingham ME, Pitlick PT, Reitz BA, Jamieson SW, Baumgartner WA, Shumway NE (1982): The durability of porcine xenograft valves and conduits in children. Circulation 66(Suppl I):172–185.

15. Fiore AC, Peigh PS, Robinson RJ, Glant MD, King H, Brown JW (1983): Valved and nonvalved right ventricular-pulmonary arterial extracardiac conduits. J Thorac Cardiovasc Surg 86:490–497.

16. Stewart S, Manning J, Alex MC, Harris P (1983):

The Hancock external valved conduit: A dichotomy between late clinical results and late cardiac catheterization. J Thorac Cardiovasc Surg 86:562–569.

17. Vergesslich KA, Gersony WM, Steeg CN, Hordof AJ, Bowman FO, Jr, Malm JR, Krongrad E (1984): Postoperative assessment of porcine-valved right ventricular-pulmonary artery conduits. Am J Cardiol 53:202–205.

18. Jonas RA, Freed MD, Mayer JE, Castaneda AR (1985): Long-term follow-up of patients with synthetic heart conduits. Circulation 72(Suppl II):77–83.

19. Downing TP, Danielson GK, Schaff HV, Puga FJ, Edwards WD, Driscoll DJ (1985): Replacement of obstructed right ventricular-pulmonary arterial valved conduits and non-valved conduits in children. Circulation 72(Suppl II):84–87.

20. Shoen FJ, Collins JJ, Cohn LH (1983): Long-term failure rate and morphologic correlations in porcine bioprosthetic heart valves. Am J Cardiol 51:957–964.

21. Murray G (1956): Homologous aortic valve segment transplants as surgical treatment of aortic and mitral insufficiency. Angiology 7:446–471.

22. Ross DN (1962): Homograft replacement of aortic valve. Lancet 2:487.

23. Barratt-Boyes BG (1964): Homograft aortic valve replacement in aortic incompetence and stenosis. Thorax 19:131–150.

24. Ross DN, Somerville J (1966): Correction of pulmonary atresia with homograft aortic valve. Lancet 2:1446–1447.

25. Moodie DS, Mair DD, Fulton RE, Wallace RB, Danielson GK, McGoon DC (1976): Aortic homograft obstruction. J Thorac Cardiovasc Surg 72:553–561.

26. Barratt-Boyes BG (1979): Cardiothoracic surgery in the antipodes. J Thorac Cardiovasc Surg 78:804–822.

27. Saravalli OA, Somerville J, Jefferson KE (1980): Calcification of aortic homografts used for reconstruction of the right ventricular outflow tract. J Thorac Cardiovasc Surg 80:909–920.

28. Kay PH, Ross DN (1985): Fifteen years' experience with aortic homograft: The conduit of choice for right ventricular outflow obstruction. Ann Thorac Surg 40:360–364.

29. Merrill WH, de Leval MR, Ball C, Macartney FJ, Taylor JFN, Stark J (1988): Homograft prosthetic heart valves. In Dunn JM (ed): "Cardiac Valve Disease in Children." New York: Elsevier, pp 436–458.

30. Spray TL, Roberts WC (1977): Structural changes in porcine xenografts used as substitute cardiac valves: Gross and histologic observations in 51

glutaraldehyde-preserved Hancock valves in 41 patients. Am J Cardiol 40:319-330.

31. Fishbein MC, Gissen SA, Collins JJ, Jr, Barsamian EM, Cohn LH (1977): Pathologic findings after cardiac valve replacement with glutaraldehyde-fixed porcine valves. Am J Cardiol 40:331-337.

32. Brown JW, Dunn JM, Spooner E, Kirsh MM (1978): Late spontaneous disruption of a porcine xenograft mitral valve: Clinical, hemodynamic, echocardiographic, and pathological findings. J Thorac Cardiovasc Surg 75:606-611.

33. Silver MM, Pollock J, Silver MD, Williams WG, Trusler GA (1980): Calcification in porcine xeno-graft valves in children. Am J Cardiol 45:685-689.

34. Thandroyen FT, Whitton IN, Pirie D, Rogers MA, Mitha AS (1980): Severe calcification of glutaral-dehyde-preserved porcine xenografts in children. Am J Cardiol 75:690-696.

35. Schoen FJ, Levy RJ (1984): Bioprosthetic heart valve failures: Pathology and pathogenesis. Cardiol Clin 2:717-721.

36. Schoen FJ, Hobson CE (1985): Anatomic analysis of removed prosthetic heart valves: Causes of failure of mechanical valves and 58 bioprostheses, 1980-1983. Hum Pathol 16:549-559.

37. Waller BF, McKay C, Van Tassel J (1991): Cath-eter balloon valvuloplasty of stenotic porcine bioprosthetic valves, Part I: Anatomic considera-tions. Clin Cardiol 14:686-691.

38. Walker WE, Duncan JM, Frazier OH, Livesay JJ, Ott DA, Reul GJ, Cooley DA (1983): Early expe-rience with Ionescu-Shiley pericardial xenograft valve: Accelerated calcification in children. J Thorac Cardiovasc Surg 86:570-575.

39. Fiddler GI, Gerlis LM, Walker DR, Scott O, Williams GJ (1983): Calcification of gluteraldehyde-preserved porcine and bovine xe-nograft valves in young children. Ann Thorac Surg 35:251-261.

40. Waller BF, McKay C, Van Tassel J, Allen M (1992): Stenotic porcine bioprosthetic valves. In Cheng TO (ed): "Percutaneous Balloon Valvuloplasty." New York: Igaku-Shoin, pp 435-459.

40a. Walley VM, Keon WJ (1987): Patterns of failure in Ionescu-Shiley bovine pericardial bioprosthetic valves. J Thorac Cardiovasc Surg 93:925-933.

40b. Wheatley D, Fisher J, Reece IJ, Spy T, Breeze P (1987): Primary tissue failure in pericardial heart valves. J Thorac Cardiovasc Surg 94:367-374.

40c. Thiene G, Bortolotti U, Valente M, Milano A, Calabrese F, Talenti E, Mazzucco A, Gallucci V (1989): Mode of failure of Hancock pericardial valve xenograft. Am J Cardiol 63:129-133.

40d. McGonagle-Wolff K, Schoen FJ (1992): Morphologic findings in explanted Mitroflow peri-cardial Bioprosthetic valves. Am J Cardiol 70:263-264.

41. Agarwal KC, Edward WD, Feldt RH (1981): Clincopathological correlates of obstructed right-sided porcine-valved extracardiac conduits. J Thorac Cardiovasc Surg 81:591-601.

42. Edward WD, Agarwal KC, Feldt RH (1983): Sur-gical pathology of obstructed, right-sided porcine-valved, extracardiac conduits. Arch Pathol Lab Med 107:400-405.

43. Waldman JD, Schoen FJ, Kirkpatrick SE, Mathew-son JW, George L, Lamberti JJ (1987): Balloon dilatation of porcine bioprosthetic valves in pul-monary position. Circulation 76:109-114.

44. Lloyd TR, Marvin WJ, Jr, Mahoney LT, Lauer RM (1987): Balloon dilation valvuloplasty of bioprosthetic valves in extracardiac conduits. Am Heart J 114:268-274.

45. Rao PS (1989): Balloon pulmonary valvuloplasty: A review. Clin Cardiol 12:55-74.

46. Ensing GJ, Hagler DJ, Seward JB, Julsrud PR, Mair DD (1989): Caveats of balloon dilation of conduits and conduit valves. J Am Coll Cardiol 14:397-400.

47. Zeevi B, Keane JF, Perry SB, Lock JE (1989): Balloon dilation of postoperative right ventricular outflow obstructions. J Am Coll Cardiol 14:401-408.

48. Unwala AA, Mintz GS, Kimbiris D (1990): Bal-loon valvuloplasty of a stenotic bioprosthesis in the pulmonary position. J Invas Cardiol 2:73-76.

49. Waldman JD, Swensson RE (1990): Therapeutic cardiac catheterization in children. West J Med 153:288-295.

50. Mullins CE, Larson LA, Neches WH, Colvin EV, Kan J (1990): Balloon dilatation of miscellaneous lesions: Results of Valvuloplasty and Angioplasty of Congenital Anomalies Registry. Am J Cardiol 65:802-803.

51. Hagler DJ (1992): Conduits and conduit valves. In Cheng TO (ed): "Percutaneous Balloon Valvuloplasty." New York: Igaku-Shoin, pp 460-467.

52. Rao PS (1988): Indications for balloon pulmonary valvuloplasty. Am Heart J 116:1661-1662.

53. Murdoch IA, Parsons JM, Anjos RD, Qureshi SA (1991): Balloon dilatation of a stenosed aortic hemograft conduit following repair of the common arterial trunk. Pediatr Cardiol 12:175-176.

54. Rao PS (1990): Balloon rupture during valvulo-plasty. Am Heart J 119:1441-1442.

55. Dev V, Shrivastava S (1989): Transverse balloon tear in valvuloplasty. Am Heart J 117:1397-1398.

56. Abele JE (1980): Balloon catheters and translumi-nal dilatation: Technical considerations. Am J Roentgenol 135:901-906.

57. Thapar MK, Rao PS (1992): Mechanism of balloon valvuloplasty/angioplasty. In Rao PS (ed): "Transcatheter Therapy in Pediatric Cardiology." New York: Wiley-Liss, Inc (in press).

58. Dev V, Shrivastava S (1990): Balloon rupture during valvuloplasty. Am Heart J 119:1441-1442.

59. Silove ED, Vogel JHK, Grover RF (1968): The pressure gradient in ventricular outflow obstruction: Influence of peripheral resistance. Cardiovasc Res 3:234-242.

60. Rao PS, Linde LM (1974): Pressure and energy in the cardiovascular chambers. Chest 66:176-178.

61. Pelikan P, French WJ, Ruiz C, Laks H, Criley JM (1988): Percutaneous double-balloon angioplasty of a stenotic modified Fontan aortic homograft conduit. Cathet Cardiovasc Diagn 15:47-51.

61a. Waldman JD, Lamberti JJ, Schoen FJ, George L, Kirkpatrick SE, Mathewson JW, Spicer RL, Grehl TM, Goodman AA (1988): Balloon dilatation of stenotic right ventricle-to-pulmonary conduit. J Cardiol Surg 3:539-566.

62. Almagor Y, Prevosti LG, Bartorelli AL, Keren G, Ferrans VJ, Jones M, Leon MB (1990): Balloon expandable stent implantation in stenotic right heart valved conduits. J Am Coll Cardiol 16:1310-1314.

62a. Hosking MCK, Benson LN, Nakanishi T, Burrows PE, Williams WG, Freedom RM (1992): Intravascular stent prosthesis for right-ventricular outflow obstruction. J Am Coll Cardiol 20:373-380.

63. Feit F, Stecy PJ, Nachamie MS (1986): Percutaneous balloon valvuloplasty for stenosis of a porcine bioprosthesis in the tricuspid valve position. Am J Cardiol 5:362-364.

64. Rao PS (1989): Balloon angioplasty and valvuloplasty in infants, children and adolescents. Curr Probl Cardiol 8:417-500.

65. Wren C, Hunter S (1989): Balloon dilatation of a stenosed bioprosthesis in the tricuspid valve position. Br Heart J 61:65-67.

66. Attubato MJ, Stroh JA, Bach RG (1990): Percutaneous double-balloon valvuloplasty of porcine bioprosthetic valves in the tricuspid position. Cathet Cardiovasc Diagn 20:202-204.

67. Chow W, Cheung K, Tai Y, Cheng C (1990): Successful percutaneous balloon valvuloplasty of a stenosed bioprosthesis. Am Heart J 119:666-668.

68. Benedick BA, Davis SF, Alderman F (1990): Balloon valvuloplasty for fungal endocarditis induced stenosis of a bioprosthetic tricuspid valve. Cathet Cardiovasc Diagn 21:248-251.

69. Rao PS (1987): Influence of balloon size in the short-term and long-term results of balloon pulmonary valvuloplasty. Texas Heart Inst J 14:57-61.

70. Calvo OL, Sobrino N, Gamallo C, Oliver J, Dominquez F, Iglesias A (1987): Balloon percutaneous valvuloplasty for stenotic bioprosthetic valves in mitral position. Am J Cardiol 60:736-737.

71. Arie S, Goncalves MTDFA, Rati MAN, Tarasoutchi F, Cardosa LF, Grinberg M, Bellotti G, Pileggi F (1989): Balloon dilatation of a stenotic dura mater mitral bioprosthesis. Am Heart J 117:201-202.

72. De Felice CA, Mullins CE, Kumpuris AG, Raizner AE (1989): Percutaneous balloon valvuloplasty of a porcine xenograft bioprosthesis in mitral position: Late hemodynamic observations. J Intervent Cardiol 2:103-107.

73. Fernandez JJ, Desando J, Leff RA, Ord M, Sabbagh AH (1990): Percutaneous balloon valvuloplasty of a stenosed mitral bioprosthesis. Cathet Cardiovasc Diagn 19:39-41.

74. Babic UU, Grujicic S, Vucinic M (1991): Balloon valvuloplasty of mitral bioprosthesis. Int J Cardiol 30:230-232.

75. McKay CR, Waller BF, Hong R, Rubin N, Reid CL, Rahimtoola SH (1988): Problems encountered with catheter balloon valvuloplasty of bioprosthetic aortic valves. Am Heart J 115:463-465.

76. Ramondo A, Gemelli M, Chioin R (1989): Balloon dilatation of porcine bioprosthetic valve in aortic position. Int J Cardiol 24:105-107.

77. Waller BF, McKay C, Van Tassel J, Allen M (1991): Catheter balloon valvuloplasty of stenotic porcine bioprosthetic valves: Part II: Mechanisms, complications and recommendations for clinical use. Clin Cardiol 14:764-772.

15

Balloon Dilatation of Other Congenital and Acquired Stenotic Lesions of the Cardiovascular System

P. Syamasundar Rao, M.D., and Mohinder K. Thapar, M.D.

Department of Pediatrics, Division of Pediatric Cardiology,
University of Wisconsin Medical School, University of Wisconsin
Children's Hospital, Madison, Wisconsin 53792-4108 (P.S.R.), and
Department of Pediatrics, Division of Pediatric Cardiology,
University of Texas Medical School, Houston, Texas 77030 (M.K.T.)

INTRODUCTION

Balloon dilatation of various congenital and acquired stenotic lesions of the heart and great vessels has been described in the previous chapters. The presentations included discussion of issues related to balloon angioplasty/valvuloplasty of isolated pulmonary valve stenosis, aortic valve stenosis, atrioventricular valve stenosis, fixed subaortic stenosis, coarctation of the aorta (both native and that following previous surgery), peripheral pulmonary artery stenosis, pulmonary stenosis associated with cyanotic congenital heart defects, stenosed Blalock-Taussig shunts, and stenotic bioprosthetic valves. There are many other obstructive lesions in the cardiovascular system, both congenital and acquired, that have not been discussed. These are either rare in occurrence or balloon dilatation techniques have not been frequently used to treat them. In this chapter, we shall review this miscellaneous group of lesions.

TRICUSPID VALVE STENOSIS

Tricuspid valve stenosis may be acquired or congenital in origin. Rheumatic fever is the most common acquired cause of tricuspid stenosis. Balloon valvuloplasty of rheumatic tricuspid stenosis has been described by several workers [1–7], was discussed in detail in Chapter 8, and will not be reviewed here. Other uncommon acquired causes are carcinoid, endomyocardial fibrosis, and systemic lupus erythematosus [8]. Mullins et al. [9] reported results of balloon dilatation in an adult patient with tricuspid stenosis caused by carcinoid heart disease. Although balloon dilatation produced some relief of pressure gradient across the tricuspid valve and symptomatic improvement, several questions were raised with regard to the significance of tricuspid stenosis and effectiveness of balloon dilatation [10]. In this section of the chapter, congenital tricuspid valve stenosis will be discussed.

Congenital tricuspid stenosis may occur alone or in association with other defects. It is most commonly associated with severe pulmonary valve stenosis or atresia with hypoplastic right ventricle [11,12]. Other lesions in which tricuspid stenosis has been reported to coexist include double-outlet right ventricle, mitral stenosis, polyvalvar disease, double-inlet left ventricle, tetralogy of Fallot, transposition of the great arteries, ventricular septal defect, Ebstein's anomaly of the tricuspid valve, and Uhl's anomaly [11]. The clinical features depend largely on the associated cardiac defects. Treatment should be directed toward the primary defect, although relief (or bypass) of tricuspid valve obstruction should be considered in the overall management of these patients.

The isolated form of tricuspid stenosis is extremely rare [11]; a recent review [13] revealed that only 15 cases of isolated tricuspid valve stenosis have been documented in the literature. Pathologically, there may be hypoplasia of the entire valve apparatus (although it may be formed normally), formation of two cusps ("mitralized") with abnormal attachments to the papillary muscle, or conversion to a sheet of valve tissue attached to short chordae and small or markedly abbreviated papillary muscle [14]. Occasionally, commissural fusion with normal annular size and preserved subvalvar apparatus may be present [15,16]. There may be moderate to severe hypoplasia of the right ventricle. Clinical features, all similar to those observed in tricuspid atresia, include cyanosis (secondary to right-to-left shunt across the interatrial communication), right atrial enlargement, left axis deviation [8], left ventricular hypertrophy, diminished or absent right ventricular forces on the electrocardiogram, and diminished pulmonary vascular markings on chest roentgenogram. This lesion is indeed difficult to distinguish from tricuspid atresia, even with cineangiography [11]. However, on two-dimensional echocardiography, the patency of the tricuspid valve may be demonstrable [11]. The treatment approach is similar to that of tricuspid atresia [17]; however, some of these patients could be treated by commissurotomy, valve excision, or valve replacement [18–20].

There are only a few instances of use of transcatheter relief of the congenital tricuspid stenosis reported [15,21–23]. In some of these reports, it is difficult to discern whether the tricuspid stenosis is congenital or acquired.

Indications

The indications for balloon valvuloplasty are difficult to define. In the presence of an inter-atrial communication, right-to-left shunt occurs, and the diastolic pressure difference across the tricuspid valve is not necessarily indicative of the degree of obstruction. In the absence of interatrial communication, it is likely that the pressure gradient is proportional to the degree of tricuspid valve obstruction. Even in this group of patients, some patients may not show diastolic gradient across the tricuspid valve [24], and provocative hemodynamic maneuvers may be necessary to unmask the occult gradient. Nonetheless, two-dimensional echocardiography may be helpful in this evaluation. When significant right-to-left shunting is present or when significant diastolic pressure gradient is present across the tricuspid valve, it may be an indication for relieving the obstruction. If commissural fusion and/or restriction of opening of the valve leaflets is demonstrated on two-dimensional echocardiography, balloon valvuloplasty is indicated.

Technique

The technique is similar to that described in Chapter 14 for balloon dilatation of bioprosthetic valve stenosis in tricuspid position. A curved (or coiled) guidewire in right ventricular apex or a straight (or J-shaped) guidewire in distal branch pulmonary arteries may be introduced for positioning the balloon valvuloplasty catheter across the tricuspid valve. A balloon size that is 20% larger than the tricuspid valve annulus [22] should be used. Single-balloon technique may be adequate in infants and younger children, while a double-balloon technique is necessary in older children and adults. It is important to measure a) simultaneous pressures from the right ventricle and right atrium and b) the cardiac index prior to and following balloon valvuloplasty. These data are used for calculation of the tricuspid valve area. Right atrial angiography (to assess the valve opening) and right ventricular angiography (to determine the presence and degree of tricuspid insufficiency) are also needed.

Results and Complications

Immediate results. In the historic report of Rubio and Limon Lason [21], the authors used a modified ureteral catheter with a wire on it to cut the tricuspid valve and produced significant relief of the obstruction. In the other reports using conventional balloon dilatation technique [15,22,23], reduction in the right atrial pressure and a fall in the gradient across the tricuspid valve were noted. Improvement in the cardiac output and calculated tricuspid valve area and, in particular, relief of symptoms of systemic venous congestion were noted.

Follow-up results. Follow-up data are scanty. In two reported instances [15,23] with 2-week and 3-month follow-up, there was continued improvement of symptoms. In one patient, the size of the right atrium diminished at follow-up, and the atrial fibrillation could easily be converted (pharmacologically) to sinus rhythm.

Complications. Reported complications are minimal with only mild increase in tricuspid insufficiency in some cases.

Mechanism

Based on the limited experience, the mechanism of balloon dilatation is by splitting the commissural fusion [15].

Comments

Congenital tricuspid stenosis is rare. The reported experience with balloon dilatation of congenital tricuspid stenosis is limited. Clinically significant (right-to-left shunt or systemic venous congestion) tricuspid stenosis is an indication for relief of obstruction. Reasonably sized, near-normal tricuspid valve annulus with fused tricuspid commissures are good candidates for balloon tricuspid valvuloplasty. There is some controversy as to whether the tips of guidewires should be positioned in the right ventricular apex or in the pulmonary artery (during balloon angioplasty). The limited experience reported thus far suggests improvement of hemodynamic parameters and clinical symptomatology. Short-term follow-up results (in only two patients) seem favorable. The complications are minimal.

With proper selection of patients, it is likely that balloon valvuloplasty will emerge as an effective alternative to surgical valvotomy or valve replacement. Experience in a larger number of patients and a longer follow-up are needed.

MITRAL VALVE STENOSIS

The most common cause of mitral stenosis is rheumatic fever. Balloon valvuloplasty of rheumatic mitral stenosis was initially described by Inoue using a specially prepared balloon [25]. Subsequently, a similar technique was applied by others, utilizing conventional single [26] and double balloons [27]. Issues related to balloon valvuloplasty of rheumatic mitral stenosis in adult patients were discussed in detail in Chapter 8. The theory and practice of balloon mitral valvuloplasty in adolescents and young adults with rheumatic mitral stenosis [26,28–32] is similar and will not be repeated. In this section of this chapter, we will review the reported experiences [28,33–35] with balloon dilatation of congenital mitral stenosis.

Congenital mitral stenosis is a rare anomaly, constituting 0.2% of all congenital heart defects [36]. The pathologic anatomy of congenital mitral stenosis is variable [37]. It may be an integral part of hypoplastic left heart syndrome, supravalvar mitral ring, parachute mitral valve, and Shone's syndrome, or the pathology may be confined to the mitral valve leaflets. There may be generalized hypoplasia of the mitral apparatus (hypoplastic left heart syndrome), supramitral stenosing ring of connective tissue (supravalvar mitral ring), attachment of all chordae tendineae to a single papillary muscle (parachute mitral valve), or a combination of abnormalities (Shone's complex). In the final type, named "typical congenital mitral stenosis" [37], the valve leaflets are thickened and fused [37]. The chordae tendineae are short, and the space between chordae may be absent [34,37]. There are two papillary muscles in the left ventricle, but the distance between them may be shortened. The latter form is also associated with other congenital malformations of the heart and include coarctation of the aorta, aortic stenosis, and subaortic stenosis [37]. To the best of our knowledge, Kveselis and associates [28] appear to be the first to use balloon dilatation technique to relieve congenital mitral valve obstruction.

Indications

Defining indications for balloon valvuloplasty for congenital mitral stenosis may be difficult because of limited application of this technique. The indications should probably be similar to those used for surgical therapy. Symptoms and signs of pulmonary venous congestion, echo-Doppler evidence for moderate to severe mitral valve stenosis, and/or cardiac catheterization evidence for significant mitral valve gradient and calculated mitral valve area less than 1 to 1.5 cm^2/m^2 may generally be considered indications for intervention. Demonstration either by echo-Doppler studies and/or angiography that the mitral valve stenosis is valvar in origin rather than due to severe hypoplasia of mitral valve annulus, subvalvar pathology (parachute), or supravalvar mitral ring is important prior to attempting balloon therapy. Mild mitral regurgitation is not a contraindication for balloon dilatation. Moderate to severe mitral insufficiency and left atrial thrombus are contraindications for balloon dilatation. Although balloon dilatation is unlikely to be successful in all cases [34,35], it should be considered in all young children (< 5 years) because of significant problems associated with mitral valve replacement in young children [38].

Technique

The technique is similar to that described in Chapter 8 for rheumatic mitral stenosis. Some important technique aspects will be pointed out. The entry into the left atrium is by a standard Brockenbrough technique using Mullins' transseptal long sheath and dilator (USCI, Bellerica, MA). Heparinization (100 units/kg body weight) is recommended in all cases. The guidewire used for positioning the balloon dilatation catheter should either be placed in the left ventricular apex [28] or in the aorta [33,34]; we prefer the latter because a more stable positioning of the balloon can be achieved with little risk of inadvertent removal of the guidewire. Positioning the guidewire into the aorta could be accomplished by the use of a flow-directed balloon catheter and/or preshaped guidewire. The size of the balloon used should probably be equal to the size of the mitral valve annulus [28] and should be no larger than 30% of the valve annulus [34]. If the valve annulus is too large for a single balloon, a double-balloon technique [22] with balloons inserted into both femoral veins and two transseptal punctures may be used. Alternatively, a specially designed double-lumen catheter (Mansfield) that allows two guidewires to be positioned into the left ventricle via a single transseptal puncture may be used. However, both balloon catheters, one at a time, should be advanced through the venous entry site and transseptal puncture [39]. When two balloons are used, effective balloon diameter [40] should be similar to mitral valve annulus. To avoid creation of atrial septal defects, some workers [41] advocate retrograde technique (femoral artery to aorta to left ventricle to left atrium), but this is unlikely to be of use in young children because of a potential for arterial injury.

Results and Complications

Immediate results. Kveselis et al. [28] and Rocchini [39] attempted balloon dilatation in three children with congenital mitral stenosis. In one 13-year-old patient, the left atrial mean pressure fell from 32 to 21 mm Hg, and the mitral valve area increased from 0.7 to 0.85 cm^2/m^2 immediately following balloon valvuloplasty. In the remaining two children, a balloon dilatation catheter could not be positioned across the mitral valve and the procedure was terminated. Alday and Juaneda [33] performed balloon dilation in a three-year-old child and reduced mitral diastolic gradient from 7 mm Hg to 1.5 mm Hg. Symptomatic improvement, decreased intensity of mitral diastolic murmur, and increase in the mitral valve orifice area by echocardiographic studies were also noted. Spevak et al. [34] reported combined experience from three children's hospitals; there were nine children, aged 0.1 to 10 years, in whom balloon valvuloplasty for congenital mitral stenosis was attempted. The mean transmitral gradient decreased from 15 ± 5 to 8 ± 7 mm Hg, and the calculated mitral valve area increased from 1.1 ± 0.5 to 1.8 ± 0.9 cm^2/m^2. In seven of the nine patients, acute reduction of the mitral valve gradient occurred. The Valvuloplasty and Angioplasty of Congenital Anomalies (VACA) Registry [35] mentions that balloon dilatation of the mitral valve was performed in 16 patients. In ten, the result was successful, while the result was unknown in five and failed in one. Ages of the patients and whether the lesion is congenital or acquired was not mentioned. Additional experience is reported in abstract form [42,43] and is encouraging.

Follow-up results. There is limited follow-up data. Kveselis et al. and Rocchini [28,39] reported that in the case of the 13 year-old patient cited above there was 6-month follow-up information; this suggested mild symptomatic and Doppler-measured hemodynamic improvement initially, but subsequently, symptoms recurred and surgical intervention was required. In the case reported by Alday and Juaneda [33], cardiac catheterization performed one month following balloon valvuloplasty revealed continued improvement in transmitral gradient and calculated mitral valve area and fall in pulmonary artery pressure. The child's exercise tolerance also improved.

Of the nine patients reported by Spevak et al. [34], two patients did not have an initial good result and required surgical replacement of the mitral valve. Of the remaining seven, five children continued to show improvement in mitral gradient by Doppler; the exact duration of follow-up for these patients was not given. The final two patients, despite improvement immediately after valvuloplasty, had recurrence of stenosis requiring surgical intervention.

Complications. Development of left atrial thrombus [28], increase in the severity of mitral regurgitation [34], and small atrial septal defects (Qp:Qs: 1 to 1.6) [34,35] have been reported. Excessive blood loss, ventricular tachycardia, hypotension, and need for intubation to treat respiratory acidosis have also been recorded [34,35].

Mechanism

The mechanism of action of balloon dilatation is likely to be splitting of the commissural fusion, although limited data [39] are available to support this contention.

Comments

The incidence of congenital mitral stenosis is very low, and experience with balloon dilatation of these lesions is limited. While generalized hypoplasia of the mitral valve, supravalvar mitral ring, and parachute mitral valve are not amenable to balloon dilatation, the so-called "typical" congenital mitral stenosis with mitral valve leaflet fusion can be successfully balloon-dilated. Signs of pulmonary venous congestion with significant diastolic gradient across the mitral valve and diminished mitral valve area (< 1.0 cm/m²) are indications for intervention. If the echo-Doppler studies support the diagnosis of "typical" congenital mitral stenosis, balloon dilatation may be an excellent option, especially in view of poor results for valve replacement in young children (< 5 years). Transseptal catheterization of the left atrium, positioning of the balloon(s) across the mitral valve over a previously introduced guidewire (with the tip positioned in the ascending aorta), and use of a balloon(s) with an

inflated diameter equivalent to the mitral annulus are required. Although the experience
reported is limited, a little more than half of
the children show clinical and hemodynamic
improvement immediately after valvuloplasty.
The duration of follow-up is short and is
available in a small number of patients. Some
children, despite initial improvement, develop
restenosis, requiring surgical intervention.
Complications appear to be few.

Based on available data, balloon valvuloplasty is a useful technique in relieving congenital
mitral stenosis if the basic pathology is limited
to valve leaflets (fusion). Use of this technique
in a larger number of patients and detailed
follow-up studies to document long-term effectiveness of this technique are needed prior to
making any definitive recommendations.

TRUNCAL VALVE STENOSIS

Truncus arteriosus is an uncommon congenital cardiac anomaly and accounts for approximately 0.7% of all congenital heart defects [36]. Stenosis of the truncal valve is rare
and is found to be present in 6 to 11% of
truncus arteriosus cases [44,45]. The pathology
of truncal valve stenosis is not well described;
it may be due to thickened, fibrotic, myxomatous leaflets, or due to valve leaflet fusion.
Truncal valve stenosis can be present with
unicuspid, bicuspid, tricuspid, or quadri-
cuspid valve leaflets [44–47].

Associated truncal valve stenosis is likely to
increase symptoms of heart failure of truncus
arteriosus. Although there are no established
criteria for intervention, a peak-to-peak gradient of approximately 50 mm Hg may be considered a reasonable indication for balloon
valvuloplasty. Antegrade introduction of a
catheter from the femoral vein to right ventricle, and from there into the truncus across the
ventricular septal defect and truncal valve is
feasible [47], and such a route is preferable to
retrograde approach. Ballerini and associates
[47] used a balloon that is 80% of truncal valve
annulus. Perhaps the size of the balloon

should not exceed the valve annulus size for
fear of producing an increasing truncal valve
regurgitation. In the single reported instance
[47], the truncal valve gradient was reduced
from 45 mm Hg to 25 mm Hg immediately
after balloon valvuloplasty, which decreased
further to 15 mm Hg eight days after the
procedure. There were no complications in the
single case reported [47]. Although Ballerini et
al. [47] performed balloon valvuloplasty in a
neonate with truncal valve stenosis in an attempt to postpone surgical intervention, this
was not feasible despite reduction of the gradient, and the infant required surgical intervention.

While there is limited experience, we feel
that it is appropriate to attempt balloon
valvuloplasty in symptomatic infants if the
truncal valve gradient is in excess of 50 mm
Hg, with the hope that valvuloplasty may help
alleviate symptoms and optimize the timing for
surgical correction. If balloon valvuloplasty is
chosen, the balloon size should be no larger
than truncal valve annulus.

DUCTUS ARTERIOSUS

The ductus arteriosus in the fetus is a large
vascular structure that connects the pulmonary
artery to the aorta and is responsible for transfer of the desaturated right ventricular blood
into the descending aorta from which the
blood makes its way into the placenta (for
oxygenation) by way of the umbilical arteries.
In the fetus, the ductus is kept widely open by
the locally produced and circulating prostaglandins. Within hours after birth, ductal constriction takes place, and the ductus is functionally closed by 10 to 15 hours of age. This
appears to be related to direct action of the PO_2
on the ductal musculature. There also appears
to be an indirect contribution of prostaglandins in that the ductal muscle becomes less
responsive to prostaglandins with increasing
gestational age. Anatomic closure of the ductus
occurs by endothelial destruction, subintimal
layer proliferation, and connective tissue pro-

liferation within two to three weeks of age. While the postnatal closure of ductus arteriosus is beneficial for infants with normally formed hearts, it is quite detrimental to the neonates with certain types of congenital heart defects. Ductal-dependent cardiac defects are listed in Table I. Even in infants with these defects, the ductus arteriosus spontaneously closes in the majority. Hitherto, surgical shunts (for conditions with ductal-dependent pulmonary flow) and corrective or palliative bypass surgical procedures (for conditions with ductal-dependent systemic circulation) have been used to treat these infants. More recently, intravenous prostaglandin E_1 or E_2 infusion and oral prostaglandin E_2 administration have been undertaken (48–50) to keep the ductus patent. While prostaglandins are useful in stabilizing the infants, they cannot be used indefinitely. Therefore, nonsurgical transcatheter means of maintaining ductal patency would be of value. In this section of this chapter, we will review both the experimental and clinical experience reported with balloon dilatation and stenting of ductus arteriosus.

Balloon Dilatation

Lund and his associates [51] performed *in vitro* balloon dilatation of ductus arteriosus in postmortem specimens from piglets and human neonates. They also carried out this procedure *in vivo* in newborn pigs, aged 2 to 13 days. They demonstrated that the technique of balloon dilatation of the ductus is feasible and that the functionally closed ductus could be made patent with resultant significant left-to-right shunts. The dilated lumen of the ductus varied from 3 to 5 mm. Pathologic examination revealed splitting of the internal elastic lamina, radial tears of the media, and preservation of the adventitia. They concluded that balloon angioplasty of ductus arteriosus has a potential utility in the palliation of ductal-dependent congenital heart defects. In a later study [52], they examined long-term patency of the ductus dilated by balloon angioplasty techniques. They balloon-dilated ductus arteriosus in eight piglets, aged 12 to 16 days. In six of the eight animals, ductal patency was demonstrated for periods of up to six months. In the remaining two piglets, the ductus was closed by thrombus formation. However, the period of follow-up was short; it was six months in only one animal and was two to six weeks in the remaining piglets. Histologic study revealed intimal and medial tears at various stages of healing. It was concluded that this is a good laboratory preparation for study of left-to-right shunts at ductal level and felt that clinical usefulness of the technique of balloon dilatation of ductus arteriosus is unclear. Suárez de Lezo et al. [53] performed balloon

---

TABLE I. Ductus-Dependent Cardiac Defects

A. Ductus-dependent pulmonary blood flow
  1. Pulmonary atresia with intact ventricular septum
  2. Pulmonary atresia with ventricular septal defect
  3. Severe tetralogy of Fallot
  4. Complex cyanotic heart disease with pulmonary atresia or severe stenosis
  5. Tricuspid atresia
  6. Critical pulmonary stenosis
  7. Ebstein's anomaly of the tricuspid valve
  8. Hypoplastic right ventricle

B. Ductus-dependent systemic blood flow
  1. Interruption of the aortic arch
  2. Severe coarctation of the aorta syndrome
  3. Hypoplastic left heart syndrome
  4. Critical aortic stenosis

dilatation of ductus arteriosus in three post-mortem human heart specimens secured from neonates who died from noncardiac causes. Five-millimeter deflated balloons were positioned in the ductus and were inflated at 8 atm of pressure for 15 seconds. Three such inflations were performed in each specimen. Disruption of intima and fragmentated and disorganized fibers in the media without loss of integrity of ductal wall were observed.

To the best of our knowledge, Corwin et al. [54] were the first to report clinical application of balloon dilatation of ductus arteriosus. This was in an infant with interrupted aortic arch. They used a 5 Fr Berman angiographic catheter, which was advanced from the main pulmonary artery into the descending aorta via the ductus arteriosus. The balloon was inflated with 1.0 ml of gas and pulled back from the descending aorta into the main pulmonary artery across the ductus arteriosus; this maneuver was performed three times. Although no postdilatation angiograms were shown, they report an increase of descending aortic, nonphasic mean pressure from 42 mm Hg to a phasic pressure of 62/36 mm Hg. The procedure improved the infant's clinical status and abolished metabolic acidosis, and the infant underwent surgical palliation three hours later. At surgery, the wall of the ductus arteriosus was found to be hemorrhagic. Corwin and his coworkers postulated that the hemorrhage in the ductal wall may have interfered with ductal constriction, thus causing its patency. They concluded that additional data are needed to ascertain whether mechanical dilatation of ductus is useful in keeping the ductus open.

Suárez de Lezo and associates (53) performed balloon dilatation of a constricted ductus arteriosus in an 8-day-old infant with hypoplastic left heart syndrome. They used a 4 Fr coronary dilatation catheter, positioned the 3.7-mm balloon across the ductus arteriosus from the main pulmonary artery, and inflated the balloon twice at 5 atm of pressure for 10 seconds each time. The descending aortic pressure increased, the pressure gradient across the

ductus was abolished, and the angiographic ductus size increased following balloon angioplasty. In addition, clinical and blood gas values improved. However, 18 hours later, the neonate sustained cardiac arrest, presumably due to basic cardiac defect (hypoplastic left heart syndrome). At necropsy, the ductus was found to be patent, and microscopic examination revealed fragmentation of the internal elastic layer and muscular media with areas of focal edema. The adventitia was not torn. These authors concluded that balloon angioplasty is a complementary alternative to prostaglandin therapy of neonates with ductus-dependent congenital heart defects and suggested balloon angioplasty of stenotic ductus for palliation prior to surgical procedure(s).

We performed balloon dilatation of the ductus arteriosus [55] in two neonates, ages 14 and 21 days (weights, 2.1 and 2.9 kg), with severe congestive heart failure secondary to aortic coarctation and large ventricular septal defect. A 4 Fr and 5 Fr balloon dilatation catheters, carrying 4.2- and 5.0-mm balloons, respectively, were used. The balloons were inflated with diluted contrast material to approximately 4 to 7 atm of pressure, and the "waisting" of the balloon was eliminated (Fig. 1). Each balloon inflation lasted for 5 seconds. A total of four balloon inflations, 5 minutes apart, were performed. Immediately after balloon angioplasty, the descending aortic pressure increased and the pressure gradient across the ductus decreased (Fig. 4, Chapter 10). Angiographic improvement was also noted (Fig. 5, Chapter 10). More importantly, the femoral pulses, which had been either absent or markedly reduced, became readily palpable, and the congestive heart failure improved. No immediate surgical intervention was required. One infant, though improved clinically, had signs of recoarctation and a large interventricular shunt six months following balloon angioplasty, and she, therefore, was restudied. At cardiac catheterization, a peak-to-peak pressure gradient of 30 mm Hg across the coarctation was found. There was a large ventricular septal defect and a small patent

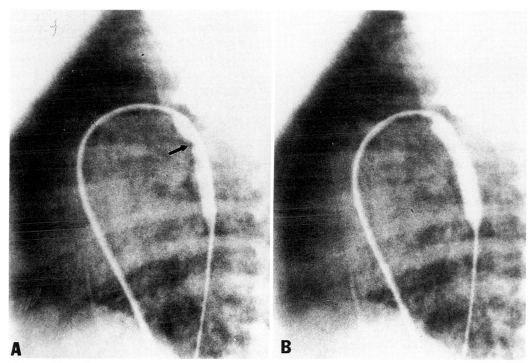

Fig. 1. The balloon dilatation catheter was passed into the descending aorta from the main pulmonary artery via the patent ductus arteriosus. Note "waisting" of the balloon (A) during the initial phases of balloon inflation, which disappeared (B) on further inflation of the balloon. (Reproduced from Rao and Solymar [55], with permission of the publisher.)

ductus arteriosus on angiography. The infant underwent successful resection of coarctation and ductal ligation. The second infant was seen one month after angioplasty in good clinical condition, but was lost for subsequent follow-up. Prompt improvement of the pressure gradient across the coarctation is similar to that observed following conventional transfemoral artery, retrograde balloon angioplasty of aortic coarctation [55].

The mechanism of action may be explained as follows: Postnatal development of coarctation has been postulated to be the result of constriction of the ductus arteriosus [56,57]. Blood flow from the isthmus of the aorta into the descending aorta around the posterolateral shelf of coarctation is facilitated by an open ductus (Fig. 2A). When the ductus arteriosus closes (Fig. 2B), this bypass mechanism is no

longer available, and acute aortic obstruction follows quickly with consequent symptomatology [56,57]. If the ductus is made to dilate, as has been done with prostaglandin E1 infusion [58,59], the symptoms of aortic obstruction can be relieved. Balloon dilatation of ductus, as outlined above, allows passage of blood from aortic isthmus into the descending aorta (Fig. 2A), bypassing the posterolateral shelf of the aortic coarctation, and it may be an alternative method to relieve aortic obstruction. Subsequent constriction of the ductus, as in our first patient, may cause recoarctation that may be dealt with either by surgery or by transfemoral retrograde arterial balloon coarctation angioplasty. The latter procedures can be undertaken when the infant is older, weighs more, and is not acutely ill. An additional advantage is saving the femoral artery for later

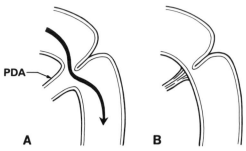

Fig. 2. Diagrammatic portrayal of the flow from the aortic isthmus to the descending aorta in coarctation of the aorta: **A,** with open ductus, and **B,** with closed ductus. See the text for discussion. (Reproduced from Rao and Solymar [55], with permission of the publisher.)

use. We recommended use of this technique in neonates if the femoral artery could not be cannulated [55], and suggested that a repeat catheterization in six months may be warranted, especially if there is an associated significant-sized ventricular septal defect.

To the best of our knowledge, there are no reports of balloon dilatation in infants with cyanotic heart defects with pulmonary oligemia (Table I).

In conclusion, balloon dilatation of stenotic ductus arteriosus has been attempted in animal models, postmortem human specimens, and human neonates with ductal-dependent systemic flow. In human studies, systemic perfusion improved in patients with interrupted aortic arch (54), hypoplastic left heart syndrome [53], and severe aortic coarctation [55]. Improvement in the first two conditions seem to be related to allowing unrestricted flow from the main pulmonary artery into the descending aorta across the dilated ductus arteriosus. In the third (coarctation), this improvement may be as described for the first two conditions and/or by a mechanism that we previously postulated [55]: relief of the aortic obstruction is by facilitation of blood flow from the isthmus of the aorta into the descending aorta around the posterolateral shelf of coarctation by an open ductus (Fig. 2A).

Although no definitive recommendations

can be made because of limited data, it would seem reasonable to use balloon dilatation of ductus in an attempt to stabilize a sick infant with metabolic acidosis secondary to hypoplastic left heart syndrome or interrupted aortic arch (or even critical aortic stenosis). Perhaps prostaglandin infusion may serve the same purpose. Clinical improvement lasting for several months in neonates with severe coarctation [55] would suggest that balloon dilatation of ductus can be considered as an alternative to surgery when conventional retrograde arterial balloon coarctation angioplasty cannot be performed for technical reasons. However, the long-term patency of the dilated ductus remains unclear.

Ductal Stents

As reviewed in the preceding section, long-term patency of the ductus by balloon dilatation appears uncertain. Stenting of the ductus is a logical extension of transcatheter methodology, especially in view of usefulness of stent implantation in coronary, renal, and peripheral arteries [60–64], branch pulmonary arteries [65,66], and venae cavae [65-68]. Coe and associates [69] demonstrated in a newborn lamb model that it is feasible to implant tubular mesh (Palmaz-Schatz) stents into the ductus arterios by the venous and retrograde arterial routes. They implanted stents in six lambs by the venous route, and in two lambs by the retrograde arterial route. No embolizations occurred. Only one of the six stents placed by the venous route was partially pulled back into the pulmonary artery. When the stent patently was examined by aortography and/or by Doppler echocardiography, three weeks to two months after implantation, all of them were patent. Pathologic examination revealed that the stents were patent in all animals and that there was a small thrombus in one of the stents. Coe's data show that stent delivery and release could be undertaken with relative ease and that continued ductal patency was present up to three months following implantation. They concluded that this method could be used to maintain ductal blood flow in neonates with ductal-dependent cardiac defects, thus avoiding thoracotomy. They also suggested that the size of shunts may be increased, although no such data are provided. Others [70] have also shown the feasibility of stent placement in lamb models to maintain ductal patency. However, when Lloyd and Markowitz [71] implanted serpentine wire (Gianturco-Roubin) stents in three piglets, thrombosis occurred in all three animals within one hour of implantation. This was so despite pretreatment with heparin. The authors concluded that thrombus formation precludes use of this type of stent as an alternative to surgery. Based on the limited data [69–71], it appears that serpentine wire (Gianturco-Roubin) stents are more thombogenic than tubular mesh (Palmaz-Schatz) stents.

Gibbs et al. [72] used stents to maintain ductal patency in two neonates with pulmonary atresia. They used Palmaz-Schatz stainless steel stents mounted on 4-mm coronary balloon angioplasty catheters. Both 15- and 7-mm segments of the stent were utilized. Multiple procedures were required because of technical difficulties and a long segment of ductus in their patients with right aortic arch and left ductus arteriosus. Severe and significant complications occurred during and following stent implantation. Both infants died, one at five weeks and the other at nine days after stent implantation, although the cause of death may not be related to stent placement. Nonetheless, these workers [72] demonstrated the successful stenting of the ductus arteriosus, which remained patent and provided pulmonary blood flow with good oxygen saturations in the neonates with pulmonary atresia. These authors concluded that it is feasible to maintain an open ductus by stenting in neonates with pulmonary atresia, thereby providing balanced central perfusion to both lungs, and that this stenting technique may prove to be an attractive alternative to aortopulmonary shunt operations.

Stenting of the ductus has also been utilized by Ruiz (quoted by Rosenthal and Qureshi [73]) in neonates with hypoplastic left heart syndrome; six patients had the procedure performed, and in three of these, stenting served as a bridge to transplantation. The other three infants died while awaiting transplantation.

The work in animal models and the limited experience in human neonates suggest that ductal stenting is feasible and effective. However, these procedures are technically demanding. Further refinement of the techniques and of the materials used in stent deployment are needed. Additional clinical trials are required to determine the efficacy and safety of stents prior to adopting wide usage.

PATENT FORAMEN OVALE

Interatrial communication with shunting across it is highly beneficial in some congenital cardiac defects. Most important of these is transposition of the great arteries (TGA) with intact ventricular septum. In TGA, the aorta arises from the right ventricle and the pulmonary artery from the left ventricle so that the circulation is parallel instead of the normal circulation in series. The systemic venous blood does not become oxygenated and the pulmonary venous blood does not reach the systemic circulation. Intracardiac mixing is essential for patient survival. These infants will present with severe cyanosis in the first few days of life and will not survive [74] unless treated promptly. Prior to 1966, the treatment of choice was surgical atrial septostomy, which, at that time, carried considerable mortality. In 1966, Rashkind and Miller [75] described a technique of nonsurgical enlargement of the patent foramen ovale during cardiac catheterization. A deflated balloon catheter is advanced from the right atrium into the left atrium across the patent foramen ovale, and the balloon is inflated with diluted radiopaque liquid and rapidly pulled back across the foramen ovale, rupturing the lower margin of the atrial wall below the patent foramen ovale. This procedure, Rashkind's balloon atrial septostomy, results in better mixing at the atrial level, increases the systemic arterial oxygen saturation, and decreases the mean pressure gradient across the interatrial septum. Once palliated with this procedure, these infants could later undergo total surgical correction. For further discussion of the issues related to this procedure, the reader is referred to Chapter 2.

There are other lesions in which an adequate interatrial opening may be of benefit. These include obstructive lesions of the ventricular inflow (or outflow) on the right (tricuspid atresia and pulmonary atresia with intact ventricular septum) or on the left (mitral atresia, aortic atresia, and hypoplastic left heart syndrome) side and total anomalous pulmonary venous connection. The usefulness of balloon atrial septostomy in the palliation of tricuspid atresia [76,77], pulmonary atresia with intact ventricular septum [78,79], mitral atresia [80,81], hypoplastic left heart syndrome [82], and total anomalous pulmonary venous connection [83,84] has been demonstrated.

The original concept and subsequent success of balloon septostomy are based on the fact that the lower margin of the patent foramen ovale is very thin and membranous and can be torn by forcefully withdrawing a balloon (filled with diluted contrast material) from the left atrium to the right atrium. Beyond the neonatal period, the lower margin of the patent foramen ovale is thick and muscular [85,86] and cannot be ruptured by balloon atrial septostomy; this has been the reason for failure of this procedure in older infants and children [85-87]. To circumvent this problem, Park and his associates [88,89] developed a catheter with a built-in, retractable blade (knife) to cut the lower margin of the foramen ovale (septum primum of the fossa ovales). The foramen ovale can then be further enlarged by balloon septostomy. Since Park's report on his clinical experience [89] with this technique, reports of the collaborative study [90], ours [91,92], and others [93-96] have been published. The success rate has ranged between 70 to 90% [90,97]. For further discussion of this technique, the reader is referred to Chapter 3. Although a larger experience with the technique and availability of different sizes

of blade catheters and long introducer sheaths have improved the success rate, adequate septostomy has not been possible in patients with small and hypoplastic left atria.

Mitchell, Sideris, and their associates [98,99], based on their success in producing large atrial septal defects by static balloon dilatation in animal models, wondered why static balloon dilation of the atrial septum could not be performed instead of dynamic balloon atrial septostomy. To the best of our knowledge, the first human application of this technique was reported by Shrivastava and colleagues [100], they successfully performed balloon dilatation of atrial septum in a 5-month-old infant with complete transposition of the great arteries.

The procedure involves advancing a 5 Fr multi-A2 catheter (Cordis) or any other type of end-hole catheter from the right atrium into the left atrium and then into a left pulmonary vein. An exchange guidewire (we prefer extra stiff Amplatz wire) is positioned in the pulmonary vein through the catheter. The catheter is removed and exchanged with a balloon angioplasty catheter. The balloon is inflated to 3 to 5 atmospheres of pressure, taking care not to inadvertently dilate the pulmonary vein. The balloon inflation is repeated twice. The duration of inflation is recommended to be approximately 5 seconds with a five-minute interval between dilatation. "Waisting" of the balloon during initial phases of balloon inflation, which disappears as the balloon is completely inflated, indicates that the foramen ovale is at least stretched beyond its initial size. Lack of "waisting" in the subsequent balloon inflations suggests that there was some enlargement of the foramen ovale. Recording of oxygen saturations, pressures across the atrial septum, and echographic, angiographic, and/or balloon-sizing [101-103] prior to and immediately after static balloon dilatation are necessary to assess effectiveness of the procedure.

There are no data to indicate the most appropriate size of the balloon that should be used in this procedure; 8 to 20-mm diameter balloons have been used [35,100,104-107].

Based on theoretical considerations with other lesions [108], a balloon that is three to four times the size of the patent foramen ovale (by echo) may be a good choice. The balloon, however, should not be larger than the estimated size of the atrium septum, measured on a pre-catheterization echocardiogram. It should be mentioned that the currently available balloon catheters are bulky and that miniaturization of these catheters may make the technique easier.

In 1988, we performed balloon dilatation of the patent foramen ovale in an infant with transposition of the great arteries, large ventricular septal defect, and severe valvar and sub-valvar pulmonic stenosis [106]. The immediate results, with improvement of atrial shunting, are gratifying, and follow-up results up to three years was good. There was echo-Doppler-demonstrable atrial septal defect, and at the time of corrective surgery three years later, a good-sized atrial defect was found. Soon, other reports [35,104–107] appeared. In the report of the VACA Registry [35], three infants with hypoplastic left heart syndrome were cited to have undergone static balloon dilatation of the patent foramen ovale; short-term results were successful. A young adult patient with primary pulmonary hypertension underwent balloon dilatation with a 12-mm balloon following Brockenbrough needle puncture of the atrial septum [104]; this produced excellent palliation with relief of symptoms in this patient. Webber and associates [105] reported producing adequate interatrial communication by balloon dilatation; the diagnoses in these patients, respectively, were pulmonary atresia with intact ventricular septum, mitral atresia, and double-outlet right ventricle with subpulmonic ventricular septal defect.

As can be seen by the above presentation, there is a limited but favorable experience with this technique. Experience in a larger number of patients with follow-up information may provide more definitive information on the safety and efficacy of this technique. Based on our own experience and this review, we would continue to recommend conventional Rashkind's balloon atrial septostomy for the newborn infants requiring adequate interatrial communication. In older infants and children, blade atrial septostomy and balloon (static) dilatation are choices. If the left atrium is large or normal in size, blade atrial septostomy should be considered. However, if the left atrium is small in size or if the pediatric cardiologist is unfamiliar with blade septostomy technique, balloon dilatation should be tried.

In conclusion, blade atrial septostomy and static balloon dilatation of the patent foramen ovale are excellent adjuncts to Rashkind's balloon atrial septostomy technique in the transcatheter enlargement of interatrial communication. When the cardiologists are not familiar with blade septostomy technique [106], or if the left atrium is small and hypoplastic, static balloon dilatation technique may be useful in enlarging a restrictive interatrial communication. Further studies to document safety and efficacy of this technique are essential prior to recommending it for general use.

SUBVALVAR PULMONIC STENOSIS

Subvalvar pulmonic stenosis occurs most commonly either as an integral part of tetralogy of Fallot or in association with severe and longstanding valvar pulmonic stenosis. However, "isolated" obstructive lesion of the right ventricular infundibulum and obstructive anomalous muscle bundles in the trabecular component of the right ventricle, so-called "double-chamber right ventricle," can also occur.

Infundibular obstruction in tetralogy of Fallot is not amenable to balloon dilatation [109,110]. The reader is referred to Chapter 13 for further treatment of this subject. Infundibular reaction secondary to longstanding, severe valvar stenosis, though not relieved by balloon dilatation, does regress with time after successful relief of valvar stenosis [111–114]. The reader is referred to Chapter 6 for further discussion on issues related to this subject. The authors are of the opinion that balloon dilatation of subvalvar obstruction should not be independently attempted in the above two conditions. Adequate balloon valvuloplasty of valvar stenosis should suffice.

Balloon dilatation of isolated subvalvar pulmonic stenosis is rarely attempted [35,115]. VACA Registry [35] lists two patients as having undergone balloon dilatation, and the result in both cases was unsuccessful. However, no details were given. Vacek and Goertz [115] balloon-dilated subpulmonic membranous stenosis in a 22-year-old woman with congenitally corrected transposition of the great arteries (ventricular inversion). They used a 20-mm diameter balloon and reduced the peak-to-peak gradient across the subpulmonic membrane from 85 mm Hg to 34 mm Hg. At the six-week follow-up reexamination, the Doppler instantaneous gradient remained unchanged at 33 mm Hg. This patient's subpulmonic membrane is located in the morphologic left ventricle and is similar to discrete membranous subaortic stenosis of the normally located morphologic left ventricle. In view of the reported success in balloon dilatation of subaortic membranes [116–118], it is not surprising that the authors achieved good results. Such discrete, membranous obstructions are likely to respond to balloon dilatation, and therefore, are good candidates for balloon angioplasty. To the best of our knowledge, isolated, muscular infundibular stenosis of the morphologic right ventricle has not been successfully relieved by balloon dilatation.

A double-chamber right ventricle most commonly coexists with a ventricular septal defect, although it can occur with an intact ventricular septum. An anomalous muscle bundle in association with an apical muscle shelf is likely to be responsible for right ventricular mid-cavity obstruction. Because the entire obstruction is muscular, it is unlikely that balloon dilatation will be effective in relieving the obstruction. However, Chandrashekar et al. [119] attempted balloon dilatation in a 21-year-old man with double-chamber right ventricle. They used a 20-mm diameter balloon and re-

duced the intracavitary peak gradient from 125 mm Hg to 75 mm Hg. Symptomatic improvement occurred. The patient was recatheterized one year following balloon dilatation, and a residual gradient of 73 mm Hg, not significantly different from the immediate postdilatation gradient, was found. Cardiac indices remained unchanged. Repeat dilatation with two 20-mm-diameter balloons did not produce a further fall in gradient. Because of a significant residual gradient, surgical correction was recommended. Thus, these authors [119] were able to document partial relief of obstruction following balloon dilatation. The mechanism of relief is not clear; perhaps stretching of the muscle or rupture of a tenacious muscular band forming a part of the muscular ring of obstruction is the most likely cause.

Although there is no theoretical basis for favorable effect of balloon dilation, severe obstructions (suprasystemic pressure in the proximal chamber) may be dilated in an attempt to reduce the gradient, which would make these patients better risk candidates for anesthesia and surgery.

SUPRAVALVAR PULMONIC STENOSIS

Stenosis of the main pulmonary artery may occur as an isolated anomaly, or it may coexist with other structural cardiac defects [36] such as valvar pulmonic stenosis, tetralogy of Fallot, and others. It may be present in patients with rubella syndrome, William's syndrome, and other syndromes [36]. Supravalvar pulmonic stenosis may also develop at the site of anastromosis in the neopulmonary artery following arterial switch procedure for transposition of the great arteries [120–124], or it may be a residua after removal of the pulmonary artery band [125]. There is only a limited experience in the balloon dilatation of supravalvar pulmonary artery stenotic lesions [35,108,125–130], and it will be reviewed here. The reader is referred to Chapter 12 for discussion of the role of transcatheter techniques in the treatment of peripheral pulmonary artery stenosis.

Indications and Technique

The indications for balloon angioplasty of supravalvar pulmonic stenosis should, in our opinion, be similar to those recommended for valvar pulmonic stenosis [131]: moderate to severe peak-to-peak systolic pressure gradient (≥ 50 mm Hg) across the narrowed area in the face of normal cardiac index. The technique is similar to that described for valvar pulmonary stenosis (Chapter 6) and branch pulmonary artery stenosis (Chapter 12). Although there are no definitive guidelines, the size of the balloon should be at least two times the diameter of the narrowest site of obstruction [129].

Results

Schranz et al. [126] successfully balloon-dilated supravalvar pulmonary stenosis in a single patient who developed it following arterial switch procedure; a 76 mm Hg peak-to-peak systolic pressure gradient across the supravalvar obstruction was reduced to 30 mm Hg after balloon angioplasty with 10-mm balloon catheter. We [108] reported hemodynamic and angiographic data in one patient who developed supravalvar pulmonary artery stenosis, and that data will be included in the presentation of our total experience in this lesion to be discussed later in this section of this chapter. Zeevi et al. [125] attempted balloon angioplasty of postarterial switch supravalvar pulmonary artery stenosis in five children, 5 to 58 months (mean, 18 months) after arterial switch procedure, and reduced the peak-to-peak gradient from 72 ± 11 mm Hg to 44 ± 15 mm Hg (p < 0.01); there was 1 to 75% gradient reduction. Based on scrutiny of individual results, their assessment was that only one patient had a successful result with reduction of peak-to-peak systolic pressure gradient from 79 mm Hg to 20 mm Hg. In the remaining four patients, the residual gradients were high, ranging from 40 to 58 mm Hg (mean, 50 mm Hg) and represented 1% to 33% gradient reduction. Three of these four patients underwent surgical relief 0 to 6 months after angioplasty. The VACA Registry recorded one patient as having had balloon dilatation, but the result was stated to be unknown [35]. Saxena and associates [127] attempted balloon dilatation of supravalvar pulmonary stenosis following arterial switch procedure in eight children. In three patients, the procedure could not be undertaken because a balloon catheter could not be positioned across the stenotic lesion. In the remaining five children, the balloon dilatation procedure was performed, but there was no improvement in pressure gradient (59 ± 17 mm Hg vs. 56 ± 13 mm Hg). Ratio of right ventricular to femoral artery peak systolic pressure did not change, nor was there any improvement in angiographic appearance. The ratio of the balloon diameter to the narrowest segment of stenosis was 1.6 to 2.3 (median, 2.0). Three of these children with ratios ≤ 2.0 (1.6, 1.7, and 2.0, respectively) underwent repeat balloon dilatation with larger balloons (new balloon to stenotic segment ratios were 2.2, 2.3, and 3.3), but again, there was no improvement in peak gradient (60, 60, and 65 mm Hg vs 60, 55, and 70 mm Hg, respectively). The authors [127] concluded that the lack of success in their series is attributable to a small pulmonary annulus with consequent multiple levels of stenosis and distortion of the main pulmonary artery.

Zeevi and associates [125] employed balloon dilatation in two patients with residual supravalvar pulmonary stenosis following removal of a previously placed pulmonary artery band. They used balloons that were 1.7 and 2.2 times the diameter of the stenotic segment. The peak-to-peak systolic pressure gradient was reduced from 60 and 65 mm Hg to 38 and 35 mm Hg, respectively. The right ventricle to aortic peak systolic pressure ratio decreased, respectively, from 0.75 and 0.72 to 0.5 and 0.4, but the percent gradient reduction was 37% and 42%. These authors [125] interpreted data as partially successful balloon dilatation.

Suarez de Lezo et al. [130] used balloon dilatation in seven patients, aged 1 to 10 years (4 ± 3 years), with isolated discrete (membranous) supravalvar pulmonary stenosis and compared the results with those of valvar pulmonary stenosis. They selected the balloon size on the basis of the size of the pulmonary valve annulus; they utilized a balloon/annulus ratio of 1.02 ± 0.2. The peak gradient across the stenotic area decreased from 83 ± 42 mm Hg to 24 ± 12 mm Hg ($p < 0.01$). Follow-up at a mean of 19 months revealed residual gradients of 20 ± 12 mm Hg, not significantly changed ($p > 0.1$) when compared to immediate postdilatation values. Both the immediate and follow-up results were comparable to those after balloon dilatation of valvar pulmonic stenosis. No complications were reported. The authors concluded that isolated supravalvar pulmonary stenosis can be effectively treated with balloon dilatation and that the results are comparable to those observed in children with valvar pulmonary stenosis.

We have attempted balloon dilatation in four children (includes three patients previously reported by us [108,129]), ages one, four, six, and 19 years, and reduced the peak-to-peak systolic gradient from 61 ± 7 mm Hg to 21 ± 14 mm Hg ($p < 0.01$) (Fig. 3). There were excellent results in three children, and in the fourth, the gradient reduction was minimal (67 mm Hg vs 42

mm Hg). Two of these children manifested supravalvar pulmonary stenosis 4 and 15 years following surgical pulmonary valvotomy, respectively, and it is not clear whether the supravalvar stenosis was native or developed secondary to surgery. The remaining two children exhibited pulmonary artery narrowing 9 and 12 months following arterial switch procedure for transposition of the great arteries, respectively. Angiographic (Fig. 4) and pressure gradient (Fig. 5) relief was impressive. Both these children had discrete (Fig. 4) postoperative obstruction. No follow-up data are available for these children.

Comments

Based on the limited experience thus far documented, it appears that discrete narrowing at the suture lines (Fig. 4) in the neopulmonary artery is likely to be relieved by balloon dilatation [108,125,126,129], while diffuse constrictions secondary to anteroposterior flattening or shrinkage and retraction of the pericardial patch used in the enlargement of the neopulmonary artery are unlikely to respond to balloon angioplasty [125,127,128]. These data led us to conclude [128,129] that supravalvar pulmonic stenosis that develops following surgery can be relieved by balloon dilatation if it is a discrete narrowing, and that balloon angioplasty should probably not be attempted if the obstruction is diffuse. Discrete, membranous congenital obstructions of the pulmonary artery [130] can also be successfully dilated. More diffuse congenital narrowing may not be suitable for balloon dilation, although there are no published data to evaluate this issue. Both the native and postoperative pulmonary artery obstruction that do not respond to conventional balloon dilatation may be successfully dilated with a high-pressure balloon in a manner similar to branch pulmonary artery stenotic lesions [132]. Alternatively, stents [60–68] may be useful in keeping the stenotic pulmonary artery lesions open. Further refinement in stent deployment techniques and clinical trials are necessary prior to

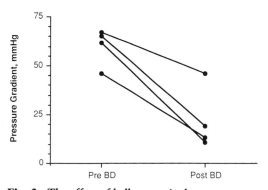

Fig. 3. The effect of balloon angioplasty on pressure gradients in four patients with supravalvar pulmonary stenosis. In three patients, the residual gradients were minimal, while in the fourth, there was significant residual gradient. BD, balloon dilatation.

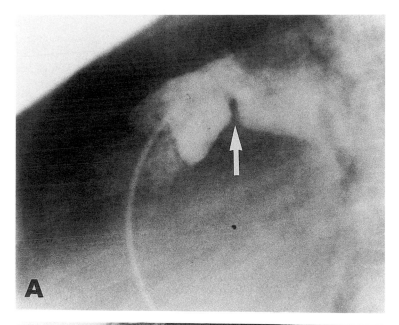

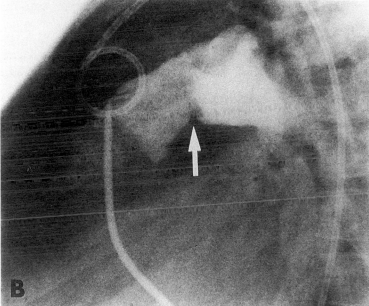

Fig. 4. Cineangiographic frames from lateral views of pulmonary arteriograms showing supravalvar pulmonary stenosis (arrow) following arterial switch operation (**A**), which improved markedly following angioplasty (**B**). (Reproduced from Rao [108], with permission of the publisher.)

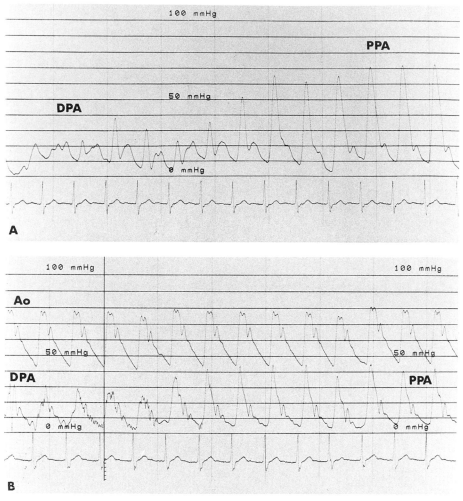

Fig. 5. Pressure pullback tracings across the supravalvar stenosis, showing a significant pressure gradient **(A)**, which diminished markedly following balloon angioplasty **(B)**. Aortic pressure is also shown in B. Ao, aorta; DPA, distal pulmonary artery; PPA, proximal pulmonary artery. Reproduced from Rao [108], with permission of the publisher.)

considering stenting as an alternative to surgical correction.

STENOSIS OF THE AORTA

Although congenital coarctation of the aorta is the most common obstructive lesion of the aorta, especially in infancy and childhood, there are many other types of stenoses of the aorta along its course. These may be congenital or acquired in origin, and include congenital abdominal aortic coarctation, atherosclerosis, Takayasu's arteritis, neurofibromatosis, and postsurgical stenosis (narrowing of anastomotic aortic sites or graft stenosis). These stenotic lesions have been dilated by several workers [133–147] with good results. The principles of dilatation techniques used, results, and complications are similar to those in native and postoperative aortic recoarctations and will not be discussed here. The reader is referred to Chapter 10, dealing with native coarctation, Chapter 11, dealing with aortic recoarctation, and to the published reports [133–147] for details.

BAFFLE OBSTRUCTION FOLLOWING MUSTARD/SENNING PROCEDURE

Systemic Venous Obstruction

Vena caval obstruction following venous switch procedures for transposition of the great arteries (Mustard and Senning operations) have been well documented [148–160]. The reported incidence of the obstruction varied between 13 to 59% (148–159), although surgical revision was required in a much smaller percent of patients. The obstructive lesions appear to have occurred irrespective of the institution where the operation was performed [148–160] and have been seen in early series [148–152] as well as in more recent series [153–159]. However, the systemic venous obstruction appears to occur more frequently with the Mustard procedure than with the Senning procedure [158,159] and is more common when Dacron was used for intraatrial baffle than when autologous pericardial patch was used [148,160]. Superior vena caval obstruction appears to occur more frequently than inferior vena caval obstruction; combined superior and inferior vena caval obstruction appears to be even less common.

Symptoms from obstruction are more likely when both vena cavae are obstructed than when only one vena cava is obstructed because of decompression of the segment proximal to the obstruction by the azygos venous system. Systemic venous congestion is the most common presentation of the vena caval obstruction; however, many children may be asymptomatic. Presentation as protein-losing enteropathy [161–163] or as chylothorax [164,165] has been reported, but on rare occasion.

Although surgical relief of baffle obstruction, when severe, has been the procedure of choice in the past, balloon dilatation has been employed more recently [22,35,163,165–168]. In this section of this chapter, we will review the published data on balloon dilatation of vena caval obstruction following Mustard and Senning procedures.

Indications and technique. Indication for balloon dilatation is the presence of clinical signs of systemic venous obstruction in association with an angiographically demonstrable stenotic lesion and pressure gradient across the site of obstruction. Although the most usual manifestations of vena caval obstruction are edema, evidence for chest wall collateral circulation, and hepatomegaly or signs of cerebral irritation (depending upon whether inferior vena caval or superior vena caval component is involved), occasionally vena caval obstruction may present with signs of protein-losing enteropathy [161-163] or chylothorax [164,165]. If there is adequate decompression via the azygos systems, there may not be any signs of systemic venous obstruction. While it is clear that symptomatic systemic venous obstruction should be relieved by balloon dilatation, it is not established that stenotic lesions with good collateral circulation bypassing the obstruction should be relieved. However, the authors of this chapter are of the opinion that such obstructions should be balloon-dilated if the obstruction is detected by routine cardiac catheterization or by echo-Doppler studies.

The technique of balloon dilatation is similar to that used for other obstructive lesions. Because of multiple prior catheterizations and surgical procedures, femoral venous access may not be possible in some patients. An internal jugular venous approach may have to be used in such cases. The size of the balloon should be at least twice the size of the narrowest diameter of the obstructed area [167]. After positioning the balloon catheter across the site of narrowing, the balloon should be inflated at low pressure to assure that "balloon waisting" is produced. If there is no "waisting," progressively larger balloons should be chosen until "balloon waisting" is visualized. Higher pressure inflations should then be applied until the "waist" is abolished. Sometimes balloons that are four times or larger than the narrowest segment may have to be used to produce adequate dilatation. Tips of guidewires and catheters should not be manipulated over the freshly dilated segments.

Results. Although the initial experience with balloon dilatation of the obstructed superior limb of the Mustard baffle (called "mid-cavity" obstruction) in a single patient was not encouraging [166], subsequent experience [22,35,163–165,167–169] has shown promise. Waldman and associates [166] performed balloon dilatation of superior baffle obstruction in a 3.5-year-old patient two years after a Mustard operation for transposition of the great arteries. Two 6-mm balloons (effective diameter, 9.8 mm), introduced via right and left basilic veins were used, and a mean pressure gradient of 16 mm Hg was reduced to 8 mm Hg. In addition, clinical improvement occurred. Three months later, symptoms recurred and cardiac catheterization revealed a return of the gradient. Therefore, a repeat balloon dilatation, again with two balloons (6 and 12 mm; effective diameter, 14.7 mm), was performed, and the gradient fell to 2 mm Hg. Restudy seven months later revealed a gradient of 14 mm Hg and angiographic narrowing. Waldman and his coworkers concluded that balloon dilatation may prove useful, although their initial experience is not encouraging and serial follow-up is necessary to identify transient from sustained relief of obstruction.

Lock and his colleagues [167] balloon-dilated two superior limb and two inferior limb Mustard baffle obstructions in four children aged 3 to 12 years and reduced the mean gradient across the obstructions from 14 ± 10 mm Hg to 5 ± 4 mm Hg. The stenotic segment increased from 3.3 ± 2.2 mm to 8.4 ± 5.6 mm. The size of the balloon used was 2.5 to 15 times the size of the stenotic segment. In three children, there was clinical improvement, and in the fourth (the obstruction was thought to be "dynamic"), tricuspid valve replacement was required. Clinical follow-up

was available in three children, and repeat catheterization was performed in two children six and nine months after balloon dilatation. Improved gradient persisted at follow-up. It was concluded that postoperative baffle obstructions can be successfully managed with balloon dilatation and that large balloons should be used to effect relief of obstruction. Benson et al. [168] used balloon dilatation to improve superior vena caval obstruction that developed 24 hours after a Senning procedure for transposition of the great arteries in a 3-month-old girl. The mean gradient across the stenotic segment decreased from 19 mm Hg to 10 mm Hg, and angiographic improvement in the size of the stenotic segment occurred. More importantly, substantial clinical improvement was observed within 12 hours of the procedure. Follow-up one year later did not reveal clinical evidence for superior vena caval obstruction. The authors were concerned about dilating a fresh suture line, but they had chest tubes in place and the surgical team was on stand by to deal with any adverse effects of dilatation of fresh anastomosis. Mullins and associates [22] balloon-dilated venae caval obstructions in three patients after a Mustard or Senning procedure. They used a double-balloon technique. The combined diameter of the two balloons chosen was 1.5 times the diameter of the normal cava proximal to the obstruction. The average gradient decreased from 20 mm Hg to 2 mm Hg, and dramatic reduction of edema of the upper body (in two patients with superior caval obstruction) or lower body (in one patient with inferior caval obstruction) occurred. No follow-up was reported.

Kirk et al. [163] used balloon dilatation technique to relieve protein-losing enteropathy (PLE) in two patients. The PLE developed 5 and 10 years after Mustard operations. The cause of PLE was obstruction of both superior and inferior limbs of the Mustard baffle. Dilatation of inferior baffle in one child and both baffles in the other child resulted in marked improvement in edema, the return of serum albumin to normal, and resolution of PLE.

Clinical follow-up in one child four months later revealed no recurrence. The authors conclude that balloon dilatation should be considered as an alternative to surgery in relieving caval obstruction following the Mustard operation. The report from the VACA Registry [35] listed 22 baffle obstructions that were dilated; 15 (68%) were categorized as successful. The result was failure in one (5%) or unknown in six (27%) patients. No further details or follow-up results were given. Rheuban and Carpentier [169] in a review on interventional catheterization published pre- and postdilatation

angiographic frames of an obstructed inferior baffle of the Mustard operation. There was an impressive angiographic improvement.

We used balloon dilatation in two children, of which one has previously been reported [165]. The first was an 11-month-old infant with transposition of the great arteries who underwent a Mustard operation at nine months of age. Approximately eight weeks following surgery, the infant presented to the local physician's office with tachypnea and dyspnea and a left lung opacity (Fig. 6B) on a chest roentgenogram. [This infant had a nor-

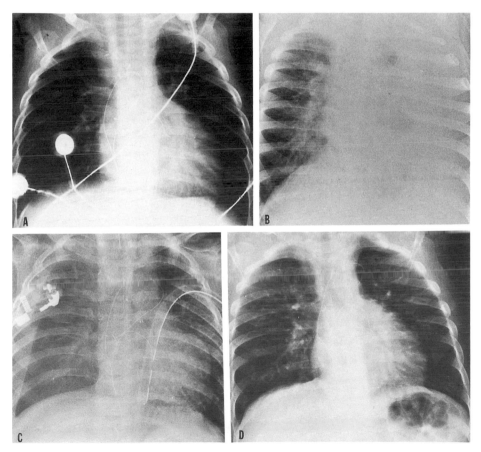

Fig. 6. Anteroposterior view of a chest x-ray one week following Mustard operation **(A)**, showing a normal-sized heart with clear lung fields. Eight weeks following surgery **(B)**, left hemithorax density developed; this was interpreted as pleural effusion, which on tapping was found to be a chylous effusion. After chest tube drainage of left pleural effusion, right pleural effusion **(C)** developed. Three months following balloon angioplasty, chest x ray **(D)** shows clear lung fields.

TABLE II. Pressure Gradients Across and Sizes of Obstructed Mustard Baffle Prior to and Immediately After Balloon Angioplasty and at Follow-Up[a]

Site	Before angioplasty			After angioplasty			At 6-month follow-up		
Pressures (mm Hg)[b]									
SVC	a-22	v-21	m-20	a-12	v-14	m-12	a-6	v-7	m-6
SVA	a-8	v-9	m-5	a-9	v-13	m-8	a-5	v-7	m-4
IVC	a-12	v-13	m-12	a-9	v-10	m-8	a-6	v-7	m-5
Gradients (mm Hg)									
Superior limb		m-15			m-4			m-2	
Inferior limb		m-7			m-0			m-1	
Angiographic size (mm)[c]									
Superior limb		3.8			7.4			7.8	
Inferior limb		2.8			7.1			8.0	

[a]Reproduced from Rao and Wilson [165], with permission of the publisher.
[b]IVC, inferior vena cava; SVA, systemic venous atrium; SVC, superior vena cava. a, 'a' wave; v, 'v' wave; m, mean.
[c]Average of posteroanterior and lateral view diameters.

mal chest x-ray at the time of discharge from the hospital following the Mustard operation (Fig. 6A)]. Pleural tap revealed chylous effusion, and a chest tube was placed. Despite a medium-chain triglyceride diet, chest tube drainage continued. In addition, a right pleural effusion (Fig. 6C) developed that required a chest tube as well. An echo-Doppler study revealed well-functioning ventricles, no pericardial effusion, and a narrowed upper pole of the Mustard baffle with turbulent flow across it. The inferior pole of the baffle was not visualized, although the inferior vena appeared dilated. Cardiac catheterization revealed a significant pressure gradient between the vena cavae and the systemic venous atrium (Table II). Angiography revealed obstruction of both superior (Fig. 7A) and inferior (Fig. 8A) limbs of the baffle; they respectively measured 3.8 and 2.8 mm (Table II). A 15-mm-diameter balloon on an 8-French catheter was initially positioned across the superior pole of the baffle (Figure 9A), and balloon angioplasty (Fig. 9B) was performed with three successive inflations

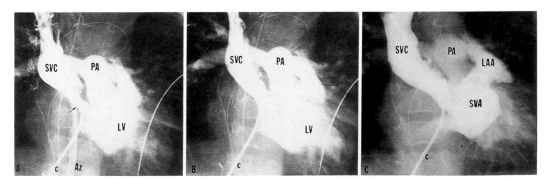

Fig. 7. Superior vena caval (SVC) cineangiogram in posteroanterior view, showing significant narrowing (arrow) of the superior limb of the Mustard baffle (**A**), which improved significantly following balloon angioplasty (**B**). The improvement persisted at a six-month follow-up angiogram (**C**). Az, azygos vein; c, catheter; LAA, left atrial appendage; LV, left ventricle; PA, pulmonary artery.

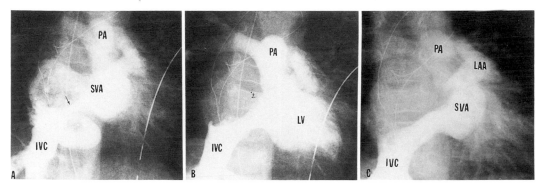

Fig. 8. Selected frame of an inferior vena caval (IVC) cineangiogram in posteroanterior view, showing narrowed (arrow) inferior limb of the Mustard baffle (**A**). Note significant improvement immediately following (**B**) and six months after (**C**) angioplasty. LAA, left atrial appendage; LV, left ventricle; PA, pulmonary artery; SVA, systemic venous atrium.

at 4, 5, and 6 atm of pressure of 10-second duration each. Superior vena caval angiography (Fig. 7B) and pressure pullback (Table II) across the dilated baffle were recorded. Balloon angioplasty of the inferior limb of the baffle (Fig. 10A, B), a pressure pullback tracing (Table II), and inferior vena caval angiography (Fig. 8B) were performed in a similar manner. No complications were encountered during the procedure. Chest tube drainage stopped over the next 24 hours and the chest tubes were removed. There was no further accumulation of pleural fluid. Repeat chest film three months later (Fig. 6D) did not show recurrence of

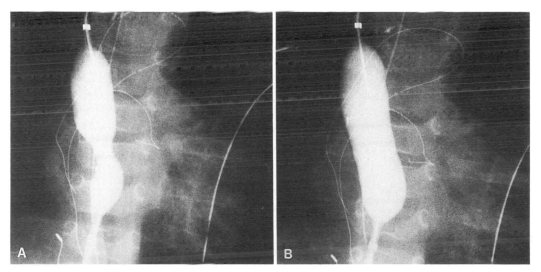

Fig. 9. Selected frames from posteroanterior views of cineradiography of the balloon dilatation catheter positioned across the narrowed superior limb of the Mustard baffle. Note "waisting" of the balloon (**A**) during the initial phases of balloon inflation, which disappeared (**B**) following full inflation. No balloon "waisting" was observed during the second and third balloon inflations. (Reproduced from Rao and Wilson [165], with permission of the publisher.)

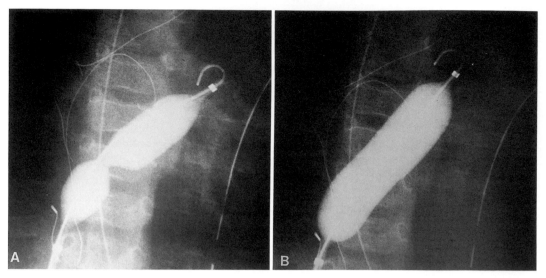

Fig. 10. Same as Figure 9, except that the balloon catheter was positioned across the inferior limb of the Mustard baffle. (Reproduced from Rao and Wilson [165], with permission of the publisher.)

chylothorax. Repeat cardiac catheterization performed six months following angioplasty revealed continuing relief of the pressure gradient across the balloon-dilated baffle obstructions (Table II), and no restenosis was observed on angiography (Figs. 7C,8C). Clinical follow-up, including a chest x-ray 1.5 years following balloon angioplasty, did not show recurrence of chylothorax.

The second patient was a 15-year-old young man who had a Mustard operation for transposition of the great arteries when he was two years of age. He was minimally symptomatic, and echo-Doppler studies (Fig. 11a, b) showed evidence for obstruction of the inferior limb of the Mustard baffle. Cardiac catheterization revealed 5 mm Hg mean pressure gradient across the inferior baffle and angiographic narrowing (Fig. 12A). Balloon angioplasty was performed with a 15-mm-diameter balloon. The mean pressure gradient decreased to 3 mm Hg, and angiographic improvement (Fig. 12B) was noted. Follow-up echo-Doppler studies (Fig. 11c, d) six months after angioplasty revealed persistent relief of obstruction.

Comments. Review of the literature suggests that baffle obstruction following the venous switch procedure is well documented. Obstruction to either superior or inferior baffle may occur without symptoms. Obstruction of both limbs of the baffle is rare, as are chylothorax and protein-losing enteropathy. Balloon dilatation can be successfully performed, but the failure of relief of obstruction has also been noted. There is inadequate data to evaluate the cause of failure of balloon angioplasty. The dynamic nature of the obstruction [167] and perhaps use of small balloons or very compliant venous structures that will stretch but not tear during angioplasty are possible causes. Adequate-sized balloons, 3 to 4 times the size of the obstructed segment, may reduce the chances for failure. Sometimes this may necessitate use of a double-balloon technique. Though it is based on limited experience, we recommend balloon angioplasty as a therapeutic procedure of choice for baffle obstruction following venous switch procedures for transposition of the great arteries. For obstructions that cannot be successfully relieved by balloon angioplasty, stenting [68] may be useful.

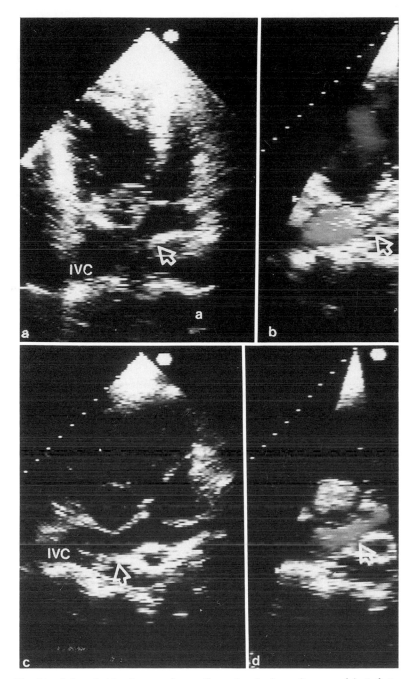

Fig. 11. Selected video frames of a two-dimensional echocardiogram of the inferior limb of the Mustard baffle (**a**) in a 15-year-old child, showing obstructed area (arrow). Color flow mapping (**b**) shows that flow acceleration and turbulence start at this point, confirming hemodynamic significance of two-dimensional visualized narrowing. Also, note dilated inferior vena cava (IVC). Similar video frames (**c** and **d**) are from the same patient, obtained six months after balloon dilatation. Note wider opening on two-dimensional echocardiographic frame (c) and lack of flow acceleration and turbulence (d).

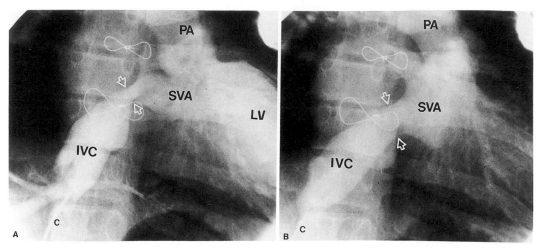

Fig. 12. Selected frame of an inferior vena caval cineangiogram in posteroanterior view, showing narrowed inferior pole of the Mustard baffle **(A)**. Note significant improvement immediately following balloon dilatation **(B)**. This is the same patient as in Figure 9. C, catheter; LV, left ventricle; PA, pulmonary artery; SVA, systemic venous atrium.

Pulmonary Venous Obstruction

Obstruction to pulmonary venous return has also been reported following atrial switch procedures for transposition of the great arteries [149,150,154,160,170-174]. Pulmonary venous obstruction appears to occur less frequently than systemic venous obstruction [149,150,154,160]. Pulmonary venous obstruction is also less common following the Senning procedure than after the Mustard operation [154,171,175], a pattern similar to that observed with systemic venous obstruction. Surgical relief of the obstruction is generally recommended in symptomatic patients. However, recently, balloon dilation [172-174] has been employed to relieve the pulmonary venous stenosis.

Indications and technique. Symptoms of pulmonary venous obstruction such as shortness of breath, cough, and pulmonary edema on a chest roentgenogram are indications for intervention. Echo-Doppler evidence for obstruction, catheter demonstration of pressure gradient across the pulmonary venous atrium, and angiographic demonstration of discrete narrowing are necessary prior to attempting balloon dilation.

The access to the pulmonary venous atrium is via the arterial system. Retrograde passage of a catheter from the femoral artery into the right ventricle, from there across the morphologic tricuspid valve into the neo-left atrium, and from there into the pulmonary vein across the obstruction is initially necessary to determine the hemodynamic and angiographic significance of the obstruction. A guidewire should then be positioned into a pulmonary vein via this catheter and the catheter exchanged for a balloon dilatation catheter. The size of the balloon should be at least three to four times the size of the narrowest segment of pulmonary venous atrium [172]. Because of the need for a large balloon and because the balloon catheters have to be positioned via arterial route, two small balloons are usually required [172-174]. Heparinization throughout the procedure is recommended.

Results and complications. To the best of our knowledge, Cooper and associates [172] were the first to report the use of balloon dilatation to relieve pulmonary venous obstruction that develops after venous switch procedure for transposition of the great arteries. They presented three children who developed pulmonary venous obstruction, 3, 7, and 14 years following a Mustard procedure, respectively. In the 3-year-old child, the procedure was unsuccessful, and the child was sent to surgery one month later. In the other two children, mean pressure difference across the pulmonary venous pathway obstruction was reduced from 6 and 12 mm Hg to 2 and 2 mm Hg, respectively. Angiographic improvement of the narrowing occurred immediately after the procedure, and the Doppler-assessed gradient across the obstruction one day following the procedure decreased. In one of these children, Doppler reassessment revealed recurrence of stenosis six months later, and the child underwent repeat balloon angioplasty, using a double-balloon technique. Two 15-mm-diameter balloons were used. There was angiographic, hemodynamic, and echo-Doppler improvement of obstruction. There was sustained clinical improvement six months after the second balloon dilatation procedure. In the remaining child, clinical and Doppler evidence for improvement were observed at a 3-month follow-up visit. Coulsen et al. [173] used this procedure in one 18-month-old child who developed obstruction ten months after a Senning operation. Two 5-mm-diameter (effective diameter, 8.2 mm) balloons were used to dilate a 4-mm stenotic segment, and a gradient of 13 mm Hg was reduced down to 5 mm Hg. Angiographic and echo-Doppler improvement were also observed. Echo-Doppler (5 months after procedure) and clinical (9 months after the procedure) follow-up suggested sustained improvement. Zeevi and associates [174] presented a 10-month-old infant who developed pulmonary venous obstruction two months after a Mustard procedure. Two 8-mm ultra-thin balloon catheters were used, and a 15 mm Hg gradient was reduced to 4 mm Hg. The size of constriction increased by angiography. Clinical and echo-Doppler improvement continued at an 8-month follow-up visit.

Hematoma formation [172] in one patient and development of staphylococal endocarditis in another [174] patient occurred.

Comments. Pulmonary venous obstruction, though not as common as systemic venous obstruction, has been observed following both the Mustard and Senning procedures. Hitherto, surgical relief of obstruction is the treatment of choice. The risk of repeat surgery is high [176], and surgery may not completely relieve the obstruction [176]. Because of these reasons, the balloon dilatation technique is attractive. Successful balloon dilatation with relief of symptoms and pressure and angiographic relief of obstruction have been observed. However, some failures are also noted. Use of retrograde arterial technique is needed to position a balloon(s) across the stenotic lesion. Balloons that are three to four times as large as the stenotic lesion are required to produce effective balloon dilatation. Despite limited experience, balloon angioplasty seems to emerge as a procedure of choice in relieving pulmonary venous obstruction following venous switch procedure for transposition of the great arteries.

SUPERIOR VENA CAVAL STENOSIS

Apart from venous switch procedures for transposition of the great arteries, just discussed, superior vena caval obstruction can also be caused by thrombosis, fibrosis, compression, and invasion [177]. Neoplastic disease accounts for the majority of superior vena caval syndrome cases. Superior vena caval obstruction can also be induced by transvenous endocardial pacing catheters [178-181]. The clinical manifestations are similar to those described in the preceding section and include swelling of the face, neck, and upper body. Cerebral edema and upper airway compromise may occur in severe forms of the disease [182]. Superior vena caval obstruction caused by neoplasms is most likely to respond to chemotherapy and radiation. In most other types of obstruction, surgical intervention [180-183] is generally recommended. With recent interest and experience with balloon dilatation techniques, some workers [180,181,183-190] have applied these techniques to relieve vena caval obstruction.

Indications and Technique

Presence of clinical signs of superior vena caval obstruction is an indication for intervention. Angiographic demonstration of the discrete obstruction may be necessary to identify the lesions that are likely to respond to balloon dilatation.

Balloon dilatation catheters may be inserted percutaneously via the femoral vein, although some authors used antecubital vein. Balloon dilatation may also be performed via a percutaneous jugular venous approach, especially if the femoral venous access is not possible. Although there are no definitive guidelines based on experience with balloon dilatation of other stenotic lesions, a balloon that is three to four times the diameter of the narrowest segment of obstruction is likely to be necessary to produce adequate dilatation. The balloon diameter should not exceed 1.5 times the superior vena caval diameter.

Results and Complications

Youngston et al. [184] attempted balloon dilatation of fibrotic obstruction of the superior vena cava in a 75-year-old woman but was not successful in relieving the obstruction. Surgery was required to relieve the obstruction. The size of the balloon used was not mentioned nor were any other technical aspects detailed. Rocchini and associates [185] presented a 15-month-old child with superior vena caval obstruction caused by an organized thrombus that developed after multiple operations for a mixed type of total anomalous pulmonary venous connection. There was almost complete obstruction of the vena cava, and a 6-mm balloon dilatation catheter was used for angioplasty. A 30-mm Hg gradient across the obstruction was reduced to 16 mm Hg, and there was angiographic improvement. Improvement of facial swelling and cyanosis was observed over the hour following balloon dilatation. However, the infant died 14 hours after dilatation;

the death did not seem to be related to the procedure and was thought to be secondary to pulmonary venous obstruction. Autopsy revealed findings suggesting that the superior vena caval obstruction is related to organized thrombus and that the mechanisms of relief of obstruction appear to be due to disruption of vena cava interna. Montgomery et al. [186] reported successful balloon dilatation in an adult patient of superior vena caval stenosis caused by endocardial pacing catheters. Symptoms did not recur during a 10-month follow-up. Subsequently, several other workers [181,187,189,190] have reported successful dilatation of superior vena caval obstruction secondary to pacing catheters. Ali et al. [1988] balloon-dilated, using a double-balloon technique, stenotic superior vena cava in a 52-year-old man. The gradient across the stenosis was reduced from 16 to 4 mm Hg, and symptoms improved. The VACA Registry [35] mentions a single case of superior vena caval stenosis (following repair of total anomalous pulmonary venous connection) in which balloon dilatation was successfully used.

Comments

Superior vena caval obstruction is secondary to multiple etiologies. When the cause is neoplastic infiltration or compression, treatment of the primary problem by chemotherapy and/or radiation is the treatment of choice unless obstruction is severe and symptomatic. In such a case, palliation with balloon dilatation may be attempted. Obstruction secondary to organizing thrombus and sclerosis of any origin may be amenable to balloon angioplasty. Acute thrombosis should be treated with thrombolytic agents. With increasing use of transvenous pacemakers, superior vena caval obstruction is found more frequently. Again, acute thrombotic occlusions should be treated with thrombolytic agents, and chronic obstruction by balloon angioplasty.

Although the reported experience is limited, balloon angioplasty seems to be a reasonable alternative to surgery in relieving superior vena caval obstruction. In patients with stenotic lesions not amenable to balloon dilatation, stenting [68] in a manner discussed in the previous section may be an option and should be considered.

INFERIOR VENA CAVAL OBSTRUCTION

Inferior vena caval obstruction may be produced by a variety of causes [191–193], including liver tumors and abscess, cystic disease of the liver, retroperitoneal abdominal tumors, metastatic carcinomatous disease, myeloproliferative disorders, hypercoagulable states, polycythemia vera, congenital membranous or diffuse obstruction of the inferior vena cava, thrombosis, and more recently, liver transplantation [194,195]. These causes are in addition to atrial switch procedures for transposition of the great arteries described in the preceding section of this chapter. Obstruction of the inferior vena cava with or without additional hepatic vein obstruction causes hepatomegaly, ascites, varicosity of the thoracoabdominal wall and/or legs, dependent edema, and hepatic cirrhosis. This constellation of findings is commonly referred to as Budd-Chiari syndrome. Conventional treatment options include surgical relief of the obstruction by direct attack on the lesion (transatrial membranotomy), excision of the obstructed position of the inferior vena cava, or bypass of the obstruction by cavoatrial shunts. These procedures carry considerable risk and are associated with recurrence of obstruction. Because of these reasons, when balloon dilatation techniques became available, they were applied to relieve inferior vena caval obstructive lesions [167,196–210].

Indications and Technique

Budd-Chiari syndrome or inferior vena caval obstruction caused by infiltrative or mass lesions should be treated by appropriate treatment of the primary disease process. Intraluminal obstructive lesions are likely to respond to balloon dilatation techniques. Patients with inferior vena caval obstruction severe enough to cause Budd-Chiari syndrome-type symptoms are candidates for relief of obstruction by balloon dilatation.

The technique of dilatation involves placing a guidewire across the site of obstruction, and then, in the superior vena cava from the femoral venous route, positioning a balloon dilatation catheter across the area of obstruction over the guidewire already in place, and inflating the balloon to eliminate the balloon "waisting." No definitive guidelines are available with regard to the size of the balloon that should be used. Based on experience with dilating other vascular lesions, the balloon diameter should be two to four times the diameter of the stenotic lesion. Perhaps the balloon size should not exceed 1.5 times the size of the inferior vena cava. While there is some communication between the inferior vena cava and the right atrium in most cases, there are instances in which there may be complete obstruction without any forward flow through the inferior vena cava [206,208,210]. In such cases, simultaneous inferior vena caval and right atrial contrast injection should be performed to visualize the length of the obstructed segment [206,208]. Such angiographic markers and/or performing the procedure under ultrasonic guidance [206] are useful in traversing completely or almost completely occluded lesions. Use of a stiff guidewire [206] or the Brockenbrough technique [208,210] have been advocated. Subsequently progressive enlargement of stenotic lesion with balloon catheters carrying increasing sizes of balloons may have to be performed in order to position an appropriate-sized balloon catheter(s) across the obstruction. Sometimes, this may necessitate introduction of two or three balloons simultaneously [206]. Sometimes the obstruction may be secondary to, or completed by, thrombi. In such cases, infusion of streptokinase or other thrombolytic agents directly into the inferior vena cava for a prolonged time [210] may be necessary prior to successfully performing the balloon angioplasty. Because of significant incidence of embolism following relief of the obstruction, all patients should be completely heparinized immediately prior to the procedure and anticoagulation should be continued after the procedure with Coumadin and/or platelet-inhibiting drugs.

Dilatation of associated [198] or isolated [211] hepatic venous obstruction may be necessary in some cases.

Results

Despite failure of the initial attempt [196] to balloon- dilate the caval obstruction, subsequent experience [197-199,201-210] is rewarding. Occasional failures of the procedure are still observed [200]. In the majority of the patients, prompt reduction of the pressure gradient across the obstruction and angiographic improvement have been observed. Rapid diuresis, disappearance of edema, ascitis, and thoracoabdominal varicosity, and improvement of liver function have been observed [197-199,201-210].

Balloon dilatation procedure is applicable not only to congenital membranous or segmental lesions of the inferior vena cava but also to postoperative anastomotic stenosis [167,199] and obstruction of conduits [207] previously placed to bypass caval obstruction.

The follow-up results have been sparse, and the available follow-up results are for only a few months. Residual or recurrent stenosis [198,200,202] has been reported. Repeat dilatation is feasible and has been performed with success [202].

Pulmonary embolism secondary to dislodgement of caval thrombi has been reported following balloon dilatation of inferior vena caval obstructions. Therefore, it is important to use thrombolytic agents and/or anticoagulation prior to, during, and following the procedure.

Comments

Inferior vena caval obstruction causing Budd-Chiari-type symptoms has been well documented, although this appears to be a disease that manifests in adulthood. Congenital and thrombotic lesions as well as postoperative lesions have been observed to respond to balloon

dilatation techniques. Appearance of clinical symptoms of inferior vena caval obstruction is an indication of transcatheter intervention. While the technique of dilatation is simple in most cases, it can be very difficult and complicated when there is complete or almost complete obstruction. A combination of thrombolytic agents, the Brockenbrough technique, and progressive dilatation with increasing balloon sizes may be necessary in some of these cases. Dramatic hemodynamic, angiographic clinical improvement is noted in most cases. Failures have been reported. Thromboembolic complications should be anticipated, and appropriate pretreatment with thrombolytic agents followed with anticoagulation during and after dilatation procedure should be considered in all cases. Recurrence and redilatation with success has been documented.

Based on the available data, it is concluded that balloon dilatation of congenital, thrombotic, and postsurgical obstructive lesions of the inferior vena cava is feasible, effective, and safe. Although there are no comparative data, in view of significant mortality, morbidity, and recurrence associated with surgical management, balloon dilatation should be considered as an effective alternative to surgical therapy. For lesions that restenose, a consideration for stent placement [68] may also be given.

PULMONARY VEIN STENOSIS

Stenotic lesions of the pulmonary veins and of the connecting vein of the total anomalous pulmonary venous connection, as well as postoperative obstruction of the common pulmonary vein-to-left atrial anastomotic site, will be discussed in this section. Pulmonary venous chamber obstruction association with venous switch operation for transposition of the great arteries was discussed in a previous section.

Congenital Stenosis of the Pulmonary Vein

Congenital stenosis of the pulmonary veins is a rare disease [212]. At least half of the patients have associated cardiac defects. The prognosis is poor. However, when two or more pulmonary veins are unaffected, the prognosis is likely to be better [212]. Pulmonary venous stenosis may be a discrete lesion, confined to its junction with the left atrium, or it may be diffuse, involving the entire pulmonary vein (diffuse hypoplasia of the pulmonary vein) [213]. The former is likely to be amenable to intervention. In addition to signs and symptoms of associated cardiac defects, signs of pulmonary venous obstruction and markedly elevated pulmonary artery pressure, not explained by other associated defects, are present. Selective cineangiograms with injection of contrast material into the pulmonary vein are necessary to demonstrate the anatomy. Surgical pulmonary venoplasty is the recommended treatment of choice for relief of the obstruction. Based on limited data [212], the results of surgery appear better in children over 3.5 years than in younger children, although this may, in part, be related to natural selection and severity of the disease process. Driscoll et al. [212] attempted balloon angioplasty in three patients, ages 17, 2, and 16 months, with 5, 6, and 7-mm-diameter balloons, respectively. In the first patient, the mean pulmonary venous pressure in the left upper and left lower pulmonary veins decreased from 63 and 33 mm Hg to 10 and 18 mm Hg, respectively, after balloon dilatation. There was clinical improvement as well. However, four weeks later, there was recurrence and return to predilatation pressures and angiographic appearance. In the second patient, balloon dilatation decreased mean pulmonary venous pressure from 65 to 25 mm Hg in the left lower pulmonary vein, and the angiographic appearance improved. The patient, however, died 36 hours later, presumably due to sepsis. Autopsy revealed a patent left pulmonary vein. In the final patient, pulmonary venous pressures following balloon dilatation were not given, but pulmonary artery pressure decreased (68 vs 45 mm Hg), and

systemic arterial pressure increased (75 vs 83 mm Hg). There was also angiographic improvement, but no clinical improvement occurred. Because of marginal results, the authors were not enthusiastic about the effectiveness of balloon dilatation in this disease entity and speculated that balloon dilatation simply stretches the area of stenosis without rupturing the intima. Lock and associates [167] attempted balloon dilatation of stenotic pulmonary veins in two patients. In one infant, the right lower lobe pulmonary vein was dilated percutaneously, while in the other, the left lower lobe pulmonary vein was dilated at surgery. In both patients, there was no improvement. In addition, the first patient developed acute hemoptysis and required emergency intubation. She died one month later. At postmortem examination, no evidence for intimal tear was observed in the dilated vein. The VACA Registry [35] lists five patients as having had undergone balloon dilatation of pulmonary vein stenosis; three were reported to have successful results. In one, it failed, and in the final case, the result is unknown. No details were given. Detailed histologic studies by Lucas and associates [214] revealed that stenotic pulmonary veins do not have a clearly identifiable media or adventitia, and that the wall thickness at the site of stenosis is less than that in pulmonary or systemic arteries. These histologic findings suggest that stretching of the thin venous wall occurs without tearing elastic elements of the pulmonary vein. However, studies of Driscoll and Lock were performed in the early 80s, and the current technology with high-pressure inflation balloons and thin-walled balloons may produce better results. In unsuccessful cases, stents [60–68] may have a role. Further clinical trials to establish safety and effectiveness are needed.

Pulmonary Veno-Occlusive Disease

Pulmonary veno-occlusive disease is an uncommon but well-documented disease [215–218] with narrowing of the pulmonary veins and venules causing pulmonary venous and pulmonary arterial hypertension. The disease is caused by sclerosing mediastinitis of unknown etiology or infiltration secondary to carcinomatous disease. Obstruction of other thoracic structures or even abdominal structures has been observed. The pathology includes obliterative fibrosis of the intima of the pulmonary vein and dilated pulmonary lymphatics [215]. Clinical and laboratory features are those of pulmonary venous and pulmonary arterial hypertension. Hemodynamic studies show pulmonary hypertension and elevated pulmonary arterial wedge pressure with normal left atrial and left ventricular end-diastolic pressures. Selective catheterization and angiography of pulmonary veins confirm the diagnosis. If the pulmonary venous obstruction is focal and discrete, it may be amenable to balloon dilatation [219]. Massumi and associates [219] reported a 35-year-old woman with pulmonary veno-occlusive disease, in whom the authors performed balloon dilatation (with a 7-mm balloon) of three pulmonary veins at surgery and demonstrated a fall in the wedge pressure (40 vs 20 mm Hg) and slight angiographic improvement. Transvenous balloon dilatation of two of the pulmonary veins was performed three months later, again showing angiographic improvement. Clinical evaluation three months later suggested good results. However, nine months after transcatheter angioplasty, the patient died with cyanosis and congestive heart failure. These authors have shown [219] that balloon dilatation in veno-occlusive disease is feasible if it is focal and have suggested that balloon angioplasty is a nonsurgical palliative alternative to this otherwise fatal disease.

Obstructed Total Anomalous Pulmonary Venous Connection

Obstruction of the anomalous vein connecting the common pulmonary vein with the systemic vein is present in almost all cases of the infradiaphragmatic type of total anomalous pulmonary venous connection, while such obstruction may be present in approximately half of the supradiaphragmatic type of connection [214]. In the infradiaphragmatic type, the obstructive elements are the long connecting vein (and stenotic lesions in this vein), hepatic microcirculation, and rarely, ductus venosus. If the major or sole obstruction is at the ductus venosus level, it can be potentially dilated; temporary relief of obstruction may make the patient a better candidate for total surgical correction. To our knowledge, there are no reported cases of balloon dilatation of this structure. The considerations for feasibility and effectiveness are similar to those described in the section of this chapter dealing with patent ductus arteriosus.

In the supradiaphragmatic type, the obstruction may be extrinsic or intrinsic [214,220]. The extrinsic obstruction is due to the entrapment of the anomalous connecting vein between the left or right main stem bronchus and the ipsilateral pulmonary artery, termed "hemodynamic vise" [221]. This type of obstruction is not likely to be affected by balloon dilatation techniques. Intrinsic obstructions or constrictions can occur at virtually all sites and have been reviewed elsewhere [214,220]. The nonobstructed portions of the anomalous veins resemble pulmonary veins histologically. The intima is separated from media by an internal elastic lamina, whereas the media and adventitia are not separated by external elastic lamina. Thus, there was no clear distinction between media and adventia; in addition, the media-adventia is thin. The sites of obstruction may be single or multiple, and they may be discrete, or a short ($\sim$ 1 cm) segment may be involved. Histologically, there is thickening of the media-adventitial portion; the intima may be normal, moderately hypertrophied, or markedly thickened [214]. The pulmonary venous-like histology of the obstructed portion of the connecting vein makes these lesions less likely to respond to balloon dilatation. Lock and associates [167,214] attempted balloon dilatation in three cases, and in none of these was there any improvement. All three children died hours to months following the procedure. Rey al. [222] reported balloon angioplasty of stenosis of the vertical vein (at its junction with the left innominate vein), which reduced pulmonary venous pressure (26 vs 14 mm Hg), decreased right ventricle/pulmonary artery systolic pressure (90 vs 60 mm Hg), increased left ventricular pressure (70 vs 95 mm Hg), and produced angiographic improvement. The pulmonary edema and heart failure abated, and the infant improved clinically. The infant was referred to surgical correction ten days later.

While the opinion of the authors of this chapter and that of others [214,222] is that total surgical correction is still the treatment of choice for total anomalous pulmonary venous connection, balloon dilatation may have a role in stabilizing the infant prior to surgery. Balloon dilatation, if successful, is likely to result in less pulmonary edema and lower right ventricular/pulmonary arterial pressure and may make the patients better

risk candidates for surgery than prior to dilatation. Therefore, it may be prudent to balloon-dilate the obstructed connecting vein at the time of diagnostic catheterization preceding surgery. Further experience with this mode of therapy is needed prior to making this recommendation definitive.

Obstruction of Anastomotic Site Following Repair of Total Anomalous Pulmonary Venous Connection

Stenosis of the anastomosis of the common pulmonary vein with the left atrium following repair of total anomalous pulmonary venous connection can occur. This will produce increased pulmonary venous pressure, pulmonary edema, and elevated pulmonary artery pressure. Surgical revision of the anastomotic site is currently the treatment of choice. The role, if any, of balloon dilatation of this postoperative stenosis is not elucidated. We have performed balloon dilatation in one patient with modest success. This is a 4-year-old child at the time of balloon angioplasty. She had repair of total anomalous pulmonary venous connection of the infradiaphragmatic type in the neonatal period. The common pulmonary

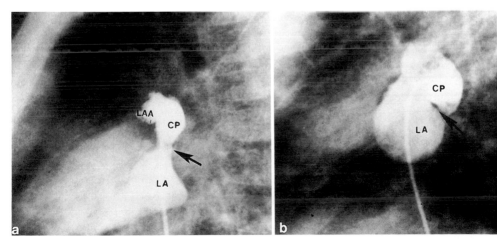

Fig. 13. Selected cineangiographic frames from a lateral view of cineangiograms, showing narrowed site (arrow) of previous anastomosis between common pulmonary vein (CP) and left atrium (LA), which is markedly improved (arrow) following balloon dilatation (b). In (a), the common pulmonary vein is partially opacified along with left atrial appendage (LAA). In b, the entire common pulmonary vein was opacified.

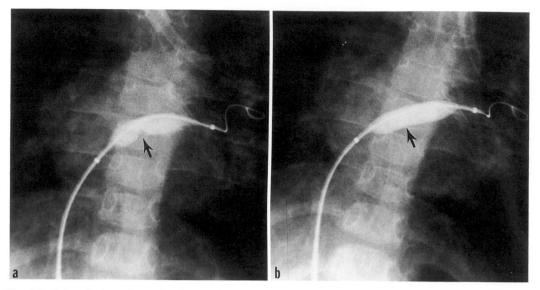

Fig. 14. Selected cineradiographic frame of the balloon positioned across the stenosed common pulmonary vein-to-left atrial anastomosis during the initial phase of balloon inflation, showing "waisting" (arrow) of the balloon (**a**), which is abolished after full inflation of the balloon (**b**).

vein was anastomosed to the left atrium. She developed progressive signs of pulmonary venous obstruction with increased diastolic Doppler flow velocity (2.9 m/s) across the anastomotic area. At cardiac catheterization, a mean gradient of 18 mm Hg was detected across the site of surgical anastomosis, and there was angiographic narrowing (Fig. 13a). A 7 Fr catheter carrying a 10-mm balloon was positioned across the obstructed area (Fig. 14a), and the balloon was inflated at 5 atm of pressure with disappearance of the "waist" (Fig. 14b). Attempts to advance a larger balloon catheter were not successful. However, there was a decrease in mean pressure gradient from 18 to 12 mm Hg and angiographic improvement (Fig. 13b). The child improved clinically, and the diastolic Doppler flow velocity decreased to 1.5 m/s. Two years later, she underwent successful surgical revision of anastomotic site. This experience would lead us to suggest that postoperative narrowings of this type are amenable to balloon dilatation. However, it is not established that balloon dilatation should be the initial treatment option.

BALLOON DILATATION OF A PULMONARY ARTERY BAND

Muller and Dammann devised pulmonary artery constriction by a band as a procedure to palliate infants and children with pulmonary overcirculation [223]. Pulmonary artery banding decreases the pulmonary artery pressure and flow, helps abate symptoms of congestive heart failure, and allows the child to grow to a suitable size and age so that a corrective operation could be performed safely. In the early era of cardiac surgery, banding of the pulmonary artery has been widely used. With the advent of hypothermic circulatory arrest and successful application of open heart surgical procedures to neonates and small infants, the use of a pulmonary band has decreased. Despite this, there are occasions when it would be advantageous to use a pulmonary artery band. However, there are disadvantages to the use of a fixed band, in that: a) it has to be removed via thoracotomy; b) its removal may increase mortality and morbidity of the corrective procedure; and c) pulmonary artery obstruction may progress rapidly, forcing earlier than anticipated correction or additional palliation with shunt procedures. Some of these disadvantages may be circumvented if the effects of pulmonary artery constriction could be partially or completely reversed. With this in mind, Vince, Rocchini, Lindberg, Smevik, Bjornstad, and their colleagues [224–231] devised a variety of reversible pulmonary artery bands that could be dilated (enlarged) by transcatheter methods.

Vince and colleagues [224,225,229] tested two types of prosthetic bands in animal models. The first was a cotton umbilical tape pleated with 8-0 silk sutures, while the other was a stainless steel, fatigued helix encased in a siliconized rubber tubing sealed with silicone type-A medical adhesive. They demonstrated that the bands can be placed around the pulmonary artery, significant stenosis can be maintained across the bands for a prolonged period of time, and the bands can later be balloon-dilated transvenously, relieving the obstruction. They felt that the stainless steel, fatigued helix prosthesis is more reliable. They have further shown in the animal model [229] that the latter prosthesis can be dilated serially. They finally performed clinical trials with this prosthesis [231] and demonstrated that these bands could be placed around the pulmonary artery of children; the success rate and complications with placing bands are similar to those of conventional bands. At the time of the corrective procedure, it was easier to completely remove the dilatable bands than conventional bands. In one child, successful balloon dilatation of the band could be performed. The authors concluded that greater dexterity is required to apply dilatable bands, that dilatable bands perform banding function in a manner similar to that of conventional fixed bands, and that it is feasible to balloon-dilate the bands when required.

Rocchini et al. [226] used absorbable suture material (Vicryl) as pulmonary artery bands in 1-week-old mongrel puppies and produced sig-nificant gradients across the bands. Six months later, they balloon-dilated and produced a reduction of gradient across the band site and an increase in the size of the band site. Restudy two months after balloon dilatation revealed persistent relief of obstruction at the band site. There was no damage to the pulmonary artery noted after the animals were sacrificed. They [226] concluded that it is feasible to create a pulmonary artery band that could be reversed later by transcatheter balloon dilatation. To the best of our knowledge, clinical application of this technique has not been reported.

Lindberg, Smevik, and their colleagues [227,228] applied a Dacron tape around the pulmonary artery and secured the tape with a 5.0 Prolene suture in vitro in a human heart-lung specimen and in vivo in dogs. In the human model, they were able to show that these bands could be successfully dilated [228] with balloon catheters at 2.4 atm. In the dog model [227], they were able to show that effective banding could be produced with this method, and that balloon dilatation could be successfully performed with significant reduction in gradient; this reduction is comparable to that obtained by surgical removal of the band. They concluded that this method may be useful in selected patients. Indeed, they later applied this technique to two children [230], aged six months and four years, and showed that balloon-debanding relieved the obstruction. They concluded that effective banding with this technique is feasible, that balloon-debanding without additional surgery is possible, and that this method has potential for general use.

Though there is limited experience with the above-described methods, several groups of workers, as described above, showed the feasibility and effectiveness of reversible bands. It seems appropriate to perform further clinical trials. The technique may be useful in selected patients whose ventricular septal defects are likely to close spontaneously and in patients in whom total surgical correction should be postponed because of the complexity of their cardiac defect.

OTHER OBSTRUCTIVE LESIONS

In addition to the above-discussed stenotic lesions, there are other lesions that can be balloon-dilated. Coronary artery stenosis that may develop after Kawasaki disease [232,233] can be relieved by balloon angioplasty. Two of the three cases had successful outcomes, while the third patient died as a result of left coronary artery obstruction secondary to balloon rupture during angioplasty with high inflation pressure. With careful attention to the technique, it may be possible to dilate these lesions percutaneously.

Cor triatriatum dexter is a rare congenital cardiac anomaly in which a membranous obstruction is present in the right atrium. Clinical presentation includes systemic venous congestion, hepatic dysfunction, and coagulopathy. In one such rare case, Savas et al. [234] employed a double-balloon technique and dilated the membranous obstruction. Decrease in pressure gradient across the membrane, angiographic improvement, increase in systemic arterial oxygen saturation, and augmentation of cardiac output occurred following balloon dilatation. There was significant clinical improvement as well. Thus, it seems that it is feasible to dilate these membranous obstructions via catheters.

SUMMARY AND CONCLUSIONS

Commonly seen stenotic lesions of the heart and great vessels in which balloon dilatation procedures have been used frequently were discussed in the preceding chapters. Less common lesions and lesions in which balloon dilatation has not been extensively used in the past are discussed in this chapter. By and large, indications for balloon intervention are similar to those used for surgical intervention. The technique involves positioning an appropriate-sized balloon catheter across the stenotic lesion

and inflating the balloon two or three times. Generally, the size of the balloon chosen is similar to the valve annulus diameter for the valvar obstructions and two or more times the size of the vascular stenotic lesions. In the latter, the balloon should not generally exceed 1.5 times the size of the adjacent normal vessel. The immediate results are good in several of the disease entities and marginal in others. There is paucity of information with regard to the long-term follow-up results. Complications are minimal. There are no data comparing surgical versus balloon therapy. The consensus of the interventional cardiologists has been to advocate these procedures if there is not significant risk for balloon dilatation because of the lack of need for anesthesia, thoracotomy, cardiopulmonary bypass, and prolonged hospitalization with these procedures. Additional advantages cited are no residual scar of the operation, less psychological trauma, and less expense. For vascular lesions not amenable to balloon dilatation, use of stents may become a treatment option. Much data is needed to support this contention.

REFERENCES

1. Al Zaibag M, Ribeiro P, Al Kasab SA (1987): Percutaneous balloon valvotomy in tricuspid stenosis. Br Heart J 57:51–53.
2. Khalilullah M, Tyagi S, Yadav BS, Jain P, Choudhry A, Lochan R (1987): Double-balloon valvuloplasty of tricuspid stenosis. Am Heart J 114: 1232–1233.
3. Ribeiro PA, Al Zaibag M, Al Kasab S, Idris M, Halim M, Abdullah M, Shahed M (1988): Percutaneous double balloon valvotomy for rheumatic tricuspid stenosis. Am J Cardiol 61:660–662.
4. Rico Blázquez J, Sobrino Daza N, Calvo Orbe J, Maté Benito I, Oliver Ruiz J, Sobrino Daza JA (1988): Percutaneous transluminal valvuloplasty in tricuspid valve stenosis: A case report. Rev Esp Cardiol 41:636–638.
5. Shrivastava S, Radhakrishnan S, Dev V (1988): Concurrent balloon dilatation of tricuspid and calcific mitral valve in a patient with rheumatic heart disease. Int J Cardiol 20:133–137.
6. Bourdillon PDV, Hookman LD, Morris SN, Waller BF (1989) Percutaneous balloon valvuloplasty

for tricuspid stenosis: hemodynamic and pathologic findings. Am Heart J 117:492-495.

7. Goldenberg IF, Pedersen W, Olson J, Madison JD, Mooney MR, Gobel FL (1989): Percutaneous double balloon valvuloplasty for severe tricuspid stenosis. Am Heart J 118:417-419.

8. Keefe JF, Wolk MJ, Levine HJ (1970): Isolated tricuspid valve stenosis. Am J Cardiol 25:252-257.

9. Mullins PA, Hall JA, Shapiro LM (1990): Balloon dilatation of tricuspid stenosis caused by carcinoid heart disease. Br Heart J 63:249-250.

10. Dalvi B (1991): Balloon dilatation of tricuspid stenosis caused by carcinoid heart disease. Br Heart J 65:113.

11. Rao PS (1990): Tricuspid valve abnormalities other than tricuspid atresia. In Long WA (ed): "Fetal and Neonatal Cardiology." Philadelphia: W.B. Saunders, pp 541-550.

12. Van Mierop LHS, Kutsche LM, Benjamine EV (1989): Ebstein's anomaly. In Adams FH, Emmanouilides GC, Riemenschneider TA (eds), "Heart Disease in Infants, Children, and Adolescents." Baltimore: Williams and Wilkins, pp 361-370.

13. Loya YS, Mashru MR, Patil RB, Karbhase JN, Sharma S (1989): Isolated tricuspid stenosis: A case report with review of literature. Indian Heart J 41:270-273.

14. Bharati S, McAllister HA, Tatooles CJ, Miller RA, Weinberg M Jr, Bucheleres HG, Lev M (1976): Anatomic variations in underdeveloped right ventricle related to tricuspid atresia and stenosis. J Thorac Cardiovasc Surg 72:383-400.

15. Lokhandwala YY, Rajani RM, Dalvi BV, Kale PA (1990): Successful balloon valvotomy in isolated congenital tricuspid stenosis. Cardiovasc Intervent Radiol 13:354-356.

16. Riker WL, Potts WJ, Grana L, Miller RA, Lev M (1963): Tricuspid stenosis or atresia complexes: A surgical and pathologic analysis. J Thorac Cardiovasc Surg 45:423-433.

17. Rao PS (1990): Tricuspid atresia. In Long WA (ed): "Fetal and Neonatal Cardiology." Philadelphia: W.B. Saunders, pp 525-540.

18. Trace HD, Bailey CP, Wendkos MH (1954): Tricuspid valve commissurotomy with a one-year follow-up. Am Heart J 47:613-617.

19. Dimich I, Goldfinger P, Steinfeld L, Lukban SB (1973): Congenital tricuspid stenosis: Case treated by heterograft replacement of the tricuspid valve. Am J Cardiol 31:89-94.

20. Smith MD, Sagar KB, Mauck HD, Cowley MJ, Lower RR (1982): Surgical correction of congenital tricuspid stenosis. Ann Thorac Surg 34:329-332.

21. Rubio V, Limon Lason R (1954): Treatment of pulmonary valvular stenosis and of tricuspid stenosis using a modified catheter. Second World Congress on Cardiology, Washington DC, Program Abstracts II, p 205.

22. Mullins CE, Nihill MR, Vick GW III, Ludomirsky A, O'Laughlin MP, Bricker JT, Judd VE (1987): Double balloon technique for dilation of valvular or vessel stenosis in congenital and acquired heart disease. J Am Coll Cardiol 10:107-114.

23. Chen CR, Lo ZX, Huang ZD, Cheng TO (1988): Concurrent percutaneous balloon valvuloplasty for combined tricuspid and pulmonic stenosis. Cathet Cardiovasc Diagn 15:55-60.

24. Ribeiro PA, Al Zaibag M, Al Kasab S, Hinchcliffe M, Halim M, Idris M, Abdullah M, Shahed M (1988): Provocation and amplification of the transvalvular pressure gradient for rheumatic tricuspid stenosis. Am J Cardiol 61:1307-1311.

25. Inoue K, Owaki T, Nakamura T, Kitamuri F, Miyamoto N (1984): Clinical applications of transvenous mitral commissurotomy by a new balloon catheter. J Thorac Cardiovasc Surg 87:394-402.

26. Lock JE, Khalilullah M, Shrivastava S, Bahl V, Keane JF (1985): Percutaneous catheter commissurotomy in rheumatic mitral stenosis. N Engl J Med 313:1515-1518.

27. Al Zaibag MA, Ribeiro PA, Al Kasab S, Al Fagih MR (1986): Percutaneous double-balloon valvotomy for rheumatic mitral valve stenosis. Lancet 1:757-761.

28. Kveselis DA, Rocchini AP, Beekman R, Snider AR, Crowley D, Dick M, Rosenthal A (1986): Balloon angioplasty for congenital and rheumatic mitral stenosis. Am J Cardiol 57:348-350.

29. Arora R, Nair M, Rajagopal S, Sethi KK, Mohan JC, Nigam M, Khalilullah M (1989): Percutaneous balloon mitral valvuloplasty in children and young adults with rheumatic mitral stenosis. Am Heart J 118:883-887.

30. Shrivastava S, Dev V, Vasan RS, Das G, Rajani M (1991): Percutaneous balloon mitral valvuloplasty in juvenile rheumatic mitral stenosis. Am J Cardiol 67:892-894.

31. Fawzy ME, Ribeiro PA, Dunn B, Galal O, Muthusamy R, Shaikh A, Mercer E, Duran CMG (1992): Percutaneous mitral valvotomy with Inoue balloon catheter in children and adults: Immediate results and early follow-up. Am Heart J 123:462-465.

32. Natarajan D, Sharma VP, Sharma SC (1992): Percutaneous mitral valvotomy by Inoue catheter in young patients with mitral stenosis. Am Heart J 123:541-543.

33. Alday LE, Juaneda E (1987): Percutaneous balloon dilatation in congenital mitral stenosis. Br Heart J 57:479-482.

34. Spevak PJ, Bass JL, Ben-Shachar G, Hesslein P,

Keane J, Perry S, Pyles L, Lock JE (1990): Balloon angioplasty for congenital mitral stenosis. Am J Cardiol 66:472–476.

35. Mullins CE, Latson LA, Neches WH, Colvin EV, Kan J (1990): Balloon dilatation of miscellaneous lesions: Results of Valvuloplasty and Angioplasty of Congenital Anomalies Registry. Am J Cardiol 65:802–803.

36. Keith JD (1978): Prevalence, incidence and epidemiology. In Keith JD, Rowe RD, Vlad P (eds): "Heart Disease in Infancy and Childhood," 3rd Ed. New York: Macmillan, pp 6, 789–801.

37. Ruckman RN, Van Praagh R (1978): Anatomic types of congenital mitral stenosis: Report of 49 autopsy cases with considerations of diagnosis and surgical implications. Am J Cardiol 42:592–601.

38. Spevak PJ, Freed MD, Castaneda AR, Norwood WI, Pollack P (1986): Valve replacement in children less than 5 years of age. J Am Coll Cardiol 8:901–908.

39. Rocchini AP (1992): Congenital mitral stenosis. In Cheng TO (ed): "Percutaneous Balloon Valvuloplasty." New York: Igaku-Shoin, pp 214–220.

40. Rao PS (1987): Influence of balloon size on short-term and long-term results of balloon pulmonary valvuloplasty. Texas Heart Inst J 41:57–61.

41. Babic VV, Pejcic P, Djurisic Z, Vucinic M, Grujicic SM (1986): Percutaneous transarterial balloon valvuloplasty for mitral valve stenosis. Am J Cardiol 57:1101–1104.

42. Grifka RG, Nihill MR, Mullins CE (1990): Percutaneous transseptal double balloon valvuloplasty for congenital mitral stenosis, abstract ed. Am J Cardiol 66:522.

43. Perry SB, Spevak PJ, Keane JF, Lock JE (1990): Balloon valvuloplasty for congenital mitral stenosis (abstract). Circulation 82(Suppl III):584.

44. Bharati S, McAllister HA, Rosenquist GC, Miller RA, Tatooles CJ, Lev M (1974): The surgical anatomy of truncus arteriosus communis. J Thorac Cardiovasc Surg 64:501–510.

45. Calder L, Van Praagh R, Van Praagh S, Sears WP, Corwin R, Levy A, Keith JD, Paul MH (1976): Truncus arteriosus communis: Clinical, angiocardiographic, and pathologic findings in 100 patients. Am Heart J 92:23–38.

46. Butto F, Lucas RV Jr, Edwards JE (1986): Persistent truncus arteriosus: Pathologic anatomy in 54 cases. Pediatr Cardiol 7:95–101.

47. Ballerini L, Cifarelli A, Di Carlo D (1989): Percutaneous balloon dilatation of stenotic truncal valve in a newborn. Int J Cardiol 23:270–272.

48. Elliot RB, Starling MB, Neutze JM (1975): Medical manipulation of the ductus arteriosus. Lancet 1:140–142.

49. Olley PM, Coceani F, Bodach E (1976): E-type prostaglandins: A new emergency therapy for certain cyanotic congenital heart malformations. Circulation 53:728–731.

50. Coe JY, Silove ED (1979): Oral prostaglandin E_2 in pulmonary atresia. Lancet 1:1297–1298.

51. Lund G, Cragg A, Rysavy J, Castaneda F, Salomonowitz E, Vlodaver Z, Castaneda-Zuniga W, Amplatz K (1983): Patency of the ductus arteriosus after balloon dilatation: An experimental study. Circulation 68:621–627.

52. Lund G, Rysavy J, Cragg A, Salomonowitz E, Vlodaver Z, Castaneda-Zuniga W, Amplatz K (1984): Long-term patency of the ductus arteriosus after balloon dilatation: An experimental study. Circulation 69:772–774.

53. Suárez de Lezo J, Lopez-Rubio F, Guzmán J, Galán A, Herrera N, Arizón J, Sancho M, Pan M, Franco M, Fernández R, Zapatero M, Vallés F (1985): Percutaneous transluminal angioplasty of stenotic ductus arteriosus. Cathet Cardiovasc Diagn 11:493–500.

54. Corwin RD, Singh AK, Karlson KE (1981): Balloon dilatation of ductus arteriosus in a newborn with interrupted aortic arch and ventricular septal defect. Am Heart J 102:446–447.

55. Rao PS, Solymar L (1988): Transductal balloon angioplasty for coarctation of the aorta in the neonate: Preliminary observations. Am Heart J 116:1558–1562.

56. Rudolph AM, Heymann MA, Spitzras V (1972): Hemodynamic considerations in the development of narrowing of the aorta. Am J Cardiol 30:514–525.

57. Talner NS, Berman MA (1975): Postnatal development of obstruction in coarctation of the aorta: Role of ductus arteriosus. Pediatrics 56:562–569.

58. Heymann MA, Berman W Jr. Rudolph AM, Whitman V (1979): Dilatation of ductus arteriosus by prostaglandin E_1 in aortic arch anomalies. Circulation 59:169–173.

59. Heymann MA (1981): Pharmacologic use of prostaglandin E_1 in infants with congenital heart disease. Am Heart J 101:837–843.

60. Palmaz JC, Kopp DT, Hayashi H, Schatz RA, Hunter G, Tio FO, Garcia O, Alvarado R, Rees C, Thomas SC (1987): Normal and stenotic renal arteries: Experimental balloon-expandable intraluminal stenting. Radiology 164:705–708.

61. Palmaz JC, Richter GA, Noeldge G, Schatz RA, Robinson PD, Gardiner GA Jr, Becker GJ, McLear GK, Denny DF, Jr, Lammer J, Paolini RM, Rees CR, Alvarado R, Heiss HW, Root HD, Rogers W (1988): Intraluminal stents in atherosclerotic iliac artery stenosis: Preliminary report of a multicenter study. Radiology 168:727–731.

62. Schatz RA (1989): A review of vascular stents. Circulation 79:445-462.

63. Levine MJ, Leonard BM, Burke JA, Nash ID, Salifan RD, Diver DJ, Baim DS (1990): Clinical and angiographic results of balloon-expandable intracoronary stents in right coronary artery stenosis. J Am Coll Cardiol 12:332-339.

64. Schatz RA, Baim DS, Leon M, Ellis SG, Goldberg S, Hirschfeld JW, Cleman MW, Cabin HS, Walker C, Stagy J, Buchbinder M, Teirstein PS, Topol EJ, Savage M, Perez JA, Curry RC, Whitworth H, Sousa JE, Tio F, Almagol Y, Ponder R, Penn IM, Leonard B, Levine SL, Fish RD, Palmaz JC (1991): Clinical experience with the Palmaz-Schatz coronary stent: Initial results of a multicenter study. Circulation 83:148-161.

65. Mullins CE, O'Laughlin MP, Vick GW III, Mayer DC, Myers TJ, Kearney DL, Schatz RA, Palmaz JC (1988): Implantation of balloon-expandable intravascular grafts by catheterization in pulmonary arteries and systemic veins. Circulation 77:188-199.

66. Rocchini AP, Meliones JN, Beekman RH, Moorehead C, London M (1992): Use of balloon-expandable stents to treat experimental peripheral pulmonary artery and superior vena caval stenosis: Preliminary experience. Pediatr Cardiol 13: 92-96.

67. Soloman N, Wholey MH, Jarmolowski CR (1991): Intravascular stents in the management of superior vena cava syndrome. Cathet Cardiovasc Diagn 23:245-252.

68. Chatelain P, Meier B, Friedli B (1991): Stenting of superior vena cava and inferior vena cava for symptomatic narrowing after repeated atrial surgery for D-transposition of the great vessels. Br Heart J 66:466-468.

69. Coe JY, Olley PM (1991): A novel method to maintain ductus arteriosus patency. J Am Coll Cardiol 18:837-841.

70. Moore JW, Kirby WC, Lovelt EJ, O'Neill JT (1991): Use of an intravascular endoprosthesis (stent) to establish and maintain short term patency of the ductus arteriosus in newborn lambs (abstract): J Am Coll Cardiol 17:19A.

71. Lloyd TR, Markowitz MA (1992): Transcatheter stenting of the ductus arteriosus: Evaluation as an alternative to surgical shunts. J Invasive Cardiol 4:167-172.

72. Gibbs JL, Rothman MT, Rees MR, Parsons JM, Blackburn ME, Ruiz CE (1992): Stenting of the arterial duct: A new approach to palliation for pulmonary atresia. Br Heart J 67:240-245.

73. Rosenthal E, Qureshi SA (1992): Stent implantation in congenital heart disease (editorial). Br Heart J 67:211-212.

74. Liebman J, Cullum L, Belloc N (1969): Natural history of transposition of the great arteries: Anatomy and birth and death characteristics. Circulation 40:237-262.

75. Rashkind WJ, Miller WW (1966): Creation of an atrial septal defect without thoracotomy. JAMA 196:991-992.

76. Rashkind WJ, Waldhausen JA, Miller WW, Friedman S (1969): Palliative treatment in tricuspid atresia: Combined balloon atrial septostomy and surgical alteration of pulmonary blood flow. J Thorac Cardiovasc Surg 57:812-818.

77. Rao PS, Covitz W, Moore HV (1992): Principles of palliative management of patients with tricuspid atresia. In Rao PS (ed): "Tricuspid Atresia," 2nd ed. Mt. Kisco, NY: Futura, pp 297-320.

78. Shams A, Fowler RS, Trusler GA, Keith JD, Mustard WT (1971): Pulmonary atresia with intact ventricular septum: Report of 50 cases. Pediatrics 47:370-377.

79. Rao PS (1985): Comprehensive management of pulmonary atresia with intact ventricular septum. Ann Thorac Surg 40:409-413.

80. Mickell JJ, Mathews RA, Park SC, Lenox CC, Fricker J, Neches WH, Zuberbuhler JR (1980): Left atrioventricular valve atresia: Clinical management. Circulation 61:123-127.

81. Rao PS, Kulungara RJ, Moore HV, Strong WB (1981): Syndrome of single ventricle without pulmonary stenosis but with left atrioventricular valve atresia and interatrial obstruction: Palliative management with simultaneous atrial septostomy and pulmonary artery banding. J Thorac Cardiovasc Surg 81:127-130.

82. Sinha SM, Rusnak SL, Sommers HM, Cole RB, Muster AJ, Paul MH (1968): Hypoplastic left heart syndrome—Analysis of thirty autopsy cases in infants with surgical considerations. Am J Cardiol 21:166-173.

83. Serrato M, Bucheleres HG, Bicoff P, Miller RA, Hastreiter AR (1968): Palliative balloon atrial septostomy for total anomalous pulmonary venous connection in infancy. J Pediatr 73:734-739.

84. Mullins CE, El-Said GM, Neches WH, Williams RL, Vargo TA, Nihill MR, McNamara DG (1973): Balloon atrial septostomy for total anomalous pulmonary venous return. Br Heart J 35:752-757.

85. Korns ME, Garabedian HA, Lauer RM (1972): Anatomic limitation of balloon atrial septostomy. Hum Pathol 3:345-349.

86. Meng CCL, Wells CR, Valdes-Dapena M, Arey JB, Black IFS, O'Riordan AC (1973): The anatomy of the foramen ovale in relation to balloon atrial septostomy, abstracted. Pediatr Res 7:304.

87. Leanage R, Agnetti A, Graham G, Taylor J, Macartney FJ (1981): Factors influencing survival after balloon atrial septostomy for complete trans-

position of the great arteries. Br Heart J 45:559–572.

88. Park SC, Zuberbuhler JR, Neches WH, Lenox CC, Zoltun RA (1975): A new atrial septostomy technique. Cathet Cardiovasc Diagn 1:195–201.

89. Park SC, Neches WH, Zuberbuhler JR, Lenox CC, Mathews RA, Fricker RJ, Zoltun RA (1978): Clinical use of blade septostomy. Circulation 58:600–606.

90. Park SC, Neches WH, Mullins CE, Girod DA, Olley PM, Falkowski G, Garibjan VA, Mathews RA, Fricker RJ, Beerman LB, Lenox CC, Zuberbuhler JR (1982): Blade atrial septostomy: Collaborative study. Circulation 66:258–266.

91. Rao PS, Mardini MK (1983): Atrial septostomy without thoracotomy: The experience with transcatheter knife atrial septostomy. King Faisal Specialist Hosp Med J 3:165–171.

92. Rao PS (1984): Transcatheter blade atrial septostomy. Cathet Cardiovasc Diagn 10:335–342.

93. Lin AE, DeSesa TG, Williams RG (1986): Balloon and blade atrial septostomy facilitated by two-dimensional echocardiography. Am J Cardiol 57:273–277.

94. Perry SB, Lang P, Keane JF, Jonas RA, Saunders PS, Lock JE (1986): Creation and maintenance of an adequate interatrial communication in left atrioventricular valve atresia or stenosis. Am J Cardiol 58:622–626.

95. Rich S, Lam W (1988): Atrial septostomy as palliative therapy for refractory primary pulmonary hypertension. Am J Cardiol 51:1560–1561.

96. Ali Khan MA, Bricker JT, Mullins CE, Al Yousef S, Nihill MR, Vargo TA (1991): Blade atrial systostomy: Experience with first 50 procedures. Cathet Cardiovasc Diagn 23:257–262.

97. Park SC, Neches WH (1993): Blade atrial septostomy. In Rao PS (ed): "Transcatheter Therapy in Pediatric Cardiology." New York: Wiley-Liss, pp 17–27.

98. Mitchell SE, Kan JS, Anderson JH, White RI Jr, Swindle MM (1986): Atrial septostomy: Stationary angioplasty balloon technique, abstracted. Pediatr Res 20:173A.

99. Sideris EB, Fowlkes JP, Smith JE, Sideris SE, Gulde RE (1988): Why atrial septostomy and not foramen ovale angioplasty? Abstracts of Cardiology and Cardiovascular Surgery: Interventions. 18th Annual Symposium of the Texas Heart Institute, 1988, p 36.

100. Shrivastava S, Radhakrishnan S, Dev V, Singh LS, Rajani M (1987): Balloon dilatation of atrial septum in complete transposition of great artery—A new technique. Indian Heart J 39:298–300.

101. King TD, Thompson SL, Steinor C, Mills NL (1978): Measurement of atrial septal defect during cardiac catheterization: Experimental and clinical trials. Am J Cardiol 41:537–542.

102. Rao PS, Langhough R (1991): Relationship of echographic, shunt flow, and angiographic size to the stretched diameter of the atrial septal defect. Am Heart J 122:505–508.

103. Forfar JC, Godman MJ (1985): Functional and anatomical correlates in atrial septal defect: An echocardiographic study. Br Heart J 54:193–200.

104. Hausknecht MJ, Sims RE, Nihill MR, Cashion WR (1990): Successful palliation of primary pulmonary hypertension by atrial septostomy. Am J Cardiol 65:1045–1046.

105. Webber SA, Culham JAG, Sandor GGS, Patterson MWH (1991): Balloon dilatation of restrictive interatrial communications in congenital heart disease. Br Heart J 65:346–348.

106. Rao PS (1992): Static balloon dilatation of restrictive atrial septal defects. J Saudi Heart Assoc 4:55–58.

107. Galal O, Al-Fadley F (1992): Balloon dilatation of a restrictive interatrial communication in a two month old infant with mitral atresia. J Saudi Heart Assoc 4:78–81.

108. Rao PS (1989): Balloon angioplasty and valvuloplasty in infants, children and adolescents. Curr Probl Cardiol 14:417–500.

109. Rao PS, Brais M (1988): Balloon pulmonary valvuloplasty for congenital cyanotic heart defects. Am Heart J 115:1105–1110.

110. Rao PS, Wilson AD, Thapar MK, Brais M (1992): Balloon pulmonary valvuloplasty in the management of cyanotic congenital heart defects. Cathet Cardiovasc Diagn 25:16–24.

111. Engle ME, Holswade GR, Goldberg HP, Lukas DS, Glenn F (1958): Regression after open valvotomy of infundibular stenosis accompanying severe valvar pulmonic stenosis. Circulation 17:862–873.

112. Fontes VF, Esteves CA, Eduardo J, Sousa JEMR, Silva MVD, Bembom MCB (1988): Regression of infundibular hypertrophy after pulmonary valvuloplasty for pulmonic stenosis. Am J Cardiol 62:977–979.

113. Thapar MK, Rao PS (1989): Significance of infundibular obstruction following balloon valvuloplasty for valvar pulmonic stenosis. Am Heart J 118:99–103.

114. Rao PS, Thapar MK (1991): Development of infundibular obstruction following balloon pulmonary valvuloplasty. Am Heart J 121:1839–1840.

115. Vacek JL, Goertz KK (1990): Balloon valvuloplasty of a subpulmonic membrane. Am Heart J 119:1419–1421.

116. Suarez de Lezo J, Pan M, Sancho M, Herrera N,

Arizon J, Franco M, Concha M, Valles F, Romanos A (1986): Percutaneous transluminal balloon dilatation for discrete subaortic stenosis. Am J Cardiol 58:619-621.

117. Lababidi Z, Weinhaus L, Stoeckle H, Walls JT (1987): Transluminal balloon dilatation for discrete subaortic stenosis. Am J Cardiol 59:423-425.

118. Rao PS, Wilson AD, Chopra PS (1990): Balloon dilatation for discrete subaortic stenosis: Immediate and intermediate-term results. J Invasive Cardiol 2:65-71.

119. Chandrashekar YS, Anand IS, Wahi PL (1990): Balloon dilatation of double-chamber right ventricle. Am Heart J 120:1234-1236.

120. Sidi D, Planche C, Kachaner J, Bruniaux J, Villain E, Le Bidois J, Piechaud JF, Lacour-Gayet F (1987): Anatomic correction of simple transposition of the great arteries in 50 neonates. Circulation 75:429-435.

121. Norwood WI, Dobell AR, Freed MD, Kirklin JW, Blackstone EH, and the Congenital Heart Surgeons' Society (1988): Intermediate results of the arterial switch repair: A 20-institution study. J Thorac Cardiovasc Surg 96:854-863.

122. Brown WJ, Mee RB (1988): Early results for anatomic correction of transposition of the great arteries and for double-outlet right ventricle with subpulmonary ventricular septal defect. J Thorac Cardiovasc Surg 95:230-239.

123. Wernovsky G, Hougen TJ, Walsh EP, Sholler GF, Colan SD, Sanders SP, Parness IA, Keane JF, Mayer JE Jr, Jonas RA, Castaneda AR, Lang P (1988): Midterm results after the arterial switch operation for transposition of the great arteries with intact ventricular septum: Clinical, hemodynamic, echo, angiographic and electrophysiologic data. Circulation 77:1333-1344.

124. Di Donato RM, Wernovsky G, Walsh EP, Colan SD, Lang P, Wessel DL, Jonas RA, Mayer JE Jr, Castaneda AR (1989): Results of the arterial switch operation for transposition of the great arteries with ventricular septal defect. Circulation 80:1689-1705.

125. Zeevi B, Keane JF, Perry SB, Lock JE (1989): Balloon dilatation of postoperative right ventricular outflow obstructions. J Am Coll Cardiol 14:401-408.

126. Schranz D, Jüngst BK, Huth R, Stopfkuchen R, Erbel R, Oelert H (1988): Pulmonary stenosis after arterial switch operation for complete transposition of the great arteries: Report of a successful balloon dilatation. Z Kardiol 77:743-745.

127. Saxena A, Fong LV, Ogilve BC, Keeton BR (1990): Use of balloon dilatation to treat supravalvar pulmonary stenosis developing after anatomical correction for complete transposition. Br Heart J 64:151-155.

128. Rao PS (1992): Balloon dilatation of supravalvar pulmonary stenosis after arterial switch procedure for complete transposition. Br Heart J 67:204-205.

129. Rao PS (1992): Pulmonary stenosis. In Cheng TO (ed): "Percutaneous Balloon Valvuloplasty." New York: Igaku-Shoin, pp 365-420.

130. Suárez de Lezo J, Medina A, Pan M, Romero M, Hernández E, Pavlovic D, Melián F (1993): Balloon valvuloplasty/angioplasty: The Spanish experience. In Rao PS (ed): "Transcatheter Therapy in Pediatric Cardiology." New York: Wiley-Liss, pp. 471-492.

131. Rao PS (1988): Indications for balloon pulmonary valvuloplasty. Am Heart J 116:1661-1662.

132. Gentles TL, Lock JE, Perry SB (1992): High pressure balloon angioplasty of pulmonary artery stenosis, abstracted. J Am Coll Cardiol 19:24A.

133. Velasquez G, Castaneda-Zuniga W, Formanek A, Zollikofer C, Barreto A, Nicoloff D, Amplatz K, Sullivan A (1980): Nonsurgical aortoplasty in Leriche syndrome. Radiology 134:359-360.

134. Grollman JH, Del Vicario M, Mittak AK (1980): Percutaneous transluminal abdominal aortic angioplasty. Am J Roentgen 134:1053-1054.

135. Martin EC, Diamond NG, Casarella WJ (1980): Percutaneous transluminal angioplasty in non-atherosclerotic disease. Radiology 135:27-33.

136. Mitchell SE, Kadir S, Kaufman SL, Chang R, Williams GM, Kan JS, White RI Jr (1983): Percutaneous transluminal angioplasty of aortic graft stenosis. Radiology 149:439-444.

137. Heeney D, Bookstein J, Daniels E, Warmath M, Horn J, Rowley W (1983): Transluminal angioplasty of the lower abdominal aorta: Report of 6 cases in women. Radiology 148:81-83.

138. Saddekni S, Sinderman KW, Hilten S, Sos TA (1980): Percutaneous transluminal angioplasty of non-atherosclerotic lesions. Am J Roentgen 135:975-982.

139. Srur MF, Sos TA, Saddekni S, Cohn DJ, Rozenblit G, Wetter EB (1985): Intimal fibromuscular dysplasia and Takayasu arteritis: Delayed response to percutaneous transluminal renal angioplasty. Radiology 157:657-660.

140. Khalilullah M, Tyagi S, Lochan R, Yadav BS, Nair M, Gambhir DS, Khanna SK (1987): Percutaneous transluminal balloon angioplasty of the aorta in patients with aortitis. Circulation 76:597-600.

141. Sharma S, Rajani M, Kaul U, Talwar KK, Dev V, Shrivastava S (1990): Initial experience with percutaneous transluminal angioplasty in the management of Takayasu's arteritis. Br J Radiol 63:517-522.

142. Gu SM, Lin G, Yi R, Li JM, Zhou J, Pan WM

(1988): Transluminal catheter angioplasty of abdominal aorta in Takayasu's arteritis. Acta Radiol 29:509-513.

143. Yakes WF, Kumpe DA, Brow SB, Parker SH, Lattes RG, Cook PS, Haas DK, Gibson MD, Hopper KD, Reed MD, Cox HE, Bourne EE, Griffin DJ (1989): Percutaneous transluminal aortic angioplasty: Techniques and results. Radiology 172:965-970.

144. Yagura M, Sano I, Akioka H, Hayashi M, Uchida H (1984): Usefulness of percutaneous transluminal angioplasty for aortitis syndrome. Arch Intern Med 144:1465-1468.

145. Park JH, Han MC, Kim SH, Oh BH, Park YB, Seo JD (1989): Takayasu arteritis: Angiographic findings and results of angioplasty. Am J Roentgen 153:1069-1074.

146. Kumar S, Mandalam KR, Rao VR, Subramanyam R, Gupta AK, Joseph S, Unni M, Rao AS (1989): Percutaneous transluminal angioplasty in nonspecific aorta-arteritis (Takayasu's disease): Experience of 16 cases. Cardiovasc Intervent Radiol 12:321-325.

147. Dev V, Shrivastava S, Rajani M (1990): Percutaneous transluminal balloon angioplasty in Takayasu's aortitis: Persistent benefit over two years. Am Heart J 120:222-224.

148. Stark J, Silove ED, Taylor JFN, Graham GR, Kirklin JW (1974): Obstruction to systemic venous return following the Mustard operation for transposition of the great arteries. J Thorac Cardiovasc Surg 68:742-749.

149. Godman MJ, Friedli B, Pasternac A, Kidd BSL, Trusler GA, Mustard WT (1976): Hemodynamic studies in children four to ten years after Mustard operation for transposition of the great arteries. Circulation 53:532-538.

150. Takahashi M, Lindesmith GG, Lewis AB, Stiles QR, Stanton RE, Meyer BW, Lurie PR (1976): Long-term results of the Mustard procedure. Circulation 56(Suppl II):85-90.

151. Sutherland CO, Henken DP, Nichols GM, Dhindsa DS, Bonchek LI, Meneshe VD, Rahimtoola SH, Starr A, Lees MH (1975): Postoperative hemodynamic and electrophysiologic evaluation of the interatrial baffle procedure. Am J Cardiol 35:660-666.

152. Wyse RKH, Haworth SC, Taylor JFN, Macartney FJ (1979): Obstruction of superior vena caval pathway after Mustard's repair. Br Heart J 42:162-167.

153. Mahoney L, Turley K, Ebert P, Heymann M (1982): Long-term results after atrial repair of transposition of the great arteries in early infancy. Circulation 66:253-258.

154. Marx GR, Haugen TJ, Norwood WI, Fyler DC,

Castaneda AR, Nadas AS (1983): Transposition of the great arteries with intact ventricular septum: Results of Mustard and Senning operation in 123 consecutive patients. J Am Coll Cardiol 1:476-483.

155. Bink-Boelkens MTE, Bergstra A, Cromme-Dijkhuis AH, Eygelaar A, Landsman MJ, Mooyaart EL (1989): The asymptomatic child a long time after the Mustard operation for transposition of the great arteries. Ann Thorac Surg 47:45-50.

156. Bender HW, Stewart JR, Merrill WH, Hamman JW Jr, Graham TP Jr (1989): Ten years' experience with Senning operation for transposition of the great arteries: Physiological results and late follow-up. Ann Thorac Surg 47:218-233.

157. Backer CL, Ilbawi MN, Ohtake S, DeLeon SY, Muster AJ, Paul MH, Benson DW Jr, Idriss FS (1989): Transposition of the great arteries: A comparison of the results of the Mustard procedure versus the arterial switch. Ann Thorac Surg 48:10-14.

158. Kaulitz R, Stumper OF, Geuskens R, Sreeram N, Elzengo NJ, Chan CK, Burns JE, Godman MJ, Hess J, Sutherland GR (1990): Comparative valve of the precordial and transesophageal approaches in the echocardiographic evaluation of atrial baffle function after an atrial correction procedure. J Am Coll Cardiol 16:686-694.

159. Bender HW Jr, Graham TP Jr, Boucek JR Jr, Walker WE, Boerth RG (1980): Comparative operative results of the Senning and Mustard procedures for transposition of the great arteries. Circulation 62(Suppl I):197-203.

160. Reul GJ, Jr, Cooley DA, Sandiford FM, Hallman GL (1974): Complications following the contoured Dacron baffle in correction of transposition of the great arteries. Surgery 76:946-954.

161. Moodie DS, Feldt RH, Wallace RB (1976): Transient protein-losing enteropathy secondary to elevated pressures and caval obstruction after the Mustard procedure. J Thorac Cardiovasc Surg 72:379-382.

162. Krueger SK, Burney DW, Ferlic RM (1977): Protein-losing enteropathy complicating the Mustard procedure. Surgery 81:305-306.

163. Kirk CR, Gibbs JL, Wilkinson JL, Wilson N, Dickinson DF, Qureshi SA (1988): Protein-losing enteropathy caused by baffle obstruction after Mustard's operation. Br Heart J 59:69-72.

164. Cumming GR, Ferguson CC (1975): Obstruction of superior vena cava after the Mustard procedure for transposition of the great arteries: Conservative management of chylothorax. J Thorac Cardiovasc Surg 70:242-247.

165. Rao PS, Wilson AD (1991): Chychothorax, an unusual complication of baffle obstruction follow-

ing Mustard operation: Successful treatment with balloon angioplasty. Am Heart J 123:244–248.

166. Waldman JD, Waldman J, Jones MC (1983): Failure of balloon dilatation in mid-cavity obstruction of the systemic venous atrium after the Mustard operation. Pediatr Cardiol 4:141–144.

167. Lock JE, Bass JL, Castaneda-Zuniga W, Fuhrman BP, Rashkind WJ, Lucas RV Jr (1984): Dilatation angioplasty of congenital or operative narrowings of venous channels. Circulation 70:457–464.

168. Benson LN, Yeatman L, Laks H (1985): Balloon dilatation for superior vena caval obstruction after Senning procedure. Cathet Cardiovasc Diagn 11:63–68.

169. Rheuban KS, Carpentier MA (1988): Diagnostic cardiac catheterization, angiography, and interventional catheterization. In Lake CL (ed): "Pediatric Cardiac Anesthesia." Norwalk, CT: Appleton & Lange, p 67.

170. Stark J, Tynan M, Aschraft KW, Aberdeen E, Waterston DJ (1972): Obstruction of pulmonary veins and superior vena cava after Mustard operation for transposition of the great arteries. 45(Suppl I):116–120.

171. Smallhorn JF, Gow R, Freedom RM, Trusler GA, Olley P, Pacquet M, Gibbons J, Vlad P (1986): Pulsed Doppler echocardiographic assessment of pulmonary venous pathway after Mustard or Senning procedure for transposition of the great arteries. Circulation 73:765–774.

172. Cooper SG, Sullivan ID, Bull C, Taylor JFN (1989): Balloon dilatation of pulmonary venous pathway obstruction after Mustard repair for transposition of the great arteries. J Am Coll Cardiol 14:194–198.

173. Coulsen JD, Jennings RB Jr, Johnson JD (1990): Pulmonary venous obstruction after Senning procedure: Relief by catheter balloon dilatation. Br Heart J 64:160–162.

174. Zeevi B, Berant M, Zalzstein E, Blieden LC (1992): Balloon dilation of pulmonary venous pathway obstruction in an infant after the Mustard procedure. Cathet Cardiovasc Diagn 25:135–139.

175. Pacifico A (1983): Concordant transposition—Senning operation. In Stark J, de Leval M (eds): "Surgery for Congenital Heart Disease." London: Grune & Stratton, pp 345–352.

176. Stark J (1989): Reoperation after Mustard and Senning operations. In Stark J, Pacifico A (eds): "Reoperations in Cardiac Surgery." London: Springer Verlag, p 205.

177. Bettman MA, Steinberg I (1983): Superior vena cava. In Abrams HL (ed): "Abrams Angiography." Boston: Little, Brown & Co., pp 924–935.

178. Pauletti M, Pingitove R, Contini C (1979): Supe-

rior vena cava stenosis at site of insertion of two pacing electrodes. Br Heart J 42:487–489.

179. Matthews DM, Forfar JC (1979): Superior vena caval stenosis: A complication of transvenous endocardial pacing. Thorax 34:412–413.

180. Blackburn T, Dunn M (1988): Pacemaker induced superior vena cava syndrome: Consideration of management. Am Heart J 116:893–896.

181. Goudevenos JA, Reid PG, Adams PC, Holden MP, Williams DO (1989): Pacemaker induced superior vena cava syndrome: Report of four cases and review of literature. PACE 12:1890–1895.

182. Stanford W, Doty DB (1986): The role of venography and surgery in the management of patients with superior vena cava obstruction. Ann Thorac Surg 41:158–163.

183. Doty DB, Baker WH (1976): Bypass of superior vena cava with spiral vein graft. Ann Thorac Surg 22:490–493.

184. Youngston GG, McKenzie FN, Nichol PM (1980): Superior vena cava syndrome: Case report. Am Heart J 99:503–505.

185. Rocchini AP, Cho KJ, Byrum C, Heidelberger K (1982): Transluminal angioplasty of superior vena cava obstruction in a 15-month-old child. Chest 82:506–508.

186. Montgomery JH, D'Souza VJ, Dyer RB, Formanek AG, Prabhu SH (1985): Nonsurgical treatment of superior vena cava syndrome. Am J Cardiol 56:829–830.

187. Sherry CS, Diamond NG, Meyers TP, Martin RI (1986): Successful treatment of superior vena cava syndrome by venous angioplasty. Am J Roentgen 147:834–835.

188. Ali MK, Ewer MS, Balakrishnan PV, Ochoa DA, Morice RC, Raizner AE, Lawrie GM (1987): Balloon angioplasty of superior vena cava obstruction. Ann Intern Med 107:856–857.

189. Walpole HT, Lovett KE, Chuang VP, West R, Clements SD Jr (1988): Superior vena cava syndrome treated by percutaneous transluminal balloon angioplasty. Am Heart J 115:1303–1304.

190. Grace AA, Sutters M, Schofield PM (1991): Balloon dilatation of pacemaker induced stenosis of the superior vena cava. Br Heart J 65:225–226.

191. McNulty JG (1977): The Budd-Chiari syndrome of hepatic venous obstruction. In McNulty JG (ed): "Radiology of Liver." Philadelphia: W.B. Saunders, pp 306–312.

192. Mitchell MC, Boitnott JK, Kaufman S, Cameren JL, Maddrey WC (1982): Budd-Chiari syndrome: Etiology, diagnosis and management. Medicine 61:199–218.

193. Victor S, Jayanthi V, Madangopalan N (1987): Coarctation of inferior vena cava. Trop Gastroenterol 8:127–142.

194. Cardella JF, Castaneda-Zuniga WR, Hunter D, Young A, Amplatz K (1988): Angiographic and interventional radiology considerations in liver transplantation. Am J Roentgenol 146:143–153.

195. Wozney P, Zajko AB, Bron KM, Point S, Starzl TE (1986): Vascular complications after liver transplantation in a 5-year experience. Am J Roentgen 147:657–663.

196. Hirooka M, Kimura C (1970): Membranous obstruction of the hepatic portion of inferior vena cava: Surgical correction and aetological study. Arch Surg 100:656–663.

197. Eguchi S, Tekeuchi Y, Asano K (1974): Successful balloon membranotomy for obstruction of the hepatic portion of the inferior vena cava. Surg 76:837–840.

198. Meier WL III, Waller RM III, Sones PJ Jr (1981): Budd-Chiari web treated by percutaneous transluminal angioplasty. Am J Roentgen 137:1257–1258.

199. Yamada R, Sato M, Kawabata M, Nakatsuka H, Nakamura K, Kobayashi N (1983): Segmental obstruction of the hepatic inferior vena cava treated by transluminal angioplasty. Radiology 149:91–96.

200. Bar-Meir S, Rubinstein Z, Miller HI (1984): Failure of balloon membranotomy of the inferior vena cava. Isr J Med Sci 20:618–621.

201. Sawada S, Oshima T, Kato T, Kubota Y, Tanaka Y (1985): Budd-Chiari syndrome treated by percutaneous transluminal angioplasty: Report of a use. Acta Radiol Diagn 26(Fasc 1):25–27.

202. Murphy FB, Steinberg HV, Shires GT III, Martin LG, Bernadino ME (1986): The Budd-Chiari syndrome: A review. Am J Roentgen 147:9–15.

203. Sparano J, Chang J, Trasi S, Bonanno C (1987): Treatment of the Budd-Chiari syndrome with percutaneous transluminal angioplasty. Am J Med 82:821–828.

204. Rose BS, Van Aman ME, Simon DC, Sommer BG, Ferguson RM, Henry ML (1988): Transluminal balloon angioplasty of infrahepatic caval anastomotic stenosis following liver transplantation: Case report. Cardiovasc Intervent Radiol 11:79–81.

205. Hosie KB, Bolia A, Watkin DFL (1988): Treatment of Budd-Chiari syndrome by percutaneous transluminal angioplasty. Lancet 2:158–159.

206. Yamazaki Y, Eguchi S, Terashima M, Maruyama Y, Yazawa M, Fujita Y, Tsukada K (1988): Inferior vena caval obstruction: Transvenous instrumental membranotomy. Cardiovasc Intervent Radiol 11:18–20.

207. Dev V, Kaul U, Jain P, Reddy S, Sharma S, Pandey G, Rajani M (1989): Percutaneous transluminal balloon angioplasty for obstruction of the suprahepatic inferior vena cava and cavo-atrial graft stenosis. Am J Cardiol 64:397–399.

208. Loya YS, Sharma S, Amrapurkar DN, Desai HG (1989): Complete membranous obstruction of inferior vena cava: Case treated by balloon dilatation. Cathet Cardiovasc Diagn 17:164–167.

209. Cheng TO (1991): Membranotomy for Budd-Chiari syndrome (letter). Ann Thorac Surg 51:521–522.

210. Sharma S, Loya S, Daxini BV (1992): Percutaneous balloon membranotomy combined with prolonged streptokinase infusion for management of inferior vena cava obstruction. Am Heart J 123:515–518.

211. Uflacker R, Fracisconi CF, Rodriquez MP, Amaral NM (1984): Percutaneous transluminal angioplasty of hepatic veins: Treatment of Budd-Chiari syndrome. Radiology 153:641–642.

212. Driscoll DJ, Hesslein PS, Mullins CE (1982): Congenital stenosis of individual pulmonary veins: Clinical spectrum and unsuccessful treatment by transvenous balloon dilatation. Am J Cardiol 49:1767–1722.

213. Nakib A, Moller J, Kanjuh V, Edwards J (1967): Anomalies of the pulmonary veins. Am J Cardiol 20:77–90.

214. Lucas RV Jr, Lock JE, Tandon R, Edwards JE (1988): Gross and histologic anatomy of total anomalous pulmonary venous connections. Am J Cardiol 62:292–300.

215. Heath D, Segal N, Bishop J (1966): Pulmonary veno-occlusive disease. Circulation 34:242–247.

216. Weisser L. Wyler F (1967): Pulmonary veno-occlusive disease. Arch Dis Child 42:322–327.

217. Nasser WK, Feigenbaum H, Fisch C (1967): Clinical and hemodynamic diagnosis of pulmonary venous obstruction due to sclerosing mediastinitis. Am J Cardiol 20:725–729.

218. Rosenthal A, Vawter G, Wagenvoort CA (1973): Intrapulmonary veno-occlusive disease. Am J Cardiol 31:78–83.

219. Massumi A, Woods L, Mullins CE, Nasser WK, Hall RJ (1981): Pulmonary venous dilatation in pulmonary veno-occlusive disease. Am J Cardiol 48:585–589.

220. Rao PS, Silbert DR (1974): Superior vena caval obstruction in total anomalous pulmonary venous return. Br Heart J 36:228–232.

221. Elliott LP, Edwards JE (1962): The problem of pulmonary venous obstruction in total anomalous pulmonary venous connection to the left innominate vein. Circulation 25:913–915.

222. Rey C, Marache P, Francart C, Dupuis C (1985): Percutaneous balloon angioplasty in an infant with obstructed total anomalous pulmonary venous return. J Am Coll Cardiol 6:894–896.

223. Muller WH Jr, Dammann FJ Jr (1952): The treatment of certain congenital malformations of the heart by creation of pulmonary artery stenosis to reduce pulmonary artery hypertension and excessive pulmonary blood flow: A preliminary report. Surg Gynecol Obstet 95:213-219.

224. Vince DJ, Culham G, Taylor GP (1987): Development of a prosthesis for banding of an artery capable of staged dilatation by intraluminal balloon dilator: An experimental investigation. J Thorac Cardiovasc Surg 93:628-635.

225. Vince DJ, Culham G, Taylor GP (1987): Balloon-dilatable arterial banding prosthesis: Experimental study. Radiology 164:141-144.

226. Rocchini AP, Gundry SR, Beekman RH, Gallagher KP, Heidelberger K, Bove E, Behrendt DM, Dysko RC, Rosen K (1988): A reversible pulmonary artery band: Preliminary experience J Am Coll Cardiol 11:172-176.

227. Lindberg H, Smelvik B. Bjørnstad PG, Rian R, Foerster A, Tjønneland S, Sørland S, Sponheim S (1988): Balloon dilatation of pulmonary artery banding in dogs: An experimental study. Cardiovasc Intervent Radiol 11:150-154.

228. Smevik B, Lindberg H, Tjønneland S, Bjørnstad PG, Sørland SJ, Foerster A (1988): Technical note: In vitro balloon dilatation of the banded pulmonary artery. Cardiovasc Intervent Radiol 11:155-156.

229. Vince DJ, Culham JAG (1989): A prosthesis for banding the main pulmonary artery, capable of serial dilatation by balloon angioplasty. J Thorac Cardiovasc Surg 97:421-427.

230. Bjørnstad PG, Lindberg HL, Smevik B, Rian R, Sørland SJ, Tjønneland S (1990): Balloon debanding of the pulmonary artery. Cardiovasc Intervent Radiol 13:300-303.

231. Vince DJ, Culham JAG, LeBlanc TG (1991): Human clinical trials of the dilatable pulmonary artery banding prosthesis. Can J Cardiol 7:339-342.

232. Echigo (1988): PTCA. In Abstracts of the 3rd International Kawasaki Disease Symposium, Tokyo, p 64.

233. Ino T, Nishimoto K, Akimoto K, Park I, Shimazaki S, Yabuta K, Yamaguchi H (1991): Percutaneous transluminal coronary angioplasty for Kawasaki disease: A case report and literature review. Pediatr Cardiol 12:33-35.

234. Savas V, Samyn J, Schreiber TL, Hauser A, O'Neill WW (1991): Cor triatriatum dexter: Recognition and percutaneous transluminal correction. Cathet Cardiovasc Diagn 23:183-186.

16

Catheter Closure of the Ductus Arteriosus

Lee Benson, M.D. F.R.C.P.(C.)

Department of Pediatrics, The Variety Club Cardiac
Catheterization Laboratories, The Hospital for Sick Children,
University of Toronto School of Medicine, Toronto,
Ontario M56 1X8, Canada

INTRODUCTION

An increasing number of acquired and congenital lesions of the heart and circulation are becoming amenable to percutaneous catheter-directed therapies [1,2], supplementing or avoiding the need for surgical intervention. It seems appropriate that the lesion whose surgical therapy ushered in the era of surgical management for congenital heart defects would find itself ideally suited for nonsurgical intervention.

HISTORICAL CONSIDERATIONS

Surgical ligation of the ductus arteriosus was initially suggested by John Munro [3] to the Philadelphia Academy of Surgery in 1907. However, it was 31 years later when the first surgical attempt was undertaken by Graybiel et al. [4] in a 22-year-old girl with bacterial endocarditis. Although surviving the procedure, the patient died of complications of the infection. Gross and Hubbard [5] of Boston performed the first successful ligation of the ductus in a 7-year-old child with chronic heart failure, thus inaugurating the modern era of surgery for congenital heart defects. Within a few years many surgeons were duplicating this feat. In 1965, Jones [6] reported on a 25 year experience, with one

death among 431 patients with an uncomplicated ductus (mortality = 0.2%), and a similar rate (0.5%) was reported by Panagopoulos et al. [7] in 1971, underscoring that ductal surgery had become commonplace, safe, and effective. In 1967, Porstmann et al. [8] were the first to develop a technique in which a polyvinyl alcohol plug was pulled into the patent ductus arteriosus from the arterial side, using an arterial-transductal-venous guidewire. More than 300 patients, mainly adults, have been treated with this method [9-12]. It is technically complicated, requiring a large-gauge sheath to be placed into the femoral artery and the formation of a femoral artery-ductal-femoral vein wire loop; this approach has not been found suitable for infants and small children. Other devices, such as polyvinyl alcohol umbrellas with steel wires or umbrella-sponge plugs, have been used in dogs to close artificial patent ductus arteriosus from either the arterial or venous circulations [13,14]. In 1979, Rashkind and Cuaso [15] successfully inserted, from a femoral arterial entry, a foam-covered wire hooked prosthesis into six infants, the smallest weighing 3.5 kg. Since those initial clinical applications, experience from a multicenter clinical trial [16] has defined the setting in which successful catheter occlusion can take place; improved equip-

Transcatheter Therapy in Pediatric Cardiology, pages 321–333
© 1993 Wiley-Liss, Inc.

ment has led to its use as an effective alternative to surgery.

ANATOMIC CONSIDERATIONS PERTINENT TO CATHETER OCCLUSION

Details concerning the embryology and morphology of the persistently patent ductus arteriosus have been excellently reviewed by Olley [17]. Although tissue samples of persistently patent ductus arteriosus are seldom available, several observations have been made in this setting. Gittenberger-de-Groot [18] found the presence of an unfragmented wavy subendothelial elastic lamina to be associated with many, but not all, patients combined with an increase in elastic tissue within the media. Intimal cushions, common in the functionally closed ductus, were sparse. The quantity of elastic tissue appeared not to correlate with the duration of ductal patency or associated cardiac malformations. Such abnormal elastic tissue was regarded as a primary prenatal abnormality and persistent ductal patency its consequence. In an earlier study, Bakker [19] similarly noted an increase in elastic tissue and applied the term *aortification* to the persistent ductus.

The angiographic appearance of the isolated ductus varies considerably. Although the majority tend to have a funnel or conical shape due to ductal smooth muscle constriction at the pulmonary artery insertion, narrowings in the middle or aortic ends have been observed [20–23]. Using the narrowest end of the ductus as a landmark, Krichenko et al. [20] identified five groupings (Fig. 1). Within groups A and B, the relationship of the pulmonary artery insertion to the trachea allowed further division into three subgroups (useful for percutaneous transvenous catheter closure; see below). In group A (Fig. 2A), the narrowest segment was at the pulmonary insertion, with a well-defined ampulla at the aortic end, while in group B (Fig. 3A) the ductus was short and narrowed at the aortic insertion. Group C (Fig.

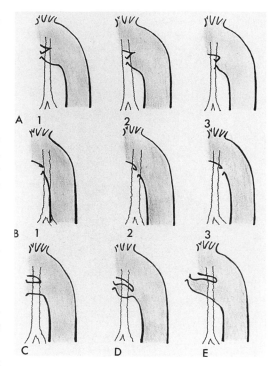

Fig. 1. Schematic representation of observed variability in ductal configuration in relationship to the tracheal air shadow.

3B) consisted of a tubular ductus without constriction, group D (Fig. 3C) a ductus with multiple constrictions, and group E (Fig. 3D) a grouping of bizarre configurations, where the ductus had an elongated conical appearance with the constriction remote from the anterior border of trachea. Without exception, the isolated ductus extends anterosuperiorly from the anterior margin of the descending aorta to the superior margin of the pulmonary artery in close proximity to the orifice of the left pulmonary artery and passes obliquely from right to left as shown in the frontal projection in Figure 2B.

The distribution of ductal sizes, measured from the narrowest segment in 200 procedures performed at The Hospital for Sick Children, Toronto, and the frequencies in the various subgroups referred to above, are shown in Figure 4. For that population, the average

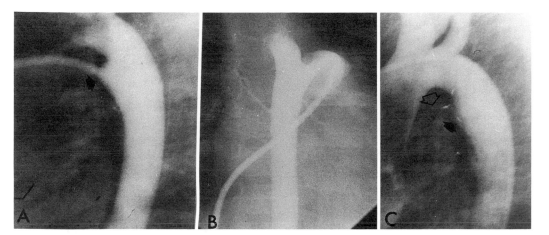

Fig. 2. A: Lateral aortogram. Arrow indicates pulmonary–ductal insertion. **B:** Anteroposterior aortogram through ductus, showing inferosuperior angulation of the ductus. **C:** Occluded ductus. Arrows indicate distal (filled) and proximal (open) arms.

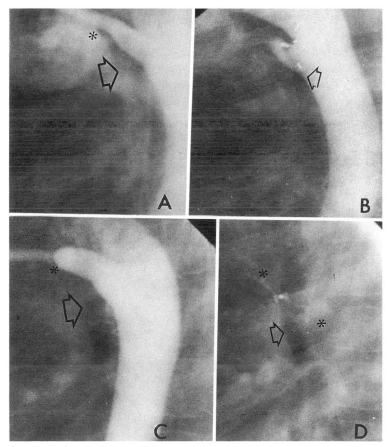

Fig. 3. A–D: Various types of ductal configurations, from the lateral aortogram. Arrows denote anterior air shadow; stars, areas of ductal construction.

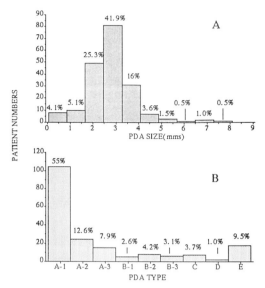

Fig. 4. A, B: Distribution of patent ductus arteriosus (PDA) sizes and types seen at The Hospital for Sick Children.

ductal size was 2.7 ± 1.0 mm (range, 0.5–8.0 mm), with the most frequently encountered group being A (>65%).

CATHETER OCCLUSION TECHNIQUES

Two transcatheter occlusion techniques have been applied in humans: 1) the polyvinyl plug [8–11], devised by Porstmann and others, which has had extensive clinical application both in Europe and Japan [9,12]; and 2) the umbrella occluder disk system pioneered by Rashkind et al. [16]. A 5 or 6 Fr triple-lumen catheter with a detachable silicone double-balloon has been described by Warnecke et al. [24], and, although it is a promising approach, it has thus far not had extensive clinical trials. Recently, Magal et al. [25] described a device consisting of a small nylon sack that could be filled with segments of guidewire, fixed with a distal flexible crossbar, and delivered in a 10 Fr catheter system. The Porstmann technique (described below) is primarily applicable to older adolescents and adults, as it requires the entry of a large French sized plug into the

femoral artery. Rashkind's device, with the technique of placement through a transvenous delivery system as described by Bash and Mullins [26], is more applicable to younger children (see below) but is not large enough to be used with a ductus larger than 9 mm.

The Rashkind Technique

The fates of both a properly positioned or an embolized device were initially studied in animal models [16,27]. In the former [16], it was found that by 3 months postimplantation both aortic and pulmonary ends were completely sealed and the foam matrix incorporated into the endothelium. In five animals the prosthesis was deployed into the pulmonary artery, where it became embedded in the vessel wall and endothelization began. Neither the lumen of the distal artery nor its side branches were affected in any manner.

The occluder consists of two open-pore medical grade polyurethane foam disks (USCI Angiographic Systems, Billerica, MA) mounted on two opposing three-arm spring assemblies, resembling two opposing umbrellas (Fig. 5). The individual arms are attached to a central spring mechanism in such a way that the

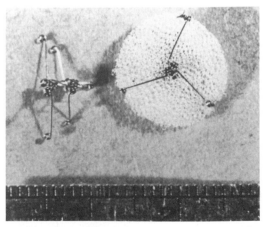

Fig. 5. The Rashkind ductus occluder with (right) and without (left) foam on metal arms. (Reproduced from Rashkind et al. [16], with permission of the publisher.)

individual arms (0.005 inch stainless steel) are 120° apart and each opposing umbrella arm 60° apart. When released, the arms spring perpendicular to the catheter shaft and thus self-seal without the need of a hooking device. An elliptical eyelet is built into the center of the occluder proximal arms to act as an attachment mechanism (Fig. 6). Each arm ends in a little 'eye' to prevent the distal end from perforating the vessel wall. Two double-disk prostheses are available in 12 and 17 mm diameters, the latter made with four wire arms (0.010 inch stainless steel) per disk but with the same spring and attachment mechanism.

The occluder delivery catheter system (Fig. 6) has an internal mechanism composed of a fine central core wire enclosed in a coiled spring delivery guidewire. The distal end of the wire is welded to a sleeve, with the central core wire passing through the length of the coiled spring wire and exiting the tip. The tip of the core wire ends in a polished knuckle that can be retracted within the sleeve by manipulating a slide plunger mechanism at the end of the

catheter and can be locked within the sleeve by a small slot on the plunger. The entire system is contained in an 85 cm long 8 Fr delivery catheter. The distal end of the delivery catheter is tipped with a thin-walled stainless steel tubular pod 1.7 cm long, also 8 Fr in size, although the larger device comes with an 11 Fr delivery pod on the same catheter French size. Prior to loading the umbrella onto the catheter, a small bend can be made on the core wire to prevent it from springing into the foam matrix of the device upon release. Loading the umbrella occluder to the catheter is accomplished by placing the knuckle on the central wire of the catheter into the eyelet on the occluder and retracting the wire into the sleeve. The two disks of the umbrella are then folded into the delivery pod, using a clear plastic loader depicted in Figure 7.

Method of closure. Although ductal closure can be accomplished with the catheter delivery system as described above from either venous or arterial entry, the use of a long sheath placed across the ductus from the

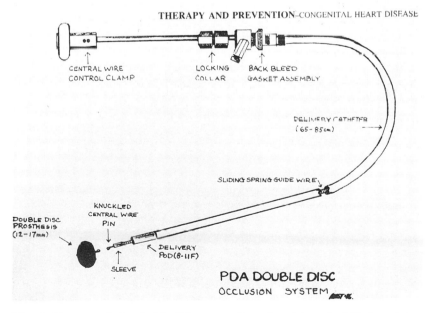

Fig. 6. Ductus occluder double disk system. (Reproduced from Rashkind *et al.* [16], with permission of the publisher.)

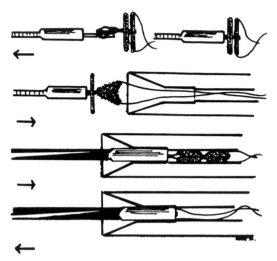

Fig. 7. Technique for loading the occluder onto the delivery catheter using a clear plastic loader. (Reproduced from Rashkind et al. [16], with permission of the publisher.)

venous circulation has achieved considerable clinical application and is the method of choice [16,26]. The clinical diagnosis should always be confirmed noninvasively prior to catheterization by two-dimensional and color-Doppler echocardiography, with particular emphasis placed on detecting associated lesions that could complicate the procedure (e.g., azygous continuation of the inferior cava), require an additional interventional procedure (such as balloon pulmonary valvotomy), or preclude catheter closure (e.g., an additional lesion that requires surgical intervention or the presence of pulmonary vascular disease). The procedure is ideally suited for patients weighing 8–10 kg or more and should not be performed in infants under 6 kg (particularly if the large diameter device need be deployed).

Special attention should also be directed to the transverse arch and isthmal region, where an unsuspected coarctation may be present. There is considerable variation in procedural details as practised among medical centers (i.e., the use coincident arterial cannulation, the number and type of angiograms, and so forth);

however, the essentials of the technique as presently applied at the Hospital for Sick Children, Toronto, are described below. The majority of procedures can be performed in an out-patient setting with discharge the afternoon of study [28].

As with any intravascular prosthetic device placement, particular care must be given to sterile technique, with endocarditis coverage given before and after the procedure. Acute bacterial endarteritis has occurred in both experimental and clinical settings when such coverage was not applied [27,29]. Our general approach has been to perform such procedures under general anesthesia, particularly with infants and children, although routine pre-catheterization sedation can be supplemented with ketamine (1 mg/kg, i.v. or i.m.) just prior to implantation.

From a percutaneous right femoral venous entry, a complete right heart catheterization with oximetry and pressure measurements is obtained in room air and the ductus crossed from its pulmonary artery end. If the pulmonary artery pressures are elevated, an 8 Fr balloon tipped side-hole catheter can be inflated within the ductus while measuring systemic and pulmonary artery pressures and saturations and administering 100% oxygen to assure that pulmonary vascular resistance is not elevated (particularly important in the older infant and child). Finally, if there is any question regarding an associated mild coarctation of the aorta, a balloon occlusion descending aortogram can be performed (Fig. 8).

Occasionally, the ductus may be found too small to cross with an 8 Fr catheter or a long sheath (o.d. 9 Fr) and may safely be dilated with progressively larger French sized catheters or a 4 mm balloon. Rarely, cannulation of the ductus from its pulmonary end is not possible. Retrograde arterial cannulation from the arterial ampulla into the pulmonary artery with an end-hole catheter (5 or 6 Fr), positioning (and retrieving) an exchange guidewire into the pulmonary artery or vena cava, and exteriorizing out the femoral vein (forming a femoral artery–

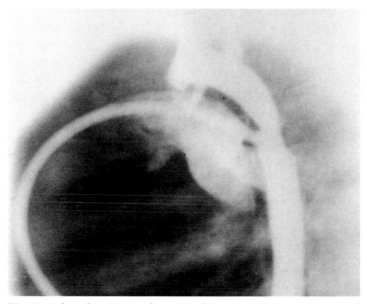

Fig. 8. A lateral angiogram from an infant with a ductus arteriosus and unsuspected mild coarctation, outlined by balloon occlusion aortography.

ductal–femoral vein loop) will facilitate venous–ductal cannulation [30].

The configuration of the ductus is identified in its anteroposterior and lateral projections from a descending aortogram using a 6, 7, or 8 Fr end- and side-hole angiographic transvenous catheter (Fig. 2A,B). A 260 cm long (0.035 inch) exchange guidewire is placed in the descending aorta and the catheter removed. A preshaped (to the sweep of the right ventricular outflow tract) long sheath and dilator is placed over the guidewire and maneuvered through the right heart, across the ductus, and into the descending aorta [26] (Fig. 9, 1). The dilator and wire are removed from the sheath and replaced with a loaded and locked Rashkind catheter delivery system. The delivery catheter is advanced within the sheath until the pod reaches the right atrium–tricuspid valve area, where the delivery wire is advanced to expel the occluder from the pod and into the sheath (Fig. 9, 2). The occluder is slowly advanced to the tip of the sheath (within the aorta) and the distal arms of the device opened by retracting the sheath back over the catheter held stationary. With the distal arms fully expanded, the catheter–sheath complex is pulled back to engage the ampulla of the ductus (Fig. 9, 3). Once the distal arms engage

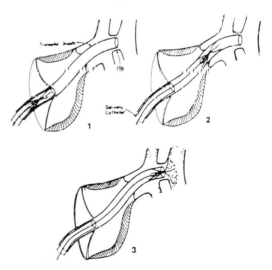

Fig. 9. Schematic of long sheath technique for delivery of the occluder system through the right heart for ductal occlusion. See text for explanation. (Reproduced from Lock et al. [2], with permission of the publisher.)

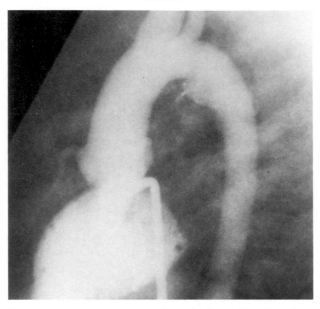

Fig. 10. Left ventriculogram after ductal occlusion. Note how the device sits with distal arms in aorta.

the ampulla, further retraction will fold the distal arms upon themselves as the occluder approaches the ductal–pulmonary artery insertion, the position of which is estimated from the lateral angiogram using the tracheal air shadow as an internal marker. With the central wire and delivery catheter fixed, the sheath is further retracted, allowing the proximal disk to spring open, securing the device within the ductus, straddling the ductal–pulmonary artery insertion (Fig. 2C). While maintaining gentle traction on the system, the release mechanism is activated, releasing the device within the ductus, and the sheath delivery system removed (Fig. 10). Postprocedure, a two-dimensional color Doppler study can be performed in the laboratory or prior to discharge. Follow-up is in 6 months and endocarditis prophylaxis continued. In those without Doppler evidence of residual shunting at that time, prophylaxis is not needed.

As mentioned above, two sizes of devices are available: 12 and 17 mm diameters. For a ductus 3.5 mm or less in narrowest diameter (at the pulmonary artery–ductal insertion) a 12 mm device should be used and, for up to 9 mm, the

17 mm device (the latter requiring placement of an 11 Fr long sheath–dilator delivery system). A ductus greater than 9 mm requires larger devices than are yet available for this technique.[1]

Clinical studies. A number of clinical series [16,28,29,31–33] have been published reporting several hundred patients. Successful implantation was accomplished in the majority (>90%) with elimination of clinical signs of left-to-right shunting. Within the first 48 hours, few patients retain ductal murmurs with correct placement, although a number may have residual shunts without murmurs (Doppler evidence of shunting, particularly over the superior aspect of the device [Fig. 11]) [29,34]. These residual shunts appear to be more frequent with the use of the 17 mm device [29], although ductal morphology appears not to be predictive of those who may have persistent shunting. Attempts to improve closure rates by soaking the device in a thrombin solution or

---

[1]Recent modifications now allow loading and delivery of the 12 mm device through a 6-Fr sheath and the 17 mm device via an 8-Fr sheath.

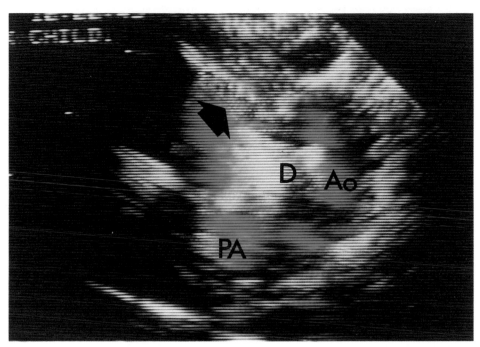

Fig. 11. Color Doppler after ductal occlusion. D, ductal occluder; blue color blood flow in aorta (Ao) and pulmonary artery (PA). Note turbulent flow (yellow streak, arrow) of small residual shunt left to right.

by pushing on the proximal arms of the device with a balloon-tipped catheter [28] have not been helpful in the Toronto experience (Vitiello, unpublished observations). Embolization to both systemic and pulmonary circulations have been encountered, with several patients requiring surgical referral. Catheter retrieval has been accomplished in both situations with snares, baskets, or grasping forceps. Care must be taken to retract the device fully into a long sheath (11 Fr) to avoid the arms catching on right heart structures [16,27,31].

From January 1985 through June 1990, at The Hospital for Sick Children/Toronto General Hospital, 200 procedures have been performed on 190 patients using the transvenous approach. Ages averaged 6.7 ± 9 (0.9–44.6) years; weights, 19.9 ± 15.1 (4–100) kg, and ductal diameters 2.7 ± 1.0 (0.5–8) mm. While 94% had an isolated ductus, two had associated pulmonary valve stenosis (both having percuta-

neous balloon valvotomies), and one each had an atrioventricular septal defect, a complex univentricular heart for which a Fontan procedure had been performed, an isolated small perimembranous ventricular septal defect, and left pulmonary artery stenosis. Two patients had previous surgical ligation and recannulization of their ductal lesions. Embolization occurred in four patients, one being the initial patient in the series. Three patients required surgical retrieval (two requiring cardiopulmonary bypass for intracardiac removal), and in one the device was removed with an intravascular retrieval catheter.

With pulsed and color-flow Doppler techniques, occlusion rates were evaluated in the initial 78 patients [34]. Thirty-eight percent had shunts detected 1 day after the procedure; falling to 27% at 6 months and to 25% at 1 year (two spontaneous late occlusions Fig. 12). Ten patients have undergone a second proce-

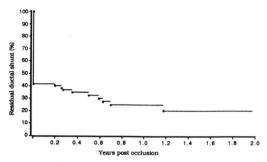

Fig. 12. Actuarial curve of residual shunt after 1 year follow-up.

dure, with successful placement of a second device in 8, giving a residual shunt rate of about 3% at 1–2 years [35]. In the latter procedures, those patients with continuous ductal murmurs have been found reoccludable (occasionally needing dilation to accommodate the sheath), while those with only echo Doppler evidence of incomplete closure have been found to have communications too small to cannulate even with a guidewire.

A few patients have demonstrated increased Doppler velocity shifts at the origin of the left pulmonary artery, presumably due to turbulance or to encroachment into the ostium of the left pulmonary artery. Follow-up studies have not demonstrated progressive obstruction to flow with estimated gradients of not more than 7 mmHg (Fig. 13). Finally, three patients (two in our studies) have experienced hemolysis after device placement, with coexistent residual shunting [36]. Two required surgical removal and ductal ligation to control the hemolytic anemia, presumably due to a residual high velocity jet hitting the proximal disk with resultant red cell destruction.

Transfemoral Plug Closure

The principle of the Porstmann method [8–12] is depicted in Figure 14. A catheter is inserted from the femoral artery across the ductus into the right heart. Either the catheter itself or an exchange length guidewire is snared from the contralateral vein and exteriorized, forming a femoral artery–ductal–femoral vein loop. This wire will serve as a guide over which to place a conical or spring guarded plug made of polyvinyl alcohol foam. The plug is introduced through a tubular applicator and threaded over the track wire. After complete closure, the guidewire track is removed from the venous side, and the plug is wedged into the ductus. The lower age limit for transfemoral plug closure is between 3 and 4 years [11]. Basically, the success of the technique depends on the ratio of the lumen of the femoral artery to that of the ductus, allowing an appropriate sized plug to be placed arterially. It is difficult to make a plug less than 3 mm, and therefore the femoral artery must be greater than 3 mm to accommodate the larger sized plastic, 20%–40% larger than the ductus. With improved cannulation materials, Sato et al. [12] believed that a ductus larger than the femoral artery could be closed; however, they may require direct arterial exposure for plug entry.

Clinical results. Several hundred cases of persistently patent ductus arteriosus have undergone occlusion with this method. In 109 cases commented on by Porstmann et al. [37], no mortality and only minor morbidity were noted. In eight cases the method was unsuccessful. In five the ductus was too large and the plug slipped into the pulmonary artery. Since the plug was still attached to the guidewire, the dislocated plug was maneuvered into the femoral vein and removed by venectomy. In the remaining three cases, because of the rigidity or small size of the ductus, the plug could not be fixed, was allowed to embolize to the aortic bifurcation, and then removed by arteriotomy.

Fig. 13. **Top:** Distal arms of the occluder in the pulmonary artery (arrows). **Middle:** Doppler signal from main pulmonary artery (MPA) to left pulmonary artery (LPA). Note slight increase in flow velocity. **Bottom:** Pulmonary arteriogram after ductal occlusion. Note mildly narrowed left pulmonary artery and distal arms of occluder in aorta.

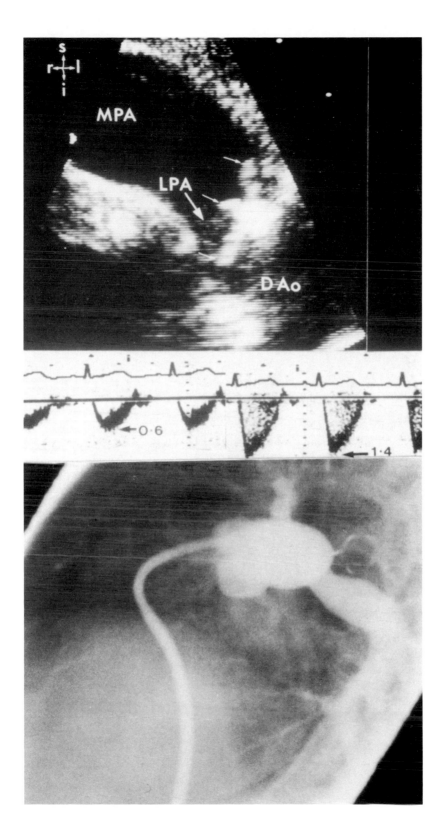

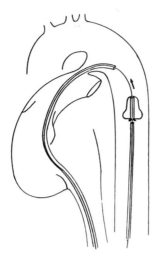

Fig. 14. Schematic representation of the Porstmann technique for plug occlusion. See text for details. (Reproduced from Sato *et al.*, with permission of the publisher.)

Disadvantages of the Porstmann technique include arterial entry with a need for arterial exposure under certain circumstances and possible arterial damage, the requirement for a transductal arterial–venous loop (venectomy for device retrieval), and the limitation on age for closure. Advantages, however, include a secured delivery system, which avoids free embolization with placement. Despite the early clinical trials and success of this approach, it remains technically complex and, except in a few medical centers worldwide, has not achieved a large clinical application. The Rashkind *et al.* approach, with Mullins' transvenous modification, has simplicity and ease of operation in its favor and, importantly, it can be used in small infants and children. Furthermore, the occluder device is of standard configuration, applicable in ductuses of variable configuration.[2]

---

[2]Editor's note: A third device is also available on a protocol basis; this is "buttoned" device and is discussed in chapter 18.

REFERENCES

1. Benson LN, Freedom RMF (1989): Interventional cardiac catheterization in congenital heart disease. In Braunwald E (ed): "Heart Disease Update." No. 4, pp 83–96.
2. Lock JE, Keane JF, Fellow KE (1987): "Diagnostic and Interventional Catheterization in Congenital Heart Disease." Boston: Martinus Nijhoff.
3. Munro JC (1907): Ligation of the ductus arteriosus. Ann Surg 46:335–338.
4. Graybiel A, Strieder JW, Boyer NH (1938): An attempt to obliterate the patent ductus arteriosus in a patient with bacterial endocarditis. Am Heart J 15:621–624.
5. Gross RE, Hubbard JP (1939): Surgical ligation of a patent ductus arteriosus. A report of first successful case. JAMA 112:729–731.
6. Jones JC (1965): Twenty-five years experience with the surgery of patent ductus arteriosus. J Thorac Cardiovasc Surg 50:149–165.
7. Panagopoulos PHG, Tatooles CJ, Aberdeen E, Waterston DJ, Bonham-Carter RE (1971): Patent ductus arteriosus in infants and children. A review of 936 operations (1946–1969). Thorax 26:137–144.
8. Porstmann W, Wierny L, Warnke H (1967): Der Verschluss des Ductus arteriosus persistens ohne Thorakotomie (vor 1 a ufige Mitterlung). Thoraxchicurgie 15:199–203.
9. Kitamura S, Sato K, Naito Y, Shimizu, Y, Fujino M, Oyama C, Nakano S, Kawashima Y (1976): Plug closure of patent ductus arteriosus by transfemoral catheter method. Chest 70:631–635.
10. Porstmann W, Wierny L, Warnke H: Der Vershlussdes Ductus arteriosus persistens ohne Thorakotomie (zweite Mitterlung). Fortschr Rontgenstr 109:133–148.
11. Porstmann W, Wierny L, Warnke H, Gerstberger G, Romaniuk PA (1971): Catheter closure of patent ductus arteriosus. Radiol Clin North Am 9:203–218.
12. Sato K, Fujino M, Kozuka T, Naito Y, Kitamura S, Makano S, Ohyama C, Kawashima Y (1975): Transfemoral plug closure of patent ductus arteriosus. Circulation 51:337–341.
13. Leslie J, Lindsay W, Amplatz K (1977): Nonsurgical closure of patent ductus arteriosus: An experimental study. Invest Radiol 12:142–145.
14. Mills ML, King TD (1976): Nonoperative closure of left-to-right shunts. J Thorac Cardiovasc Surg 72:371–378.
15. Rashkind WJ, Cuaso CC (1979): Transcatheter closure of patent ductus arteriosus: Successful use in a 3.5 kilogram infant. Pediatr Cardiol 1:3–7.
16. Rashkind WJ, Mullins CE, Hellenbrand WE, Tait

MA (1987): Nonsurgical closure of the patent ductus arteriosus: Clinical application of the Rashkind PDA Occluder System. Circulation 75:583-592.

17. Olley PM (1987): Ductus arteriosus: Its persistence and its patency. In Anderson RH, et al. (eds): "Pediatric Cardiology." pgs 931-957, Churchill-Livingstone, Edinburgh.

18. Gittenberger-de-Groot AC (1977): Patent ductus arteriosus: Most probably a primary congenital malformation. Br Heart J 39:610-618.

19. Bakker PM (1962): "Morfogense en envolutie van de ductus arteriosus." Thesis, Leiden.

20. Krichenko A, Benson L, Burrows P, Moes CAF, McLaughlin P, Freedom RM (1989): Angiographic classification of the isolated persistently patent ductus arteriosus and implications for percutaneous catheter occlusion. Am J Cardiol 63:877-880.

21. Hoffman E (1964): Die obliteration des ductus Botalli Langenbeck. Arch Klin Chir 306:289.

22. Everett NB, Johnson RJ (1951): A physiologic and anatomic study of the ductus arteriosus in dog. Anat Rec 110:103.

23. Barnard WG (1939): Pathologic changes in the wall of the ductus arteriosus. St. Thomas Hosp Rep (2nd Ser) 4:72.

24. Warnecke I, Frank J, Hohle R, Lemm W, Bucherl ES (1984): Transvenous double-balloon occlusion of the persistent ductus arteriosus: An experimental study. Pediatr Cardiol 5:79-84.

25. Magal C, Wright KC, Dupart Jr G, Wallace S, Gianturco C (1989): A new device for transcatheter closure of the patent ductus arteriosus: A feasibility study in dogs. Invest Radiol 24:272-276.

26. Bash GE, Mullins CE (1984): Insertion of patent ductus occluder by transvenous approach: A new technique. Circulation 70:(Suppl II): II-285.

27. Lock JL, Bass JI, Timil C, Rycavy JA, Lucas RV Jr (1985): Transcatheter closure of patent ductus arteriosus in piglets. Am J Cardiol 55:826-829.

28. Wessel DL, Keane JF, Parness I, Lock JE (1988):

Outpatient closure of the patent ductus arteriosus. Circulation 77:1068-1071.

29. Dyck JD, Benson LN, Smallhorn JF, McLaughlin P, Freedom PM, Rowe RD (1988): Catheter occlusion of the persistently patent ductus arteriosus: Initial experience and early followup. Am J Cardiol 62:1089-1092.

30. Benson LN, Dyck J, Hecht B (1988): Technique for closure of the small patent ductus arteriosus using the Rashkind occluder. Cathet Cardiovasc Diagn 14:82-84.

31. Latson LA, Hofschire PJ, Kugler JD, Cheatham JP, Gumbiner CH, Danford DA (1989): Transcatheter closure of patent ductus arteriosus in pediatric patients. J Pediatr 115:549-553.

32. Ali Khan MA, Mullins CE, Nihill MR, AL Yousef S, Al Oufy S, Abdullah M, Al Fagih MR, Swayer W (1989): Percutaneous catheter closure of the ductus arteriosus in children and young adults. Am J Cardiol 64:218-221.

33. Perry SB, Keane JF, Lock JE (1987): Interventional catheterization in pediatric congenital and acquired heart disease. Am J Cardiol 61:(Suppl):109G-117G.

34. Musewe NN, Benson LN, Smallhorn JS, Freedom RM (1989): Two-dimensional echocardiographic and colour-Doppler evaluation of ductal occlusion with the Rashkind prosthesis. Circulation 80:1706-1710.

35. Hosking MCK, Benson LN, Musewe N, Freedom RM (1989): Reocclusion for persistent shunting after catheter placement of the Rashkind patent ductus arteriosus occluder. Can J Cardiol 5:340-342.

36. Ladusans EJ, Murdoch I, Franciosi J (1998): Severe haemolysis after percutaneous closure of a ductus arteriosus (arterial duct). Br Heart J 61:548-550.

37. Porstmann W, Mieronymi K, Wierny L, Warnke H (1974): Nonsurgical closure of oversized patent ductus arteriosus with pulmonary hypertension. Circulation 50:376-381.

17

Transcatheter Closure of Atrial Septal Defects

Larry A. Latson, M.D.

Division of Pediatric Cardiology, University of Nebraska Medical
Center, Omaha, Nebraska 68198-2166

INTRODUCTION

The development of a safe and effective technique for transcatheter closure of atrial septal defects (ASDs) is attractive for a number of reasons. Secundum atrial septal defect is one of the more common congenital heart defects, accounting for approximately 7% of congenital cardiac defects detected clinically during childhood [1,2]. Untreated patients have an increasing incidence of arrhythmias, cardiomegaly, congestive heart failure, and pulmonary hypertension with age. Therefore, surgical therapy is generally recommended if the left to right shunt is moderate or large [3]. However, most young patients with an isolated ASD have few symptoms, and the prospect of a major open heart operation (and the resulting scar) may be very distressing to families of these often minimally symptomatic children (approximately two-thirds of whom are females). The ease of manipulation of a catheter across an ASD and the relatively large size of most patients (closure of an ASD is only rarely required in infancy) are other factors leading to the relatively early development of transcatheter devices to close this defect.

ASD OCCLUSION DEVICE OF KING AND MILLS

In 1974, King and Mills [4] developed a catheter device to close experimental ASDs. The device consisted of two independent umbrella-like components made of stainless steel and dacron. Placement of the device was accomplished through a femoral venous cutdown (the delivery catheter was quite large). The left atrial umbrella was pushed through an outer catheter that was placed in the left atrium, and an "opening cone" advanced over the obturator guidewire was needed to open the arms of this device fully. The opened umbrella was retracted against the atrial septum, and the right atrial umbrella was then delivered over the obturator guidewire that was attached to the left atrial umbrella. Pushing on the right atrial umbrella with a locking catheter forced the right atrial umbrella to open, and further pressure resulted in locking of the left and right atrial umbrellas to each other (Fig. 1). The threaded obturator guidewire was then unscrewed to release the double umbrella. In 1976, Mills and King [5] reported successful placement of a device in 5 of 10 patients in whom the procedure was attempted. The device, however, was never developed to the point of routine clinical use, perhaps because of its large size and relatively complex method of delivery.

RASHKIND ASD OCCLUSION DEVICE

Following development and early clinical trials of the Bard PDA Umbrella device, Dr. William Rashkind turned his attention to developing a device for transcatheter closure of ASDs. Several experimental devices were evaluated, and a final design was approved by the FDA for multicenter clinical trials in 1987. The initial

Transcatheter Therapy in Pediatric Cardiology, pages 335–348

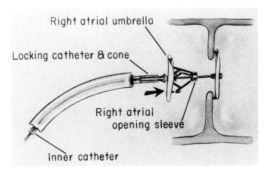

Fig. 1. King-Mills ASD Occlusion Device. The distal umbrella has been opened in the left atrium and is against the left atrial side of the septum. The right atrial umbrella is being pushed over the threaded obturator guidewire by the locking catheter and cone. Pressure on the locking catheter and cone causes expansion of the right atrial umbrella, and further pressure causes the left and right atrial umbrellas to lock together. The threaded obturator guidewire is then unscrewed and the catheters and guidewire are removed. (Reproduced from King and Mills [4], with permission of the publisher.)

Rashkind device consisted of a single self-expanding umbrella with six stainless steel arms covered by the same polyurethane foam material utilized in the Bard PDA Umbrella device (USCI Division, CR Bard, Inc., Billerica, MA). Three of the umbrella arms were tipped with sharp "fishhook-like" barbs designed to penetrate into the atrial septum and to hold the device in place. Flexible centering arms on the delivery system were designed to maintain the device in a central location with relation to the defect as the system was pulled against the atrial septum (Fig. 2).

The Rashkind ASD Occluder (USCI Division, Bard) had to be loaded into the delivery system with great care so that the hooks did not become entangled in the foam or other arms. The presence of these hooks required that the delivery system be relatively large (16 Fr). To use the device, a long transseptal sheath was placed across the ASD from the femoral

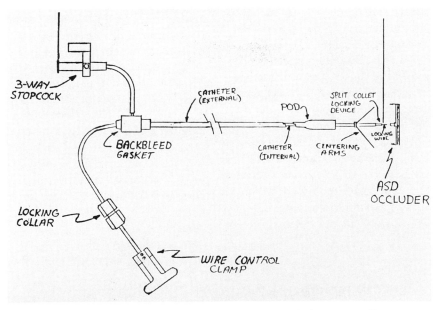

Fig. 2. Rashkind ASD Occluder. The Rashkind ASD Occluder was a self-expanding polyurethane-covered disk with six arms. Three of the arms had barbs to hold the device against the atrial septum. The ASD Occluder was attached to the locking wire and carefully folded toward the base of the centering arms. The centering arms and occluder were then withdrawn into the pod by pulling on the extension rod, which contained the locking collar and wire control clamp that activated the release mechanism.

vein and the delivery system was then advanced through the sheath. The sheath was retracted to the inferior vena cava once the delivery system was in the left atrium. The device was then advanced out of the pod, and the arms were allowed to open in the cavity of the left atrium. Once the arms attained their maximal opening, the entire delivery system was retracted. The centering arms on the delivery system ideally kept the device centered with respect to the ASD. When the arms were seen to bend against the atrial septum, a sharp tug was used to "set" the barbs of the hooked arms of the device. If the device was in the correct position, then left atrial pressure plus the hooks on the three arms kept the ASD device in position against the left atrial side of the atrial septum.

Animal studies indicated that the device could work to close experimental ASDs, but some problems were foreseen. It was found that the foam material fairly rapidly became occlusive as the pores filled with fibrin material and that fibrous attachment of any areas of contact of the foam with myocardium began within 1 week after placement of the device [6]. It was also found that embolization of the device because of incorrect positioning or purposeful release in both the left and right atria resulted in no instances of acute hemodynamic deterioration. The devices would follow the flow of blood and bend or turn to be nonobstructive unless purposely implanted in a position to obstruct flow. The device was highly successful in closing experimental ASDs in cows, but in sheep and pigs the relatively smaller atrial septum made accurate placement of the device more difficult. The animal studies indicated that one arm of the device could easily contact the roof or posterior wall of the left atrium and a hook could imbed in that position. If this occurred, then the position of the other hooks was predetermined to be incorrect (Fig. 3).

ASD closure using the Rashkind device was attempted in a small number of patients in a limited multicenter trial. The device was successfully placed in approximately two-thirds of the patients. There were no long-term complications from devices that were improperly placed or that embolized. However, the investigators felt that the large size of the delivery system and the inability to reposition the device after even one of the barbed arms contacted a structure in the heart made the device less than optimal and not acceptable for routine clinical use.

BARD CLAMSHELL SEPTAL UMBRELLA

Because of the success of the (Rashkind) hookless Bard PDA Umbrella in closing a small number of baffle leaks and small ASDs [7], the device was modified to enhance its ability to occlude septal defects. The PDA Umbrella was designed to cause an obstruction in a narrow tube. In order to use the double umbrella system as a means to close a defect in a relatively thin septum, a second spring was placed in the center of the umbrella arms to bring the tips of the arms back toward the opposing umbrella so that the device would clamp on opposite sides of a thin septum (Fig. 4). On the most recent modification of the device, the umbrellas each have four arms and are covered with dacron mesh rather than polyurethane foam. This design allows the delivery system to be reduced to 11 Fr (regardless of the length of the arms of the umbrella). Because this device has no hooks on the arms, it can be easily repositioned in the left atrium and/or removed from the body if necessary.

Studies of human pathology specimens demonstrated that the majority of ASDs are suitable in position and size for closure by the Clamshell ASD occlusion device [8]. Dr. James Lock developed the technique for using the Clamshell Septal Umbrella to close ASDs (USCI Division, Bard) and in his early animal studies the device was successful in closing six of eight experimental ASDs in lambs. Histologic studies showed that the devices were covered by endothelium in 1 to 2 months and that the dacron material became densely adher-

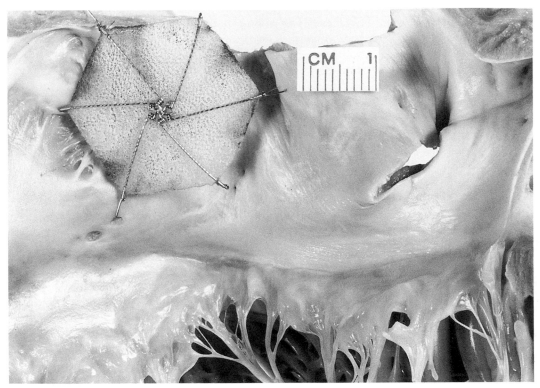

Fig. 3. Rashkind ASD Occluder pathologic specimen. View of the opened left atrium with a recently (less than 1 hour) implanted Rashkind ASD Occluder covering an experimental ASD (not shown). Barbed extensions are seen on the arms in the 3 o'clock, 7 o'clock, and 11 o'clock positions. Notice that the hook of the arm in the 3 o'clock position was caught in a fold along the posterior left atrium, and the posterior part of the device is therefore not in contact with the atrial septum.

ent to areas of contact with the atrial septum by ingrowth of fibrous tissue [8].

TECHNIQUE FOR USE OF CLAMSHELL ASD DEVICE

The Clamshell ASD occlusion device is delivered percutaneously through an 11 Fr long sheath from the femoral vein. A complete right heart catheterization is performed to evaluate the pulmonary to systemic flow ratio and pulmonary artery pressures and to rule out the possibility of anomalous drainage of any of the pulmonary veins. The catheter is passed across the ASD and into at least one right and one left pulmonary vein. Because size and location of the ASD are important in determining the most appropriate sized device to use, an angiogram with the catheter in the right upper pulmonary vein is generally recommended. The device is not suitable to close sinus venosus or ostium primum ASDs.

Although the angiogram helps to delineate the region of the atrial septal defect and the presence of tissue above and below the defect, it very often is inadequate for accurate sizing. It is important to determine the "stretched diameter" of the ASD, since this measurement has been found to correlate best with the size of the device that will be needed. An exchange length guidewire is placed in the left upper pulmonary vein, and the venous catheter is removed. A

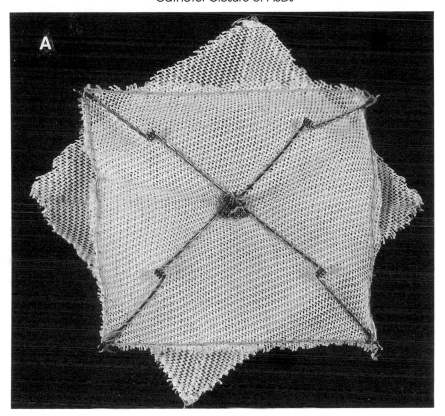

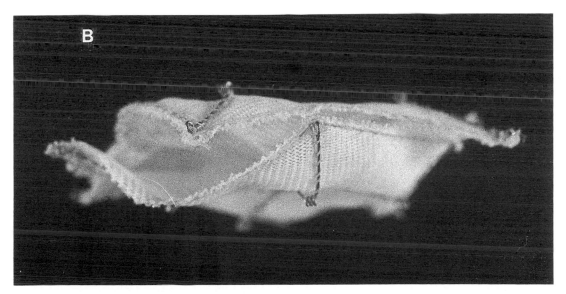

Fig. 4. Bard Clamshell Septal Umbrella. **A:** The Clamshell device is composed of two opposing umbrellas similar to the design of the Bard PDA Umbrella. A spring in the center of each arm of the device adds a second angle to bring the tip of each arm back toward the opposing umbrella. **B:** Side view of the Bard Clamshell Septal Umbrella. This view illustrates the shape of the arms of the umbrellas and why the device is called a "clamshell."

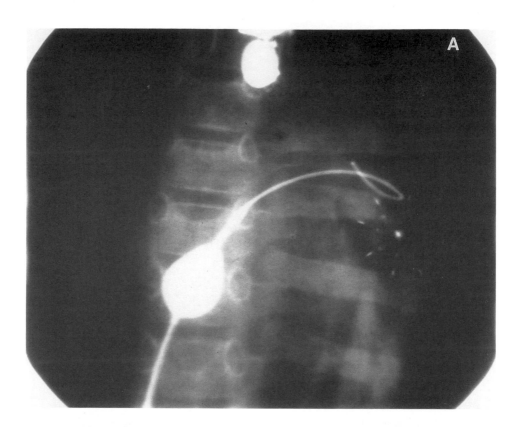

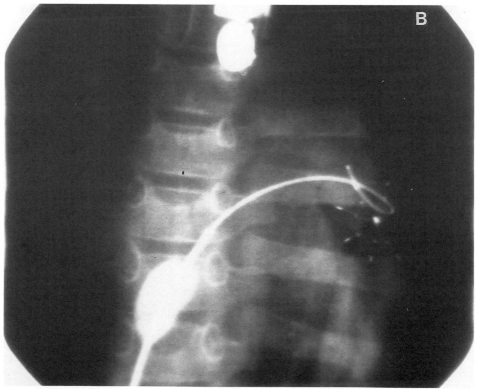

balloon-tipped catheter with a relatively soft balloon (Meditech Large Occlusion Balloon Catheter) is advanced over the guidewire to the left atrium. This balloon is inflated under fluoroscopy with a known amount of contrast material and gently pulled against the atrial septal opening (Fig. 5). If the balloon easily passes through the ASD, it is readvanced to the left atrium and filled with slightly more contrast material. A cineangiogram is recorded of the balloon as it is pulled through the ASD with just enough contrast material in it to create a "waist" in the balloon. During filming of the cineangiogram, an ASD occlusion device can be left on the patient's chest for a rough comparison of the diameter of the waist in the balloon to the fully extended diameter of the occlusion device. For a more accurate measurement, a grid can be recorded in the position of the heart without moving the imaging tubes (to be certain that the tube to image intensifier distance does not change). The position of the atrial septum as the balloon pulls through the septum is also noted for reference when the ASD occlusion device is being placed. If multiple ASDs are present, then the stretched diameter of the particular defect that the balloon catheter passes through will not give an accurate indication of the total extent of the septum involved with defects. We have found that transesophageal echocardiography is especially helpful in these patients.

The Clamshell Septal Umbrella is best suited to close small- to moderate-sized ASDs. Present devices ranged in size from 17 to 40 mm. The size (length of diagonal of one umbrella) of the Bard Clamshell Septal Umbrella to be utilized should be at least 1.6 times the stretched diameter of the ASD. Defects larger than 25 mm in stretched diameter are generally considered too large to be closed with even the 40 mm ASD device. Most such defects have very little remaining tissue around the defect (except in large adult patients), and the construction of the devices will allow even the 40 mm device to slip to the inferior portion of the ASD and not cover the defect properly.

Once it is determined that the defect is an appropriate size and in the appropriate position, the best-sized Clamshell device is selected and soaked in a saline solution as the 11 Fr long delivery sheath is positioned in the left upper pulmonary vein or left atrium over a guidewire. Because of the risk of air embolization, it is vital that careful technique be utilized to ensure that the long sheath remains completely filled with fluid and air bubbles are not allowed to be drawn into it. One technique to ensure that the sheath remains completely filled is to use a Y Adapter (USCI Pediatric TB-I) on the end of the dilator. This device provides a side port on the end of the dilator so that the space between the dilator and the guidewire can be flushed with fluid. Flushing is continued as the sheath and dilator are advanced over the guidewire and until the sheath is positioned in the left upper pulmonary vein. Continuous flushing can then continue as the dilator and guidewire are removed as a single unit. This continuous flushing should keep the long sheath completely filled with fluid during the withdrawal process.

The Clamshell Septal Umbrella is then loaded into the delivery system by using an acrylic folding block identical to the system utilized for folding the Bard PDA Umbrella.

Fig. 5. ASD sizing. **A:** A sizing balloon catheter has been advanced over a guidewire that is in the left upper pulmonary vein. A septal occlusion device has been placed on the patient's chest and is shown just below the loop in the guidewire. A transesophageal echocardiography probe is shown in the upper portion of the picture. **B:** The sizing balloon has been retracted, and a waist is shown in the center portion of the balloon as it comes through the ASD. Notice how low the atrial septum is when traction is applied to pull the balloon through the ASD. Comparison of the waist in the balloon with a radiologic grid is the most accurate way to determine the stretch diameter of the ASD.

The delivery catheter is inserted through the long sheath and fluid is continuously infused through the sidearm of the sheath as the delivery system is advanced (to prevent forming a vacuum and drawing air into the sheath behind the delivery pod). The delivery pod is advanced slowly until it is near the lower part of the right atrium (Fig. 6). The extension rod at the end of the catheter is then used to push the device out of the delivery catheter and into the long sheath, which serves as an extension of the delivery pod. The device is advanced to near the end of the long sheath and held in place by maintaining the position of the extension rod. The long delivery sheath is then slowly withdrawn to allow opening of the distal umbrella. Care must be taken not to withdraw the sheath too far, because this would allow expansion of the proximal umbrella in the left atrium. The entire sheath and the delivery system are gradually withdrawn to allow full opening of the distal arms of the umbrella in the left atrium. Care must be taken to ensure that the arms can open fully and that none of the arms are trapped in the pulmonary veins or common pulmonary venous chamber. The sheath and delivery system are then gradually withdrawn further until the arms of the distal umbrella can be seen to bend against the atrial septum.

Because of the angle of the atrial septum (relatively vertical) in relation to the angle of opening of the umbrella (relatively horizontal), the superior arms of the device will contact the atrial septum before the inferior arms of the device are in a position to contact the atrial septum. If the device is large in relation to the

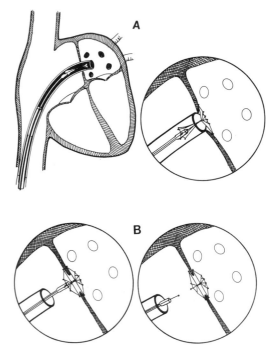

Fig. 6. Use of the Bard Clamshell Septal Umbrella to close an ASD. **A:** In the left-hand diagram, the long delivery sheath has been placed in the left atrium, and the delivery system has been advanced through the sheath. The delivery pod is shown in the low right atrium, and the folded clamshell device is near the end of the delivery sheath. In the right-hand illustration, the distal umbrella has been pushed out of the long delivery sheath and has opened in the left atrium. The umbrella has been pulled against the left atrial side of the atrial septum. **B:** In the left-hand illustration, the delivery sheath has been further withdrawn to allow expansion of the right atrial umbrella. In the right-hand illustration, the clamshell device has been released and remains in place to close the ASD. The delivery sheath and catheter can be removed from the body. (Reproduced from Lock et al. [8], with permission of the publisher.)

Fig. 7. Transesophageal echocardiography during Clamshell Umbrella placement. **A:** A properly positioned device with both umbrellas expanded. This echocardiographic plane demonstrates nearly the full length of the left atrial (LA) umbrella in close proximity to the atrial septum (arrows). The right atrial (RA) umbrella is only partially shown in this view, but it is clear that there are no arms of the device protruding through the ASD. **B:** Clamshell Umbrella in poor position. This echocardiographic image demonstrates that the left atrial umbrella has pulled through the atrial septum (arrows), and three of the arms of the device are now in the right atrium. When this occurs, the angle of the device is such that the umbrella can be seen in a "planar" view while the atrial septum is seen in cross section.

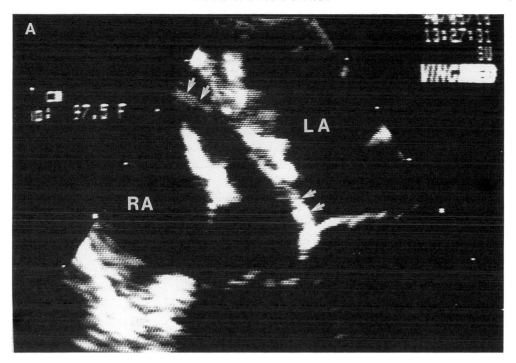

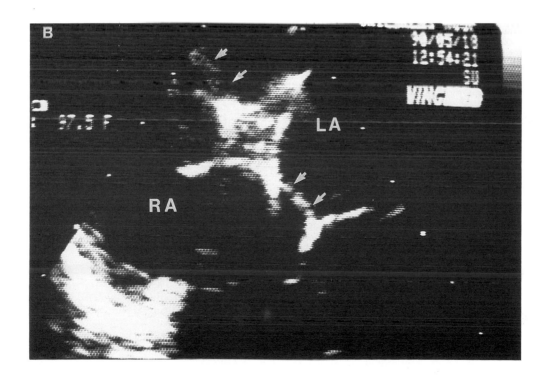

ASD, then there is little concern about pulling the device completely through the ASD. However, if the amount of tissue at the upper part of the atrial septum is relatively limited, it is quite easy to pull one or more of the top arms through. If this occurs and is unrecognized, then the device will not be oriented correctly and the risk of embolization is high. Transesophageal echocardiography is especially helpful at this point to ascertain that all of the arms of the distal umbrella are in fact in the left atrium (Fig. 7). If transesophageal echocardiography is not available, an injection of contrast into the right pulmonary artery will help to delineate the plane of the atrial septum and show the ASD occlusion device (Fig. 8).

If the ASD occlusion device is not in good position and only the distal arms of the umbrella have been extended, then simple traction on the delivery system will cause the distal arms to fold into the delivery system again. It may then be necessary to repeat the entire process to reposition the long sheath before attempting again to deploy the distal umbrella of this or a larger device.

Once the distal umbrella is in proper position against the atrial septum and held with slight tension, the sheath is slowly retracted as the device is held in place. This allows the proximal arms of the device to open in the right atrium. The position of both sets of arms can again be checked by transesophageal echocardiography or by a pulmonary arteriogram. Gentle movement of the delivery system helps to confirm that all of the arms are in contact with part of the atrial septum. If the device seems to be in proper position, then the release mechanism can be activated to release

the delivery wire from the Clamshell device. There will generally be a slight change in position of the device as the tension on the atrial septum is released. An arteriogram after injection of contrast into either the pulmonary artery or the right atrium (through the long sheath) can then be performed to see if there is evidence of a significant left-to-right or right-to-left shunt. Minimal catheter manipulation in the area of the occlusion device is recommended because of the possibility of dislodging the device early after it is placed. The cineangiogram will demonstrate the position of the ASD occlusion device in relation to the plane of the atrial septum. If the device is in good position and there is only a small amount of left-to-right shunting visible, then there is generally no reason for concern. The woven dacron mesh is relatively porous for a short period of time, and small leaks can occur in areas where the dacron material does not make good contact with the atrial septum. Many of these areas will eventually seal as tissue reaction occurs.

PROBLEMS WITH PLACEMENT OF THE CLAMSHELL ASD OCCLUSION DEVICE

As mentioned previously, if only the distal umbrella has been allowed to open, the device can easily be withdrawn into the 11 Fr long sheath if necessary. If only one or two of the arms have pulled through the ASD, then the entire system and long sheath can be advanced and the arms may bend and return to the left atrial side of the atrial septum. Slight rotation of the sheath may be sufficient to reposition the arms so that they properly engage the left

Fig. 8. Angiography during placement of the Clamshell Septal Umbrella. **A:** The left atrial umbrella has been opened and pulled against the atrial septum with slight tension. A second catheter was placed in the right pulmonary artery for an arteriogram to delineate the atrial septum. Notice the relatively horizontal orientation of the plane of the umbrella with cephalad bending of the superior (closest to the right upper pulmonary vein) arms. **B:** Levophase of a pulmonary arteriogram after release of the occlusion device. The ASD occlusion device is seen in a side view in good location along the atrial septum. The left atrium and left ventricle are filled, but little or no contrast is seen in the right atrium.

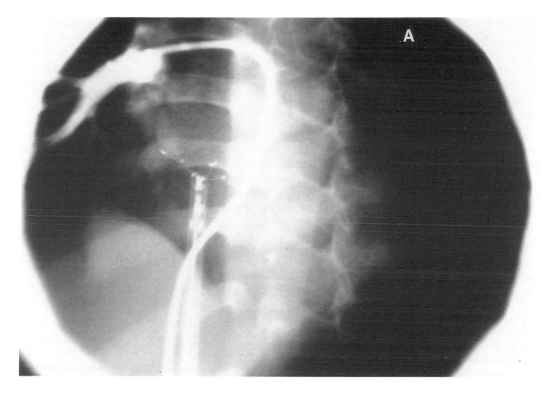

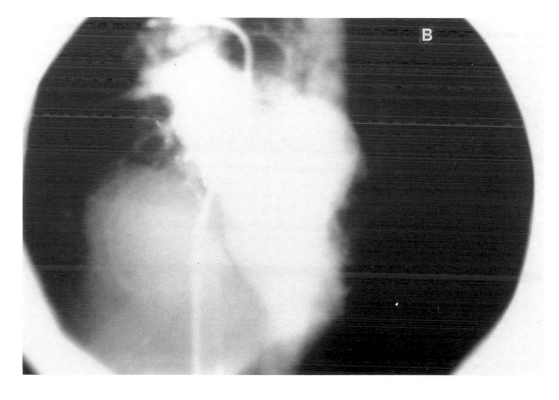

atrial side of the atrial septum. If the system cannot be easily advanced back to the left atrium, then traction on the delivery system will cause the distal arms to refold into the 11 Fr sheath and the system can be withdrawn. The device generally cannot be retracted back into the pod of the delivery system, and the device may be distorted as it is pulled out the end of the long sheath; thus a new device may be needed for a second attempt.

If both the distal and proximal arms of the device are allowed to expand before incorrect positioning is recognized (or occurs), then removal of the device can be more difficult. Simple traction on the delivery system will force the proximal arms to collapse in the opposite direction of their intended folded positions. Thus the system can usually not be fully withdrawn into the 11 Fr sheath. The entire Clamshell can then be withdrawn as much as possible into the delivery pod and then as far as possible into the delivery sheath. Care must be taken not to exert too much tension, because this will cause detachment of the Clamshell device from the safety wire. Although the arms may extend slightly past the mouth of the delivery sheath, the sheath can generally be retracted easily into the inferior vena cava and through the insertion site in the groin. If this maneuver is necessary, it is possible to maintain access to the vein when the entire system is removed. Before collapsing the Clamshell device, the delivery pod is advanced to the proximal umbrella and the long sheath is retracted until the large delivery pod is outside the end of the sheath. It is then possible to advance a guidewire through the long sheath (along side the delivery catheter), and, if the pod is out of the sheath, then the guidewire can extend through the end of the sheath and be placed high into the superior vena cava or innominate vein. The tip of the guidewire will still be in the patient's body, and a new sheath and delivery system can then be advanced into position and the entire process repeated.

If improper positioning is not recognized and the device embolizes, it most commonly will embolize to the right atrium or right ventricle. Surprisingly, the device has a marked tendency to turn in the direction to cause least resistance to blood flow. Because it is relatively flexible, even moderate pressure forces the arms to bend, and the likelihood of the device causing occlusion of either the tricuspid or pulmonary orifice appears to be quite small. Particularly if the device embolizes to the right ventricle or pulmonary artery, it is important to collapse the arms of the device completely before trying to pull it out, since the arms can become entangled in the chordae or valve apparatus if tension is applied. Therefore a larger (14 Fr) long sheath needs to be inserted. A grasping catheter (USCI Urologic grasping catheter) can then be inserted through the long sheath and manipulated to the area of the device. The device can be grasped and withdrawn into the large sheath by collapsing the arms with tension on the grasping catheter and device.

ASSESSMENT OF LONG-TERM RESULTS OF THE CLAMSHELL ASD OCCLUSION DEVICE

As of the spring of 1990, approximately 100 patients had been enrolled in an FDA-approved multicenter trial of the Clamshell ASD occlusion device. A device was successfully placed in 93% of patients. Patients in whom a device was not left in place included those who were found at catheterization to have a defect that was too large to attempt placement. The device was used in one patient to close temporarily an ASD in order to better evaluate the patient's pulmonary hypertension. Use of this device demonstrated that elimination of a small right-to-left shunt resulted in an increase in the patient's pulmonary artery pressure, and the patient was therefore not submitted to previously planned surgery.

A device embolized in three patients. The embolized device was retrieved nonsurgically in one patient in whom it had become dislodged during movement of a transvenous pacemaker lead. In the other two patients, it was removed at the time of surgical closure of an ASD that was thought to be too large for success. Two of the embolizations occurred during the catheterization procedure. One embolization to the right ventricle occurred sometime in the first month after placement of the device and was discovered at a 1 month follow-up visit. This patient had a large defect and had been subjected to vigorous chest percussion and physiotherapy (unbeknownst to the cardiologist) for an unrelated pulmonary disease.

In the first year of use of the device, there were no mortalities or long-term morbidities. There were no instances of clinically detectable thromboemboli or arrhythmias. Follow-up evaluations on all patients have been by non-invasive means. Complete closure of the ASDs has been demonstrated by color Doppler in 84% of patients in whom the device was placed. The remaining patients have demonstrated disappearance of clinical signs of a significant left-to-right shunt, and any residual defects have been thought to be small by echocardiographic criteria.[1]

INDICATIONS FOR USE OF CLAMSHELL OCCLUSION DEVICE IN PATIENTS WITH ASD

The Clamshell ASD occlusion device can be considered for use in any patient with a secundum ASD. The device is not suitable for primum or sinus venosus ASDs. It is also not appropriate for use in patients with anomalous pulmonary venous return or in patients with endocarditis or other active infections. The size of a secundum ASD is important in patient selection. Defects that are clinically and echocardiographically considered to be *large* usually do not have sufficient tissue around the defect to allow proper placement of the umbrella arms. In older patients, such defects are over 25 mm in diameter. In younger patients, the actual diameter will vary depending on the size of the patient. Defects with an echocardiographic diameter greater than two-thirds of the length of the atrial septum are less likely to be closable because of the need to use a device at least 1.6 times the diameter of the defect. In uncomplicated ASDs, the defects should be large enough that the patients would be considered surgical candidates: They should exhibit clinical findings of right ventricular enlargement, have at least mild cardiomegaly on chest x-ray, and have a Qp/Qs ratio greater than 1.5. Patients with more complex heart lesions may have other indications for closure. Those with a right-to-left shunt and a resting saturation of less than 94% might be candidates even if the defect is small. Similarly, patients who have a history of a paradoxical embolus with even a small ASD would be considered candidates for transcatheter closure [9].

The availability of a nonoperative method to close ASDs may provide increased safety and flexibility to the approach to other cardiac lesions. Certain patients undergoing complex surgical procedures such as the Fontan procedure may remain slightly cyanotic but have better cardiac output if the atrial septal patch has a small hole in it to allow decompression of the right atrium and improved cardiac output. Once these patients have recovered from surgery, the right-to-left shunt can be eliminated by electively closing the small ASD in the catheterization lab [10]. A small number of patients may also develop left-to-right shunts through the transseptal perforations used for balloon mitral valvuloplasty for congenital or rheumatic mitral stenosis. If the mitral stenosis is relieved and the patients

---

[1] Editor's note: As of the fall of 1991, breakage of the wires of the device was noted by some of the investigators [11]. For this reason the FDA suspended clinical trials of this device while awaiting further study of the problem.

are not considered to be candidates for repeat valvuloplasty, then closure of these small ASDs may also be indicated with the transcatheter technique.

SUMMARY

Transcatheter closure of ASDs has been shown to be an achievable goal. Several devices have evolved and are still under investigation. Successful development of one that could be used to close even two-thirds of congenital secundum ASDs could eliminate approximately 1,200 open heart procedures per year in the United States alone [1,2]. In addition, these devices may be able to reduce the risk of stroke in young adult patients who suffer from paradoxical emboli and may add to the options available to surgeons and cardiologists treating complex congenital cardiac defects.

ACKNOWLEDGMENTS

The author acknowledges the expert assistance of Geri Miller and Jeanine Pittman in preparation of this manuscript; Bruce McManus, M.D., Ph.D., and Rhonda Caruso in photographing several of the illustrations; and Drs. Lock, Hellenbrand, and Mullins, who are also involved in the clinical trials of the Clamshell Occluder.

REFERENCES

1. McNamara DG, Latson LA (1982): Long-term follow-up of patients with malformations for which definitive surgical repair has been available for 25 years or more. Am J Cardiol 50:560–568.
2. Roberts NK, Cretin S (1980): The changing face of congenital heart disease. Med Care 18:930–939.
3. Vick GW, Titus JL (1990): Defects of the atrial septum including the atrioventricular canal. In Garson A, Bricker JT, McNamara DG (eds): "The Science and Practice of Pediatric Cardiology." Philadelphia: Lea & Febiger, pp 1023–1054.
4. King TD, Mills NL (1974): Nonoperative closure of atrial septal defects. Surgery 75:383–388.
5. Mills NL, King TD (1976): Nonoperative closure of left-to-right shunts. J Thorac Cardiovasc Surg 72:371–378.
6. Latson LA, Sobczyk W, Kilzer K, et al. (1987): Closure of atrial septal defect with Rashkind Occluder: Rapid loss of permeability. Circulation 76:IV-265.
7. Lock JE, Cockerham JT, Keane JF, et al. (1987): Transcatheter umbrella closure of congenital heart defects. Circulation 75:593–599.
8. Lock JE, Rome JJ, David R, et al. (1989): Transcatheter closure of atrial septal defect. Experimental studies. Circulation 79:1091–1099.
9. Lechat PH, Mas JL, Lascault G, et al. (1988): Prevalence of patent foramen ovale in patients with stroke. N Engl J Med 1148-1152.
10. Bridges ND, Lock JE, Castaneda AR (1990): Fontan repair with baffle fenestration and subsequent transcatheter closure in high risk patients. JACC 15:203A.
11. Latson LA, Benson LN, Hellenbrand WE, Mullins CE, Lock JE (1991): Transcatheter closure of ASD—Early results of multicenter trial of Bard Clamshell septal occluder (Abst). Circulation 84 (Suppl II): 544.

18

Transcatheter Closure of Heart Defects: Role of "Buttoned" Devices

P. Syamasundar Rao, M.D., and E.B. Sideris, M.D.

Division of Pediatric Cardiology, University of Wisconsin Medical
School, University of Wisconsin Children's Hospital, Madison,
Wisconsin 53792-4108 (P.S.R.); Pediatric Cardiology,
Amarillo, Texas (E.B.S)

INTRODUCTION

The incidence of congenital heart defects is 0.8% of liveborn infants. Of these, 8%–13% are atrial septal defects (ASDs), 6%–11% are patent ductus arteriosus (PDA), and 20%–25% are ventricular septal defects (VSDs). These defects can be successfully repaired by closed heart (for PDA) or open heart (for ASD and VSD) surgical techniques. The mortality rate for the surgical correction is low (1%–5%), and the major complication rate is minimal. However, the morbidity associated with cardiac surgical procedures is universal, and the surgical scar is present in all. If a less invasive method of repairing these heart defects is available with mortality and complication rates similar to surgical methods, it would be advantageous and the children can be spared cardiac surgery. Pioneering works of Porstmann, King, and Rashkind have explored the potentials of transcatheter methods of closure of cardiac septal defects in replacing heart surgery and laid a foundation upon which other transcatheter methods could be developed and refined. The purpose of this chapter is to review the state of art of the transcatheter methods of closure of cardiac septal defects.

ATRIAL SEPTAL DEFECT
Evolution of Transcatheter Closure

King and associates [1–3] described experimental transcatheter closure of ASDs in dogs and described a few clinical applications of their technique. They used paired, opposed, dacron-covered, stainless steel, interlocking umbrellas collapsed into a capsule attached to the tip of a catheter. Their technique involves a complicated locking and unlocking mechanism, required to secure the paired umbrellas on both sides of the interatrial septum, with consequent system failures. A 23 Fr sheath is required for delivery of the device. This method has not been adopted by other investigators, presumably because of complicated maneuvering required for implantation of the device. It is our understanding that King and associates have become dissatisfied with their technique and are not currently pursuing their investigation in this area. Rashkind designed a single foam umbrella with miniature hooks and with an elaborate centering mechanism and applied it to both animal models and human subjects [4–6]. The device and the delivery system were also bulky and required a 16 Fr sheath for insertion. Of the 20 patients (14 children

Transcatheter Therapy in Pediatric Cardiology, pages 349–369

and 6 adults) in whom the ASD was closed, 13 closures were successful. Four children required emergency explantation of the device because of improper implantation; in those patients, the ASD was successfully closed at the time of emergency surgery. Of the remaining three incomplete closures, two required elective closure of the ASD. This technique was also used by other workers [7,8]. Hellenbrand and Mullins [7] attempted implantation of Rashkind's "hooked" device in three patients; one was a complete closure, the second a partial closure with a small residual shunt, and in the final patient elective surgical closure was performed several months later because of incomplete closure. Beekman et al. [8] applied this device in three children, with successful closure in only one child; the other two required surgical explantation of the misplaced device. Because of the difficulties associated with implantation of the hooked, single-umbrella device, Rashkind [4] introduced a double disk device. This device was later modified by Lock and associates [9] and is without hooks, uses spring tension to allow arms of the device to fold back against each other, is called a *Clamshell* device, and requires an 11 Fr sheath for insertion.

Lock et al. used this clamshell, double disk, umbrella device to close experimentally created ASDs in lambs; six of the eight umbrellas were correctly positioned [9]. Hellenbrand et al. [10] reported their initial experience with this device; they accomplished transcatheter closure of ASDs in 10 of 11 patients aged 13 months to 46 years; the single failure was in their youngest patient, an 11 kg, 13-month-old infant. General anesthesia with endotracheal intubation was utilized in all children. Residual shunt was present in only one child. The initial clinical experience of Lock et al. [11] with the Clamshell device included attempted ASD closures in 16 patients aged 1–56 years, and they were able to close the defects in 14 patients. In the remaining two patients the closure could not be performed. They concluded that further

clinical trials are warranted. They later presented a more detailed description of their results in 34 patients [12].

A "buttoned," double disk device that can be delivered via a 8 Fr sheath was developed by Sideris and associates [13]. They used these devices to close experimentally created ASDs in piglets; they were able to close 17 of the 20 defects successfully; only in the first three experiments were there any failures. They concluded that these new devices offer promise for human application. Initial clinical trials with this custom-made device were performed by Sideris et al. [14] and by Rao et al. [15,16] with good success. The advantage of this system is that the device can be delivered via an 8 Fr sheath and thus can be used in very young children, if such a need arises; indeed, we were able to close an ASD in a 3.6 kg infant successfully [15].

Indications and Contraindications

The indications for transcatheter closure are essentially the same as those for surgical closure. Secundum ASD with a pulmonary-to-systemic flow ratio (Qp:Qs) $\geq 1.5{:}1$ is generally considered an indication for surgical closure, and similar criteria are used for transcatheter closure. Because of the need for the device to hold well, it is important that a good rim of atrial septal tissue is present all around the ASD. Also, because of limitation of the size of the device that could be safely placed, defects larger than 25 mm may not be good candidates for transcatheter closure. Ostium primum and sinus venosus ASDs are contraindications for closure, as is partial anomalous pulmonary venous connection. Obstructive lesions of the right heart requiring right-to-left atrial shunt to allow egress of the right atrial blood are obvious contraindications. Similarly, an obstructive lesion of the left heart requiring left-to-right atrial shunt and pulmonary vascular obstructive disease are also contraindications. Closure of a patent foramen ovale to prevent further episodes of paradoxical embolism [17,18] has

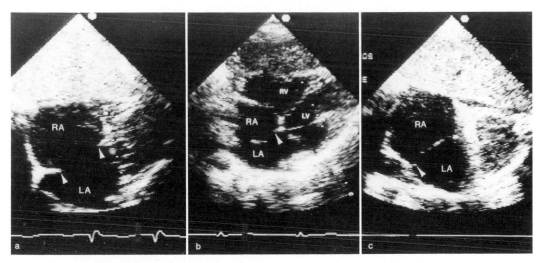

Fig. 1. Subcostal two-dimensional echocardiographic views of the atrial septum in three patients showing short rims of atrial septal tissue in the inferior and superior margins (**a**), inferior margin (**b**), or superior margin (**c**), marked with arrowheads. These defects are unlikely to be suitable for transcatheter closure because of inadequate amount of rim of atrial septal tissue to get a good hold of the device on the septum. LA, left atrium; LV, left ventricle; RA, right atrium; RV, right ventricle. (Reproduced from Rao et al. [16], with permission of the publisher.)

been performed and may become another indication for transcatheter closure [13,16].

Device Implantation

There are two types of ASD closure devices currently in clinical trials: 1) Lock's modification of Rashkind's double disk device, called a Clamshell device;[1] and 2) the "buttoned," double disk device of Sideris. Prior to implantation of either device, complete echocardiographic and Doppler study is recommended to confirm the clinical diagnosis and to exclude any other abnormalities. The size of the ASD in a subcostal view is measured and the rim of atrial septum surrounding the ASD is assessed. It is important that there is sufficient atrial septal rim to hold the device in place (Figs. 1, 2). We

also measure the size of the left atrium and interatrial septum in multiple views to have a rough assessment of the size of the structures, which will in turn give us an idea of the largest umbrella that could be used for ASD closure.

Once it is decided that a given patient's ASD is suitable for closure, the procedure and the potential risks associated with transcatheter closure are explained to the patient and/or parents, as appropriate. The procedure is performed on a protocol basis and is approved by a local institutional review board and with an FDA investigational device exemption. After obtaining appropriate informed consent, cardiac catheterization is performed and the usual hemodynamic and angiographic evaluation is performed to confirm the diagnosis and to exclude any other defects. Attempts to enter all the pulmonary veins from the left atrium are made. A cineangiogram from the right, upper pulmonary vein at its junction with the left atrium in a four-chamber (30° LAO and 30° cranial) view is performed. Having confirmed the diagnosis, balloon-sizing of the ASD

[1]At the time of this writing, the FDA had suspended clinical trials with this device, pending further study of the breakage arms.

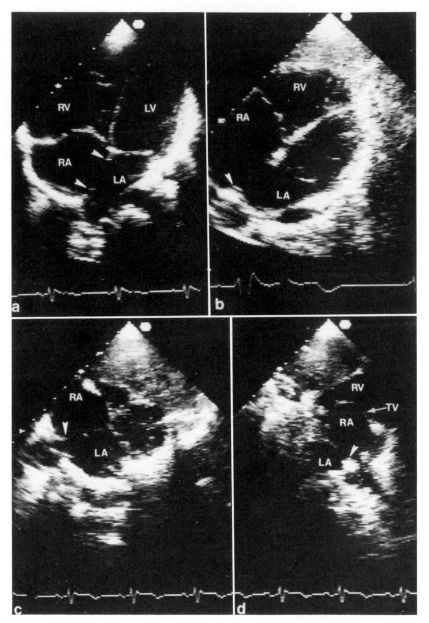

Fig. 2. Apical **(a)** and subcostal **(b)** four-chamber views of the atrial septum showing deficient atrial septal tissue (arrows); also Subcostal, four-chamber views of the atrial septum in a long-axis **(c)** and a short-axis **(d)** view of the atrial septum, also showing deficient septum in a different patient. Solid arrowheads indicate the diminutive atrial septal rims. LA, left atrium; LV, left ventricle; RA, right atrium; RV, right ventricle; TV, tricuspid valve. (Reproduced from Rao *et al.* [22], with permission of the publisher.)

[19,20,20a] is performed. We initially use the Edward atrial septostomy catheter or the Fogarty embolectomy catheter. If these balloons are too small to size the ASD, then a Meditech occlusion balloon catheter, as described elsewhere [20], is used. The stretched diameter of the ASD is thus determined. As per the current protocol, we will attempt to close the defects, if they are 25 mm or less, by stretched diameter measurement. Once the defect size is suitable, we proceed with transcatheter closure. It is generally recommended that the size of the device chosen be larger than the size of the stretched diameter of the ASD. Lock et al. [11,12] recommend a device at least 1.6 times larger than the stretched diameter of the defect. Sideris et al. [13,14] suggested a device that is 12–15 mm larger than the defect. In the initial protocol [16], we have arbitrarily chosen devices that are at least 15 mm larger than the stretched diameter of the ASD. Based on that experience [16] and on theoretical considerations, we now use a device that is approximately 5 mm larger than two times the size of the ASD, provided the left atrium can accommodate a device of that size.

Modified Rashkind (Clamshell) device. The Clamshell Septal Umbrella (USCI) consists of two opposing umbrellas, one to be positioned on either side of the atrial septum [9,11,12]. Each umbrella is composed of four steel arms, and each arm is hinged at the center of the device and is covered with a woven dacron patch. Each arm has a hinge in the center to allow the arm to fold back against itself. The hooks and centering mechanism of the original Rashkind's single-umbrella device were removed, and the device can be delivered via an 11 Fr sheath. The method of device implantation has been described in detail elsewhere [9-12]. It consists of positioning an 11 Fr sheath into the left atrium, advancing the device in the sheath so as to open the distal arms in the midleft atrium, withdrawing the device against the septum until the arms are minimally bent, and further retracting the sheath, allowing the proximal umbrella to open on the right atrial side. Once the operator is sure that the device is well-positioned, the pin–pin mechanism is activated, thus releasing the umbrellas. The procedure has been performed by fluoroscopic and/or transthoracic or transesophageal echocardiography [9–12]. The majority of these procedures are performed under general anesthesia [9-12]. Heparinization during the procedure and antibiotic administration are a part of the routine.

"Buttoned" device. The buttoned device consists of three components: the occluder, the counteroccluder, and the delivery system. The occluder is made of polyurethane foam with a Teflon-coated wire skeleton. The wire skeleton is X shaped when unfolded, and the wires are in nearly parallel position when folded and can be introduced into an 8 Fr sheath. A 2 mm string loop is attached to the center of the occluder; the loop is closed by a 1 mm knot ("button"). A radiopaque marker identifies the position of the "button." The counteroccluder is made up of rhomboid-shaped, polyurethane foam with a Teflon-coated wire skeleton. A rubber piece is sutured in its center and becomes the "buttonhole." The delivery system consists of 1) a loading wire, which is a Teflon-coated, 0.035-inch guidewire (Cook); 2) a folded 0.008 inch Nylon thread that passes through the loop in the center of the occluder; 3) an 8 Fr long sheath (Cordis); and 4) an 8 Fr end-hole catheter (pusher) that is used to advance the occluder within the sheath.

The device is implanted in the cardiac catheterization laboratory. The patient is premedicated with a mixture of demerol, phenergan, and thorazine. No general anesthesia is used. Sterile technique is used during catheterization and device implantation. The child is heparinized (100 units/kg body weight). An 8 Fr end-hole (or multi-A2) catheter carrying an 8 Fr long sheath is positioned in the left atrium. The catheter is removed and the sheath clamped to prevent back bleeding. The occluder is folded and introduced into the sheath. An 8 Fr catheter is inserted over the loading guidewire into the sheath and advanced, pushing the occluder toward the heart. When the occluder is at the tip of the sheath, verification that the tip is in the midleft atrium is made by biplane fluoroscopy. While holding the device in the midleft atrium, the sheath is gently withdrawn, allowing the occluder to spring open; it will assume its original shape. The occluder is gently pulled back against the atrial septum; once it is clear that the occluder size is appropriate to the size of the ASD, the pusher catheter is then removed. The counteroccluder is threaded (through the rubber piece; "buttonhole") over the loading wire and positioned in the sheath. The pusher catheter is reintroduced into the sheath (over the loading wire) and advanced, pushing the counter occluder toward the right atrium. The sheath is withdrawn into the midright atrium, keeping the occluder in the left atrium. The counteroccluder is then extruded out of the sheath into the midright atrium, with the counteroccluder still on the loading wire. Introduction of the 1 mm knot of the occluder ("button") through the rubber piece ("buttonhole") of the counteroccluder is then performed. This is accomplished by simultaneously (gently) pulling the occluder against the atrial septum while advancing the counteroccluder with the long sheath. Verification that the knot has been pulled through the "buttonhole" can be obtained by fluoroscopy because of the radiopaque marker on the knot (Fig. 3). If the implantation of the device is satisfactory, the loading wire is cut at the tip and pulled out, leaving the Nylon strands holding the occluder. The device is disconnected by pulling one of the two Nylon strands, thus disconnecting the implanted device from the loading system. Fifteen minutes later, oxygen saturations from the right heart chambers are obtained, and a pulmonary artery cineangiogram is performed to visualize the adequacy of the ASD closure on the levophase of the cineangiogram. Three doses of Keflex (50–75 mg/kg/day) are administered; the first dose is given in the catheterization laboratory intravenously, and the second and third doses are given 6 hours and 12

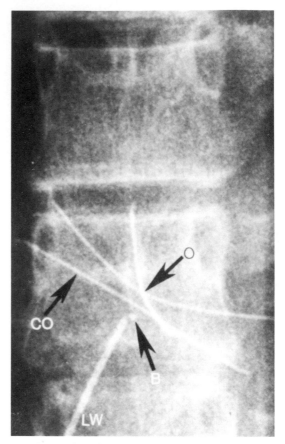

Fig. 3. Selected cineradiographic frame of the device after its implantation but before disconnecting the loading wire (LW), showing the occluder (O), counteroccluder (CO), and the radiopaque "button" (B). (Reproduced from Rao et al. [22], with permission of the publisher.)

hours after the first dose. Oral aspirin, 5–10 mg/kg/day, is begun on the day following device implantation to prevent excessive aggregation of platelets on the device. Aspirin is discontinued 6 weeks later.

Results

Although several devices, as outlined in an earlier section of this chapter, have been used for transcatheter closure of ASDs, to our knowledge only two systems are under clinical trials with FDA-approved investigational devices. Hellenbrand and associates [10] attempted

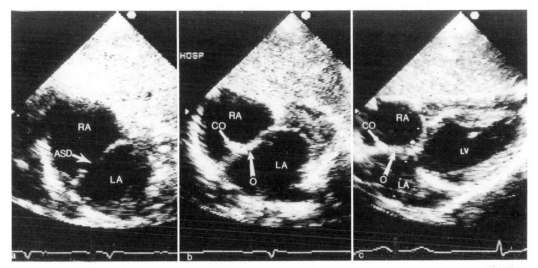

Fig. 4. Subcostal four-chamber echocardiographic views of atrial septum showing an atrial septal defect (ASD) prior to closure (**a**) and the device in place on the afternoon of (**b**) and 3 months following (**c**) the implantation of the device. The large arrows in b and c indicate the occluder (O) on the left atrial side of the atrial septum, and the smaller arrows indicate the counteroccluder (CO) on-end. LA, left atrium; LV, left ventricle; RA, right atrium. (Reproduced from Rao *et al.*[16], with permission of the publisher.)

ASD closure with the Clamshell device in 11 patients aged 13 months to 42 years; the procedure was successful in eight patients. In the three patients without initial success, the device was implanted at a subsequent catheterization. General anesthesia was administered to all patients. Transesophageal echocardiographic guidance was used in four of these patients. Immediate results were excellent; in only one patient was there a residual left-to-right shunt noted. No follow-up data were presented.

Rome *et al.* [12] reported the results of ASD closure by the Clamshell device in 34 patients. The results were mixed with those from other types of closure devices, and cannot be separated for this group.

In the multicenter clinical trial [21], approximately 100 patients were enrolled; the ASD closure with Clamshell device was successful in 93%.[2] In three patients, the device

embolized; the devices were retrieved by the transcatheter method (in one) or by surgery (in two). In one patient, embolization was discovered at a 1 month follow-up visit. Follow-up, noninvasive studies, including color Doppler studies, demonstrated complete closure in 84% of patients with successful device placement [21]. In the remaining patients, the residual defects were small.

Sideris *et al.* [14] reported application of a "buttoned" device to occlude the ASD in three children aged 4–12 years; in two, there was complete closure of the ASD, while in the remaining patient the occlusion was partial. Rao *et al.* [15,16,22] applied the technique in 12 patients (Fig. 4) aged 7 months to 45 years (weight 3.6–64 kg); the device was successfully implanted in all patients, but in one child the device dislodged from the ASD within minutes of implantation and the child was taken to

---

[2]In a recent abstract presentation (Latson L, *et al.* [1991]: Circulation 84(Suppl II):544), the experience with 400 patients in the multicenter trial was described. The results were similar but breakage of wire hinges at follow-up is of concern.

surgery where the device was removed and the ASD closed. In the remaining 11 patients after 0.5–24 months follow-up echo-Doppler studies, there was no residual shunt in nine patients and minute residual shunt in two. In the international experience, 31 patients have undergone transcatheter closure of ASDs [23], with a successful implantation rate of 90%. Further FDA-approved clinical trials with this device are underway: A preliminary analysis [24] of a total of approximately 100 patients indicates encouraging results.

PATENT DUCTUS ARTERIOSUS
Evolution of Transcatheter Closure

Porstmann and associates [25,26] have developed and utilized a technique for transcatheter closure of PDA. It involves cannulation of both a femoral artery and a femoral vein and an intracardiac maneuver that is quite complex. The prosthesis (Ivalon plug) is inserted via the artery, necessitating the use of a large-caliber artery and insertion of a large conduit into it. The PDA was successfully closed in 56 of 62 patients in whom Porstmann et al. [25] applied the technique. Because of the large size of the conduit (18 Fr) that needs to be inserted into the femoral artery, there were only five patients less than 10 years of age in the initial 62 patients. A larger experience with this device was later reported by Wierny et al. [27]. Although the Porstmann method of PDA closure has been known for more than two decades, only a few other laboratories [28–30] have applied it clinically; this is probably related to its complexity.

Mills and King [2] attempted closure of experimentally created PDAs in 10 dogs with a dumbbell-shaped plug and with a dacron-covered umbrella. In five, the PDA was successfully occluded and remained occluded 6 months later. Leslie and associates [31] used Ivalon sponge plugs sutured onto stainless steel umbrellas to close experimentally created aortopulmonary shunts in 13 mongrel dogs and successfully closed the shunt in ten dogs.

Warnecke and associates [32] used a device consisting of a 5 Fr and 6 Fr triple-lumen catheters carrying a detachable silicone double balloon at the tip to close experimentally created PDA in beagles. Successful occlusion was achieved in 15 of the 21 animals. Magal et al. [33] developed a device consisting of a Nylon sack of various sizes and shapes (with a crossbar to hold it in position) that can be filled with a segment of modified guidewire. This device can be delivered through a 10 Fr catheter and can be repositioned or retrieved before it is released. They were able to place the device across the brachiocephalic trunk in all 10 dogs in whom they attempted device placement. Follow-up angiographic and necropsy studies revealed permanent occlusion of the vessel. Echigo and colleagues [34] utilized a temperature-shape changeable, shape memory polymer (polynorbornene) in a PDA occlusion device and tested it in an in vitro PDA model. They showed that 1) this device was easily positioned across the "ductus"; 2) it expanded on exposure to hot water; and 3) it remained in place after removal of the guidewire. The device was introduced through a 12 Fr sheath in this model. To my knowledge, no clinical applications of these techniques were reported.

Rashkind et al. [35,36] devised a single foam-covered umbrella with miniature hooks (fishhooks) to close the PDA. Because of the difficulty in manipulating the prosthesis once extruded from the catheter delivery system and because of a significant incidence of incomplete closures, improper implantation, and prosthesis embolization [4], they redesigned the system, this time using a double-disk, non-hooked prosthesis [4,37]. Subsequent clinical trials by several groups of workers [7,37–42] revealed reasonably good results, with successful implantation occurring in 72%–81% of the patients [7]. Unlike with the Porstmann and the initial single-disk Rashkind occluders, a venous rather than an arterial route was used. But implantation of the devices requires 8 Fr and 11 Fr sized sheaths, depending on the size of the PDA to be occluded.

Sideris *et al.* [43] also developed a PDA device similar to the one they used for ASD closure and tested it in piglet models; in all 11 attempts they were able to occlude the PDA successfully. We have used a similar custom-made device to close PDA successfully in a child [44]. The advantage of this system lies in the fact that the device can be delivered via a 7 Fr catheter; this is quite contrary to the currently used Rashkind double-umbrella occluder, which requires an 8 or 11 Fr sheath, depending upon the size of the ductus, for delivery. Addition clinical experience with this custom-made device in six patients [44a] is encouraging. Further clinical trials will start once the FDA grants investigational device exemption.

Indications and Contraindications

The indication for ductal closure is its presence, unless it is a part of a more complex cardiac defect that is ductal dependent with regard to either pulmonary or systemic flow. Although several angiographic types of ductuses have been described [45], most are suitable for transcatheter closure. The contraindications for ductal closure include unusual ductal location, very large ductus, pulmonary vascular obstructive disease, and, as mentioned above, ductal-dependent, cyanotic congenital heart defects.

Device Implantation

Several types of PDA devices are in use. The Porstmann Ivalon plug is mostly used by Porstmann *et al.* and in the Far East, and it is usually applicable to the older patient. The Rashkind double-umbrella device and the "buttoned" device of Sideris are two other types available for PDA closure. A complete echo-Doppler study to document the diagnosis of PDA and to exclude other abnormalities is recommended. Once it is decided that the patient is suitable for closure, informed consent, as detailed in the ASD section, is obtained. Cardiac catheterization to confirm the diagnosis and to exclude other defects [42] is

performed, and the size of the ductus arteriosus is determined either by balloon inflation aortography [46] or by direct injection into the aorta at the level of PDA.

The Porstmann Ivalon plug. The occluding device consists of a radiopaque Ivalon foam, which is either prepared or selected from the stock on the basis of the size and shape of the PDA, as determined from a review of a lateral selective aortic angiogram. The plug is threaded over a guidewire and can be introduced through a tubular applicator into the femoral artery.

The procedure of device placement is described in detail elsewhere [25-30]. It consists of insertion of a catheter into the femoral artery, either percutaneously or via cutdown; advancing it into the PDA, and from there, into the right heart and inferior vena cava; and advancing a long (300 cm) guidewire through the catheter and retrieving it through the femoral vein. The Ivalon plug is then inserted over the guidewire into the femoral artery with the help of a tubular applicator. Once in the femoral artery the plug is advanced over the guidewire with the help of a pushing catheter until the plug is positioned into the ductus, the ductus closure is confirmed by contrast injection into the aorta, and removal of the guidewire is made from the venous side, taking care not to dislodge the plug. The patients are heparinized during the procedure, and the heparin effect is neutralized with protamine after the procedure is completed.

The Rashkind Double-Disk device. The device consists of two opposing, polyurethane foam-covered, three-arm spring wire disks, which can be delivered to the ductal site via either an 8 Fr or an 11 Fr sheath, depending on the size of the device. The device delivery system is composed of a fine central core wire enclosed in a coiled spring guidewire and a thin-walled, stainless steel, tubular delivery pod. The disks of the device can be folded into the delivery pod with the help of a clear plastic loader. The core wire ends in a polished knuckle that can be attached to an elliptical eyelet built into the device. Once the device is in place, it can be disconnected by dislodging the knuckle from the eyelet of the device by a slide plunger mechanism at the external end of the catheter.

The procedure is described elsewhere [37–41] and includes the following. Initially, a long sheath (8 or 11 Fr, depending on the size of the device chosen) is placed across the PDA, via the venous route, with the help of a guidewire and an appropriate-sized catheter/dilator. The dilator and wire are removed and replaced with a loaded Rashkind double-disk delivery system. The system is advanced until the pod reaches the right atrium. At this point, the device is extruded out of the pod and into the sheath. From here onward, the sheath across the ductus serves as an extension of the pod. The device is slowly advanced up to the tip of the sheath. The tip of the sheath is positioned horizontally in the aorta at the level of the ductus. The arms of the distal umbrella are opened by slowly withdrawing the sheath while holding the device catheter steady. When the distal arms are open, the entire system is pulled back such that the arms of the open umbrella engage the ampulla of the ductus. Further retraction will show slight folding of the distal arms; this is at the junction of the ductal insertion into the pulmonary artery. The latter can be marked by straight lateral angiogram and the tracheal air shadow. At this point, the sheath is withdrawn, keeping the delivery catheter fixed; this allows opening of the arms of the proximal umbrella. This should result in straddling of the device on either side of the pulmonary artery insertion of the PDA. If this position of the device is satisfactory, the device release mechanism is activated and the catheter delivery system and sheath removed.

"Buttoned" device. The "buttoned" device also consists of three major components: the occluder, the counteroccluder, and the delivery system. The occluder consists of a square-shaped, polyurethane foam mounted on a Teflon-coated wire skeleton, which can be introduced into a 7 Fr sheath. A 5–10 mm string loop is attached to the center of the occluder; the loop is closed by a 1 mm knot ("button"). The knot is identified with a radiopaque marker. The counteroccluder is also made up of a narrow strip of polyurethane foam mounted on a wire skeleton with a rubber piece sewed in its center in a manner similar to that in the ASD device. The delivery system consists of a 0.035 inch Teflon-coated wire, through which an 0.008 inch Nylon thread passes through the loop in the occluder, a 7 Fr long sheath (Cordis or USCI), and a 7 Fr end-hole catheter (pusher).

The procedure is performed in the cardiac catheterization laboratory. The patient is premedicated with a mixture of demerol, phenergan, and thorazine. General anesthesia is not used. The patient is prepared and draped, and the procedure is performed using a sterile technique. After obtaining routine pressure and oxygen saturation data to confirm the diagnosis of PDA, biplane cineangiograms are performed in posteroanterior and lateral views to demonstrate the location, size, and shape of the ductus [45,46]. Heparinization is started (100 units/kg body weight). Initially, a 5 or 6 Fr end-hole catheter is positioned in the descending aorta across the patient ductus arteriosus. An appropriate-sized (0.032–0.035 inch) guidewire is then positioned in the descending aorta, and the catheter is removed. A long 7 Fr multi-A2 catheter and a 7 Fr sheath are advanced over the guidewire, with their tips positioned in the descending aorta. The dilator and guidewire are removed and the sheath clamped to prevent back bleeding. The device is then positioned in the sheath, and a 7 Fr end-hole catheter is advanced into the sheath over the guidewire of the delivery system. Advancing this catheter within the sheath pushes the device toward the descending aorta. Once the device is across the ductus, but still within the sheath, the sheath is slowly withdrawn into the ductus, thus opening the occluder in the descending aorta at its junction with the ductus. The entire system is slowly withdrawn to ensure anchoring of the occluder on the descending aortic side of the ductus. Once in position, the sheath and the catheter are withdrawn into the main pulmonary artery. The catheter is removed while maintaining the tip of the sheath in the main pulmonary artery. The counteroccluder is then threaded over the guidewire, but within the sheath, and is delivered to the pulmonary artery side of the PDA. Buttoning of the occluder and counteroccluder is performed in a manner similar to that described for ASD closure. The radiopaque marker serves as a guide to ensure adequate buttoning. Once the occluder is adequately positioned across the PDA, the delivery system is disconnected from the device, as described in the ASD section. The sheath is then used to introduce a Berman angiographic catheter for the purpose of angiography, which is performed 15 minutes following implantation of the device; ductal closure is thereby demonstrated. Keflex and aspirin are administered, as described in the ASD section.

Results

Porstmann and associates [25–27] attempted transvascular closure of PDA by the Ivalon plug in 208 patients aged 5–62 years. They were able to close the ductus successfully in 95% of patients. These 197 successfully treated patients were followed for 1–15 years; there was no evidence for recanalization of the ductus by auscultation and phonocardiography. On follow-up, slippage of the Ivalon plug in 23 (11%) cases and arterial complications in 16 (8%) were noted. Sato and associates [29,30] reported successful closure of PDA by the Porstmann method in 83 of 87 (95%) consecutive patients. They introduced modifications to the Porstmann system so that it could not only be used for a conical-shaped ductus but also for cylindrical and window types of ductus. Follow-up evaluation 3 months to 3.6 years revealed neither dislodgement of the plug nor residual shunts. Other

investigators [28,47–50] have also used this technique. In all, Weirny [27] estimates, as of 1985, that some 800 patients have been successfully treated by the Porstmann method.

The Rashkind double-umbrella device has been used by several workers [37–41,51], and successful implantation was accomplished in more than 90% of the patients [51]. In Benson's series [51], 200 procedures were performed in 190 patients from January 1985 through June 1990; ages ranged between 0.9 and 44.6 years. Device embolization occurred in four (2%) of the patients; three underwent surgery for removal of the device; and one patient had the device retrieved by transcatheter methods. Careful echo-Doppler studies in the initial 78 patients [52] revealed residual shunt in 38% 1 day after the procedure, falling to 25% 1 year later. Placement of a second device was attempted in 10 of these children [51–53], with success in eight, giving a residual shunt rate of 3% at 1–2 years. Based on this experience, it was concluded that reimplantation with a second device is feasible in patients with residual PDA murmurs, but reimplantation is not possible if the residual shunt is only documented by echo-Doppler, without auscultatory evidence of shunt. Additional complications included mild, residual, left pulmonary artery stenosis and intravascular hemolysis; the latter requiring surgical removal of the device and ductal ligation.

The clinical experience with Sideris' "buttoned" device is limited [44,44a,54]; we have successfully closed the PDA in nine children. Echo-Doppler (Fig. 5) and angiographic (Fig. 6) documentation of the closure can easily be obtained. The patients ranged in age from 1.5 to 5 years (median 2.5 years). The weights ranged from 7.2 to 19 kg (median 9.9 kg). The pulmonary-to-systemic flow ratio was 1.3 to 3.2 (1.8 ± 0.8) prior to closure and was reduced to 1.0 in eight children and to 1.3 in the remaining child after closure. Angiographically, no ductus was visualized in five, and a small residual shunt was seen in three children. Color Doppler echographic studies

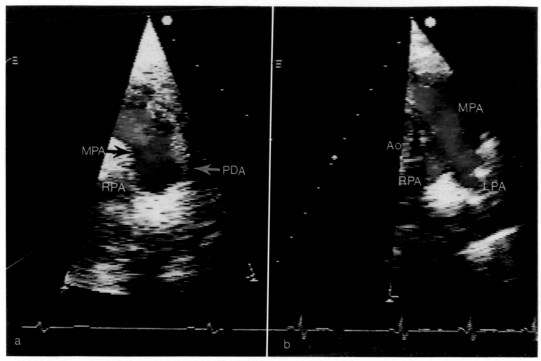

Fig. 5. Selected video frames from two-dimensional and color Doppler echocardiographic precordial short-axis views of the heart prior to **(a)** and 1 day following **(b)** transcatheter closure of patent ductus arteriosus (PDA). Note color flow disturbance in a, indicating a small to moderate-sized PDA that is no longer seen in b following transcatheter occlusion. Forward (blue) flow in the main pulmonary artery (MPA) is shown. Ao, aorta; LPA, left pulmonary artery; RPA, right pulmonary artery. (Reproduced from Rao *et al.* [44], with permission of the publisher.)

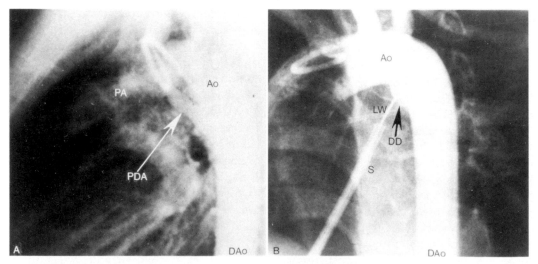

Fig. 6. Selected frames for aortic (Ao) cineangiographic views prior to **(A)** and 10 minutes following **(B)** transcatheter closure of the patent ductus arteriosus (PDA). Note PDA (arrow) in a. Aortography following occlusion but before disconnecting the loading wire (LW) revealed no opacification of the ductus; the ductus diverticulum (DD) is shown. DAo, descending aorta; S, sheath that was used to deliver the device. (Reproduced from Rao *et al.* [44], with permission of the publisher.)

showed similar results. A continuous murmur was heard in all nine children prior to transcatheter closure, which disappeared in all after transcatheter closure. There was no continuous murmur even in the three children with residual shunt detected by angiography and color Doppler echocardiography. Follow-up was available in six children, 1-12 months following the procedure. There were no complications. No shunts were seen in five children and a small residual shunt was seen in one patient. Although this limited experience with ductal closure utilizing the "buttoned" device is encouraging, further clinical trials on a larger group of patients is necessary prior to its general use.

VENTRICULAR SEPTAL DEFECT
Evolution of Transcatheter Closure

Catheter closure of VSDs in animal models was initially performed by Rashkind [5] and by Rashkind and Cuaso [55]; they used a hooked, single-disk device and a double-disk device. Lock and associates [56] attempted transcatheter closure of seven VSDs in six patients aged 8 months to 82 years. Four were postinfarction VSDs, and three were congenital VSDs. These workers used Rashkind's double-disk umbrella device. Successful closure was accomplished in six of the seven VSDs. In the seventh (which was a postinfarction VSD), the umbrella embolized into the pulmonary circuit. The same authors later reported, in abstract form [57], their experience with transcatheter closure of 14 congenital VSDs. They used Rashkind's double-disk umbrella or Clamshell device. The device was implanted accurately in all but one. The latter was extracted via the catheter, and successful transcatheter closure was performed the following day. The VSD shunt was abolished in 13 and significantly reduced in the remaining patient. The devices were delivered via an 11 Fr sheath in the Lock et al. studies (56,57). Subsequently, other reports [58,59] also appeared in the literature.

Indications and Contraindications

Indications for VSD closure are defects that not only cause significant elevation of pulmonary artery pressure and flow but also cannot be medically controlled and are at risk for causing pulmonary vascular obstructive disease. The patients with more common subaortic, perimembranous VSDs are not candidates for transcatheter closure, because these defects are very close to the aortic valve. Apical and muscular defects are more suitable for transcatheter closure. Indeed, transcatheter closure may be preferable to surgical closure because the latter frequently leaves significant residual shunt, especially when transatrial or right ventricular approaches are used. Additional contraindications for transcatheter closure are very large defects, defects located very close to aortic or mitral valves, and associated pulmonary vascular obstructive disease. Patients with cyanotic heart disease requiring an open VSD for intracardiac mixing are also not candidates for closure.

Device Implantation

The devices that can be used for VSD closure are essentially the same as those used for ASD closure. The method of implantation, however, is more complex because of the fact that it is difficult to advance the device delivery catheters directly across the VSD. A double-catheter approach [56] is necessary. In this technique, an end-hole balloon catheter (Swan-Gantz type), with the balloon partially inflated, is introduced retrogradely from the aorta into the left ventricle and from there into the right ventricle across the VSD. With the help of a soft J guidewire, the catheter is manipulated into the right atrium or into the main pulmonary artery. At this point, a long (400 cm) 0.035 inch guidewire is advanced through the tip of the catheter and the guidewire is snared from a percutaneous, right femoral venous or internal jugular venous approach, depending on the location of the VSD. The guidewire is brought out through the venous sheath. This guidewire is used to position a balloon-sizing catheter and subsequently the device carrying the catheter and device implanted, as detailed in the ASD section. For further details of the technique, the reader is referred to publications by Lock and coworkers [56,57,59].

Results

Lock and associates [56,57] attempted transcatheter closure of VSDs in 14 patients. The Rashkind double-umbrella devices or Clamshell devices were used. Successful implantation was accomplished in all but one; the latter required adjustment of the arms of the device at surgery. The shunt was abolished or significantly reduced. No long-term results have been published to date. Others [58] used the Rashkind PDA device to occlude the VSD in a patient with right-to-left ventricular shunting following a Fontan procedure. The Clamshell device was also used to close muscular VSDs in complex congenital heart defects as a part of overall management of the patients; in 12 patients Bridges et al. [59] successfully closed 21 VSDs and reduced left-to-right shunt markedly. We have used the transcatheter method with the Sideris "buttoned" device in one patient, with success.

COMPLICATIONS

Potential complications include dislodgement and embolization of the device and improper implantation. These are rare in a large series of animal experiments [1,5,9,13,43,60] and human subjects [3,7,26,29,35–51,61]. Embolization was simulated by Rashkind [4,36] in experimental animals by deliberately releasing the device at the site of implantation. The device that embolized into the descending aorta could be removed via the contralateral femoral artery [62,63] with a simple catheter snare or by a grabber or basket retrieval system. With regard to improper implantation, it is desirable to implant the device directly across the defect. This is accomplished easily; improper implantation is unlikely if care is taken

to open the device close to the defect. In the event of improper seating, the prosthesis can be removed with a snare or other types of retrieval kits [62,63]. Failing transcatheter retrieval, surgical exploration might be required to remove the device. At the same time, the cardiac defect can be repaired.

Other possible complications are cardiac perforation and arrhythmia; these have not occurred in the reported series. Air embolism is another possibility because of the large sheaths used, but adequate care to flush the systems continuously and to avoid creating a vacuum in the sheath will prevent such problems. Thromboembolism is another potential problem. This may be prevented by appropriate heparinization during the procedure and by administering platelet-inhibiting drugs following the procedure; thus far, there has not been documented evidence for thromboembolism during follow-up either in animals or in humans. Because of the potential for bacterial endocarditis [39,60], antibiotic coverage, as described in the section on device implantation is generally recommended.

Persistent residual shunt may be present in some patients at follow-up; these can be reoccluded with a second device [53]. Intravascular hemolysis may rarely be observed, which, if cannot be controlled by rest and oral iron, may require surgical removal of the device.

ADVANTAGES

Although the mortality rates for surgical closure of the defects are low, the morbidity is 100%. Psychological impact on the children and their parents is also high. Surgical closure requires a 7–10 day hospitalization, general anesthesia, thoracotomy, cardiopulmonary bypass (for ASDs and VSDs), and postoperative monitoring in the intensive care unit for 1 to several days, all of which carry risks as well as expenses. Transcatheter closure can be accomplished during a 2 day hospitalization without thoracotomy and cardiopulmonary bypass. General anesthesia is not required in some types of transcatheter closure. The transcatheter procedures are less expensive, result in no scar on the chest, and have potentially less psychologic trauma to the patient and to the parents. Despite the advantages, the questions of safety and long-term residua are not completely settled. These questions are likely to be answered by the clinical trials that are currently underway.

OTHER ISSUES
Endothelialization

Inspection of the hearts of the sacrificed animals shows endothelialization of the devices [4,8,9,13,37,39], this appears to be noticed sometime after 2 weeks following implantation. Such endothelialization is similar to that observed following patch closure of atrial and ventricular septal defects and prosthetic valve implantation. Because of complete endothelialization, there may not be a need to continue bacterial endocarditis prophylaxis unless residual leaks across the device are present.

Balloon-Sizing

The stretched diameter of the ASD by balloon-sizing is utilized by all workers [3,4,9,10,12,15,16] as a guide to the selection of the size of the device for implantation. Although measurement of the stretched diameter of the ASD by passing balloons of varying sizes, as previously described [19,20,20a], can be accomplished during cardiac catheterization, it is a cumbersome procedure and sometimes requires use of very large balloon catheters. Therefore, it is desirable to have an alternative, less cumbersome, less invasive method of measuring the ASD size that can be used for selection of the size of the device for ASD closure. To achieve this objective, we have examined echocardiographic, angiographic, and physiologic measures of ASD size in a group of 16 patients, aged 7 months to 45 years (median, 4.5 years) and compared them with the stretched diameter of the ASD to determine if any of these can predict the

stretched diameter of the ASD [20]. Although the pulmonary-to-systemic flow ratio (Qp Qs) and angiographic size have a significant ($P <$ 0.05) correlation with stretched diameter ($r =$ 0.55 and 0.54, respectively), the echo diameter has the best correlation coefficient ($r =$ 0.82, $P < 0.001$). Based on this regression equation, the stretched diameter (mm) can be estimated as $1.05 \times$ echo (mm) $+$ 5.49. Subsequently, we prospectively evaluated this formula in estimating the stretched ASD diameter by two-dimensional echocardiographic measurements obtained in two (long and short axis) subcostal views (Fig. 7) in another group of 21 patients aged 2.5–29 years (median, 4.5 years) [64]. The predicted stretched diameter calculated using the above formula was 15.7 ± 3.1 mm and is similar ($P > 0.1$) to the measured diameter, 15.3 ± 4.0 mm. The correlation (Fig. 8) between predicted and measured ASD size was excellent ($r = 0.9$, $P < 0.001$). The mean squared error was 2.4. The differences between the measured and predicted values were within 3 mm of each other in all but two patients. We concluded that the stretched diameter can be accurately estimated by the subcostal echo, which in turn may be used for selection of device size for closure of the ASD. Further validation of this method by other workers may be helpful in confirming these observations.

Selection of Device Size for Closure of ASD

All workers recommend a device size that is larger than the size of the ASD. King et al. [2] recommended that the device be at least 10–15 mm larger than the ASD diameter. Lock and associates [9,12] suggested that the device size should be 1.6 times that of the stretched diameter of the ASD. Sideris et al. [13,14] recommended a device that is 12–15 mm larger than the defect. During our initial experience [15,16], we arbitrarily chose devices that were at least 15 mm larger than the stretched diameter of the defect. But, based on theoretical considerations (Fig. 9) and on our subsequent

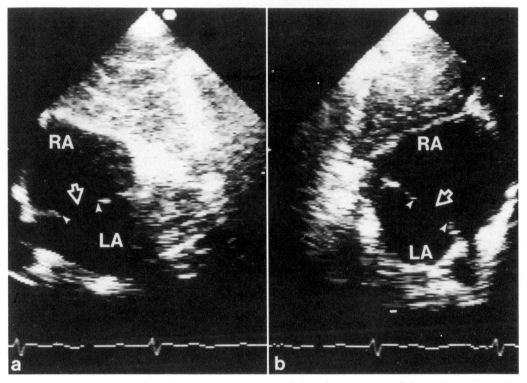

Fig. 7. Selected video frames from two-dimensional, subcostal, four-chamber views of the atrial septum in a long axis **(a)** and a short axis **(b)** view, showing the atrial septal defect (arrow). Echographic size of the atrial septal defect (ASD) is measured from the leading edge to the trailing edge in both views and averaged. LA, left atrium; RA, right atrium.

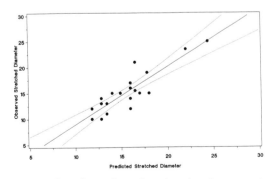

Fig. 8. The relationship of predicted and measured stretched atrial septal defect diameter is plotted. A regression line along with 95% confidence limits (dashed lines) are shown. r = 0.9, P < 0.001, and the mean squared error was 2.4. (Reproduced from Rao *et al.* [64], with permission of the publisher.)

experience [22], we suggest that the size of the device be larger than two times the size of the defect. When the device is released in the left atrium and pulled back to ensure appropriate positioning of the device on the left atrial side of the atrial septum, the device is likely to be pulled inferiorly with the center of the device toward the lower margin of the ASD (Fig. 9). Therefore, only the superior half of the device is positioned across the defect. Thus, the device should be at least two times the size of the atrial defect. To ensure some margin of safety, a device 5 mm larger than two times the size of the ASD should be chosen. A pie diagram showing device sizes required for ASD closure is depicted in Figure 10. However, this solu-

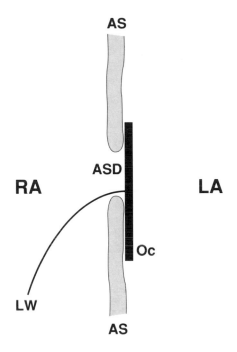

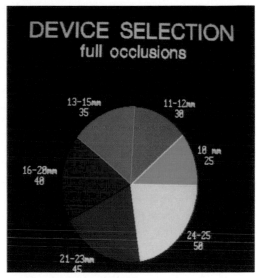

Fig. 10. A pie diagram indicating the device sizes to be used with various stretched diameters of ASD, based on 1) principles outlined in Figure 9 and 2) device implantation data from our collaborative multi-institutional study.

Fig. 9. Artist's diagram of atrial septum (AS) separating left (LA) and right (RA) atria, showing atrial septal defect (ASD). The occluder (Oc) of the device has been delivered into the LA, and, as the loading wire (LW) is gently pulled, the occluder positions itself with its center at the lower margin of the ASD. If the occluder is less than double the size of the ASD, it is likely to flip back into the RA. If the occluder is larger than two times the size of the ASD, it is likely to be held in position in the LA, as shown in the figure. (Reproduced from Rao et al. [16], with permission of the publisher.)

tion to prevent withdrawal across the ASD and to prevent residual defects may have a potential problem in that the device may be too large to be accommodated in the left atrium. In the precatheterization echocardiogram, we determine the size of the left atrium in several directions (anteroposterior, inferosuperior, left-to-right, and diagonal) and of the size of the interatrial septum, measured on the left atrial side. If the selected device (based on stretched diameter and other considerations discussed above) is larger than the size of the left atrium or interatrial septum, it may not be advisable

to implant the device because it may impinge upon the mitral valve apparatus or cause pulmonary venous obstruction.

Role of Transesophageal Echocardiography in ASD Closure

We have used fluoroscopy, transthoracic echocardiography, and occasionally transesophageal echocardiography during device implantation across the ASD. Advantages of transesophageal monitoring during device placement have been outlined [10]. Hellenbrand et al. [10] utilized transesophageal monitoring in 4 of 11 patients undergoing ASD closure with the Clamshell device; they stated that the number, size, and position of the defect(s) could be easily assessed and appropriate seating of the device can be ascertained. We have been favorably impressed with this technique, based on our experience with its use in three adult patients [23]. While there are advantages for transesophageal monitoring, it does carry additional risk and does prolong the procedures. Furthermore, general anesthesia is usually required [10] if transesophageal monitoring is utilized during device implantation. Since we perform the procedure with a sedative mixture and local xylocaine anesthesia, we have not utilized transesophageal echocardiographic guidance in children. At this time we feel that fluoroscopy and transthoracic echocardiography are adequate for implantation of the "buttoned" device in children. The advantages and disadvantages with the additional use of transesophageal monitoring are worth investigating in future studies. However, transesophageal studies of atrial septal defect patients are useful in the evaluation for their suitability for transcatheter closure, particularly in the adult and older teenage patients in whom precordial or subcostal views are not adequate for detailed study of the atrial septum.

Paradoxical Embolism

Recent studies indicated that there is a high prevalence of patent foramen ovale with transient right-to-left shunting (demonstrated by transesophageal echocardiography) among young adults with stroke [17,18]. It is hypothesized that clinically evident or latent venous thrombus may paradoxically embolize through the patent foramen ovale, causing stroke. Although there is no consensus [65], some authors [66,67] recommend surgical closure of the foramen ovale in an attempt to prevent further paradoxical embolism. It is not clear whether anticoagulant therapy alone or in combination with closure of the patent foramen ovale are the most appropriate choices in the management of these patients. If closure of patent foramen ovale is chosen, it seems to us that transcatheter closure is an effective alternative to surgical closure. We [16,22], Mills and King [2], and Rome and associates [12] have utilized this technique and achieved closure of the patent foramen ovale. No recurrence of paradoxical embolism was observed during the follow-up period, although the duration of follow-up has not been very long. We

believe that the transcatheter closure of a patent foramen ovale in this group of patients is an effective alternative to surgical closure and may have a role in the management of young adults with stroke. Further clinical trials to investigate these issues are warranted.

CONCLUSIONS

Attempts to replace surgical treatment of selected congenital heart defects with transcatheter methods began in the mid 1960s. Several types of devices and device delivery systems have been developed and refined to some degree. Safety and efficacy have been reasonably good, but most of the available devices and delivery systems are bulky and cumbersome. Some miniaturization of the devices has taken place, and some are more suitable for clinical use today than in the past. Clinical trials to examine the safety and effectiveness and further miniaturization of the devices are required prior to routine application of these techniques in the treatment of certain congenital cardiac defects.

REFERENCES

1. King TD, Mills NL (1974): Nonoperative closure of atrial septal defects. Surgery 75:383–388.
2. King TD, Thompson SL, Steiner C, Mills NL (1976): Secundum atrial septal defect: Nonoperative closure during cardiac catheterization. JAMA 235:2506–2509.
3. Mills NL, King TD (1976): Nonoperative closure of left-to-right shunts. J Thorac Cardiovasc Surg 72:371–378.
4. Rashkind WJ (1983): Transcatheter treatment of congenital heart disease. Circulation 67:711–716.
5. Rashkind WJ (1975): Experimental transvenous closure of atrial and ventricular septal defects, abstracted. Circulation 52:11–18.
6. Rashkind WJ, Cuaso CC (1977): Transcatheter closure of atrial septal defects in children, abstracted. Eur J Cardiol 8:119–120.
7. Hellenbrand WE, Mullins CE (1989): Catheter closure of congenital cardiac defects. Cardiol Clin 7:351–368.
8. Beekman RH, Rocchini AP, Snider AR, Rosenthal A (1989): Transcatheter atrial septal defect closure:

Preliminary experience with the Rashkind occluder device. J Intervent Cardiol 2:33-41.

9. Lock JE, Rome JJ, Davis R, Van Praagh S, Perry SB, Van Praagh R, Keane JF (1989): Transcatheter closure of atrial septal defects: Experimental studies. Circulation 79:1091-1099.

10. Hellenbrand WE, Fahey JT, McGowan FX, Weltin GG, Kleinman CS (1990): Transesophageal echocardiographic guidance of transcatheter closure of atrial septal defect. Am J Cardiol 66:207-213.

11. Lock JE, Hellenbrand WE, Latson L, Mullins CE, Benson L, Rome JJ (1989): Clamshell umbrella closure of atrial septal defects: Initial experience, abstracted. Circulation 80(Suppl II):592.

12. Rome JJ, Keane JF, Perry SB, Spevak PJ, Lock JE (1990): Double-umbrella closure of atrial defects: Initial clinical applications. Circulation 82:751-758.

13. Sideris EB, Sideris SE, Fowlkes JP, Ehly RL, Smith JE, Gulde RE (1990): Transvenous atrial septal occlusion in piglets using a "buttoned" double-disc device. Circulation 81:312-318.

14. Sideris EB, Sideris SE, Thanopoulos BD, Ehly RL, Fowlkes JP (1990): Transvenous atrial septal defect occlusion by the "buttoned" device. Am J Cardiol 66:1524-1526.

15. Rao PS, Sideris EB, Chopra PS (1991): Catheter closure of atrial septal defect: Successful use in a 3.6 kg infant. Am Heart J 121:1826-1829.

16. Rao PS, Wilson AD, Levy JM, Gupta VK, Chopra PS (1992): Role of "buttoned" double-disc device in the management of atrial septal defects. Am Heart J 123:191-200.

17. Lechat R, Mas JL, Lascault G, Loron P, Therod M, Khimezag M, Drobinski G, Thomas D, Grosgogreat Y (1988): Prevalence of patent foramen ovale in patients with stroke. N Engl J Med 318:1148-1152.

18. Webster MWI, Chancellor AM, Smith HJ, Swift DL, Sharpe DN, Base NM, Glasgow GL (1988): Patent foramen ovale in young stroke patients. Lancet 2:11-12.

19. King TD, Thompson SL, Mills NL (1978): Measurement of atrial septal defect during cardiac catheterization: Experimental and clinical results. Am J Cardiol 41:537-542.

20. Rao PS, Langhough R (1991): Relationship of echocardiographic, shunt flow, and angiographic size to the stretched diameter of the atrial septal defect. Am Heart J 122:505-508.

20a. Forfar JC, Godman MJ (1985): Functional and anatomical correlates in atrial septal defect: An echocardiographic analysis. Br Heart J 54:193-200.

21. Latson LA (1993): Transcatheter closure of atrial septal defects. In Rao PS (ed): "Transcatheter Therapy in Pediatric Cardiology." New York: Wiley-Liss, pp 335-348.

22. Rao PS, Wilson AD, Chopra PS (1992): Transcatheter closure of atrial septal defects by "buttoned" devices. Am J Cardiol 69:1056-1061.

23. Sideris EB, Rao PS, Lloyd TR, Beekman RH, Worms AM, Lababidi Z (1991): Transvenous occlusion at atrial septal defect by the Sideris buttoned device: Early international experience, abstracted. Circulation 84:II-544.

24. Sideris EB, Rao PS: Unpublished observations.

25. Porstmann W, Wierny L, Warnke H (1967): Der verschluss des ductus arteriosus persistens ohne thorakotomie (1, Miffeilung). Thoraxchirurgie 15:199-203.

26. Porstmann W, Wierny L, Warnke H, Gerstberger G, Romaniuk PA (1971): Catheter closure of patent ductus arteriosus: 62 cases treated without thoracotomy. Radiol Clin North Am 9:203-218.

27. Wierny L, Plass R, Porstmann W (1986): Transluminal closure of patent ductus arteriosus: Long-term results of 208 cases treated without thoracotomy. Cardiovasc Intervent Radiol 9:279-285.

28. Takamiya M (1973): Ductus closure without thoracotomy. Jpn J Thorac Surg 26:749-753.

29. Sato K, Masaoki F, Kozuka T, Nappo Y, Kitamura S, Nakano S, Ohyama C, Kawashima Y (1975): Transfemoral plug closure of patent ductus arteriosus: Experience with 61 consecutive cases. Circulation 31:337-341.

30. Kitamura S, Sato K, Naito Y, Shimizu Y, Fujino M, Oyama C, Nakano S, Kawashima Y (1976): Plug closure of patent ductus arteriosus by transfemoral catheter method: A comparative study with surgery and a new technical modification. Chest 70:631-635.

31. Leslie J, Lindsay W, Amplatz K (1977): Nonsurgical closure of patent ductus arteriosus: An experimental study. Invest Radiol 12:142-145.

32. Warnecke I, Frank J, Hohle R, Lemm W, Bucherl ES (1986): Transvenous double-balloon occlusion of the persistent ductus arteriosus: An experimental study. Pediatr Cardiol 5:79-84.

33. Magal C, Wright KC, Duprat G, Wallace S, Gianturco C (1989): A new device for transcatheter closure of patent ductus arteriosus: A feasibility study in dogs. Invest Radiol 24:272-276.

34. Echigo S, Matsuda T, Kamiya T, Truda E, Suda K, Kuroe K, Ono Y, Yazawa K (1990): Development of a new transvenous patent ductus arteriosus occlusion technique using a shape memory polymer. ASAIO Trans 36:M195-198.

35. Rashkind WJ, Cuaso CC (1979): Transcatheter closure of a patent ductus arteriosus: Successful use in a 3.5 kg infant. Pediatr Cardiol 1:3-7.

36. Rashkind WJ, Cuaso CC, Gibson R: Closure of patent ductus arteriosus in infants and small children without thoracotomy. Proceedings of the Association of European Pediatric Cardiologists. 7th Annual meeting, Madrid, Spain, 8–11 May 1979, p 67.

37. Rashkind WJ, Mullins CE, Hellenbrand WE, Tait MA (1987): Nonsurgical closure of patent ductus arteriosus: Clinical application of the Rashkind PDA occluder system. Circulation 75:583–592.

38. Wessel DL, Keane JF, Parness I, Lock JE (1988): Outpatient closure of the patent ductus arteriosus. Circulation 77:1068–1071.

39. Dyck JD, Benson LN, Smallhorn JF, McLaughlin PR, Freedom RM, Rowe RD (1988): Catheter closure of the persistently patent ductus arteriosus. Am J Cardiol 62:1089–1092.

40. Latson LA, Hofschire PJ, Kugler JD, Cheatham JP, Gumbiner CH, Danford DA (1989): Transcatheter closure of patent ductus arteriosus in pediatric patients. J Pediatr 115:549–553.

41. Khan MA, Mullins CE, Nihill MR, Al Yousef S, Aloufy S, Abdulla M, Al Fagih MR, Sawyer W (1989): Percutaneous catheter closure of the ductus arteriosus in children and young adults. Am J Cardiol 64:218–221.

42. Gelb BD, O'Laughlin MP, Mullins CE (1990): Prevalence of additional cardiovascular anomalies in patients referred for transcatheter closure of patent ductus arteriosus. J Am Coll Cardiol 16:1680–1686.

43. Sideris EB, Sideris SE, Ehly RL (1990): Occlusion of patent ductus arteriosus in piglets by a double-disc self-adjustable device, abstracted. J Am Coll Cardiol 15:240 A.

44. Rao PS, Wilson AD, Sideris EB, Chopra PS (1991): Transcatheter closure of patent ductus arteriosus with "buttoned" device: First successful clinical application in a child. Am Heart J 121:1799–1802.

44a. Rao PS, Wilson AD, Chopra PS, Smith PN, Sideris EB (1992): Transcatheter occlusion of patent ductus arteriosus with buttoned device, abstracted. Clin Res 40:759a.

45. Krichenke A, Benson L, Burrows P, Moes CF, McLaughlin P, Freedom RM (1989): Angiographic classification of the isolated persistently patent ductus arteriosus and implications for percutaneous catheter occlusion. Am J Cardiol 63:887–889.

46. Rao PS (1985): Descending aortography with balloon inflation: a technique for evaluating the size of the persistent ductus arteriosus in infants with large proximal left-to-right shunts. Br Heart J 54:527–532.

47. Furukawa S, Toriedo M, Nakayama T, Morita N,

Kahn R, Oda T, Fujii Y, Yamaki R (1977): Catheter closure of patent ductus arteriosus without thoracotomy. Kyobu Geka 30:673–677.

48. Naito Y, Shirakura R, Matsudo Y, Imura K, Hata S, Fujii Y, Sato K (1977): Plug closure of patent ductus arteriosus without thoracotomy. Experience in 50 consecutive patients with technical improvements. Kyobu Geka Gakkai Zasshi 25:1270–1277.

49. Shimizu Y, Miyamoto T, Horiguchi Y, Ozawa M, Oohashi H, Suzuki H, Suchiro S, Okamoto E, Sato K (1978): Nippon Kyobu Geka Gakkai Zasshi 26:1093–1104.

50. Bussmann WD, Sievert H, Kaltenbach M, Kohler KP (1984): Transfemoraler verschlusse des ductus arteriosus persistens. Dtsch Med Wochenschr 35:1322–1326.

51. Benson L (1993): Catheter closure of the ductus arteriosus. In Rao PS (ed): "Transcatheter Therapy in Pediatric Cardiology." New York: Wiley-Liss, pp 321–333.

52. Musewe NN, Benson LN, Smallhorn JS, Freedom RM (1989): Two-dimensional echocardiographic and color-Doppler evaluation of ductal occlusion with the Rashkind prosthesis. Circulation 80:1706–1710.

53. Hosking MCK, Benson LN, Musewe N, Freedom RM (1989): Reocclusion for persistent shunting after catheter placement of the Rashkind patent ductus arteriosus occluder. Can J Cardiol 5:340–342.

54. Rao PS, Sideris EB: Unpublished observations.

55. Rashkind W, Cuaso C (1977): Transcatheter closure of atrial and ventricular septal defects in the experimental animal, abstracted. Eur J Cardiol 5:297.

56. Lock JE, Block PC, McKay RG, Baim DS, Keane JF (1988): Transcatheter closure of ventricular septal defects. Circulation 78:361–368.

57. Goldstein SAN, Perry SB, Keane JF, Rome J, Lock JE (1990): Transcatheter closure of congenital ventricular septal defects. J Am Coll Cardiol 15:240A.

58. O'Laughlin MP, Mullins CE (1989): Transcatheter occlusion of ventricular septal defects. Cathet Cardiovasc Diagn 17:175–179.

59. Bridges ND, Perry SB, Keane JF, Goldstein SAN, Mandell V, Mayer JE Jr, Jonas RA, Easteneda AR, Lock JE (1991): Perioperative transcatheter closure of congenital muscular ventricular septal defects. N Engl J Med 321:1312–1317.

60. Lock JE, Bass JL, Lund G, Rysavy JA, Lucas RV, Jr (1985): Transcatheter closure of patent ductus arteriosus in piglets. Am J Cardiol 55:826–829.

61. Lock JE, Cockerman JT, Keane JF, Finley MP, Wakely PE, Fellows KE (1987): Transcatheter um-

brella closure of congenital heart defects. Circulation 75:593-599.

62. Rashkind WJ (1969): A cardiac catheter device for removal of plastic catheter emboli from children's hearts. J Pediatr 74:618-620.

63. Fisher RG, Ferreyro R (1978): Evaluation of current techniques for nonsurgical removal of intravascular iatrogenic foreign bodies. Am J Roentgenol 130:541-552.

64. Rao PS, Langhough R, Beekman RH, Lloyd TR, Sideris EB (1992): Echocardiographic estimation of balloon-stretched diameter of secundum atrial septal defects for transcatheter occlusion. Am Heart J 124:172-175.

65. Kase CS, Fisher M, Babilaan VL, Mohr JP (1991): Cerebrovascular disease. In Rosenberg RN (ed): "Comprehensive Neurology." New York: Raven Press, pp 97-156.

66. Shaw RC, Rudbrook A, Weiss AN, Welden CS (1976): Massive pulmonary embolism permitting paradoxical systemic arterial embolism: successful surgical management. Ann Thorac Surg 22:293-295.

67. Lascalzo J (1986): Paradoxical embolism: Clinical presentation, diagnostic strategies, and therapeutic options. Am Heart J 112:141-145.

19

Role of Embolization Therapy in the Treatment of Infants and Children

Jean S. Kan, M.D.

Division of Pediatric Cardiology, The Helen B. Taussig Children's
Cardiac Center, The Johns Hopkins University School of Medicine,
Baltimore, Maryland 21205

INTRODUCTION

Transarterial embolization techniques were first developed for neurovascular applications in the mid-1960s. Subsequently, interventional radiologists applied the methods to systemic vascular malformations. Embolization materials evaluated have included microfibrillar collagen; autologous blood clot; latex and silicone balloons; barium; bucrylate; wool and dacron coils; thrombin or aminocaproic acid–enhanced blood clot; Gelfoam particles; Ivalon particles (nonabsorbable), liquid silicone; Oxycel; and lyophilized human dura mater [1]. Embolization methods in infants and children became possible with improvements in the tools, advanced catheter techniques to allow entry into complex vacular malformations, and development of the specialty of interventional pediatric cardiology [2].

EMBOLIZATION MATERIALS

Coils

In 1975, 3 mm metalic emboli with cotton strands attached were described by Gianturco et al. [3] for occlusion of small arteries with a coiled version with wool strands for larger arteries. Subsequent modification of the coils permitted introduction through tapered tip catheters [4]. The coils are available in varied sizes. The tip of the delivery catheter is to be positioned through with a guidewire at the site where the coil is to rest. The appropriately sized coil is loaded into the catheter and pushed through with a guidewire. Coil size is selected about 25% larger than the diameter of the vessel to be occluded [2]. The coils cannot be withdrawn back out of the catheter once delivery is initiated. Multiple coils may be inserted into the vessel to be occluded. Soaking coils in thrombin has been suggested for occlusion of high flow vessels [5].

Detachable Balloons

Detachable mini-balloons made of silicone or latex have two advantages over coils. They can be test inflated and then deflated and retrieved if the placement is deemed to be not ideal. The introducing catheter can be positioned proximal to the site of placement and the balloon allowed to float, attached to the inflation catheter, to the desired site of embolization [6].

A double-balloon method has been suggested for balloon occlusion of high velocity flow vessels. An occlusion balloon is inflated in the vessel proximal to the site of occlusion and inflated to reduce flow and prevent premature detachment until the balloon is fully inflated and in a stable position [2]. Balloon size has been recommended to be 20% greater than the vessel diameter measured from the angiogram [2]. Modifications of the technique with development of a guidewire-directed detachable balloon may increase the possible applications to more difficult to reach vessels [7].

Particulate Embolic Material

Small vessels or vascular beds may be occluded with particles mixed with contrast media into a slurry and injected through the delivery catheter in 0.5–1.0 ml volumes. Injection of the slurry is followed by injection of contrast material to clear the catheter and to test for completeness of occlusion [1]. Autologous blood clot, gelfoam, and microfibrillar bovine collagen are absorbable materials that may be resorbed, resulting in incomplete occlusion. Ivalon is not resorbable and may establish more permanent occlusion [8].

Selection of the embolization material depends on the size and shape of the vascular malformation, the ability to direct the catheter to the point of desired occlusion, and the experience of the interventionalist. Combinations of embolic agents (e.g., balloon plus coils) may be used.

VASCULAR MALFORMATIONS TREATED WITH EMBOLIZATION IN INFANTS AND CHILDREN

Systemic Collateral Vessels to Pulmonary Circulation[1]

Large congenital systemic collateral vessels to the pulmonary circulation are associated with cyanotic congenital heart disease, most commonly tetralogy of Fallot with pulmonary atresia. Perry described embolization of 58 aorta pulmonary collateral vessels with Gianturco coils [5]. Complete occlusion was achieved in 42 and subtotal occlusion in 14.

Coil embolization of a large collateral vessel is shown in Figure 1. Balloon embolization may alternatively be utilized in closure of collateral vessels, as shown in Figure 2.

Bleeding Small Collateral Vessels to the Lung

Rupture of small acquired collateral vessels to the lung with resultant hemoptysis may be controlled by proximal embolization of the vessel [9]. Embolization of the source of small collaterals to the lung is demonstrated in Figure 3. Extravasation of contrast during the angiogram to confirm the site of bleeding has been noted to be unusual [9]. Caution is emphasized to define and avoid embolization of vessels from which spinal arteries originate [9].

Pulmonary Arteriovenous Malformations

Pulmonary artery to pulmonary vein fistulae are congenital malformations in the pulmonary vascular bed and may present with cyanosis or hemoptysis and may be familial (Fig. 4). Seventy-six patients with pulmonary arteriovenous malformations (PAVM) were reported by White et al. [10]. In those patients, 266 PAVMs were treated with balloon embolization alone, and 10 had placement of coils in addition to balloon placement. Some of the patients required multiple catheterizations to achieve successful occlusion. Occlusion of diffuse multiple PAVMs by coil placement only has been reported [11].

Blalock-Taussig Shunts

Balloon embolization of Blalock-Taussig shunts has been successful in experimental [12], and in clinical [13] settings. High flow velocity has presented a technical challenge. Coil embolization in a series of 14 patients resulted in complete occlusion in six and sub-

---

[1]Editor's note: Another important application of this technique is in infants with Scimilar syndrome who are in heart failure secondary to systemic arterial supply to the lung.

Dickinson et al. (Br Heart J 1982; 47:468–472) selectively occluded an aberrant artery with Gelfoam fragments. The infant rapidly improved from symptoms of heart failure.

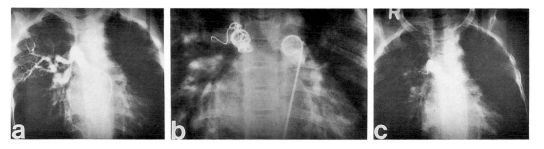

Fig. 1. a: A large systemic arterial collateral vessel to the pulmonary circulation in a young girl with severe tetralogy of Fallot. **b:** Multiple Gianturco coils inserted into the large collateral vessel. **c:** Selective injection proximal to the coils shows occlusion of the collateral vessel.

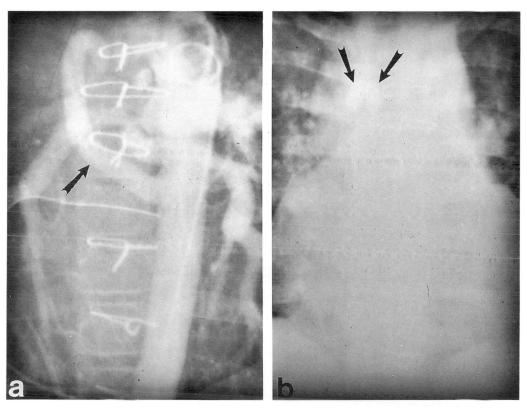

Fig. 2. a: Large collateral vessels to both lungs demonstrated on an aortogram in a girl who had congestive heart failure after the first stage of repair of tetralogy of Fallot with pulmonary atresia. The large vessel to the right lung (arrow) was occluded by two detachable balloons. **b:** Two balloons are in place in the collateral vessel (arrows). The first balloon had migrated to an area of stenosis in the collateral vessel after premature detachment. The vessel was completely occluded by placement of the second balloon.

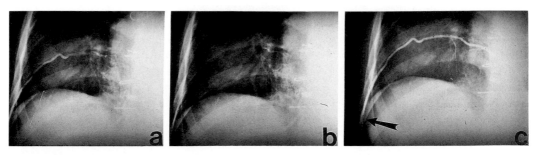

Fig. 3. Selective intercostal injection angiograms in an adolescent with massive recurrent hemoptysis following a Glenn shunt and right ventricle outflow tract reconstruction for management of pulmonary atresia and hypoplastic right ventricle. **a:** The intercostal vessel supplying the flow to the right lower lung in the area of infiltrate on chest x-ray (early phase). **b:** Late phase of the angiogram shows opacification of the lung parenchyma and the typical absence of extravasation of contrast into the lung. **c:** Following embolization with Gelfoam particles distal occlusion of the vessel was demonstrated (arrow) with no late filling of the lung. Subsequently, there was no recurrence of hemoptysis.

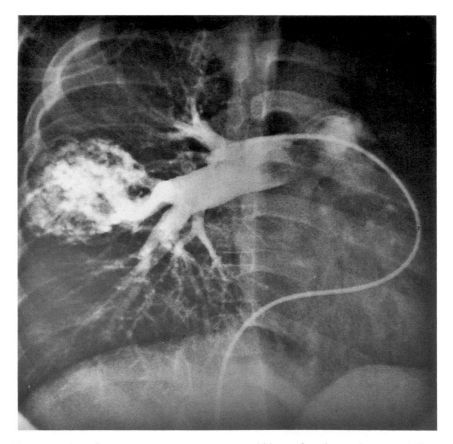

Fig. 4. Right pulmonary arteriogram in a 6-year-old boy referred to pediatric cardiology for evaluation of cyanosis and a heart murmur. The pulmonary arteriovenous malformation was subsequently managed by balloon occlusion of the feeder vessels in a collaborative procedure with interventional radiology.

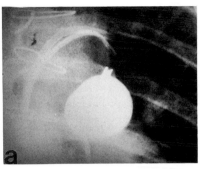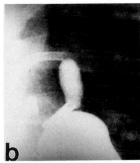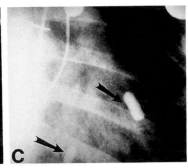

Fig. 5. Attempted double-balloon technique for detachable balloon occlusion of a Blalock-Taussig shunt that remained after total correction of tetralogy of Fallot. **a:** A large occlusion balloon is in place in the left pulmonary artery at the site of insertion of the Blalock-Taussig shunt. **b:** The detachable balloon is inflated in what appeared by cineangiography to be a tiny shunt. **c:** Despite occlusion of flow through the shunt and stable position of two detachable balloons at the time of detachment, both embolizing detachable balloons migrated into the left pulmonary artery after deflation of the large occlusion balloon (arrows).

total occlusion in five, with coil embolization to the pulmonary artery in three [5].

Systemic Arteriovenous Fistulae

Because of the skills of the interventional pediatric cardiologist, involvement in the treatment of systemic arteriovenous fistulae may be primary or collaborative. Embolization techniques are usually preferable to surgical intervention and include balloon, coil, particulate, and liquid agents [14].

Vein of Galen Malformations

Clinical congestive heart failure in neonates may involve the pediatric cardiologist in the early diagnosis and management of vein of Galen malformation. Friedman et al. [15] reported a multidisciplinary staged protocol that involved embolization and neurosurgical obliteration. Twenty-two patients who presented in the neonatal period were managed by a collaborative team from neonatology, pediatric cardiology, neuroradiology, neurosurgery, pediatric neurology, and nursing.

Coronary Artery Fistulae

Transcatheter occlusion of coronary artery fistula connection to right atrium or right ventricle has been accomplished with coil placement, balloon placement, and balloon plus coil placement [16–18].

Internal Mammary to Portal Vein

There is one report of balloon occlusion of a fistula connecting the left internal mammary artery and the portal vein in a 10-month-old infant [19].

COMPLICATIONS OF EMBOLIZATION THERAPY

Complications reported as a consequence of embolization therapy include embolization of the device (Fig. 5), pulmonary embolism [20], embolization to the systemic arterial circulation [5,10,21], chest pain [9,10], premature detachment of balloon [13], catheterization failure, vascular damage, ectopic deposition of coil, bacterial contamination of thrombus, transient pulmonary infarction [21], and fever [9]. As in any interventional procedure, the risks and benefits must be weighed to reach a decision about therapy.

REFERENCES

1. Kadir S, Kaufman SL, Barth KH, White RI (1982): "Selected Techniques in Interventional Radiology." Philadelphia: WB Saunders.

2. Mitchell SE, Kan JS, White RI (1985): Interventional techniques in congenital heart disease. Semin Roentgenol 20:290–311.

3. Gianturco C, Anderson JH, Wallace S (1975): Mechanical devices for arterial occlusion. Am J Roentgenol 124:428–435.

4. Chuany VP, Wallace S. Gianturco C (1980): A new improved coil for tapered-tip catheter for arterial occlusion. Radiology 135:507–509.

5. Perry SB, Radtke W, Fellows KE, Keane JF, Lock JE (1989): Coil embolization to occlude aortopulmonary collateral vessels and shunts in patients with congenital heart disease. J Am Coll Cardiol 13:100–108.

6. Mullins CE (1990): "The Science and Practice of Pediatric Cardiology." Philadelphia: Lea and Febiger p 2183.

7. Makita K, Furui S, Machida T, Yamauchi T, Takenaka E (1991): Wire-directed detachable balloons. Radiology 180(3):139:140.

8. White RI, Strandberg JD, Gross GS, Barth KH (1977): Therapeutic embolization with long-term occluding agents and their effects on embolized tissues. Radiology 125:677–687.

9. Kaufman SL, Kan JS, Mitchell SE, Flaherty JT, White RI Jr (1986): Embolization of systemic to pulmonary artery collaterals in the management of hemoptysis in pulmonary atresia. Am J Cardiol 58:1130–1132.

10. White RI, Lynch-Nyhan A, Terry P, Buescher PC, Farmlett EJ, Charnas L, Shuman K, Kim W, Kinnison M, Mitchell SE (1988): Pulmonary arteriovenous malformations: Techniques and long-term outcome of embolotherapy. Radiology 169:663–669.

11. Kirsch LR, Sos TA, Engle MA (1991): Successful coil embolization for diffuse, multiple arteriovenous fistulas. Am Heart J 122:245–248.

12. Gewillig M, Van der Hauwaert L (1990): Transcatheter occlusion of high flow Blalock-Taussig shunts with a detachable balloon. Am J Cardiol 65:1518–1519.

13. Florentine M, Wolfe RR, White RI (1984) Balloon embolization to occlude a Blalock-Taussig shunt. J Am Coll Cardiol 3:200–202.

14. Gerson LP (1990) Arteriovenous fistulae. "The Science and Practice of Pediatric Cardiology." Philadelphia: Lea and Febiger, pp 1471–1481.

15. Friedman DM, Madrid M. Berenstein A. Choi IS, Wisoff JH (1991): Neonatal vein of Falen malformations: Experience in developing a multidisciplinary approach using a embolization treatment protocol. Clin Pediatr 30:621–629.

16. Issenberg HJ (1990): Transcatheter coil closure of a congenital coronary artery fistula. Am Heart J 120:1441–1443.

17. Reidy JF, Tyman MJ, Quereshi S: (1990): Embolization of a complex coronary ateriovenous fistula in a 6 year old child: The need for specialized embolization techniques. Br Heart J 63:246–248.

18. Reidy JF, Anjos RT, Qureshi SA, Baker EJ, Tynan MH (1991): Transcatheter embolization in the treatment of coronary artery fistulas. J Am Coll Cardiol 18:187–192.

19. Cobby MJ, Culling W, Jordan SC, Hartnell GG (1989): Balloon embolization of a congenital arteriovenous fistula between the internal mammary artery and a portal vein radicle. Brit J Radiol 62:371–373.

20. McCarthy P, Kennedy A, Dawson P, Allison D (1991): Pulmonary embolus as a complication of therapeutic peripheral arterio-venous malformation embolization. Br J Radiol 64:177–178.

21. Remey-Jardin M, Wattinne L, Remy J (1991): Transcatheter occlusion of pulmonary arterial circulation and collateral supply: Failures, incidents and complications. Radiology 180:699–705.

20

Transcatheter Retrieval of Intravascular/Intracardiac Foreign Bodies

P. Syamasundar Rao, M.D.

Department of Pediatrics, Division of Pediatric Cardiology,
University of Wisconsin Medical School, University of Wisconsin
Children's Hospital, Madison, Wisconsin 53792-4108

INTRODUCTION

Due to the widespread use of polyethylene catheters in critically ill patients, both for monitoring and for fluid administration, inadvertent embolization of these catheters into the cardiovascular system has increased and constitutes the single largest source of intracardiac and/or intravascular foreign bodies. Fragments of guidewires and catheters dislodged during cardiac catheterization, pacing catheters, detached cerebral ventriculoatrial shunts (used for hydrocephalus), and other foreign bodies constitute a minority of intracardiac foreign bodies. The first documented episode of intravascular embolization of polyethylene catheter is that reported by Turner and Summers [1] in 1954. Initial treatment approach was by surgical removal. To the best of my knowledge, Thomas et al. [2] were the first to remove an intravascular foreign body (broken guidewire) nonsurgically. In their 1964 report, they retrieved the guidewire with a bronchoscopic forceps introduced via saphenous vein cutdown. Documentation of intracardiac foreign body removal in children, to the best of my knowledge, was first presented by Rashkind [3] in 1969. Over the years, multiple reviews of this subject have appeared in the literature, and these [4–14] are listed for use by the interested reader. In this chapter, I will review the current state of the knowledge on intravascular/intracardiac foreign bodies with

particular reference to their transluminal retrieval. There is extensive experience with this technique in adult patients. There is a limited but successful use of this technique in pediatric patients. The general principles related to intravascular foreign bodies are similar for both groups, and the ensuing presentation is equally applicable to both groups.

INTRAVASCULAR FOREIGN BODIES
Incidence

Since the first introduction by Myers [15] in 1945 of indwelling intravascular catheters, these catheters have become a common source of intravascular and intracardiac foreign body emboli. In the earlier years, severing of the polyethylene catheters by the needle tip of the introducer set was the cause of catheter embolization. More recently, after these introducer sets were replaced with new puncture systems (Seldinger technique or its modification), the embolization appears to be related to the severing of the catheter while the fixation suture is cut during catheter removal [13]. Incidence of catheter embolization is essentially unknown, but based on extensive review of published cases, Burri et al. [7] estimated it to be 0.1 % of catheters inserted. This was in 1971, and therefore, with the modification of the techniques and introduction of other sources of embolism (such as interventional cardiology

Transcatheter Therapy in Pediatric Cardiology, pages 377–392
© 1993 Wiley-Liss, Inc.

procedures), the current incidence may be quite different.

Types of Foreign Bodies

The vast majority of the intravascular foreign bodies are polyethylene catheter fragments used for pressure monitoring or intravenous infusion. In an extensive survey [10], 143 of 180 (79%) were found to be central venous pressure catheters. Other frequently reported foreign bodies in this survey were standard diagnostic cardiac catheters (3%), guidewires (3%), broken permanent pacing catheters (4%), and cerebral ventriculoatrial shunt catheters (7%) used for treatment of hydrocephalus. Other types of intracardiac foreign bodies reported in this survey, and those observed by other investigators, include femoral vein dilators [10,12], metal catheter-shapers [10], broken Swan-Ganz catheters [10], Gianturco coils [14,16–19], Kirschner wires [20], bullets [10,21,22], Kimray-Greenfield or other vena caval filters [14,23], Rashkind's patent ductus arteriosus devices [24], sapphire laser tips [14], and hemodialysis catheters [13]. The relative prevalence of various types of foreign bodies will understandably change as changes in practice of insertion and maintenance of intravenous catheters take place. This also has changed with the introduction of new catheter intervention techniques.

Sites of Foreign Bodies

Bloomfield [6] identified the determinants of lodging sites of the foreign bodies once they are released into the cardiovascular system. These include: a) site of origin of the foreign body embolus; b) length of the embolized fragment; and c) the material from which the embolus is made up of.

Sites of origin of foreign bodies. Venous embolic sites will be determined by the blood flow patterns of the right heart, while arterial emboli on the left heart blood flow pattern. A catheter embolus originating from the antecubital, subclavian, or internal jugular vein (superior vena caval drainage) usually passes through the superior vena cava into the right atrium. The leading end may lodge against the inferior aspect of the tricuspid annulus or in the right ventricular body [6]. The catheter fragment may pass through the right ventricle and embolize into the pulmonary arteries [25], but is unlikely to be lodged in the right ventricular outflow tract. It is rare that such a foreign body passes through the right atrium and down into the inferior vena cava [26,27].

Catheter emboli arising from inferior vena caval draining sites may lodge in the inferior vena cava and high in the right atrium, and on occasion, the leading end may be located in the superior vena cava or right atrium [6]. Occasionally these may paradoxically embolize into the left heart [9].

The foreign bodies released in the aorta (or left ventricle) embolize into the periphery. The factors that control the site of embolization to a specific site are not known.

Length of the foreign body. With longer catheter emboli, the trailing end is likely to remain in the superior vena cava, innominate vein, or subclavian vein [1,26]. If the catheter fragment is short, the trailing end may be in the right atrium and may swing anteriorly. If the end of the catheter is sharp, it may embed into the atrial wall, making it difficult to snare and remove. Very short emboli are likely to embolize into the pulmonary arterial tree.

Type of embolic material. The migration patterns do, to some extent, depend upon the material from which the embolic material is made. Lightweight emboli (polyethylene tubing) are likely to float and follow the direction of the blood flow unless prevented by embedding of one of the ends into the wall of the cardiac chamber. Heavy substances are likely to follow the forces of gravity and land in a dependent position [10], although they can, and do sometimes, follow the flow pattern [22].

Bloomfield's survey results [10] indicated that the proximal end is located in the right atrium in one third of the right heart emboli. Twenty-five percent were lodged in the superior vena cava, and another 25% were lodged in the pulmonary artery. Other lodging sites of the proximal end were the subclavian vein and inferior vena cava. Only rarely were the internal jugular vein, right ventricle, and umbilical vein the lodging sites on the proximal end. By contrast, the right ventricle was the most frequent (33%) site of lodgement of the distal (leading) end. The pulmonary artery (31%) and right atrium (18%) were the next most common sites for the distal end. The distal end was also found lodged in the superior vena cava (5%), inferior vena cava (5%), and hepatic vein (3.5%). The subclavian vein, internal jugular vein, and umbilical vein were the most infrequent (<1%) sites where the distal end was found.

Richardson et al. [9] analyzed 202 cases of catheter embolism reported in 62 publications and determined sites of embolism. These were the pulmonary artery (33%), great veins (25%), right ventricle (18%), right atrium (15%), and lung periphery (4%). Paradoxical embolism into the left heart occurred in 1% of cases.

The left ventricle [28] and aorta [29,30] are rare sites of intravascular emboli. But with the introduction of percutaneous transluminal coronary angioplasty (PTCA), left heart emboli, particularly in the coronary arteries [31–40], have become more frequent.

Adverse Effects of Foreign Bodies

Significant complications have been encountered with retained intravascular/intracardiac foreign bodies. These complications may be categorized into two types [12]. The first type, related to mechanical irritation, includes arrhythmia, arrest, perforation, and inflammation of the heart wall. The second type, related to thrombus formation (which in turn serves as nidus for infection), includes pulmonary embolism, bacterial or fungal endocarditis, sepsis, caval obstruction, and paradoxical embolism. The first group is likely to occur within hours of foreign body embolism, while the thrombotic complications can occur early or late [11].

Most workers identified significant mortality and morbidity related to retained intracardiac foreign bodies. Several investigators reviewed their own material or that reported in the literature and found mortality rates varying from 16 to 61% (Table I), attributable to unremoved foreign bodies [4,7,9,11,41–45]. The causes of death appear to be related to cardiac perforation, arrhythmia, pulmonary embolism, endocarditis, and sepsis [9,13]. The mortality appears to be related to the duration of the unremoved foreign body and the location of the embolus [13]. They are highest when the emboli are located in the right atrium or ventricle, and lowest when they are in the pulmonary artery [9,13].

Apart from the mortality described above, significant nonfatal complications also occur if the foreign body is not removed. In one survey [9], fatal complications occurred in one fourth

TABLE I. Mortality Rate in Patients With Retained Foreign Bodies

Authors	Year	Number of patients	Mortality, number (%)
Taylor and Rutherford	1963	11	5 (46)
Doering et al.	1967	49	8 (16)
Wellman et al.	1968	37	13 (35)
Bernhardt et al.	1970	28	17 (61)
Blair et al.	1970	30	8 (27)
Burri et al.	1970	112	45 (40)
Richardson et al.	1974	42	18 (43)
Burri and Ahnefeld	1977	57	18 (32)
Fisher and Ferreyro	1978	42	16 (38)

of the patients, and nonfatal complications were observed in one fourth. The remaining half of the patients had no major complication during the period of observation.

INDICATIONS FOR FOREIGN BODY REMOVAL

In earlier years, there has been a debate [46,47] as to whether the intracardiac foreign bodies should be removed. This is partly supported by reported incidences in which no complication was observed after retention of a foreign body [9,48–53], and in part, related to risk of open heart surgery (in earlier years) that is required to remove the foreign bodies. As discussed above, there is significant mortality and morbidity associated with retained intravascular/intracardiac foreign bodies. With the availability of less invasive techniques to remove intravascular foreign bodies and the realization that there is significant morbidity and mortality associated with unremoved intravascular foreign bodies, it is now generally recommended that most intravascular foreign bodies be removed, and that this removal be attempted by transcatheter methodology. Perhaps the exceptions for this recommendation are terminally ill patients [6,10], free-floating thrombus [14], and vascular perforation by the foreign body [14]. A relative contraindication is a foreign body that had been in for a long period of time for fear of dislodging mural thrombus [54]. Another exception is a foreign body in the periphery of the lung [9], first of all, such foreign bodies are difficult to snare, and secondly, there is little chance for significant complication associated with such foreign bodies. Thus, the majority of foreign bodies should be removed because of the potential for significant morbidity and mortality.

METHODS OF FOREIGN BODY RETRIEVAL

Prior to attempting retrieval of the foreign body, its precise location should be deter-

mined. In most cases, this can be done by obtaining plain chest x-ray films and through fluoroscopy, because the foreign body is radiopaque. If thrombus formation is suspected, angiography and/or echocardiography may be needed to localize the extent of thrombus material [12]. If the foreign body is not radiopaque, selective cineangiography [25,55] or precordial [56,57] or transesophageal echocardiography [58] may be necessary to locate the foreign body. Once localized, one of the several foreign body retrieval devices may be chosen for foreign body extraction. Most workers, at the present time, use the percutaneous femoral venous route for insertion of the retrieval device. Occasionally the internal jugular venous approach may be necessary [13] to access the foreign body. Various methods/devices that are available for foreign body retrieval will be discussed in the ensuing section of this chapter.

Loop Snare

Some authors [8,12] credit the 1969 publication of Curry [59] for the first description of the loop snare method. But careful review of the literature suggests that Steiner et al. [60] used a loop snare type of instrument in 1965 but were not successful in retrieving the foreign body. Details of the method were not described. In 1967 Massumi and Ross [61] successfully used a loop snare method and removed a catheter embolus whose proximal end was lodged in the superior vena cava and the distal end in the inflow tract of the right ventricle. They utilized a 60-cm-long polyethylene catheter with a doubled-over, 135-cm, flexible guidewire. The loop of the guidewire was used to capture and snare the foreign body, and the entire system was withdrawn through the venous entry site. In 1969 Curry [59] proposed a very similar system and described the technique in detail. However, he had not, as of that time, used the technique to retrieve intracardiac foreign bodies. Since the introduction of this technique, multiple modifications of the wire loop snare have been proposed, and include use of steel or nylon loops [62–64], wire and suture through the catheter [65–67], partial or complete removal of the central core of the guidewire [27,68–70], and introduction of a bend or crimp in the guidewire [71]. These modifications were introduced to position the wire loop in a plane that makes it easier to snare the foreign body. Other catheter snare systems, such as the right-angle snares [72,73], gooseneck nitinol snares [74], and triple-lumen catheter and loop snares [75] have also been introduced to produce a wire loop that is perpendicular to the axis of the embolized foreign body. However, the advisability of such high-tech solutions to this uncommon problem has been questioned [76].

Loop snare sets may easily be custom-fabricated from the standard cardiac catheters and guidewires that are ordinarily available in most cardiac catheterization laboratories. They are also commercially available (Cook Inc., Bloomington, IN, and Medi-tech, Watertown, MA). Cook Inc. manufactures both adult and pediatric sets. The adult set consists of a 100-cm-long, 8-Fr catheter with a 300-cm-long, 0.021-inch guidewire. The pediatric set is a 45-cm-long, 6.3-Fr catheter with a 125-cm-long, 0.018-inch guidewire. Medi-tech makes an oval loop retriever that is commercially available. The nitinol gooseneck snares (Microvena, Vadnais Heights, MN) are also commercially available in different sizes: 5, 10, 15, and 25-mm loops (Fig. 1).

The selected (or that provided by the manufacturer) guidewire is folded and introduced into the catheter. When the folded guidewire is extruded out of the catheter, a loop is formed. The size of the loop can be adjusted, as necessary, by withdrawing or advancing one of the ends of the guidewire. The loop snare

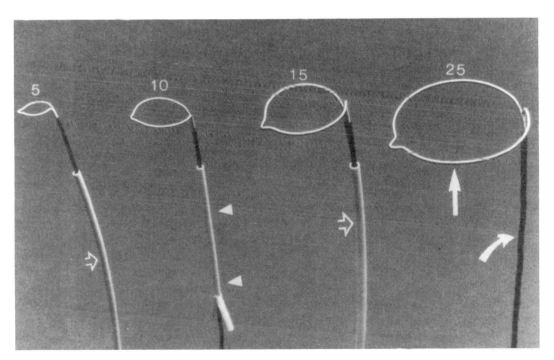

Fig. 1. Nitinol gooseneck snares (5,10,15, and 25 mm). The following are shown: gold-plated snare loop (solid straight arrow), Teflon shrink-wrap around cable (curved arrow), 4-Fr (small open arrow) and 6-Fr (large open arrow) polyethylene-guiding catheters, and "cheater" (arrow heads) for introduction of snare into catheter. (Reproduced from Yedlicka et al. [74], with permission of the publisher.)

can also be moved by manipulation of the catheter. The patient or the fluoroscope is positioned in such a manner that the foreign body is seen in its entire length and both ends are visualized. The free end of the foreign body is identified by its motion that is somewhat independent of the cardiac wall motion. It is necessary that a free end is present for application of the loop snare technique for foreign body retrieval. The loop of the retrieval system is positioned at right angles to the long axis of the foreign body. Under fluoroscopy this loop will appear closed. By appropriate motion of the loop snare systems, the foreign body is encircled. When this is accomplished, the catheter is slowly advanced, keeping the loop and foreign body stationary. The tendency for an inexperienced operator is to pull the wire loop into the catheter. This will usually result in disengaging the foreign body from the loop [6]. After the foreign body is engaged by the loop, it is trapped between the tip of the catheter and the guidewire loop by advancing the catheter. Then the entire system, including the foreign body, is withdrawn out of the body. Snaring of the proximal end should be first tried. If it is not feasible, or if it is not free, snaring of the distal end should be attempted. Sometimes it

may be difficult to engage the foreign body within the loop. Use of a redundant loop [5], a compound, convoluted loop [12], Smith's technique [77] (Fig. 2), or a curved-tip catheter [12] may be necessary. Sometimes a different route of entry may have been chosen to effect foreign body retrieval. One of the major problems is that the ordinary wire loop projects in the same direction as the foreign body. However, if the loop is at a 90° angle to the line of the foreign body, the latter may be captured easily by the loop snare. Such right-angle snare loops can either be produced by putting a crimp in the loop [71] or by designing and manufacturing such loops [74]. Although there are no controlled studies with regard to their efficacy, it is likely that a greater success may be achieved with these right-angle snares than with ordinary loop snares.

Baskets and Grasping Forceps

To the best of my knowledge, Lassers and Pickering [30] were the first to employ helical baskets for foreign body retrieval. The tip of a guidewire was broken off and was lost in the left atrium during a Brockenbrough transseptal procedure and embolized into the descending aorta. The guidewire was retrieved

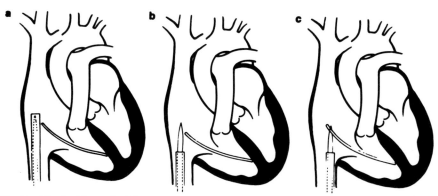

Fig. 2. The Smith method for retrieval of a foreign body if the tight, folded end of the snare loop cannot be placed within the catheter. **a:** The tip of the introducing catheter containing the snare loop is placed beyond the foreign body fragment. **b:** The catheter is withdrawn while the tight, folded end of the snare loop remains in place, forming a loop within the right atrium. **c:** The free end of the catheter fragment is gently encircled by the snare loop. (Reproduced from Gerlock and Mirfakhree [84], with permission of the publisher.)

with the help of a Dormier ureteric stone catcher (Endoscopic Instruments, Co., London), introduced retrogradely via the right femoral artery. Subsequent to this, several workers (5,13,14,16,78–88) used this and other types of helical baskets and removed various types of foreign bodies from the cardiovascular system.

There are several types of helical baskets that are commercially available from Cook, Inc. (Bloomington, IN) and Medi-tech (Watertown, MA). Multiple basket sizes are on the market. The basket consists of four parallel metallic wires, which, when extruded out of the catheter, become spirally oriented and assume the shape of a basket (Fig. 3). The basket can be opened and closed, respectively, by advancing and retracting the handle at the distal end of the catheter.

The basket catheter is introduced through a sheath and positioned at the level of the foreign body. When the basket is opened and closed, the foreign body is trapped, and the basket catheter, along with the foreign body, is removed through the sheath. The basket is particularly useful for retrieval of foreign bodies in the vessels whose diameter does not exceed that of the open basket. It may not be useful in the cardiac chambers, which are much larger

than the diameter of the basket. Sometimes the basket may be bent at its base so as to achieve directional control [12]. The baskets are particularly suited for removal of nonlinear foreign bodies such as bullets and coils [12]. The major problem with this system (apart from not being suitable for extracting foreign bodies from cardiac cavities) is the potential for cardiac perforation from the rigid tip of the helical basket. Modification of the device by converting the rigid tip into a filiform tip or by introducing it over a guidewire (over-guidewire version, Medi-tech, Watertown, MA) may have obviated this problem.

Ranniger [89] designed a grasping forceps with three pronged wires; the pronged wires approximate each other when withdrawn and open up (Fig. 3) when advanced. He used it for foreign body retrieval. Others [57,67] also have used this or similar devices. Commercial sets of this type are readily available from Medi-tech (Watertown, MA) and Microvena (Vadnais Heights, MN).

Endoscopic Forceps and Myocardial Biopsy Catheters

Thomas and associates [2] were not only the first to report the removal of an intravascular foreign body transvenously but were also the

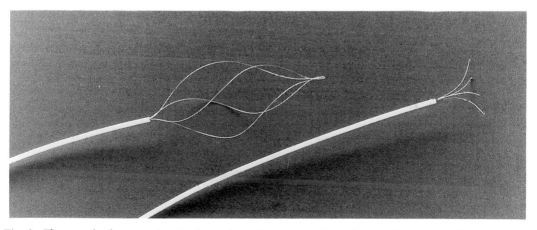

Fig. 3. Photograph of open retrieval basket and grasping forceps. (Reproduced with permission from Medi-tech, Watertown, MA.)

first to use a bronchoscopy forceps to remove it. While performing transseptal puncture in a 48-year-old woman, a 9.5-cm length of the guidewire broke off and became lodged in the right atrium and inferior vena cava. After failing to snare the wire with a hooked-end guidewire, they introduced a bronchoscopic forceps through the saphenous vein, grasped the guidewire embolus in the inferior vena cava, and removed it. Subsequently, many other workers [5,6,9,25,88,90–92] used similar bronchoscopic or other types of endoscopic forceps to retrieve intracardiac/intravascular foreign bodies.

The endoscopic instruments are generally used for removal of foreign bodies from the esophagus, tracheobronchial tree, and urinary tract. They are rigid, straight instruments with an alligator-type tip. They are most commonly introduced by cutdown through the jugular, or occasionally the saphenous/femoral, venous route. These forceps have excellent grasping capability and are most useful in retrieving foreign bodies without a free end, which precludes the use of loop snares or helical baskets for removal. The limitations are rigidity of the instrument, posing considerable risk for perforation;

short length, limiting its use to the foreign bodies within the reach of the forceps; need for cutdown in most cases; and limited maneuverability making it difficult to grasp the right atrial foreign bodies, which are usually displaced anteriorly. Initially placing a smaller-sized catheter (for example, 4-Fr catheter) to guide the introduction of the rigid forceps has been suggested [6] to circumvent the problem of perforation and vascular injury, and may be of value.

The problem of rigidity and risk of perforation and short length may be, in part, solved by using myocardial biopsy catheters to capture and remove intracardiac foreign bodies. These catheters have been successfully used [14,93,94] for retrieving intracardiac foreign bodies. They can be introduced percutaneously either via saphenous or jugular venous routes. The length, flexibility, maneuverability, and grasping capability are advantages of this method. However, perforation can occur, the catheter is expensive, and the catheters can only grasp small-diameter foreign bodies. A free end is not necessary for retrieval, but a foreign body firmly adherent to the wall of the cardiovascular chamber may not be detached with this system (Fig. 4).

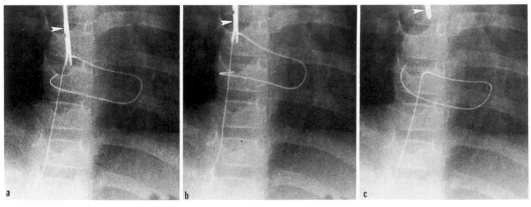

Fig. 4. Selected cineradiographic frames from the attempted retrieval of an intracardiac catheter embolus that has been in place for more than 3 years. A myocardial biopsy catheter was introduced percutaneously via right jugular vein. The radiopaque foreign body was captured by the biopsy catheter (a), and the catheter was pulled. The whole catheter and the "heart" moved upward (b). As further withdrawal proceeded, the catheter became dislodged and fell back to the original place (c). After multiple such attempts, this patient had the foreign body removed surgically. Both ends of the foreign body were found to be completely embedded into the vascular wall.

Selby and associates [95] used a new urologic retrieval forceps (Cook Urological, Spencer, IN) for removing foreign bodies in the pulmonary artery, aorta, and common iliac artery. The forceps is mounted on a flexible, 3-Fr, stainless-steel shaft and is commercially available. Two sizes, 65- and 115 cm in length, are available and are used through a sheath or a guiding catheter. This type of instrument may be useful, and is likely to obviate the disadvantages enumerated for the endoscopic and myocardial biopsy forceps.

Other Methods

While the above-described methods are most commonly used, there are other methods of foreign body retrieval that may be useful in some situations in which the earlier-described methods are not feasible. These include use of a hook guidewire [96], hook catheter [6,67,97,98], pigtail catheter [99], deflector catheter [100–102], and Fogarty catheter [28,94,103,104]. These instruments are more often used as adjuncts to the previously described methods and help reposition and dislodge the foreign body to effect retrieval by other methods [10]. Similarly, a hook catheter [105,106] or a multi-purpose catheter-guidewire set [107] may be used to capture the foreign body; the hook catheter or guidewire may then be snared with a wire loop [105] or helical basket [106,107] and the entire system, including the foreign body, removed. Another technique is a catheter pass-over technique [105], in which a guidewire is passed through the foreign body via a large-caliber catheter, the large-sized catheter is passed over the foreign body, and finally, the entire system is removed (Fig. 5). When simpler methods are not successful in retrieving the foreign body, it may be worthwhile trying a combination of methods to effect retrieval.

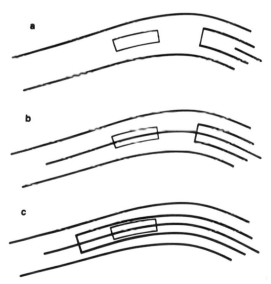

Fig. 5. Catheter pass-over technique. Foreign body fragment in a small branch of the pulmonary artery. **(a).** An introducing catheter is used to direct a guidewire into the foreign body lumen **(b)**. The introducing catheter is advanced over the foreign body fragment **(c)**, and the whole system is removed. Reproduced from Gerlock and Mirfakhree [12], with permission of the publisher.)

RESULTS

The success rate of transcatheter retrieval of intravascular/intracardiac foreign bodies approaches 90%. Bloomfield [10] performed an international survey of nonsurgical retrieval of these foreign bodies and combined them with the published reports. There were a total of 180 intravascular foreign bodies in which adequate data were available for analysis. In only 18 of these could the foreign body not be retrieved, giving a 90% success rate. Transcatheter retrieval was achieved either with a standard loop snare method or a modified version of it in two thirds of the patients. The retrieval was accomplished with helical baskets in one sixth of the patients, and with endoscopic forceps in the remaining one sixth of the patients.

More recently, Dondelinger et al. [14] analyzed 12 published reports [6,13,35,67,83, 87,105,108–112] containing six or more patients in whom transcatheter removal was attempted. There were 176 such attempts, including 12 of their own patients. The foreign bodies were successfully retrieved in 158 patients, giving, again, a 90% success rate. Thus, there appears to be a reasonably good and uniform result following transcatheter retrieval.

The reasons for failure to remove the foreign body have been examined by several workers [6,10,11,14]. These are: a) nonavailability of free ends of the foreign body to capture it with, particularly small foreign body fragments in the peripheral pulmonary artery branches or coronary arteries; b) chronically left-in foreign bodies that are firmly anchored to the vessel or cardiac chamber wall, such as permanent endocardial pacemaker leads; and c) unrecognized extravascular position of the foreign body. Failure of retrieval because the foreign body is on a different plane than the retrieval instrument can be circumvented by the use of biplane fluoroscopy and right-angled snares.

Although the reported experience of transcatheter retrieval in the pediatric patient is not as extensive as in the adult, the results have been as good as those seen in adult patients. I have attempted to gather as many reports in children as I can find; these are listed in Table II [3,5,13,14,21,57,62–64,73,77,79,81,88,95, 100,105,112–117]. As can be seen, transcatheter retrievals have been performed in neonates, children, and adolescents. All methods of removal have been utilized in the pediatric patient. However, it is difficult, based on these reports, to assess degree of success since the number of subjects in whom transcatheter retrieval was attempted is not known. With the availability of small-sized retrieval systems, there is no reason to suspect that the success rate is any different from that observed in adults.

COMPLICATIONS

In the previous reports, transcatheter retrieval of intravascular foreign bodies has not been associated with any significant complications. After an extensive international survey, Bloomfield [10] commented that there is a virtual lack of any complications. Such is also the view of Fisher and Ferreyro [11] after a survey of the literature. Transient arrhythmia has been observed by some workers [6,82,98,105]. Significant arrhythmia [69], manifested as ventricular tachycardia requiring postponement of the procedure, was noted once. If the foreign body has been present for more than a few days, thrombus may develop on the foreign body, and this thrombus may embolize during retrieval attempts. Indeed, asymptomatic pulmonary emboli have been documented [10] by pulmonary perfusion scans following retrieval of a 5-year-old permanent pacemaker catheter. Therefore, it is important that thrombus formation should be excluded if removal of a longstanding intracardiac (vascular) foreign body is attempted. Echocardiography and/or angiography may be necessary to detect thrombus formation. Injury and perforation of vessel or cardiac chamber wall is another potential complication, especially with rigid baskets and endoscopy forceps. Appropriate precautions should, therefore, be undertaken when these methods of retrieval are chosen.

PREVENTION OF FOREIGN BODY EMBOLIZATION

Embolism of foreign bodies into the cardiovascular system should be prevented. Embolization of catheters inserted for pressure monitoring and fluid administration is a preventable complication [60,118]. This complication may be prevented by strictly adhering to the manufacturer's recommendation. Accidental cutting of the tubing with the sharp needle is still possible because of inadvertent or uncontrollable motion of the patient. Because of these problems, these catheters have been, by and large, replaced with Seldinger techniques. While this method has avoided some of the embolizations, embolism continues to occur; this appears to be due to accidental cutting of the catheter while cutting the stay suture during the catheter removal. Meticulous attention to the

TABLE II. Transcatheter Retrieval of Foreign Bodies From the Cardiovascular System in Patients ≤ 20 Years Reported in the Literature

Authors	Year	Ref. no.	Age (years)	Type of foreign body	Location of foreign body[a]	Method of retrieval
Rashkind	1969	3	6	PE catheter	RA	Loop snare
Soni et al.	1970	80	14	PE catheter	LSV-RV	Basket
Tatsumi and Howland	1970	113	0.3	Holter valve	RA-RV	Loop snare
Dotter et al.	1971[b]	5	1	PE catheter	LSV-SVC	Loop snare
McSweeny and Schwartz	1971	100	5	Ventriculoatrial shunt	RA-RV	Catheter deflector
Marlon et al.	1971	62	20	Intracath	RA-RV	Modified loop snare
Bett and Anderson	1971	63	18	Intracath	SVC-RV	Nylon loop modification of loop snare
Delany and Starer	1972	114	9	Spitz-Holter valve	RV-PA	Loop snare
Fergusson	1973	64	1.4	Pudenz valve	RV	Hook wire and loop snare
Block	1973	112	3	Ventriculoatrial shunt	RA-RV	Loop snare
Harnick and Rohmer	1974	81	1.5	Pudenz valve	SVC-IVC	Basket
			7	PE catheter	LSV-RV	Basket
Fisher and Mattox	1978	115	0.2	Hyperalimentation line	IVC-RA	Loop snare
Smith	1978	77	0.02	Argyle UA catheter	DAO-UA	Loop snare
			0.005	Argyle UV catheter	HV-RA	Loop snare
Woo et al.	1979	57	16	Angiocath	IVC-RA	Grasping forceps
Zollikofer et al.	1979	73	3	Catheter plus guidewire	LSV IVC	Loop snare
			14	Hakim ventriculoatrial shunt	RA-PA	Hook catheter and loop snare
			1.6	PE catheter	LPA	Loop snare
Chung et al.	1980	116	0.07	PE catheter	RA	Loop snare
			0.12	Silastic catheter	RA	Loop snare
Shaw	1982	88	17	Silicone catheter	LSV-RV	Gastroscopy biopsy forceps
Uflacker et al.	1986	105	0.4-65	Number of children and other details are not given		
Grabenwoeger	1988	13	2	PE catheter	RA	Basket
Gaylord and Johnsrude	1989	21	17	Bullet	LPA	Basket
Selby et al.	1990	95	3	PE catheter	RPA	Retrieval forceps
			14	Detachable balloon	LCIA	Retrival forceps
Mehan et al.	1990	117	10	7-Fr catheter tip	RA	Loop snare
Dondelinger et al.	1991	14	16	PE catheter	RA	Basket

[a]When two sites are mentioned, they respectively indicate proximal and distal (leading) ends of embolic foreign body. DAo, descending aorta; HV, hepatic vein; IVC, inferior vena cava; LCIA, left common iliac artery; LPA, left pulmonary artery; LSV, left subclavian vein; PE, polyethylene; RA, right atrium; RPA, right pulmonary artery; RV, right ventricle; SVC, superior vena cava; UA, umbilical artery; UV, umbilical vein.
[b]This is personal communication to Dotter from WJ Howland.

details of the technique should prevent or at least reduce catheter embolism. Due to the potential for embolization, all indwelling plastic catheters should be radiopaque so that they can be visualized by fluoroscopy and removed by transcatheter technique in the event of inadvertent embolization.

With regard to embolism of broken catheters and guidewires during cardiac catheterization procedures, these can be prevented by careful manipulation and avoiding stress on the catheter and guidewire segments. It is also important to avoid use of bent catheters or guidewires.

Recognition of the potential for embolism each time an intravascular access is contemplated, and meticulous attention to the details of the technique of insertion, maintenance, and removal, are likely to reduce the incidence of intravascular foreign bodies.

SUMMARY AND CONCLUSIONS

Widespread use of polyethylene catheters in critically ill patients for monitoring and for fluid administration has resulted in inadvertent embolization of these catheter fragments. While recognition of the problem and modifications of the infusion/monitoring catheter systems have resulted in a decrease in catheter emboli, new sources of emboli, such as widespread use of catheter interventional procedures, have emerged. Retained intravascular foreign bodies cause serious complications of arrhythmia, perforation, thrombosis, sepsis, and death. The overall risk of serious complications or death from an unremoved intracardiac foreign body is estimated to be 16 to 61%. Because of this, and because of the availability of the transcatheter method of retrieval, all intracardiac/intravascular foreign bodies should be removed once they are detected. There are many different types of foreign body retrieval techniques. Guidewire loop snare, helical basket, and endoscopic forceps are most commonly utilized in the retrieval. The success rate for transcatheter removal of for-eign bodies is high, at 90%. The complications associated with retrieval are minimal and negligible. Prevention of embolization by meticulous attention to the technique of placing, securing, and removing intravenous catheters is of utmost importance. Due to the potential for embolization, all indwelling plastic catheters should be radiopaque so that they can be visualized by fluoroscopy and removed by transcatheter technique in the event of inadvertent embolization.

There has been extensive experience with transcatheter retrieval techniques in adult patients; there is limited but successful use of this technique in pediatric patients, including neonates and premature infants.

Initial retrieval devices were bulky, but there has been sufficient reduction in the size of the instruments to be of use in pediatric patients. Also, there are a large number of modifications of the initially described techniques so that they can be applied to effectively retrieve most intracardiac/intravascular foreign bodies.

REFERENCES

1. Turner DD, Sommers SC (1954): Accidental passage of a polyethylene catheter from cubital vein to right atrium: Report of a fatal case. N Engl J Med 251:744–745.
2. Thomas J, Sinclair-Smith BC, Bloomfield DA, Davachi A (1964): Non-surgical retrieval of a broken segment of steel spring guide from the right atrium and inferior vena cava. Circulation 30:106–108.
3. Rashkind WJ (1969): A cardiac catheter device for removal of plastic catheter emboli from children's hearts. J Pediatr 74:618–619.
4. Wellman KF, Reinhard A, Salazar EP (1968): Polyethylene catheter embolism: Review of the literature and report of a case with associated fatal tricuspid and systemic candidiasis. Circulation 38:380–392.
5. Dotter CT, Rösch J, Bilbao MK (1971): Transluminal extraction of catheter and guide fragments from the heart and great vessels; 29 collected cases. Am J Roentgenol Radium Ther Nucl Med 111:467–472.
6. Bloomfield DA (1971): Techniques of nonsurgical retrieval of iatrogenic foreign bodies from the heart. Am J Cardiol 27:538–545.

7. Burri C, Henkeneyer H, Passler HH (1971): Katheterembolien. Schw Med Wschr 101:1537–1539.

8. Hipona FA, Sciammas FD, Hublitz UF (1971): Nonthoracotomy retrieval of intraluminal cardiovascular foreign bodies: Clinical and experimental aspects. Radiol Clin North Am 9:583–595.

9. Richardson JD, Grover FL, Trinkle JK (1974): Intravenous catheter emboli: Experience with twenty cases and collective review. Am J Surg 128:722–727.

10. Bloomfield DA (1978): The non-surgical retrieval of intracardiac foreign bodies—An international study. Cathet Cardiovasc Diagn 4:1–14.

11. Fisher RG, Ferreyro R (1978): Evaluation of current techniques for nonsurgical removal of intravascular iatrogenic foreign bodies. Am J Roentgenol 130:541–548.

12. Gerlock AJ, Mirfakhraee M (1987): Retrieval of intravascular foreign bodies. J Thorac Imaging 2:52–60.

13. Grabenwoeger F, Bardach G, Dock W, Pinterits F (1988): Percutaneous extraction of centrally embolized foreign bodies: A report of 16 cases. Br J Radiol 61:1014–1018.

14. Dondelinger RF, Lepoutre B, Kurdziel JC (1991): Percutaneous vascular foreign body retrieval: Experience of an 11-year period. Eur J Radiol 12:4–10.

15. Meyers L (1945): Intravenous catheterization. Am J Nurs 45:930–933.

16. Chuang VP (1979): Nonoperative retrieval of Gianturco coils from abdominal aorta. Am J Roentgenol 132:996–997.

17. Weber T (1980): A complication with the Gianturco coil and its nonsurgical management. Cardiovasc Intervent Radiol 3:156–158.

18. Smith LP (1982): An improved method for intraarterial foreign body retrieval. Radiology 145:539.

19. Vujic I, Moore L, McWey RE (1986): Retrieval of coil after unintentional embolization of ileocolic artery. Radiology 160:563–564.

20. Ahmadi A, Zebe H, Roth E, Storch HH, Schmitz W (1976): Iatrogenic foreign bodies in heart. Thoraxchirurgie 24:213–218.

21. Gaylord GM, Johnsrude IS (1989): Split 24-F Amplatz dilator for percutaneous extraction of an intravascular bullet: Case report and technical note. Radiology 170:888–889.

22. Martire JR, Bijpuria ML, Wilson TH Jr., Wademan RL (1978): Bullet embolus: Heart to right femoral artery. South Med J 71:1435–1437.

23. Yakes WF (1988): Percutaneous retrieval of Kimray-Greenfield filter from the right atrium and placement in the inferior vena cava. Radiology 169:849–851.

24. O'Laughlin MP, Vick GW, Nihill MR, Bricker JT, Mullins CE (1987): Foreign body retrieval: Transcatheter removal of embolized patent ductus arteriosus occlusion devices and catheter pieces, abstracted. J Am Coll Cardiol 9:130A.

25. Smyth NPD, Biovin MR, Bacos JM (1968): Transjugular removal of foreign body from the right atrium by endoscopic forceps. J Thorac Cardiovasc Surg 55:594–597.

26. Hammermeister KE, Kennedy JW (1968): Removal of broken cardiac catheter. N Engl J Med 278:911.

27. Ramo BW, Peter RH, Kong Y (1968): Migration of a severed transvenous pacing catheter and its successful removal. Am J Cardiol 22:880–884.

28. Keltai M, Meier B (1987): Percutaneous retrieval of foreign body from the left ventricular cavity. Cathet Cardiovasc Diagn 13:405–406.

29. Rao VRK, Rout D, Sapra RP (1982): Retrieval of a broken catheter from the aorta without operation. Neuroradiology 22:263–265.

30. Lassers BW, Pickering D (1967): Removal of iatrogenic foreign body from aorta by means of ureteric stone catheter. Am Heart J 73:375–376.

31. Steele PM, Holmes DR Jr., Mankin HT, Schoff HV (1985): Intravascular retrieval of broken guide wire from the ascending aorta after percutaneous transluminal coronary angioplasty. Cathet Cardiovasc Diagn 11:623–628.

32. Keltai M, Bartek I, Biro V (1986): Guidewire snap causing left main coronary occlusion during coronary angioplasty. Cathet Cardiovasc Diagn 12:324–326.

33. Krone RJ (1986): Successful percutaneous removal of retained broken coronary angioplasty guidewire. Cathet Cardiovasc Diagn 12:409–410.

34. Watson LE (1987): Snare loop technique for removal of broken steerable PTCA wire. Cathet Cardiovasc Diagn 13:44–49.

35. Hartzler G, Rutherford B, McConahan D (1987): Retained percutaneous transluminal coronary angioplasty equipment components and their management. Am J Cardiol 60:1260–1264.

36. Steffanino G, Beier B, Finci L, Velebit V, von Segesser L, Faidutti B, Rutishauser W (1988): Acute complications of elective coronary angioplasty: A review of 500 consecutive procedures. Br Heart J 59:151–158.

37. Mikolich JR, Hanson MW (1988): Transcatheter retrieval of intracoronary detached angioplasty guidewire segment. Cathet Cardiovasc Diagn 15:44–46.

38. Yeon EB, Cemaletin NS, Moses JW, McCrossan J (1990): Successful percutaneous removal of retained probe balloon wire during coronary angioplasty. Am Heart J 119:1201–1205.

39. Gurley JC, Booth DC, Hixson C, Smith MD (1990: Removal of retained intracoronary percutaneous transluminal coronary angioplasty equipment by a percutaneous twin guidewire method. Cathet Cardiovasc Diagn 19:251–256.

40. Feldman RL, Trice WA, Hennemann WW III, Furst A (1990): Retrieval of a fractured USCI probe tip from a diseased coronary artery using another fixed-wire balloon catheter, the cordis orion. Cathet Cardiovasc Diagn 19:257–263.

41. Taylor F, Rutherford C (1963): Accidental loss of plastic tube into the venous system. Arch Surg 86:19–21.

42. Doering RB, Stemmer EA, Connolly JE (1967): Complications of indwelling venous catheters. Am J Surg 114:259–266.

43. Bernhardt LC, Wegner G, Mendenhall J (1970): Intravenous catheter embolization to the pulmonary artery. Chest 57:329–332.

44. Blair E, Hunziker R, Flanagan ME (1970): Catheter embolism. Surgery 67:457–461.

45. Burri C, Ahnefeld FW (1977): "Cava Katheter." Berlin: Springer Verlag, pp 55–84.

46. Decker HR (1939): Foreign bodies in the heart and pericardium. Should they be removed? J Thorac Cardiovasc Surg 9:62–79.

47. Swan H, Forsee JH, Goyette EM (1952): Foreign bodies in the heart: Indications for and technique of removal with temporary interruption of cardiac blood flow. Ann Surg 135:314–323.

48. Fair GL (1935): Foreign body in the heart: Report of a case with retention of a large needle with recovery. N Y State J Med 35:453–458.

49. Scebat L, Renais J, Meeus-Bithe L, Le Negre J (1957): Accidents, indication et contre-indications du cathetarisme des cavites droites du coeur. Arch Mal Coeur 50:943–959.

50. Shapiro S (1941): Passage of hollow needle into venous blood stream to heart, through cardiac wall and into thorax. Am Heart J 22:835–838.

51. Tulgan J, Budnitz J (1963): Prolonged survival after catheter embolus. Ann Intern Med 59:564–565.

52. Turner GG (1942): A bullet in the heart for twenty-three years. Surgery 9:832–852.

53. Lamprecht W (1965): Zur Kasuistic iatrgener intrakardialer fremdkorper. Chirurg 36:182–183.

54. Pappas G, Schoultz CA, Jr., Blount SG Jr. (1969): Fractured intracardiac transvenous pacemaker catheter—An unusual cause of pacemaker failure. Am Heart J 78:807–810.

55. McIvor ME, Kaufman SL, Stare R, Porterfield JK, Brinker JA (1989): Search and retrieval of a radiolucent foreign object. Cathet Cardiovasc Diagn 16:19–23.

56. Davies J, Alvares R, Allison DJ (1981): An intracardiac foreign body: Diagnosed non-invasively and removed non-surgically. Br J Radiol 54:987–989.

57. Woo VL, Gerber AM, Scheible W, Woo Seo K, Bookstein J, Leopold G (1979): Real-time ultrasound guidance for percutaneous transluminal retrieval of non-opaque intravascular catheter fragment. Am J Roentgenol 133:750–761.

58. Neumann HPH, Hoffmann T, Koester W, Billmann P, Kauffmann GW (1988): Extraction of an intracardiac catheter embolus using combined radiography and transesophageal echocardiography. Clin Cardiol 11:427–429.

59. Curry JL (1969): Recovery of detached intravascular catheter or guide wire fragments. Am J Roentgenol 105:894–896.

60. Steiner ML, Bartley TD, Byers FM, Krovetz J (1965): Polyethylene catheter in heart: Report of a case with successful removal. J Am Med Assoc 193:1054–1056.

61. Massumi RA, Ross AM (1967): Atraumatic, non-surgical technic for removal of broken catheters from cardiac cavities. N Engl J Med 277:195–196.

62. Marlon AM, Cohn LH, Fogarty TJ, Harrison DC (1971): Retrieval of catheter fragments: Report of two cases. Calif Med 115:61–63.

63. Bett JHN, Anderson ST (1971): Plastic catheter embolism into the right heart: A technique for non-surgical removal. Med J Aust 2:854–856.

64. Ferguson DJG (1973): Removal of an intracardiac foreign body without thoracotomy. Hawaii Med J 32:321–323.

65. Geraci AR, Selman MW (1973): Pulmonary artery emboli: Successful non-surgical removal. Ann Intern Med 78:353–356.

66. Barman PC (1974): A simple method for removal of polyethylene catheters from the pulmonary artery. J Thorac Cardiovasc Surg 65:792–794.

67. Cho SR, Tisnado J, Beachley MC, Vines FS, Alford WL (1983): Percutaneous unknotting of intravascular catheters and retrieval of catheter fragments. Am J Roentgenol 141:397–402.

68. Henley FT, Ballard JW (1969): Percutaneous removal of flexible foreign body from the heart. Radiology 92:176.

69. Hyman AL (1972): An improved snare catheter for retrieving embolized fragments of polyethylene tubing. Chest 62:98–99.

70. West RD, Charrette EJP, Parker JO (1977): Technique for removal of detached polyethylene catheters from intracardiac chambers and great vessels. Can Med Assoc J 117:1310–1311.

71. Hubert JW, Krone RJ, Shatz BA, Susman N (1980): An improved snare system for nonsurgical retrieval of intravascular foreign bodies. Cathet Cardiovasc Diagn 6:405–411.

72. Randall PPA (1972): Percutaneous removal of

iatrogenic intracardiac foreign body. Radiology 102:591-595.

73. Zollikofer C, Nath PH, Castaneda-Zuniga WR, Probst P, Barreto A, Tadavarthy SM, Amplatz K (1979): Nonsurgical removal of intravascular foreign bodies. Fortschr Rontgenstr (ROFO) 5:590-593.

74. Yedlicka JW Jr., Carlson JE, Hunter DW, Castaneda-Zuniga WR, Amplatz K (1991): Nitinol gooseneck snare for removal of foreign bodies: Experimental study and clinical evaluation. Radiology 178:691-693.

75. Furui S, Yamauchi T, Makita K, Takeshita K, Irie T, Tsuchiya K, Sawada S, Nakamura H, Okazaki M (1992): Intravascular foreign bodies: Loop-snare retrieval system with a three-lumen catheter. Radiology 182:283-284.

76. Hartnell GG (1991): Homemade snare for removal of foreign bodies (letter). Radiology 181:903-904.

77. Smith PL (1978): Umbilical catheter retrieval in the premature infants. J Pediatr 93:449-502.

78. Shander D (1970): Removal of embolized polyethylene catheter using a ureteral stone catheter. Chest 57:348-349.

79. Edelstein J (1970): Atraumatic removal of a polyethylene catheter from superior vena cava. Chest 54:381-383.

80. Soni CJ, Osatinsky M, Smith T, Vega S, Vela JE (1970): Nonsurgical removal of polyethylene catheter from right cardiac cavities. Chest 57:398-399.

81. Harnick E, Rohmer J (1974): Atraumatic retrieval of catheter fragments from the central circulation of children. Eur J Cardiol 1:421-422.

82. Pickering E, Gaasch WH (1975): Nonsurgical removal of intracardiac polyethylene catheter emboli. J Am Osteopath Assoc 74:489-491.

83. Aldridge HE, Lee J (1977): Transvascular removal of catheter fragments from the great vessels and heart. Can Med Assoc J 117:1300-1302.

84. Gerlock AJ Jr., Mirfakhraee M (1985): Foreign body retrieval. In "Essentials of Diagnostic and Intervention Angiographic Techniques." Philadelphia: W.B. Saunders.

85. Ransdale DR, Arumugam N, Pidgeon JW (1985): Removal of fractured pacemaker electrode tip using Dotter basket. P A C E 8:759-760.

86. Singer J, Joyce P, Brems J (1989): Basket removal of intraatrial catheter after liver transplantation: Technical note. Cardiovasc Intervent Radiol 12:230-231.

87. Kuffer G, Gebauer A, Antes G, Rath M (1981): Percutane transluminale ent fernung embolisierter-katheterteile. Fortschr Rontgenstr 135:691-694.

88. Shaw TRD (1982): Removal of embolized catheters using flexible endoscopy forceps. Br Heart J 48:497-500.

89. Ranniger K (1968): Instrument for retrieval of intravascular foreign bodies. Radiology 91:1043-1044.

90. Markkula H, Baer G, Heldt C, Isotalo J, Väyryen J (1974): Entfernung eines abgeschnittenen V. subclavia-katheters aus dem rechten herzen mit hilfe einer urologischen fabzange. Anaesthesist 23:232-233.

91. King JF, Manley JC, Zeft HJ, Auer JE (1976): Nonsurgical removal of foreign body from right heart: A new percutaneous approach. J Thorac Cardiovasc Surg 71:785-786.

92. Millan VG (1978): Retrieval of intravascular foreign bodies using a modified bronchoscopic forceps. Radiology 129:587-589.

93. Kurita A, Kanazawa M, Kanie T, Kimura E, Nakayama R, Shoji T (1972): Successful removal of a foreign body from the caval veins by use of endomyocardial bioptome. Jpn Heart J 13:464-469.

94. Bashour TT, Banks T, Cheng TO (1974): Retrieval of lost catheters by a myocardial biopsy catheter device. Chest 66:395-396.

95. Selby JB, Tagtmeyer CJ, Bittner GM (1990): Experience with new retrieval forceps for foreign body removal in the vascular, urinary, and biliary system. Radiology 176:535-538.

96. Wendth AJ, Cross VF, Moriarty DJ, Vitale P, Lopez F (1972): Retrieval of an intracardiac foreign body. Angiology 23:329-337.

97. Maxwell DD, Anderson RE (1972): Transfemoral retrieval of an intracardiac catheter fragment, using a simple hook-shaped catheter. Radiology 103:213-214.

98. Rossi P (1979): "Hook catheter" technique for transfemoral removal of foreign body from right side of the heart. Am J Roentgenol 109:101-106.

99. Khaja F, Lakier J (1979): Foreign body retrieval from the heart by two catheter technique. Cathet Cardiovasc Diagn 5:263-268.

100. McSweeny WJ, Schwartz DC (1971): Retrieval of a catheter foreign body from the right heart using a guide-wire deflector system. Radiology 100:61-62.

101. Gerlock AJ (1975): Guidewire deflector system removal of catheter foreign body retained in the right heart for six months. J Trauma 9:830-832.

102. Nemcek AA Jr., Vogelzang RL (1987): Modified use of the tip-deflecting wire in manipulation of foreign bodies. Am J Roentgenol 149:777-779.

103. Swersky RB, Reddy K, Hamby RI (1975): Balloon catheter technique for removing foreign bodies from heart and great vessels. N Y State J Med 75:1077-1079.

104. Mathur AP, Pochaczersky R, Levowitz BS, Feraru F (1971): Fogarty balloon catheter for removal of catheter fragment in subclavian vein. J Am Med Assoc 217:481.
105. Uflacker R, Luma S, Melichar AC (1986): Intravascular foreign bodies: Percutaneous retrieval. Radiology 160:731-735.
106. Grabenwoeger F, Dock W, Pinterits F, Appel W (1988): Fixed intravascular foreign bodies: A new method for removal. Radiology 167:555-556.
107. Foster CJ, Brownlee WC (1988): Percutaneous removal of ventricular pacemaker electrodes using a Dormier basket. Int J Cardiol 21:127-134.
108. Rossi P, Passariello R, Simonetti G (1980): Intravascular iatrogenic foreign body retrieval. Ann Radiol 23:286-290.
109. Weber J, Sartor K (1980): Perkutane Entfernung intravasaler Fragmente von Infusions Angiographieund Liquor-Drainagekathetern mittels Fangschlingentechnik. Chirurg 51:711-716.
110. Kappenberger L, Tartini R, Steinbrunn W (1985): Transluminale Entfernung endovasaler Fiemdkörper. Schweiz Med Wochenschr 115:258-260.
111. Erdmann E (1988): Perkutane transfemorale Fremdkörperentfernung aus dem Herzen oder aus großen Gefäßen. Dtsch Med Wochenschr 113:1594-1597.
112. Block P (1973): Transvenous retrieval of foreign bodies in the cardiac circulation. J Am Med Assoc 224:241-242.
113. Tatsumi T, Howland WJ (1970): Retrieval of a ventriculoatrial shunt catheter from the heart by a venous catheterization technique: Technical note. J Neurosurg 32:593-596.
114. Delany DJ, Starer F (1972): Recovery of catheters lost in vascular system. Br Med J 1:510.
115. Fisher RG, Mattox KL (1978): Percutaneous extraction of an embolized sialastic hyperalimentation catheter fragment from a 4-kilogram infant. South Med J
116. Chung KJ, Chernoff HL, Leope LL, Kreidberg MB (1980): Transfemoral snaring of broken catheters from the right heart in small infants. Cathet Cardiovasc Diagn 6:331-335.
117. Mehan VK, Lokhandwala YY, Kale PA (1990): Use of a coronary guiding catheter to direct a snare in removal of a retained catheter fragment. Cathet Cardiovasc Diagn 21:294-295.
118. Ross AM (1970): Polyethylene emboli: How many more?. Chest 57:307-308.

21

Transcatheter Ablation in the Treatment of Childhood Dysrhythmia

Paul C. Gillette, M.D., Christopher L. Case, M.D., and Vicki L. Zeigler, R.N., M.S.N.

South Carolina Children's Heart Center, Medical University of South Carolina, Charleston, South Carolina 29425

INTRODUCTION

Tachydysrhythmia may be treated by four modalities. Medication remains the first approach in most cases. Direct surgical ablation of the arrhythmogenic substrate remains the gold standard of definitive nonpharmacologic therapy. Device treatment (pacemaker and defibrillator) and catheter ablation are other treatment modalities. In this chapter we discuss catheter ablation as it relates to pediatric arrhythmias. We do not focus on minute details of technique, since they are changing so rapidly.

Catheter ablation was introduced in 1982 by Schienman et al. [1] and Gallagher et al. [2]. It was put forth mainly as a treatment for chronic refractory atrial fibrillation. The technique involved a direct current discharge from a catheter electrode to a large back paddle. Energies of ≥ 200 W seconds were used. The intent was to create complete atrioventricular (AV) block and to implant a permanent pacemaker. The optimal ablation would completely destroy the bundle of His at its junction, with the AV node resulting in an escape rate that could support the patient if the pacemaker failed.

The technique was expanded to treat any dysrhythmia that used the bundle of His as part of a reentry circuit or in which the tachydysrhythmia could be confined to the atrium by His bundle ablation [3]. Thus AV node reentry, orthodromic reentry in Wolff-Parkinson-White, His bundle automatic focus, atrial automatic focus, and supraventricular tachycardia all underwent His bundle ablation.

Later, other structures, including atrial automatic foci [4], accessory connection [5], Maheim fibers [6], and ventricular myocardial [7] sites that included not only the right atrium and ventricle but also the coronary sinus [8] and left atrium and ventricle, were ablated. The forms of energy used for catheter ablation have also expanded to include radiofrequency [9] laser, microwave, and cryothermia [10]. Lower energy DC ablation with special catheters and discharge waveforms have also been used.

The success of large series of adults has been approximately 64% for producing complete AV block with a small percentage improved by accidental modification of AV node conduction [11]. Major complications both acute and subacute have also arisen in a few percent [12,13]. Cardiac perforation at the time of ablation occurs in about 1% of cases of His bundle ablation. It leads to tamponade but can often be treated by pericardial aspiration or surgical drainage. Late sudden death is another uncommon complication. The exact cause is not known. It is possible, however, that an arrhythmogenic substrate is created by the electrical discharge. A variety of dysrhythmias may be created acutely, including ventricular

Transcatheter Therapy in Pediatric Cardiology, pages 393–399
© 1993 Wiley-Liss, Inc.

ectopy, tachycardia, and junctional automatic tachycardia.

CATHETER ABLATION IN PEDIATRIC PATIENTS (FIGS. 1-3)

Catheter ablation was first applied to pediatric patients with junctional automatic ectopic tachycardia (JET) [14], a dysrhythmia with a 50% mortality with standard management. The arrhythmogenic substrate is an irritative focus in the bundle of His based on electrophysiologic and histopathologic studies. One case had previously been treated by surgical cryoablation [15]. Two infants who had medically refractory JET were ablated using 5 WS/kg. In each the tachycardia was eliminated and an atrial sensing ventricular pacemaker implanted. In the first patient AV conduction resumed but the tachycardia did not. The third case attempted was a 1-day-old neonate with JET. He had been detected *in utero* since his sister had died of JET. He had severely compromised myocardial function. A good His bundle recording could not be obtained, and after two attempts at catheter ablation he was taken to the operating room for surgical ablation, where he expired. Radiofrequency ablation of the bundle of His has also been used successfully in another infant with JET [16].

His bundle ablation has also been used in children for other arrhythmias that involve the

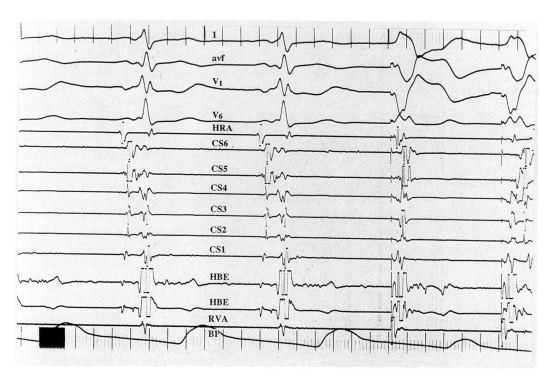

Fig. 1. Surface ECG leads 1, AVF, V1, and V6 recorded simultaneously with a high right atrial electrogram, six coronary sinus electrograms, two His bundle electrograms, a right ventricular apex electrogram, and femoral artery blood pressure. Shown are two sinus beats and two ventricular paced beats. The sinus beats indicate Wolff-Parkinson-White syndrome with short PR interval and delta wave and very short conduction between the electrode pairs 5 and 6, between left atrium and left ventricle. The second beat of ventricular pacing, which is without fusion, shows very rapid ventriculoatrial conduction in the same area.

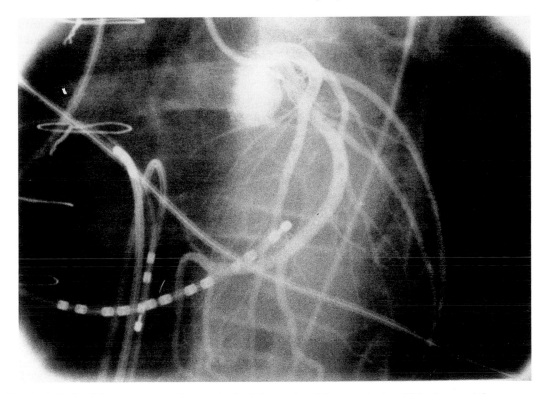

Fig. 2. Selective left coronary arteriogram in the left anterior oblique projection. This shows a left coronary artery with normal left anterior descending and circumflex branches. The circumflex branch ends parallel to the coronary sinus electrode catheter. Three descending branches take off from the circumflex. Also shown are His bundle right ventricular apex and a high right atrial catheter. An ECG electrode passes behind the patient diagonally.

bundle in reentry such as Wolff-Parkinson-White and the permanent form of junctional reentry (PJRT) [7]. His bundle ablation has also been used for AV node reentry in children with success. His bundle ablation therefore is an accepted mode of therapy for certain supra-ventricular tachyarrhythmias in children.

Ablation of the arrhythmogenic substrate has also been reported in children, including atrial automatic foci [4]. The results have been less successful than His bundle ablation. Only three of five atrial automatic tachycardias were ablated and only one of four accessory pathways in PJRT. Only one of four accessory pathways were successfully ablated in another series [17]. No serious complications have been reported in pediatric series.

In the last 18 months we have performed radiofrequency catheter ablation on 125 pediatric patients. The substrates ablated included manifest and concealed Wolff-Parkinson-White, atrial automatic tachycardias, AV node reentry SVT, atrial flutter, and automatic ventricular tachycardia. Overall, a 92% success rate has been found. No serious complications or death has occurred.

INDICATIONS

The indications for catheter ablation have changed dramatically in the last few years. The indications for radiofrequency catheter ablation are the same as those for surgery: 1) life-threatening dysrhythmias, such as syncope related to atrial flutter, fibrillation, or SVT in a patient with Wolff-Parkinson-White; 2) med-

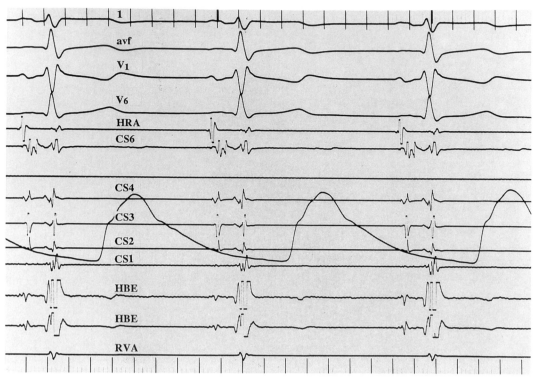

Fig. 3. Postablation surface electrogram showing normal PR interval without delta wave, high right atrial, five coronary sinus bipolar electrograms, His bundle electrogram, right ventricular apex electrogram, and femoral artery blood pressure. The atrioventricular conduction time in coronary sinus pair 6, which had been very short, is now normal. Coronary sinus pair 5, in which the ablation took place, was no longer able to record. Tracing is now normal.

ical failure or intolerance in a patient with non-life-threatening tachycardia (usually medical failure is declared after two drugs; we now make it our practice to offer radiofrequency ablation at the same time as a type I drug, e.g., flecoinide); 3) paitent/parent preference (some patients prefer to take the risk of radiofrequency ablation over the problems of a successful long-term medication); 4) life-threatening potential in an asymptomatic patient (this controversial indication would include a short

antegrade refractory period of the accessory connection in Wolff-Parkinson-White or a rapid response to induced atrial fibrillation in Wolff-Parkinson-White); and 5) cardiomyopathy due to a tachycardia.[1]

ENERGY SOURCES

Radiofrequency (RF) ablation is being used with increasing frequency in adults. It offers the advantage of not creating a pressure wave

[1]Editors note: This type of "arrhythmia-induced cardiomyopathy" will respond favourably if the ventricular rate is brought down; this is irrespective of whether the reduction in ventricular rate is achieved by drug treatment, by surgery, or by transcatheter ablation (Rao PS, Najjar HN: Congestive cardiomyopathy due to chronic tachycardia: resolution of cardiomyopathy with antiarrhythmic drugs. In J Cardiol 17:216–220, 1987).

as DC ablation does. It thus may be less likely to perforate. It has the disadvantage (or advantage) of creating a smaller lesion. His bundle and accessory connection ablation have been performed in adults and children.

Radiofrequency catheter ablation using an atrial approach has been very effective in infants and children. For left-sided pathways a transseptal puncture is used if a patent foramen ovale is not present. We have found this technique successful in 95% of 50 such patients, including several infants. There has been no mortality or significant complications in our series.

Accessory connection ablation has been performed either from the coronary sinus or with a bipolar approach from the left atrium (or coronary sinus) to the left ventricle. Sudden death and left ventricular aneurysm have been reported with the ventricular approach using direct current [20,21].

Modification of the AV node has also been reported using radiofrequency as well as DC ablation in adults. This approach could be useful in atrial arrhythmias. Destruction of the slow pathway between the mouth of the coronary sinus and the tricuspid valve annulus can cure AV node reentry in over 85% of cases using radiofrequency energy. There is a very low risk of AV block using this technique. Lesions in this area may also prevent recurrences of atrial flutter in patients with otherwise normal hearts.

Cryoablation is the technique of choice of surgeons when they prefer not to perform a sharp dissection [18]. It has been used for posterior septal accessory connections and AV node reentry in children from an endocardial approach. It has also been combined with epicardial dissection for free wall and posterior septal accessory connection. Cryothermia lesions are extremely discrete with sharp edges and thus are thought to be less arrhythmogenic. We are currently testing a cryocatheter that uses the Joule-Thompson effect. Expanding nitrous oxide cools the tip to −60° to −70°C. In our

first series we were able to create complete AV block in four of five swine with a transvenous femoral vein approach with an 11 Fr cryocatheter [10]. The fifth animal developed 2:1 AV block. Follow-up was 1 hour. Histologically the lesions were in the proximal bundle of His and were very discrete. No damage to surrounding structures was found. Further studies showed that an 8 Fr catheter with a large hoof-shaped tip was as effective at producing acute AV block as the 11 Fr round tip catheter, while a smaller tipped 8 Fr was not. Chronic studies have shown only 40% complete AV block at 6 weeks after ablation with the 8 Fr catheter. An additional 40% have AV node modification, while in 20% conduction returns to normal [22]. Histologically most of the AV node and proximal bundle of His is destroyed, but a deep rim is left in cases with partial block.

Echocardiography with color Doppler has not shown any significant tricuspid, aortic, or mitral insufficiency either acutely or chronically. Acutely the fibrinogen level decreases about 30%, but no other blood cells or factors change statistically. At 6 weeks postprocedure all blood cells and factors have normalized. No animal has developed sudden death or arrhythmia during 6 weeks of follow-up. Atrial arrhythmia induction protocols have not produced any arrhythmias at the time of procedure or 6 weeks later. Swine under general anesthesia frequently develop ventricular arrhythmia under stimulation in the resting state, so postprocedure stimulation protocols have not been done.

Cryoablation appears to offer promise as the ablation technique of the future; however, significant problems remain to be overcome. Lasers have also been used to ablate the bundle of His in animals. They create discrete lesions and appear to cause little damage to other cardiac structures. They may improve in the future. Other energy sources have also been used, but the effectiveness and complication rates remain to be determined.

CONCLUSIONS

Catheter ablation of arrhythmogenic substrates offer promise of nonsurgical treatment of tachyarrhythmias in children. Improved energy sources will surely bring this technique to its promise in the decade of the 1990s. Improvement in catheter mapping techniques will also be necessary to allow refined small lesions. Techniques that will damage only the arrhythmogenic substrate and not other cardiac structures and advances in interventional techniques of catheterization will have a positive influence on this field. It is likely that in the early twenty-first century totally noninvasive techniques of mapping and ablation will become possible.

ACKNOWLEDGMENTS

This work was supported by grant 1R01HL3842-01 from the National Heart, Lung, and Blood Institute.

REFERENCES

1. Scheinman M, Morady F, Hess DS, Gonzales R (1982): Catheter induced ablation of the atrioventricular junction to control refractory supraventricular arrhythmias. JAMA 248:851–855.
2. Gallagher JJ, Svenson RH, Kasell JH, German LD, Bardy GH, Broughton A, Critelli (1982): Catheter technique for closed-chest ablation of the atrioventricular conduction system. A therapeutic alternative for the treatment of refractory supraventricular tachycardia. N Engl J Med 306:194–200.
3. Scheinman MM, Evans-Bell T (1984): Catheter ablation of the AV junction: A report of the percutaneous mapping and ablation registry. Circulation 70:1024–1029.
4. Gillette PC, Wampler DG, Garson A, Zinner A, Ott D, Colley D (1985): Treatment of atrial automatic tachycardia by ablation procedures. J Am Coll Cardiol 6:405–409.
5. Morady F, Scheinman MM, Winston SA, DiCarlo LA, Davis JC, Griffin JC, Ruder M, Abbott JA, Eldar M (1985): Efficacy and safety of transcatheter ablation of posteroseptal accessory pathways. Circulation 72:170–177.
6. Gillette PC, Zinner A (1987): The use of fulguration in the treatment of tachydysrhythmias in children.

In "Ablation of Cardiac Arrhythmias." New York: Futura.
7. Evans GT, Scheinman MM (1986): Catheter ablation for control of ventricular tachycardia: A report of the percutaneous cardiac mapping and ablation registry. PACE 9:1391–1395.
8. Fisher JD, Bordman R, Kim SG, Matos JA, Brodman LE, Wallerson D, Waspe LE (1984): Attempted non-surgical electrical ablation of accessory pathways via the coronary sinus in the Wolff-Parkinson-White syndrome. J Am Coll Cardiol 4:685–694.
9. Huang SK, Bharati S, Graham AR, Lev M, Marcus FI, Odell R (1987): Closed chest catheter dessication of AV junction using radiofrequency-energy. A new method of catheter ablation. J Am Coll Cardiol 9:349–358.
10. Gillette PC, Harold M, Swindle MM, Thompson R, et al. (1990): Chronic cryocatheter block and modification of atrioventricular conduction, abstracted. PACE 13:499.
11. Evans GT, Scheinman MM (1987): The percutaneous cardiac mapping and ablation registry: Summary of results. PACE 10:1395–1399.
12. Bardy GH, Ivey TD, Coltorti F, Stewart RB, Johnson G, Green L (1988): Developments, complications and limitations of catheter-mediated electrical ablation of posterior accessory atrioventricular pathways. Am J Cardiol 61:309–316.
13. Hartzler GO, Giorgi LV, Diehl AM, Hamaker WR (1985): Right coronary spasm complicating electrode catheter ablation of a right lateral accessory pathway. J Am Coll Cardiol 6:250–253.
14. Gillette PC, Garson A Jr, Porter CJ, et al (1983): Junctional automatic ectopic tachycardia: New proposed treatment by transcatheter His bundle ablation. Am Heart J 106(4):619–623.
15. Gillette PC, Garson A, Hesslein PS, Karpawich PP, et al. (1981): Successful surgical treatment of atrial, junctional and ventricular tachycardias in infants and children. Am Heart J 102:984–991.
16. Van Hare GF, Velvis H, Langberg JJ (1990): Successful transcatheter ablation of congenital junctional ectopic tachycardia in a ten-month-old infant using radiofrequency energy. PACE 13:730–735.
17. Bromberg BI, Dick M (1987): Transcatheter electrical ablation of accessory pathways in children. J Am Coll Cardiol 9:2:36A.
18. Case CL, Crawford FA, Gillette PC, Ross BA, Zeigler VL (1988): Successful surgery for atrioventricular reentrant tachycardia in a small child. Am Heart J 116:1:187–189.
19. Oslizlok P, Case CL, Gillette PC (1990): Successful transcatheter ablation of an accessory connection in a child following failed surgery: An ideal case? Am Heart J 119:6:1424–1426.
20. Jordaens L, Vallaeys J, D'Hoore P, Cuvelier C,

Clement DL (1990): Pathology in a patient with sudden death 3 months after successful ablation of the AV-Node with a single low-energy shock. RBM 12:143.

21. Mabo P, Druelles P, DePlace C, Paillard F, LeBreton H, Oaubert C (1990): Left ventricle (LV) aneurysm and left circumflex artery–LV fistula after DC ablation of a left lateral accessory pathway. RBM 12:151.

22. Gillette PC, Swindle MM, Thompson R, Gaymes C, Fyfe DA, M Harold (1990): Can permanent complete AV block be produced by transvenous catheter cryoablation? RBM 12:143.

22

Balloon Valvuloplasty/Angioplasty: International Experience

P. Syamasundar Rao, M.D.

Department of Pediatrics, Division of Pediatric Cardiology, University of Wisconsin Medical School, University of Wisconsin Children's Hospital, Madison, Wisconsin 53792-4108

Although balloon dilatation techniques involving congenital valvar and vascular stenotic lesions originated in the United States, these techniques were rapidly adopted in many other countries on all continents. The use of these methods had to await the availability of dilatation catheters and acceptance of the concepts in the respective countries. Parenthetically, it should be noted that some catheters not available for use by the U.S. worker are readily available to workers abroad. Some of these non-U.S. workers have made significant contributions to the understanding, new applications, and refinement of the balloon valvuloplasty/angioplasty procedures in the pediatric patient. In addition, the material from abroad adds to the total experience of these relatively new procedures. With this in mind, I have conceived this (these) chapter(s) to describe the experience from workers abroad. Several more than the authors contributing to chapters 22a through 22f were invited to report their experience with balloon valvuloplasty/angioplasty. However, presumably because of time constraints, some of the authors either declined to contribute or were unable to provide their chapters by the time the book went into press.

Dr. Fontes from São Paulo, Brazil, not only describes his personal experience at Instituto "Dante Pazzanese" de Cardiologia in São Paulo but also summarizes the results of workers from other institutions in Curitiba, Rio de Janeiro, and São Paulo. Dr. Wren from New Castle upon Tyne, England, presents the British experience. The author discusses his series from Freeman Hospital combined with the data from his colleagues at the Hospital for Sick Children in London. In addition, he summarizes the published studies from other institutions in the United Kingdom. Lo and his associates discuss their balloon dilatation series performed at Grantham Hospital/University of Hong Kong, Hong Kong. Drs. Shrivastava and Dev review the balloon valvuloplasty/angioplasty experience at All India Institute of Medical Sciences in New Delhi, India, and state that interventional procedures of such type are being performed at at least six other institutions in India; they also present some of the published data from other investigators. Dr. Ali Khan concentrates on balloon pulmonary valvuloplasty performed by him and his colleagues at Riyadh Armed Forces Hospital in Saudi Arabia, although they have had experience with dilating other stenotic lesions in the cardiovascular system. Some of the data on balloon dilatation performed at King Faisal Specialist Hospital and Research Center, Riyadh, Saudi Arabia, has been included in the chapters prepared by the editor of this book and therefore need not be separately enumerated. Finally, Dr. Suarez de Lezo and his associates describe the Spanish experience. They combine the data from Hospital Reina

Transcatheter Therapy in Pediatric Cardiology, pages 401–402
© 1993 Wiley-Liss, Inc.

Sofia in Cordoba and Hospital del Pino in Las Palmas de Gran Canaria for the purpose of discussion. They also summarize the published work from other institutions in Spain.

The editor believes that the chapters to follow on the international experience enrich the presentations in previous chapters dealing with individual lesions.

22a

Balloon Valvuloplasty/Angioplasty: The Brazilian Experience

Valmir F. Fontes, M.D.

Division of Pediatric Cardiology and Hemodynamic Laboratory,
Institute Dante Pazzanese of Cardiology, Ibirapuera,
São Paulo, SP 4012 Brazil

INTRODUCTION

Pulmonary valvuloplasty was introduced to Brazil in 1983 by the Institute Dante Pazzanese of Cardiology, São Paulo [1]. All over the world, this method has been accepted as a treatment of choice for congenital pulmonary stenosis [2–8]. The satisfactory results obtained with this technique encouraged us since 1986 to extend the method to native coarctation and recoarctation of the aorta.

This chapter reports the Institute Dante Pazzanese of Cardiology experience (Fig. 1). The results of other four Institutions in our country are also discussed.

PULMONARY VALVULOPLASTY

The experience of the Institute Dante Pazzanese of Cardiology is based on 253 patients with pulmonary stenosis who underwent balloon pulmonary valvuloplasty.

Selection of Patients and Balloon Sizes

The basic indication for pulmonary valvuloplasty has been a peak systolic pressure gradient above 50 mmHg between the right ventricle and main pulmonary artery. We have also considered the size of pulmonary valve annulus as well as valve leaflet morphology as seen by angiography. Results were poor in both dysplastic pulmonary valves and underdeveloped pulmonary annulus. In our experience,

pulmonary stenosis with severe infundibular hypertrophy (Fig. 2) also had a favorable prognosis. This hypertrophy regresses some months after valvuloplasty [9–12]. The management of neonates with severe pulmonary stenosis has been dificult due to right heart dilatation and severity of obstruction. In pulmonary stenosis associated with obstructive lesion of left heart, it is advisable to treat both congenital defects at the same time. It is also possible to perform a balloon dilatation of a stenotic pulmonary valve and to occlude a patent ductus arteriosus or an interatrial communication using the Rashkind or other occluder systems.

When Kan et al. [2] introduced pulmonary valvuloplasty in 1982, they recommended a balloon diameter 1–2 mm smaller than the valve annulus diameter. Following this recommendation most institutions all over the world started to perform pulmonary valvuloplasty with small balloons. When follow-up hemodynamic studies were performed, residual gradients were observed in most of the cases. Because of this, balloon selection criteria were modified, and balloons 20%–40% larger than the valve annulus diameter were chosen.[1]

---

[1]Editors note: The reader is referred to Chapter 6 (this volume) for further discussion on selections of balloon sizes for pulmonary valvuloplasty.

Transcatheter Therapy in Pediatric Cardiology, pages 403–419

"Dante Pazzanese" Institute of Cardiology
Balloon Valvuloplasty/Angioplasty
Overall Experience
350 Procedures

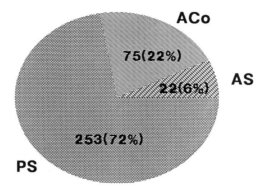

Fig. 1. Pie diagram showing overall experience at the Institute Dante Pazzanese of Cardiology.

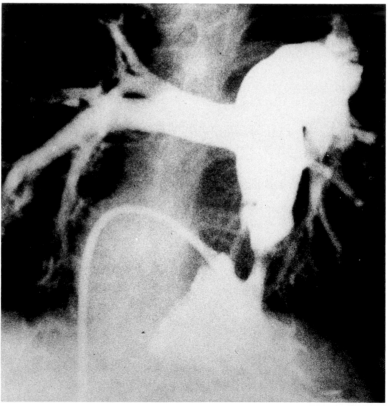

Fig. 2. Selected cineangiographic frame from a right ventriculogram in a 5-year-old boy with severe pulmonic valve stenosis showing marked infundibular hypertrophy.

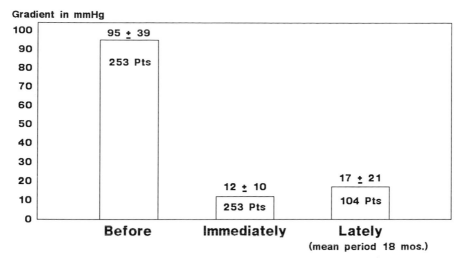

Fig. 3. Bar graph showing the behavior of the mean systolic pressure gradient in 253 patients (before and after valvuloplasty) and in 104 patients after a mean follow-up period of 18 months.

Patient Population and Immediate Results

From March 1983 to July 1992, 253 patients with pulmonary stenosis underwent balloon valvuloplasty. The patients' ages ranged from 2 months to 61 years (mean age 9 years). There were 136 males. The diagnosis of pulmonary stenosis was based on the clinical, radiologic, electrocardiographic, ecocardiographic, and cardiac catheterization findings. A patent foramen ovale was present in 185 patients. Ten were cyanotic at rest due to a right-to-left shunt at the atrial level. Other associated malformations included tricuspid valve stenosis in one patient and aortic valve stenosis in other. In both of these patients additional obstructive lesions were dilated during the same procedure. The systolic pressure gradient between right ventricle and pulmonary artery decreased from 95 ± 39 mmHg (mean ± SD) to 12 ± 10 mmHg immediately after balloon valvuloplasty (Fig. 3). Ninety-five of 253 patients had suprasystemic right ventricular systolic pressure, and for this reason they constitute a special group of patients. The systolic gradient through pulmonary valve decreased from 129 ± 38 mmHg to 12 + 10 mmHg

immediately after pulmonary valvuloplasty (Fig. 4). Infundibular systolic pressure gradient was present in 62 of these patients and ranged from 14 to 185 mmHg. Angiography performed immediately after pulmonary valvuloplasty showed that the infundibular narrowing appeared more severe in this group of patients (Fig. 5) than in patients with less severe obstruction.

Complications

Minor. Hematoma developed in eight patients at the femoral vein puncture site due to prolonged bleeding; one of them needed blood transfusion. There were two femoral vein thromboses. Bradycardia has developed in 22.8% of patients during balloon inflation and ventricular ectopics beats without hemodinamic disturbance in 8%. One patient had trivial hemoptysis shortly after valvuloplasty, probably because the guidewire had perforated the pulmonary artery. Balloon rupture was seen in 16 patients.

Major. A 1-year-old baby with suprasystemic right ventricular pressure had excellent relief of obstruction after valvuloplasty, but developed coagulation disturbance and pro-

Gradient in mmHg

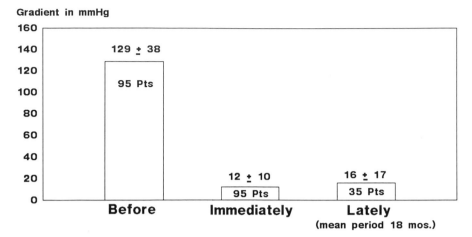

Fig. 4. Bar graph depicting the mean systolic pressure gradient in a group of patients with suprasystemic pressure in the right ventricle and infundibular reaction before, immediately after, and a mean period of 18 months after valvuloplasty.

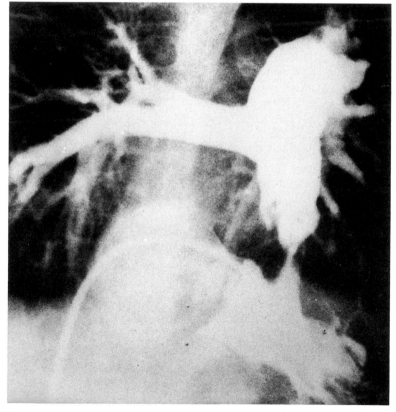

Fig. 5. Right ventriculogram from the same patient shown in Figure 2 (immediately following balloon dilatation), showing more severe infundibular narrowing during ventricular systole.

longed bleeding that required replacement therapy. Ventricular fibrillation occurred, and this patient died 2 hours after valvuloplasty. Two other patients with suprasystemic right ventricular pressure and severe infundibular hypertrophy developed low cardiac output after the procedure, but were controlled with the use of medications.

Follow-Up Results

Mean hospitalization time was 24 hours, and patients were followed thereafter with clinical, radiological, electrocardiographic, echocardiographic, and hemodynamics evaluation. One hundred four patients had cardiac cateterization 18 months (mean) after the procedure (range, 3–38 months). Residual mean systolic gradient was 17 ± 21 mmHg.

In nine patients residual gradients were high, between 40 to 90 mmHg. Seven of these patients were sucessfully redilated. In two patients with a dysplastic pulmonary valve the valvuloplasty was not effective, and they underwent successful surgery. Thirty-five of 95 patients in the suprasystemic right ventricular pressure group had a follow-up catheterization (Fig. 4). The mean time follow-up in this group was 16 months, and the mean systolic pressure was 16 ± 17 mmHg. None of these patients had infundibular pressure gradient.

The angiography showed an excellent valve opening in 95 patients as well as better valve cusp motion. In those patients with previous infundibular hypertrophy, regression of the hypertrophy was observed (Figs. 6 and 7).

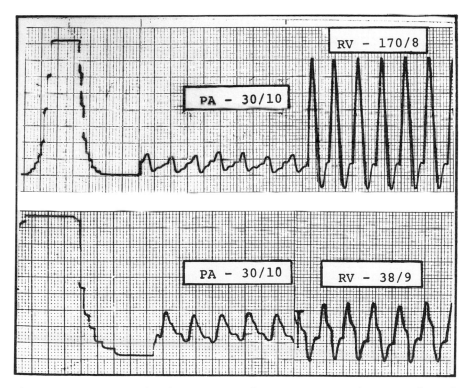

Fig. 6. Pressures measured in the same patient shown in Figures 2 and 5. Top: Peak systolic pressure gradient of 140 mmHg. Bottom: 18 months after the dilatation with only an 8 mmHg pulmonary valvar gradient.

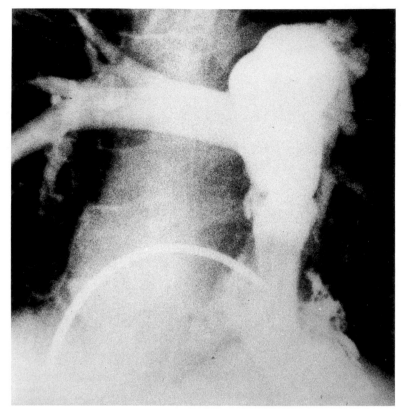

Fig. 7. Right ventriculogram from the same patient depicted in Figures 2, 5, and 6, 18 months after valvuloplasty. Note marked regression of the infundibular hypertrophy.

Valve competence was evaluated clinically and by two-dimensional echocardiography. Mild pulmonary insuficiency was noted in 30% of patients.

In summary, from March 1983 to July 1992, 253 patients with pulmonary stenosis underwent balloon valvuloplasty. The patients' ages ranged from 2 months to 61 years (mean age 9 years). The peak systolic pressure gradient across the pulmonic valve ranged from 47 to 260 mmHg (95 $\pm$ 39 mmHg) prior to the valvuloplasty and fell to 0–55 mmHg (12 $\pm$ 10 mmHg) immediately after dilation (P < 0.001). Repeat catheterization at a mean follow-up period of 18 months (3–38 months) showed a mean systolic pressure gradient of 17 $\pm$ 21 mmHg. A residual gradient ranging from 40 to 90 mmHg was noted in nine patients. Two patients had dysplastic pulmonary valve, and they underwent surgical repair. Successful redilatation was performed in seven patients. As a major complication, a 1-year-old baby died 2 hours after the procedure due to coagulation disturbance and ventricular fibrillation. Pulmonary regurgitation was noted in 30% of the cases. Infundibular hypertrophy that was present prior to valvuloplasty regressed at follow-up, indicating that infundibular hypertrophy is reversible.

We conclde that balloon valvuloplasty is the procedure of choice in patients with isolated pulmonary valve stenosis. The method is simple, safe, and effective.

SUMMARY OF BALLOON VALVULOPLASTY/ANGIOPLASTY FROM OTHER INSTITUTIONS IN BRAZIL

1. From May 1987 to March 1992, 115 patients with pulmonary valve stenosis underwent balloon valvuloplasty at the Hospital de Cardiologia de Laranjeiras, Rio de Janeiro, under the direction of Drs. Marco Aurélio Santos, and Luiz Carlos Simões. The material was divided into two groups based on balloon-to-pulmonary valve annulus ratio: Group I, 46 patients, had a balloon/annulus ratio of <1.0 (mean, 0.89). The mean gradient before valvuloplasty was 92 mmHg, and it regressed to 31 mmHg after the procedure (63% reduction).

Group II, 69 patients, had a balloon/annulus ratio of >1.0 (mean 1.30). The mean gradient before valvuloplasty was 89 mmHg and was reduced to 27 mmHg immediately after valvuloplasty, with a gradient reduction of 67%. In both groups the results were statistically significant ($P < 0.001$) and are independent of balloon/annulus ratio. There was no significant difference ($P > 0.1$) between the mean pressure gradients before valvuloplasty in groups I and II (92 and 89 mmHg).

Sixty eight patients were followed for a period of 12–58 months, and two-dimensional and Doppler echocardiography were performed to assess the gradient between right ventricle and pulmonary artery. Thirty patients with a mean balloon/annulus ratio of 0.89 were followed for 29 months. The pulmonary valvar peak pressure gradient seen by Doppler echocardiography was 90 mmHg before and 32 mmHg at follow-up, with a gradient reduction of 67.4%. Thirty eight patients with a balloon/annulus ratio of 1.30 were followed for 31 months. These patients had a mean gradient of 91 mmHg before and 22 mmHg at

follow-up, with a gradient reduction of 76.0%. A comparative analysis of the results from both groups (balloon/annulus ratios <1.0 and >1.0) using the Mann Whitney test, showed that, when the follow-up results are compared, the valvuloplasty was more efective in group II than in group I.[2]

Complications included hematoma in one case, edema in three patients, and transient hemiparesia in two patients. We conclude that pulmonary valvuloplasty is a safe and effective method. Better results have been obtained at follow-up evaluation in the group with a balloon/annulus ratio of >1.0.

2. Fifty-six patients with pulmonary valve stenosis underwent balloon valvuloplasty at the Hospital Evangélico, Curitiba, under the direction of Dr. Antoninho Krichenko. The mean pressure gradient was 80 ± 40 mmHg before and 20 ± 2 mmHg immediately after valvuloplasty. A postdilatation hemodynamic study 10 ± 7 months after valvuloplasty was performed in 30 cases. Five patients had successful repeat valvuloplasty. There were no complications.

3. From July 1986 to March 1992, eighty six patients with pulmonary valve stenosis underwent balloon catheter valvuloplasty at the Escola Paulista de Medicina, São Paulo, under the direction of Dr. Antonio Carlos C. Carvalho. Fifty seven patients were males and 29 females. The patients' ages ranged from 5 days to 62 years (mean age 12 ± 14). Cyanosis was present in 9 cases and disapeared immediately after valvuloplasty in 8 patients. The right ventricular peak systolic pressure was reduced from 95 ± 64 mmHg to 34 ± 30 mmHg immediately after valvuloplasty. The mean systolic gradient across the pulmonary valve fell from 84 ± 16 mmHg to 24 ± 12 mmHg immediately after valvuloplasty. Infundibular systolic gradient was found in 39 pa-

---

[2]Editor's note: These data are consistent with the results previously published by us (Rao: Texas Heart Inst. J 14:57–61, 1987; and Rao: Br Heart J 60: 507–511, 1988). While immediate results are similar with both small and large balloons, the follow-up results are better when balloons larger than valve annulus are used.

tients and ranged from 10 to 130 mmHg. Repeat catheterization was obtained in 23 patients after a mean follow-up period of 14 months. No infundibular gradient was detected at follow-up.

4. From October 1984 to May 1992, 235 patients with pulmonary valve stenosis underwent balloon valvuloplasty at the Instituto do Coração da Faculdade de Medicina da Universidade de São Paulo, São Paulo, under the direction of Dr. Miguel A. Rati, and Dr Luiz Junya Kagita. They were divided into three groups, based on age at valvuloplasty: group I, twenty-one patients aged 4-11 months,: group II, one hundred and seventy patients aged 1-12 years; and group III, forty four patients aged 13-34 years. The associated malformations included interatrial communication in three cases, supravalvar pulmonary stenosis in four, persistent ductus arteriosus in one, and tricuspid insufficiency in one.

In group I, the mean systolic gradient across the pulmonary valve was reduced from 87 to 29 mmHg. Unsuccessful dilatation occurred in three cases. Two of them underwent surgical valvotomy. Two patients developed restenosis and were dilated 2 and 3 years after the first valvuloplasty, respectively.

In group II the mean systolic gradient was reduced from 84 to 20 mmHg in 165 patients. Dilatation was not successful in eight patients. This was due to dysplastic pulmonary valve in four patients, and in the other four it was due to supravalvar stenosis. Late follow-up evaluation showed restenosis in two patients, and these were successfully redilated 2 years after the first procedure.

In group III the valvuloplasty was effective in 41 patients. The mean systolic gradient was reduced from 100 to 26 mmHg.

Complications included prolonged bleeding in two cases in group I, and blood transfusions were required. In group II one patient had a transient stroke. Tricuspid insufficiency occurred in another patient. In group III one patient had a stoke with full recovery after 3 months. In conclusion, pulmonary valvulo-plasty is an effective method in treating pulmonary valve stenosis.

5. Five patients with stenosis aortopulmonary anastomosis following Jatene surgery underwent transluminal angioplasty at the Instituto do Coração da Faculdade de Medicina da Universidade de São Paulo, São Paulo, under the direction of Dr. Miguel Antonio N. Rati. Six patients with transposition of the great arteries submitted to Jatene surgery presented in the postoperative period with supravalvar pulmonary stenosis at the previous anastomotic site. In three patients successful percutaneous transluminal angioplasty was performed 6 months to 1 year after surgery. Pressure gradients decreased from 75 to 10 mmHg, 83 to 25 mmHg, and 111 to 23 mmHg, respectively, with clear cut improvement in the angiographic narrowing. In two patients partial relief of the stenosis was achieved. Balloon angioplasty should be considered as an alternative to the surgical correction of stenosed pulmonary trunk following Jatene surgery.

AORTIC STENOSIS

Transluminal balloon valvuloplasty has been utilized in the treatment of congenital aortic stenosis since 1984, when Lababidi et al. [13] reported the safety and efficacy of the procedure. This technique has been used in neonates, infants, children, and adult populations [14-20]. The effectiveness of the procedure may vary according to the anatomic type of valve. According to Perry et al. [16], in the pediatric group the obstruction is almost always due to stenosis of congenitally bicommissural or unicommissural valves. Sholler et al. [21] subsequently studied valvular morphology by two-dimensional echocardiograms. Stenotic aortic valves were classified according to the number of commissures (uni- or bicommissural), thickness of the cusps, and domed valve thin shape during systole. Better results were observed in patients with bicommissural valves and domed valves. Aortic regurgitation was common with unicommissural valves. In newborn subjects with critical valvular aortic stenosis the balloon valvuloplasty was a high-risk procedure due to congestive heart failure and other associated malformations.

Patient Selection and Balloon Size

In general, children with congenital valvular aortic stenosis with transaortic peak systolic pressure gradients in excess of 50 mmHg are considered for balloon valvuloplasty. The valve morphology and annulus size are important factors and should be evaluated before procedure.

The percutaneous transfemoral approach was the technique utilized for our initial experience. The ideal balloon size was considered to be about 90% of the valve annulus diameter. Oversized balloons may cause damage to the left ventricular outflow tract and mitral valve and aortic regurgitation.

Patient Population and Immediate Results

Transluminal balloon aortic valvuloplasty was performed in 22 patients with congenital aortic stenosis. The patients' ages ranged from 3 to 23 years, with a mean age of 9 years. There were 17 male and 5 female patients. The anatomy of the valve was bicommissural and domed in 14 (Fig. 8) and unicommissural in 8. Before the procedure seven patients (3 uni- and 4 bicommissural) had grade I aortic regurgitation.

Mean aortic valve gradients were 83 ± 29 mmHg before valvuloplasty, which decreased to 29 ± 15 mmHg after the procedure. Left ventricle pressures fell from 177 ± 28 mmHg to 94 ± 17 mmHg after dilatation (Fig. 9A, B).

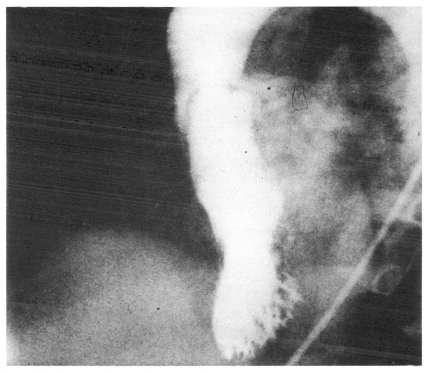

Fig. 8. Left ventriculogram in a 3-year-old patient with aortic stenosis showing central flow. The valve leaflets are thickened and domed, and they appear bicommissural. This appears to be an appropriate case for balloon dilatation.

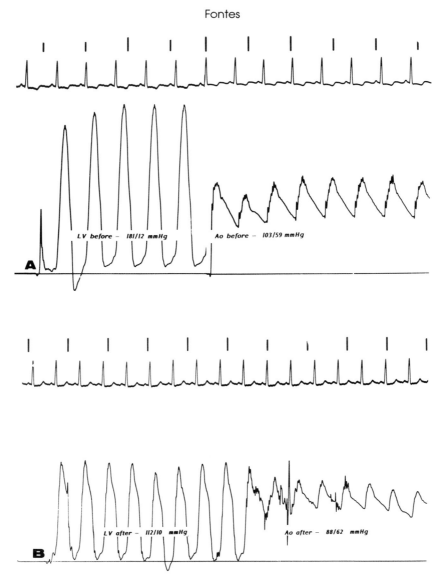

Fig. 9. A: Left ventricular (LV) and aortic (AO) pressures measured before valvuloplasty in the patient depicted in Figure 8 showing a systolic gradient of 78 mmHg. **B:** Note pressure gradient reduction immediately after valvuloplasty. The residual peak systolic gradient was 24 mmHg.

Better excursion of the valve cusps (Fig. 10) was observed after valvuloplasty. Substantial increases in aortic regurgitation occurred in 3 of 8 (37%) unicommissural valve patients. In two patients of bicommissural valves, aortic regurgitation did not increase after procedure. In seven cases the aortic valve remained com-petent (Fig. 11). Two other patients developed very slight aortic regurgitation.

Follow-Up Results

The mean follow-up period was 45 months (range, 1–74 months). Twelve patients were asymptomatic, 9 complained of dyspnea on

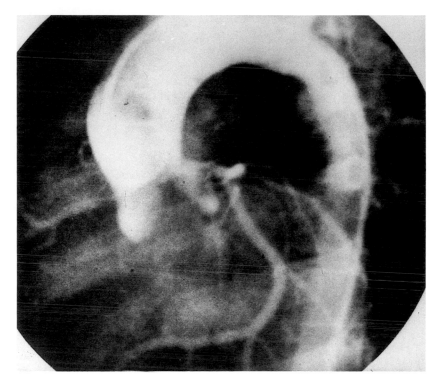

Fig. 10. Aortogram immediately after valvuloplasty in ventricular systole exhibiting excellent opening of the stenotic valve and better excursion of the cusps.

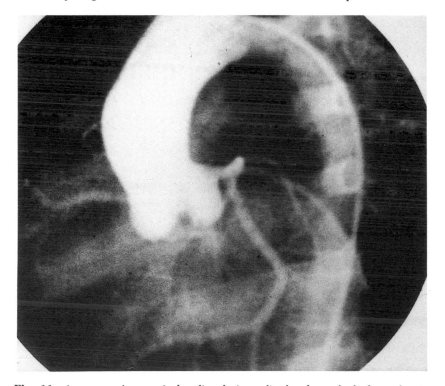

Fig. 11. Aortogram in ventricular diastole immediately after valvuloplasty showing competence of the aortic valve.

exertion, and one patient died of an unknown cause 2 months after valvuloplasty. Two patients with unicommissural valves and significant aortic regurgitation postvalvuloplasty developed enlargement of the heart and showed electrocardiographic findings of severe left ventricular hypertrophy and abnormalities of T waves. Probably they will be candidates for aortic valve replacement very soon. Follow-up catheterization was performed in only one patient, and a residual peak systolic pressure gradient of 28 mmHg and slight aortic regurgitation was observed.

In summary, 22 patients with aortic stenosis, aged 3–23 years, underwent aortic valvuloplasty. The peak systolic gradient across the valve varied from 50 to 140 mmHg (84 ± 29) prior valvuloplasty and from 0 to 57 mmHg (22 ± 15) immediately after dilatation. At clinical follow-up between 1 and 74 months, the systolic thrill had disappeared and the systolic murmur had become softer. Diastolic murmur was present in 10 patients; two of them developed enlargement of the left ventricle and left ventricular hypertrophy. A hemodynamic study after dilatation was carried out in one patient, and the systolic gradient across the valve was similar to that immediately after dilatation (28 mmHg), and the aortic valve showed slight regurgitation. One of the patients died suddenly. The follow-up of our patients is limited; long-term evaluation will provide a better comparison basis with surgical alternatives. As Sholler et al. [21] have demonstrated, the results depend on the valvular morphology. A unicommissural valve may be at increased risk of developing aortic regurgitation. However, we feel that satisfactory results can be achieved in the pediatric age group with bicommissural valves.

AORTIC COARCTATION

Balloon angioplasty has been considered a nonsurgical alternative for the treatment of aortic coarctation after animal model studies,

pathologic correlative studies, and human studies [22–30]. The world experience has shown that dilatation was accomplished by rupture of the intimal and medial layers of the arterial wall. Thus a potential consequence in the late follow-up period would be aneurysmal formation, specially if the patient has native coarctation. This subject is still controversial. Nevertheless, based on our own experience we feel it is feasible to obtain good results if the cases are well selected.

Selection of Patients and Balloon Sizes

Several factors are important for the success of balloon angioplasty. First is the morphology of the coarctation segment. This segment must be central and with wasting of the aortic wall in all directions (Fig. 12). When the coarctation is an asymmetric lesion with

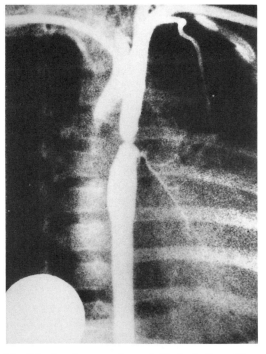

Fig. 12. Aortic coarctation suitable for balloon dilatation. Note central location of the aortic coarctation. This type of coarctations is likely to respond favourably to balloon angioplasty.

a distorted shape, having a marked intraarterial shelf and very thin walls, the case may be unsuitable for angioplasty (Fig. 13). In such cases the risk of complete rupture of the intimal and medial layers of the arterial wall may lead to aneurysmal formation. Second is the patient's age. After the fourth decade the risk for aortic dissection and aneurysmal formation is very high due to inherent degenerative abnormalities of the aortic wall. In our experience the best age to undergo balloon aortoplasty is pediatric. During the first months of life, especially in the neonatal period, the incidence of recoarctation is very high, 50% according the literature [31,32]. However, recoarctation can be redilated. Third, the size of the balloon is an important factor. This should be equal to the aortic diameter at the level of the origin of the left subclavian artery or 1-2

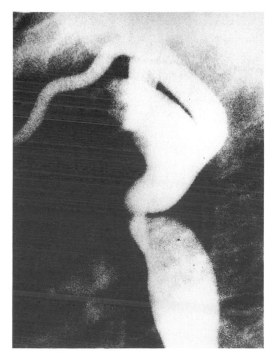

Fig. 13. Asymmetric aortic coarctation with a distorted shape. This type is unlikely to achieve a favorable result following balloon dilatation.

mm smaller.[3] The frequency of aortic aneurysm related to balloon size is probably due to utilization of oversized balloons, and this may represent the major reason for rupture of the medial layer of the aortic wall. The adventitial layer alone may not tolerate the systemic pressure and will respond with dilatation and aneurysm formation.

According Wren et al. [32] the basic cause of aneurysm formation in the cases reported by Cooper et al. [33] and Marvin et al. [34] was the use of oversized balloons. Isner et al. [35] observed a very high incidence of cystic medial necrosis within the coarcted segments and suggested that these abnormalities are potential contributors to aneurysm formation.

Patient Population and Immediate Results

From September 1986 to July 1992, 75 balloon dilatation procedures were performed in 70 patients with coarctation of the aorta. There were 51 male and 24 female patients aged 28 days to 49 years (67% of the cases were under 10 years). In 59 patients, native coarctation was present. In the remaining cases, 11 coarctations had occurred after previous surgical repair and 5 after balloon dilatation. Seventeen patients had associated abnormalities: Ventricular endocardial fibroelastosis was found in four, ventricular septal defect in two, subaortic stenosis in two, patency of the arterial duct in one, and univentricular atrioventricular connection in one.

All patients after clinical assessment and conventional laboratory studies (electrocardiogram; chest X-ray; M-mode, two-dimensional, and Doppler echocardiographic) underwent cardiac catheterization to confirm the clinical diagnosis and to consider balloon dilatation. The angiographic study was performed with the catheter positioned at the level of left sub-

[3]Editor's note: For detailed discussion of balloon size used for balloon coarctation angioplasty, the reader is referred to Chapters 4 and 10 (this volume).

clavian artery; 10° right anterior oblique and left lateral projections were used. A left ventricular angiogram was also performed to assess the ventricular septum, mitral valve, and abnormalities of the left ventricular outflow tract. The size of the balloon chosen for aortoplasty was similar to a 1–2 mm smaller than the aorta at the level of the origin of left subclavian artery.

Percutaneous transfemoral balloon angioplasty was performed in 68 patients. In six less than 2 months old a cut-down of the left axillary artery was utilized. In another 7-month-old child a cut-down and dissection of the right femoral artery was employed.

Medi-Tech balloon dilatation catheters were utilized. The systolic gradient across the coarctation site was 47 ± 20 mmHg before aortoplasty, and it was reduced to 7 ± 8 mmHg immediately after the procedure. The aortic diameter at the coarctation site was 6 ± 3 mm before dilatation and has expanded to 11 ± 5.2 mm after aortoplasty. Angiographic studies showed excellent relief of obstruction in the majority of the cases.

Early Complications

Delayed bleeding occurred in 8 patients and resolved when antagonists to heparin were administered. There was occlusion of the right femoral artery in one case, and this patient required a femoropopliteal bypass surgery. A 2-month-old baby had an occluded left axillary artery with spontaneous recanalization. Cerebrovascular accident was noted in one case. Angiographic study showed slight dissection of the aortic intima. A 2-month-old patient developed recoarctation 6 months later. During the second dilatation, the balloon catheter could not be removed because of severe spasm of the femoral artery, and in spite of the use of vasodilator an emergency surgical procedure was required. Two balloons ruptured during angioplasty; no adverse effects were observed.

Follow-Up Results

Clinical follow-up was available in 60 patients between ages 4 and 66 months, with a mean period of 44 months after angioplasty. Fifty-eight patients were asymptomatic. Two patients complained of fatigue and dyspnea, respectively, on exertion. The femoral pulse was normal in 57 patients, slightly decreased in one, and absent in two. Of the last three patients, one required an operation to close a large ventricular septal defect at 6 months after dilatation, and five required redilatation 6

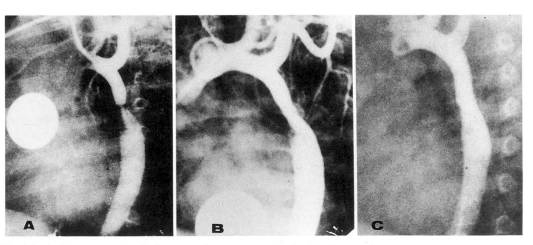

Fig. 14. A: Severe coarctation before aortoplasty. **B:** Immediately after the procedure. **C:** 12 months after dilatation. Excellent relief of coarctation was observed both immediately after (B) angioplasty and at follow-up (C).

months after the initial angioplasty. The blood pressure was normal in 57 patients. Postangioplasty catheterization was performed in 21 patients at a mean of 14 months after the procedure. The angiographic studies performed showed excellent relief of the dilated segment in 16 patients (Fig. 14). Five patients had recoarctation, and all of them underwent successful repeat dilatation (Fig. 15). The recoarctation has occurred only in patients under 1 year old. A fusiform dilatation suggestive of aneurysm formation was found in one patient.

In summary, from September 1986 to July 1992, seventy five balloon dilatation procedures were performed in 70 patients with aortic coarctation. Sixty-seven percent of the patients were under 10 years of age. The mean systolic coarctation gradient was 47 ± 20 mmHg before angioplasty, and it was reduced to 7 ± 8 mmHg after the procedure.

The coarctation diameter increased from 6 ± 3 to 11 ± 5 mm after dilatation. At presentation 67 of the 70 patients were hypertensive. After dilatation, at a mean period of 44 months, 59 of the 70 were normotensive. Five patients had recoarctation 6 months after the first dilatation and all of them, respectively, underwent successful repeat angioplasty. One patient who was considered inadequate for redilatation developed an aneurysm at the coarctation site.

Our experience has proved that balloon angioplasty is an effective method for treating patients with coarctation of the aorta. Adequate selection in terms of morphology of the coarctation, the size of the balloon catheter, and the experience of the hemodynamic team are crucial factors to the success of the procedure. The late follow-up and the natural history data thus far have been favorable in our experience.

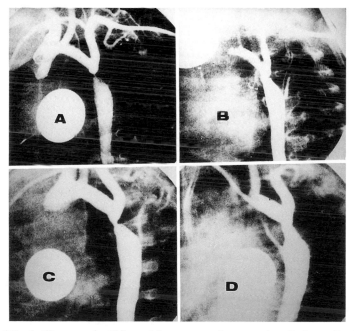

Fig. 15. A: Two-month-old boy with severe aortic coarctation; **B:** Immediately after dilatation. **C:** Recoarctation 6 months after aortoplasty. **D:** Immediately after redilatation. Note improvement immediately after balloon angioplasty (B), which recoarcted at follow-up (C). This was successfully redilated (D).

REFERENCES

1. Fontes VF, Sousa JEMR, Pimental FO WA, Büchler JR, Silva MVD, Bembom MCLB (1983): Valvoplastia pulmonar com cateter-balão. Apresentação de um caso. Arq Bras Cardiol 41:49-52.

2. Kan JS, White RI Jr, Mitchell SE, Gardner TJ (1982): Percutaneous balloon valvuloplasty: A new method for treating congenital pulmonary valve stenosis. N Engl J Med 307:540-542.

3. Lababidi ZA, Wu J, Walls J (1983): Percutaneous balloon pulmonary valvuloplasty. Am J Cardiol 52:560-562.

4. Pepine CJ, Gessner IH, Feldman RL (1982): Percutaneous balloon valvuloplasty for pulmonic valve stenosis in the adult. Am J Cardiol 50:1442-1445.

5. Rocchini AP, Kveselis DA, Crowley D, Dick M, Rosenthal A (1984): Percutaneous balloon valvuloplasty for treatment of congenital pulmonary valvar stenosis in children. J Am Coll Cardiol 3:1005-1012.

6. Kan JS, White Jr RI, Mitchell SE, Anderson JH, Gardner TJ (1984): Percutaneous transluminal balloon valvuloplasty for pulmonary valve stenosis. Circulation 69:554-560.

7. Rao PS (1986): Transcatheter treatment of pulmonary stenosis and coarctation of the aorta: Experience with percutaneous balloon dilatation. Br Heart J 56:250-258.

8. Tynan M, Baker EJ, Rohmer J (1985): Percutaneous balloon pulmonary valvuloplasty. Br Heart J 53:520-524.

9. Fontes VF, Esteves CA, Sousa JEMR, Silva MVD, Bembom MCB (1988): Regression of infundibular hypertrophy after pulmonary valvuloplasty for pulmonic stenosis. Am J Cardiol 62:977-978.

10. Fontes VF, Sousa JEMR, Esteves CA, Silva MVD, Cano MN, Maldonado G (1988): Pulmonary valvuloplasty experience of 100 cases. Int J Cardiol 21:335-342.

11. Mullins CE, Ludomisky A, O'Laughlin MP, Vick GW, Murphy Jr DJ, Huhta JC, Nihill MR (1988): Balloon valvuloplasty for pulmonic valve stenosis—two-year follow-up: Hemodynamic and Doppler evaluation. Cathet Cardiovasc Diagn 14:76-81.

12. Rao PS, Fawzy ME, Solymar L, Mardini MK (1988): Long-term results of balloon pulmonary valvuloplasty of valvar pulmonic stenosis. Am Heart J 115:1291-1296.

13. Lababidi Z, Wu J, Walls JT (1984): Percutaneous balloon aortic valvuloplasty: Results in 23 patients. Am J Cardiol 53:194-197.

14. Lababidi Z, Weinhaus L (1986): Successful balloon valvuloplasty for neonatal critical aortic stenosis. Am Heart J 112:913-916.

15. Wren C, Sullivan I, Bull C, Deanfield J (1987): Percutaneous balloon dilatation of aortic valve stenosis in neonates and infants. Br Heart J 58:608-612.

16. Perry SB, Zeevi B, Keane JF, Lock JE (1989): Interventional catheterization of the left lesions, including aortic and mitral valve stenosis and coarctation of the aorta. Cardiol Clin 7:341-349.

17. Choy M, Beekman RH, Rocchini AP (1987): Percutaneous balloon valvuloplasty for valva aortic stenosis in infants and children. Am J Cardiol 59:1010-1015.

18. Mario C Di, Beatt K, Feyter P, Brand M, Essed C, Serruys CE (1987): Percutaneous aortic balloon dilatation for calcific aortic stenosis in elderly patients: Immediate haemodynamic results and short term follow-up. Br Heart J 58:644-652.

19. Cribier A, Savin T, Berland J (1987): Percutaneous transluminal balloon valvuloplasty of adult aortic stenosis. Report of 92 cases. J Am Coll Cardiol 9:381-388.

20. Ferguson III J, Riuli EP, Massumi A, Treistman B, Edelman SK, Harlan MV, Brasier SE, Murgo JP (1990): Balloon aortic valvuloplasty. The Texas Heart Institute Experience. Clin Invest 17:23-30.

21. Sholler GF, Keane JF, Perry SB Sanders SP, Lock JE (1988): Balloon dilation of the aortic stenosis: Results and influence of technical and morphological features on outcome. Circulation 78:351-360.

22. Lock JE, Niemi T, Burke BA, Einzig S, Castaneda-Zuniga WR (1982): Transcutaneous angioplasty of experimental aortic coarctation. Circulation 66:1280-1286.

23. Lock JE, Castaneda-Zuniga WR, Bass JL, Foker JE, Amplatz K, Anderson RW (1982): Balloon dilation of excised aortic coarctation. Radiology 143:689-691.

24. Ho SY, Sommerville J, Yip WCL, Anderson RH (1988): Transluminal balloon dilation of ressected coarcted segments of thoracic aorta: Histological study and clinical implications. Int J Cardiol 19:99-105.

25. Lock JE, Bass JL, Amplatz K, Fuhman BP, Castaneda-Zuniga W (1983): Balloon dilation angioplasty of aortic coarctations in infants and children. Circulation 68:109-116.

26. Lababidi Z (1983): Neonatal transluminal balloon coarctation angioplasty. Am Heart J 106:752-753.

27. Lababidi Z, Daskalopoulos DA, Stoeckle Jr H (1984): Transluminal balloon coarctation angioplasty: Experience with 27 patients. Am J Cardiol 54:1288-1291.

28. Fontes VF, Sousa JEMR, Büchler JR, Pimental FO WA, Assis SF, Esteves CA, Silva MVD (1987): Aortoplastia com cateter-balão no tratamento da coartação da aorta. Arq Bras Cardiol 49:159-163.

29. Rao PS, Naijar HN, Mardini MK, Solymar L, Thapar M (1988): Balloon angioplasty for coarcta-

tion of the aorta: Immediate and long-term results. Am Heart J 115:657–665.

30. Fontes VH, Esteves CA, Braga SLN, Silva MVD, Silva MAP, Sousa JEMR (1990): It is valid to dilate native aortic coarctation with a balloon catheter. Int J Cardiol 27:311–316.

31. Mossman RA, Velho FP, Achutti AC, Schimiedt MI, Goldoni MA, Petracco JB (1986): Angioplastia transluminal percutânea. Um novo método para tratamento da coartação da aorta. Arq Bras Cardiol 47:49–51.

32. Wren C, Peart I, Bain H, Hunter S (1987): Balloon dilatation of unoperated aortic coarctation: Immediate results and one year follow-up. Br Heart J 58:369–373.

33. Cooper RS, Ritter SB, Rothe WB, Chen CK, Griepp R, Golinko RJ (1987): Angioplasty for coarctation of the aorta: Long-term results. Circulation 75:600–604.

34. Marvin WJ, Mahoney LT, Rose EF (1986): Pathological sequelae of balloon dilatation angioplasty for unoperated coarctation of the aorta in children, abstracted. J Am Coll Cardiol 7:117A.

35. Isner JM, Donaldson RF, Fulton D, Bhan I, Payne DD, Cleveland RJ (1987): Cystic medial necrosis in coarctation of the aorta: A potencial factor contributing to adverse consequences observed after percutaneous balloon angioplasty of coarctation sites. Circulation 75:689–695.

22b

Balloon Valvuloplasty/Angioplasty: The British Experience

Christopher Wren, M.D.

Department of Paediatric Cardiology, Freeman Hospital, Newcastle upon Tyne NE7 7DN, England

INTRODUCTION

The introduction of balloon dilatation procedures to the United Kingdom was dependent on the availability of equipment developed and produced in the United States. Because of this, early experience relied heavily on the experimental and early clinical work of American investigators. Once the materials were available, however, the technique was taken up with enthusiasm and has been applied to palliation or treatment of many forms of congenital heart disease. British workers have been particularly interested in applying the technique to relief of coarctation of the aorta and to palliation of cyanotic heart disease.

Our indications for treatment and the details of the techniques used differ little from those in the United States and elsewhere. In most medical centers balloon dilatation has become the accepted treatment for pulmonary valve stenosis, and it is also widely used in palliation of aortic stenosis and relief of recurrent coarctation of the aorta. In other conditions, such as tetralogy of Fallot and unoperated coarctation of the aorta, long-term programs are in progress for careful assessment of the role of balloon dilatation. This chapter assesses the British experience of balloon dilatation and considers indications, technical details, immediate and long-term results, and complications for each of the major lesions treated.

BALLOON DILATATION AS AN ALTERNATIVE TO SURGERY

Pulmonary Valve Stenosis

The speed with which balloon dilatation became the treatment of choice for pulmonary valve stenosis was a measure of its efficacy and safety. No surgical pulmonary valvotomy for treatment of classic pulmonary stenosis has been performed in this center or in many others since the first balloon dilatation. Initial results have been so encouraging that the threshold for treatment has fallen, and many children with moderate valve stenosis now undergo balloon dilatation. The contemporaneous introduction of Doppler echocardiography for assessment of severity means that most patients now have a single admission for assessment and treatment. Experience from very long follow-ups of surgical pulmonary valvotomy shows that the prognosis is excellent, and it seems likely that balloon valvotomy will produce equally good long-term results [1,2].

The lower threshold for treatment is variable. A Doppler pulmonary artery velocity of >3.5 m/s is usually taken as an indication for catheterization, and balloon dilatation will usually be performed even if the valve gradient at catheter is only around 30 mmHg. All of our procedures are performed under general anesthesia, and the out-patient Doppler ultrasound may be a better measure of the severity of pulmonary stenosis than the hemodynamics at the time of catheterization.

Transcatheter Therapy in Pediatric Cardiology, pages 421–432
© 1993 Wiley-Liss, Inc.

Our technique is very similar to that described and employed elsewhere. We use a short balloon (3–4 cm) with a diameter roughly 130% of the pulmonary valve diameter, and two balloons are used if a 23 mm balloon is too small. The technique has been used in infants and neonates; we have not experienced particular problems in neonates except that crossing the valve is sometimes more difficult. If prostaglandin is used to maintain ductal patency, balloon inflation is well tolerated. However, if the ductus has closed the procedure may be more difficult. Qureshi et al.. [3] reported the death of an 11-week-old infant after balloon dilatation and suggested that serial dilatation with progressively larger balloons (beginning with a 3 mm coronary angioplasty balloon) may be safer in this situation. In a later report from the same center, which probably includes many of the same patients, Ladusans et al. [4] attempted pulmonary valve dilatation in 15 neonates and were successful in 11 (73%). Satisfactory relief of stenosis persisted during a mean follow-up of 2 years in seven patients, while the other four required a second procedure (balloon or surgery). Despite the dysplastic nature of the valves in this age group, balloon dilatation seems to be more effective than it is in older children with pulmonary valve dysplasia.

Early in our experience we found that balloon dilatation of dysplastic pulmonary valve stenosis produced no reduction in gradient. Such children have small valve rings with myxomatous, "space-occupying" valve leaflets and do not have cusp fusion, so it is not surprising that pulmonary valve dilatation is ineffective. Similar experience has subsequently been reported [5–7].[1]

We have also performed balloon dilatation of pulmonary stenosis in 15 adults aged 17–74 years (median, 35 years), using a single balloon in eight and two 20 mm balloons in seven patients with a valve anulus larger than 25 mm. The transvalvar pressure drop was reduced from 60–130 mmHg (mean, 92) to 10–30 mmHg (mean, 24). Each procedure was performed under local anesthesia and was well tolerated. In one patient successful dilatation was achieved despite calcification of the pulmonary valve, and there has been no evidence of recurrence in follow-ups of more than 12 months. Two patients had significant residual infundibular pulmonary stenosis immediately after balloon dilatation, but follow-up with Doppler echocardiography has shown resolution of the right ventricular hypertrophy and the subpulmonary stenosis, similar to that reported in younger patients. Interestingly, several patients reported an improvement in well-being afterwards, despite having been asymptomatic beforehand.

Tetralogy of Fallot

After achieving successful relief of pulmonary stenosis it was logical to extend the technique to other forms of right ventricular outflow obstruction. There has been a particular interest in this country in palliation of tetralogy of Fallot, and the largest experience has been in Liverpool and in Guy's Hospital, London. The series began in late 1983 and is now extensive [8–10]. The balloon diameter used has been approximately 150% of the measured pulmonary valve ring, but neither balloon size nor any other variable can at present predict the likely response. The procedure may precipitate a hypercyanotic spell, and urgent palliative surgical shunting has sometimes been necessary. Occasionally serious damage to the right

---

[1]Editor's note: While the results of balloon valvuloplasty of dysplastic pulmonary valves are not as good as with non-dysplastic pulmonary valves, some authors (Marantz [7] and Rao [Am Heart J 116:1168–1176]) have reported reasonably good results. Based those reported by us and by Marantz [7], I would recommend balloon valvuloplasty as a first-option procedure for relief of pulmonary stenosis even with angiographic features of pulmonary valve dysplasia; a balloon that is 1.4–1.5 times the size of pulmonary valve anulus is recommended. For further discussion on this subject, the reader is referred to Chapter 6 (this volume).

ventricular outflow may be produced [11]. The mechanism of relief of stenosis is uncertain. One might expect the outflow morphology to have a bearing on the effectiveness of the procedure, with better results in those with predominant valve stenosis and less effect when there is more infundibular stenosis, but this has not been borne out so far. Assessment of the effectiveness of the procedure is sometimes difficult. Although there may be a measurable rise in systemic oxygen saturation, the main improvement is often subjective.

There has been no formal comparison of balloon dilatation of tetralogy of Fallot with surgical palliation. Aortopulmonary shunting is known to relieve symptoms and to promote pulmonary artery growth, and early reports suggest that balloon dilatation can do the same [12]. However, a report of surgical findings at subsequent repair failed to demonstrate any growth of the pulmonary valve or main pulmonary artery [13]. Twenty-seven patients who had previously undergone balloon dilatation of the right ventricular outflow underwent operative repair of tetralogy of Fallot 3–39 months (mean, 16 months) later. Two had had aortopulmonary shunts prior to balloon dilatation, and five required a shunt subsequently. Evidence of previous balloon dilatation was found at operation in 74%. The most common finding was an abnormality of the pulmonary valve—split leaflets in 33% and detachment of leaflets in 30%. In no case had the valve split along the commissures. In 19% there was a posterior split of the pulmonary anulus and pulmonary artery. There was no relationship between the ratio of balloon diameter to pulmonary valve diameter and the morphologic findings. The authors concluded that balloon dilatation of tetralogy of Fallot did not induce pulmonary annular growth and did not reduce the need for transannular patching.

Pulmonary Atresia

Qureshi et al. [14] have recently extended the technique of balloon dilatation to pulmonary valve atresia by using a catheter-guided hot-tip laser to cross the atretic valve before introducing the balloon catheter. The valve could be crossed in six of seven patients and was dilated with balloons 5–8 mm in diameter. This is an exciting new development that may offer an alternative to palliative aortopulmonary shunting and may improve the prospects of a biventricular circulation in the long term.

Aortic Valve Stenosis

The introduction of balloon dilatation for management of children with aortic stenosis has been more cautious than in those with pulmonary valve stenosis. Aortic stenosis is generally a progressive problem, and it has long been recognized that surgical valvotomy is only palliative. Because many patients will require a second or third surgical operation, there are obvious attractions in replacing the initial operation with a balloon catheter procedure. Early experience has shown that balloon dilatation of aortic stenosis in children can be accomplished safely, with satisfactory reduction in gradient and no significant worsening of aortic regurgitation. Early results compare favorably with those from surgical palliation, and in many centers in the United Kingdom balloon dilatation is now the treatment of choice.

The indication for treatment is similar to that for operation. Intervention is advised in the presence of symptoms, resting or exercise-induced ECG abnormalities, and a catheter gradient >60–70 mmHg. Experience over the past 2–3 years has led to a slightly lower threshold for intervention, as the safety and efficacy of the procedure suggest that there may be advantages in reduction of valve gradient of children with moderately severe stenosis in the absence of symptoms and ECG changes.

We usually cannulate both femoral arteries, one for the balloon catheter and the other to introduce a catheter to measure the valve gradient before the balloon catheter is withdrawn completely. Heparin is always used. We have found it helpful to position a right ventricular pacing wire, not so much to cover any small risk of temporary atrioventricular block as to prevent postectopic pauses by pacing just below the sinus rate. Occasionally the large left ventricular stroke volume after a postectopic pause will eject the catheter before dilatation can be accomplished. We use a longer balloon than in patients with pulmonary valve stenosis, 8 cm in older children and young adults and 5 cm in younger children. This stabilizes the position in the aorta and prevents ejection of the balloon before dilatation is accomplished. The balloon diameter is chosen to be equal to the diameter of the aortic valve, and two balloons are used only if the aortic valve is larger than 20 mm.

In a combined series with colleagues at The Hospital for Sick Children, Great Ormond Street, we performed balloon dilatation of aortic stenosis in 33 consecutive children aged 16 months to 17 years [15]. The pressure gradient was reduced from a mean of 71 ± 30 (± SD) to 28 ± 18 mmHg. New aortic regurgitation was produced in nine patients (27%)—grade I/IV in eight and grade II/IV in one—and preexisting aortic regurgitation was exacerbated in two patients (22%) (an increase from grade I/IV to grade II/IV). One patient suffered a serious vascular complication (avulsion of the iliac artery) when the balloon catheter became entangled with a pressure monitoring catheter introduced from the contralateral femoral artery. At repeat cardiac catheterization in 24 patients 2-19 (mean 9) months later the residual pressure drop was similar (35 ± 20 immediately and 31 ± 20 mmHg at follow-up). Repeat dilatation was performed in two patients with good effect. Balloon dilatation provides effective palliation of congenital aortic stenosis in children in the short to medium term and is now used as first line treatment.

Critical neonatal aortic stenosis is an altogether more difficult problem. Valve morphology is severely abnormal, and left ventricular function is usually poor, with left ventricular hypoplasia or dilatation and endocardial fibroelastosis. Some of these neonates have a very poor outlook whatever form of treatment is employed. Our experience with neonatal and early infant aortic stenosis [16] now extends to 24 patients, with follow-ups of up to 5 years. Details are given in Figure 1. The overall survival rate is only 54%. Four of 11 deaths (36%) were related to the balloon procedure, and six (55%) followed surgery of the aortic valve or coexisting mitral valve disease. Patients enrolled in our series were at particularly high risk: Four were considered unsuitable for surgery, three had significant stenosis despite recent surgery, and three also had severe mitral valve disease on presentation. A reduction in valve gradient in this situation is encouraging, but relief of heart failure is the main indication of success. In the presence of severe heart failure we have even documented an increase in the valve gradient following balloon dilatation as cardiac function has improved. Several long-term survivors still have significant valve stenosis as measured by Doppler but are not in heart failure.

The procedure is technically difficult. Introduction of the balloon catheter into the femoral artery risks damage to the vessel, but smaller catheters on thinner shafts and increasing experience have reduced this problem. Occasionally it may not be possible to cross the valve with a guidewire. One or two of those with very poor ventricular function may not tolerate occlusion of the outflow. A report by Ladusans et al. [17] of six neonates, three of whom had been detected by prenatal ultrasound, highlights the technical difficulties. In two patients the balloon could not be advanced beyond the aortoiliac junction, and both patients died shortly after the procedure. In one case the valve could not be crossed by the balloon catheter, and the patient died after a surgical valvotomy. In three patients balloon dilatation was accomplished safely, but all three died within 3 weeks from severe left ventricular dysfunction.

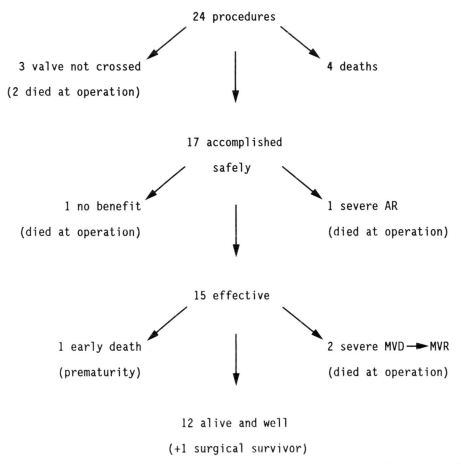

Fig. 1. Results of balloon dilatation of neonatal and early infant critical aortic valve stenosis. AR, aortic regurgitation; MVD, mitral valve disease; MVR, mitral valve replacement.

The results of balloon dilatation of neonatal aortic stenosis must, of course, be compared with the results of surgery. One of the difficulties of assessing surgical reports is to know which patients were included and which were rejected. Our series included patients who were refused for surgery because ventricular function was thought to be too poor or ventricular size too small. Most surgical series only report patients undergoing an operation and therefore give an overoptimistic view. However, realistic surgical series show just as great a difficulty with treatment [18–20]. The choice between balloon dilatation and surgical valvotomy is best decided individually in each insti-

tute. It seems likely that similar results will be achieved whatever mode of treatment has been employed [21]. The smallest, sickest babies with the most dysplastic valves and poorest ventricular function will continue to have a poor prognosis.

Recognition of aortic valve stenosis in the fetus implies a very poor outlook, as there is almost invariably severe left ventricular dysfunction. Because of this Maxwell et al. [22] attempted interuterine balloon dilatation of the aortic valve in two fetuses at 28 and 31 weeks gestation. One fetus died the next day and the other died 5 weeks after premature delivery. This report shows that the procedure is technically feasible, but whether it will improve the prognosis of fetal aortic stenosis remains to be seen.

Coarctation of the Aorta

Following reports of successful dilatation of experimental animal coarctation and of excised human coarctation segments, there was considerable enthusiasm for balloon angioplasty of coarctation. It was soon shown that dilatation of coarctation can be accomplished safely and effectively in children older than 12 months, but early results in neonates and infants were disappointing, with a high incidence of early recoarctation and of femoral arterial problems—experience confirmed more recently by Redington et al. [23]. Balloon angioplasty of vascular lesions achieves its effect by disruption of the intima and media of the vessel, leaving the adventitia intact. This has led to anxieties about the long-term effects, particularly the risk of late development of aortic aneurysm. Because of this, balloon dilatation of unoperated coarctation remains an experimental procedure, and it will be some time before its role in clinical practice is established.

The results of surgical treatment of coarctation in children older than 12 months are good, with low morbidity and mortality rates and a fairly high success rate. Restenosis is relatively uncommon (depending on how it is defined), and there are few reports of long-term complications, although these are now coming to light in series with longer follow-ups, especially after patch aortoplasty. The results of balloon dilatation must be compared with those from surgery, as this is the established treatment, but unfortunately few surgical patients have been subjected to the same intensive scrutiny as those now undergoing balloon dilatation, with immediate, early, and late reinvestigation by catheterization and angiography. Consequently we do not know the residual pressure gradient at catheterization in patients undergoing resection of coarctation or the incidence of "aneurysm" in surgical series. Until that information is available the risks

and benefits of balloon dilatation of unoperated coarctation of the aorta cannot be compared directly with surgical results. However, a preliminary report of 21 children undergoing surgical repair of coarctation and 27 treated by balloon dilatation [24] concluded that surgical repair and balloon dilatation yielded similar results in terms of residual pressure gradient and aneurysm formation in short-term follow-up.

Balloon dilatation of unoperated coarctation has been practiced in this center since 1984. It has been applied to patients from ages 1 year to early adulthood (the oldest being 32 years), and initial results are encouraging. All procedures are performed under general anesthetic, and patients are heparinized. An aortogram is performed, and the diameter of the coarctation and of the proximal aorta is measured, using a marker catheter to correct for magnification. We use a single balloon in most cases, choosing its diameter to be no larger than the proximal aorta but more than twice the minimum coarctation diameter (see below). All patients receive postoperative treatment with an oral β-blocker for 1 month.

Early in our experience the procedure was offered as an alternative to surgery in consecutive patients, and almost all patients or their parents opted for balloon dilatation [25]. We have seen only two aneurysms (which occurred in two of our first three patients), but we are concerned by the incidence of mild residual stenosis measured at follow-up [26]. In our series, and in others recently reported, the residual pressure drop across the site of the coarctation was less than 10 mmHg in most patients when measured under sedation or general anesthesia. However, the pressure gradient was abolished altogether in only a few patients, and even a small residual gradient implies some residual obstruction to blood flow. This may contribute to hypertension in the long term and is of particular concern because follow-up of coarctectomy patients has shown that even those with normal blood pressure and good operative results have identifiable residual abnormalities of left ventricular function. Our current indications for balloon dilatation of coarctation have been modified by experience. It seems possible to predict the likely outcome from the angiographic appearance, and this has influenced patient selection. A lower residual gradient will be achieved in those with "milder" stenosis (as a percentage narrowing) and when the coarctation is symmetrical. Tight and/or eccentric lesions have less chance of being abolished.

Aneurysm remains an uncommon problem in short- and medium-term follow-ups. Our first report included two aneurysms, one occurring immediately and one at 12 months [25]. In both cases the balloon used was more than 3.5 times larger than the coarctation. Since then we have seen no further aneurysms despite a continuing program with restudy at 12 months. We also found higher residual gradients when the balloon was less than twice the diameter of the coarctation. One would expect a larger balloon to produce better relief of coarctation at the expense of a higher risk of aneurysm. However, numbers in both our series and in other published reports are too small to prove that this association is real. Added variables are the anatomy of the lesion, possible histologic abnormalities of the aortic wall, and our lack of knowledge of how to select optimal balloon diameter. It is still not clear whether the balloon should be selected from the diameter of the coarctation (often very difficult to measure exactly despite multiple angiographic projections) or derived from the proximal aortic diameter (which is in itself variable, as proximal hypoplasia is common). Currently we use a balanced approach, trying to select a balloon roughly 2.5 times the minimum coarctation diameter and yet no larger than the proximal aorta.[2]

Balloon dilatation of coarctation will continue to be performed in a few centers with careful assessment of long-term results. A well-designed direct comparison with surgical treatment using the same invasive follow-up is urgently needed. Until the remaining questions are resolved balloon dilatation of unoperated coarctation will remain an experimental procedure.

BALLOON DILATATION OF POSTOPERATIVE STENOSES
Recoarctation of the Aorta

While the controversy surrounding balloon dilatation of unoperated coarctation remains unresolved, the situation regarding treatment of postoperative residual or restenosis is clearer. The results of the catheter technique have to be compared with the outcome of surgery. The morbidity and mortality rates of reoperation are higher than for a first operation and the outcome is less good, so there has been greater incentive to find a more effective treatment with lower risk. It seems that balloon dilatation can provide this, and the technique is now recommended as treatment of choice [27].

In a joint study with our colleagues at The Hospital for Sick Children, we performed balloon dilatation in 44 patients a mean of 4 years postoperatively [28]. Their ages ranged from 2 months to 20 years and their weights from 2 to 72 kg. Two-thirds of patients had had an operation in the neonatal period. The indication for treatment was clinical evidence of recoarctation with a catheter gradient of 15 mmHg or more and discreet narrowing on the angiogram at the site of repair. The balloon diameter was chosen to be just smaller than the proximal aorta. We found that balloon dilatation reduced the pressure gradient from a mean of 37 ± 16 to 14 ± 11 mmHg and increased the coarctation to aorta ratio from

---

[2]Editors note: Some workers use a balloon that is no larger than the diameter of the descending aorta at the level of diaphragm. See Chapter 10 (this volume) for further discussion.

0.45 ± 0.14 to 0.85 ± 0.16. The ascending aortic pressure was reduced from 120 ± 25 to 113 ± 20 mmHg, and the descending aortic pulse pressure rose from 22 ± 7 to 36 ± 8 mmHg. The type of surgery (end-to-end anastomosis, subclavian flap, patch aortoplasty, or multiple operations) had no influence on the results. One patient developed a small aneurysm immediately after dilatation.

At follow-up there was no overall change in the angiographic diameter of the dilated segment, but there was a further small reduction in the pressure gradient. Angiographically no change was apparent in the patient with an aneurysm, but new aneurysms were seen in two patients (10% of those undergoing follow-up). Aneurysm development seemed not to be related to balloon diameter or to balloon-to-coarctation ratio, but contributing factors could not be identified because of the small numbers involved. Since this report an 8-year-old boy undergoing balloon dilatation of recoarctation with a previous patch repair sustained a rupture of the aorta at the site of dilatation and died [29]. Thus the procedure is not without risk. However, in view of the difficulties of reoperation, there seems to be a developing consensus that balloon dilatation is the treatment of choice for postoperative residual or recoarctation [27]. Our study also found that vascular complications (particularly femoral artery occlusion) occurred only in patients weighing less than 10 kg, and in some circumstances it may be appropriate to defer reinvestigation until that weight is achieved.

Two particular situations deserve special mention. Occasionally it may be impossible to wean a patient with complex congenital heart disease from ventilation after cardiac surgery because of residual coarctation. Balloon dilatation may expedite extubation [28].

Second, recoarctation in the presence of a ventricular septal defect offers the alternative of a transvenous approach via the ventricular septal defect with an anterograde approach to the coarctation, thus avoiding percutaneous femoral artery puncture in a small infant. We have adopted this technique in two small infants awaiting cardiac surgery, in each case using a coronary dilatation balloon (diameter 3-4 mm) in view of the small size (Fig. 2). Good relief of coarctation was achieved.

Atrial Baffle Stenosis After the Mustard Operation

Late problems developing after the Mustard operation include systemic and pulmonary venous obstruction at the site of baffle placement. We have encountered five such patients aged 6-15 years, two with superior caval obstruction and three with inferior caval obstruction. Superior caval obstruction in one patient needed serial dilatation, as there was almost complete occlusion at the first study. Balloons were introduced via the femoral vein for inferior caval obstruction and from an infraclavicular subclavian approach for superior caval obstruction as the superior cava could not be entered from below. Very large balloons were needed (e.g., 18 mm diameter for 4 mm stenosis and 23 mm diameter for 5 mm stenosis). There has been persistent improvement in all cases in up to 4 years follow-up, although one patient later developed pulmonary venous obstruction that required reoperation.

Pulmonary venous obstruction is a more difficult problem. Cooper et al. [30], from The Hospital for Sick Children, attempted balloon dilatation for relief of pulmonary venous obstruction in three children following Mustard operations. The balloon diameter was chosen to be three or four times the minimum diameter measured on echocardiography. The balloon was passed over a guidewire retrogradely via the aortic valve and tricuspid valve to the pulmonary venous atrium. One patient tolerated the procedure very poorly so that it was ineffective and was not repeated. In the other two there was marked hemodynamic and angiographic improvement associated with resolution of pulmonary edema. Pulmonary venous balloon dilatation is an attractive alternative to reopera-

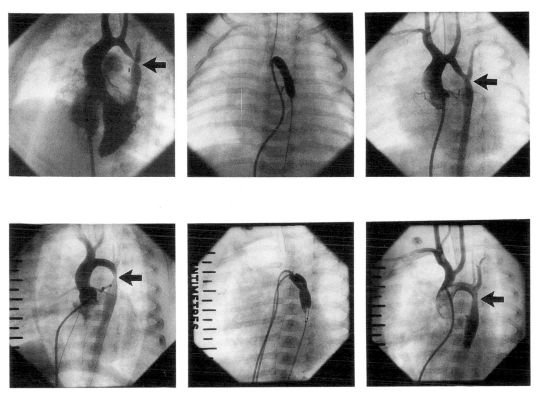

Fig. 2. Transvenous balloon dilatation of severe residual coarctation (arrows) in association with a ventricular septal defect. **Top:** Angiographic appearance before (left) and after (right) balloon dilatation with a single 4 mm coronary angioplasty balloon (center) in a premature baby with Shone's syndrome. **Bottom:** Angiographic appearance before (left) and after (right) balloon dilatation using two 3 mm coronary angioplasty balloons (center) introduced through the ventricular septal defect.

tion, but only time will tell if it can produce a lasting improvement.

Aortopulmonary Shunts

Classic and modified Blalock-Taussig shunts are widely used for palliation of cyanotic congenital heart disease. Early shunt failure is usually related to thrombosis and may respond to streptokinase infusion or revision of the operation. Late problems include shunt stenosis, and, unless the patient is suitable for definitive repair, the main approach until recently has been a second shunt rather than reoperation on the first shunt. However, if the angiogram shows a discrete stenosis balloon, then dilatation may be an appropriate alterna-

tive [31,32]. The balloon diameter is chosen to be roughly equal to the shunt diameter on the angiogram. The balloon is usually introduced retrogradely via the femoral artery. Postdilatation reassessment may be difficult, as there is often no convincing increase in systemic saturation despite an angiographic improvement. However, there is often an impressive subjective improvement in symptoms of cyanosis, fatigue, and effort intolerance. At best this technique extends the duration of palliation, but it seems to be safe and is effective in selected patients, offering an alternative to further palliative surgery.

Balloon dilatation of other aortopulmonary shunts may be more problematic. Gibbs *et al.*

[33] performed balloon dilatation of a Waterston shunt anastomosis in a 13-year-old with pulmonary atresia and ventricular septal defect. Initial inflation with an 8 mm balloon produced no waisting, so a 12 mm diameter balloon was employed. The pulmonary artery pressure rose from 15 ± 11 to 42 ± 30 mmHg, and the systemic arterial saturation rose from 79% to 96%. Acute pulmonary edema developed within a few hours and was rapidly fatal. At autopsy the Waterston anastomosis was enlarged to around 10 mm by a tear on its inferior aspect extending from the aorta to the proximal right lower lobe pulmonary artery, but there was no hemorrhage or extravasation. The authors suggest that in this situation failure to produce waisting of the balloon does not necessarily imply too small a balloon diameter.

Supravalvar Pulmonary Stenosis

Supravalvar stenosis of the pulmonary artery is one of the main postoperative problems in patients who have undergone anatomic repair of transposition of the great arteries ("switch" operation). Saxena et al. [34] attempted balloon dilatation in five patients with supravalvar pulmonary stenosis on eight occasions but were unable to reduce the right ventricular pressure or to improve the angiographic appearance. They attribute their lack of success to the smallness of the pulmonary valve anulus, multiple levels of stenosis, and distortion of the main pulmonary artery.

Bioprosthetic Valves

Balloon dilatation of a stenosed bioprosthesis in the tricuspid valve position was employed in a 19-year-old girl in an attempt to avoid reoperation [35]. The patient had previously undergone repair of tetralogy of Fallot with tricuspid valve replacement following infective endocarditis and a further valve replacement after valve failure. Balloon dilatation of the bovine pericardial valve was performed twice, and, although it produced a dramatic reduction in right heart failure on each occasion, the effect

only lasted for 3–6 months. Tricuspid valve replacement was eventually undertaken, and the valve leaflets were found to be very stiff with calcific vegetations on both surfaces. There was no evidence of the previous balloon dilatations, and the mechanism of the temporary reduction of the stenosis is unclear.

CONCLUSIONS

The introduction of balloon dilatation has transformed the practice of pediatric cardiology over the last few years. Its rapid acceptance is a measure of its safety and efficacy. The next few years will probably see further refinements of technique and further applications. The procedure is already accepted for treatment of pulmonary valve stenosis, aortic valve stenosis, and recoarctation. Further experience will show whether it is effective in balloon dilatation of pulmonary arterial stenosis, subaortic stenosis, and pulmonary venous obstruction following the Mustard operation. Trials in hand will determine whether palliative balloon dilatation of the right ventricular outflow tract in tetralogy of Fallot will induce symmetric pulmonary arterial growth making subsequent repair easier. Comparative studies of surgical treatment and balloon dilatation of unoperated coarctation will establish the place of the latter.

REFERENCES

1. Sullivan ID, Robinson PJ, Macartney FJ, Taylor JFN, Rees PG, Bull C, Deanfield JE (1985): Percutaneous balloon valvuloplasty for pulmonary valve stenosis in infants and children. Br Heart J 54:435–441.
2. Tynan M, Baker EJ, Rohmer J, Jones ODH, Reidy JF, Joseph MC, Ottenkamp J (1985): Percutaneous balloon pulmonary valvuloplasty. Br Heart J 53:520–524.
3. Qureshi SA, Ladusans EJ, Martin RP (1989): Dilatation with progressively larger balloons for severe stenosis of the pulmonary valve presenting in the late neonatal period and early infancy. Br Heart J 62:311–314.
4. Ladusans EJ, Qureshi SA, Parsons JM, Arab S, Baker EJ, Tynan M (1990): Balloon dilatation of

critical stenosis of the pulmonary valve in the neo-nates. Br Heart J 63:362-367.

5. Di Sessa TG, Alpert BS, Chase NA, Birnbaum SE, Watson DC (1987): Balloon valvuloplasty in chil-dren with dysplastic pulmonary valves. Am J Cardiol 60:405-407.

6. Musewe NN, Robertson MA, Benson LN, Smallh-orn JF, Burrows PE, Freedom RM, Moes CAF, Rowe RD (1987): The dysplastic pulmonary valve: Echocardiographic features and results of balloon dilatation. Br Heart J 57:364-370.

7. Marantz PM, Huhta JC, Mullins CE, Murphy DJ, Nihill MR, Ludomirsky A, Yoon GY (1988): Results of balloon valvuloplasty in typical and dysplastic pulmonary valve stenosis: Doppler echocardio-graphic follow-up. J Am Coll Cardiol 12:476-479.

8. Sreeram N, Saleem M, Jackson M, Peart I, McKay R, Arnold R, Walsh K (1991): Results of balloon pulmonary valvuloplasty as a palliative procedure in tetralogy of Fallot. J Am Coll Cardiol 18:159-165.

9. Qureshi SA, Kirk CR, Lamb RK, Arnold R, Wilkin-son JL (1988): Balloon dilatation of the pulmonary valve in the first year of life in patients with tetralogy of Fallot: A preliminary study. Br Heart J 60:232-235.

10. Qureshi SA, Ladusans EJ, Parsons JM, Baker EJ, Tynan MJ (1989): Efficacy of percutaneous balloon dilatation of the pulmonary outflow tract as pallia-tion of tetralogy of Fallot, abstracted. Br Heart J 61:482.

11. Lamb RK, Qureshi SA, Arnold R (1987): Pulmo-nary artery tear following balloon valvoplasty in Fallot's tetralogy. Int J Cardiol 15:347-349.

12. Parsons JM, Ladusans EJ, Qureshi SA (1989): Growth of the pulmonary artery after neonatal bal-loon dilatation of the right ventricular outflow tract in an infant with the tetralogy of Fallot and atrioven-tricular septal defect. Br Heart J 62:65-68.

13. Battistessa SA, Robles A, Jackson M, Miyamoto S, Arnold R, McKay R (1990): Operative findings after percutaneous pulmonary balloon dilatation of the right ventricular outflow tract in tetralogy of Fallot. Br Heart J 64:321-324.

14. Qureshi SA, Rosenthal E, Tynan M, Anjos R, Baker EJ (1991): Transcatheter laser assisted pulmonic valve dilatation in pulmonic valve atresia. Am J Cardiol 67:428-431.

15. Sullivan ID, Wren C, Bain H, Hunter S, Rees PG, Taylor JFN, Bull C, Deanfield JE (1989): Balloon dilatation of the aortic valve for congenital aortic stenosis in childhood. Br Heart J 61:186-191.

16. Wren C, Sullivan I, Bull C, Deanfield J (1987): Percutaneous balloon dilatation of aortic valve ste-nosis in neonates and infants. Br Heart J 58:608-612.

17. Ladusans EJ, Parsons JM, Qureshi SA, Baker EJ,

Tynan MJ (1989): Results of percutaneous balloon dilatation for critical aortic stenosis in neonates with severe endocardial fibroelastosis, abstracted. Br Heart J 61:470.

18. Gundry SR, Behrendt DM (1986): Prognostic fac-tors in valvotomy for critical aortic stenosis in in-fancy. J Thorac Cardiovasc Surg 92:747-754.

19. Pelech AN, Dyck JD, Trusler GA, Williams WG, Olley PM, Rowe RD, Freedom RM (1987): Critical aortic stenosis. J Thorac Cardiovasc Surg 94:510-517.

20. Hammon JW, Lupinetti F, Maples MD, Merrill WH, Frist WH, Graham TP, Bender HW (1988): Predictors of operative mortality in critical valvular aortic stenosis presenting in infancy. Ann Thorac Surg 45:537-540.

21. Zeevi B, Keane JF, Castaneda AR, Perry SB, Lock JE (1989): Neonatal critical aortic stenosis: Surgery vs. balloon dilation. Circulation 80:831-839.

22. Maxwell D, Allan L, Tynan MJ (1991): Balloon dilatation of the aortic valve in the fetus: A report of two cases. Br Heart J 65:256-258.

23. Redington AN, Booth P, Shore DF, Rigby ML (1990): Primary balloon dilatation of coarctation of the aorta in neonates. Br Heart J 64:277-281.

24. Boucek MM, Ruttenberg HD, Orsmond GS, Veasy LG, Shaddy RE, Sturtevant J, McGough EC (1988): Results of balloon coarctation angioplasty versus surgical repair in children, abstracted. Am J Cardiol 62:508.

25. Wren C, Peart I, Bain H, Hunter S (1987): Balloon dilatation of unoperated aortic coarctation: Immedi-ate results and one year follow up. Br Heart J 58:369-373.

26. Wren C, Hunter S (1988): Balloon angioplasty for relief of aortic coarctation. Cardiol Board Rev 5:126-134.

27. Huhta JC (1989): Angioplasty for recoarctation. J Am Coll Cardiol 1:420-421.

28. Cooper SG, Sullivan ID, Wren C (1989): Treatment of recoarctation: Balloon dilatation angioplasty. J Am Coll Cardiol 14:413-419.

29. Balaji S, Oommen R, Rees PG (1991): Fatal aortic rupture during balloon dilatation of recoarctation. Br Heart J 65:100-101.

30. Cooper SG, Sullivan ID, Bull C, Taylor JFN (1989): Balloon dilatation of pulmonary venous pathway obstruction after Mustard repair for transposition of the great arteries. J Am Coll Cardiol 14:194-198.

31. Qureshi SA, Martin RP, Dickinson DF, Hunter S (1989): Balloon dilatation of stenosed Blalock-Taussig shunts. Br Heart J 61:432-434.

32. Parsons JM, Ladusans EJ, Qureshi SA (1989): Bal-loon dilatation of a stenosed modified (poly-tetrafluoroethylene) Blalock-Taussig shunt. Br Heart J 62:228-229.

33. Gibbs JL, Wilson N, Da Costa P (1988): Balloon dilatation of a Waterston aortopulmonary anastomosis. Br Heart J 59:596–597.

34. Saxena A, Fong LV, Ogilvie BC, Keeton BR (1990): Use of balloon dilatation to treat supravalvar pulmonary stenosis developing after anatomical correction for complete transposition. Br Heart J 64:151–155.

35. Wren C, Hunter S (1989): Balloon dilatation of a stenosed biprosthesis in the tricuspid valve position. Br Heart J 61:65–67.

22c

Balloon Valvuloplasty/Angioplasty: The Hong Kong Experience

Roxy N.S. Lo, M.B.B.S. F.R.C.P., D.C.H., Maurice P. Leung, M.B.B.S., M.R.C.P., D.C.H., and K.C. Lau, M.B.B.S., F.R.C.P., D.C.H.

Department of Paediatrics, University of Hong Kong, The Grantham Hospital, Hong Kong

INTRODUCTION

Interventional cardiac catheterization in children in Hong Kong was introduced in April 1986, when Professor Robert M. Freedom of Toronto, who was then Visiting Professor at the University Department of Paediatrics, demonstrated balloon dilatation for congenital pulmonary valve stenosis in two patients. Further exposure to the field was obtained when one of us (R.N.S.L.) spent several months in 1987 with Dr. James Lock at Children's Hospital in Boston. At present, all interventional catheterizations are performed by the authors at The Grantham Hospital, with back-up support from the cardiothoracic surgical unit.

TABLE I. Interventional Catheterization in Pediatrics, April 1986 to March 1991, Grantham Hospital, Hong Kong

Valvuloplasty	
Pulmonary stenosis	68
Aortic stenosis	10
Mitral stenosis	1
Tricuspid stenosis	1
Pulmonary stenosis in complex CHD[a]	2
Angioplasty	
Coarctation of aorta	13
Pulmonary artery stenosis	2
Coil embolization	
Modified Blalock-Taussig shunt	4
Total	101

[a]CHD, Congenital heart defects.

From April 1986 to March 1991 101 therapeutic cardiac catheterizations were performed (Table I). The majority of procedures (68%) were done for relief of pulmonary valve stenosis. This review presents our results and experience with transcatheter therapy in children in Hong Kong.

TECHNIQUE

Diagnosis of the cardiac lesions was made by the usual clinical, electrocardiographic, x-ray, and combined two-dimensional and Doppler echocardiographic examinations. Assessment of severity of pulmonary or aortic stenosis was by continuous-wave Doppler estimation of gradient. Cardiac catheterization with the aim of balloon valvuloplasty was performed if the gradient was 50 mmHg or more or if the valve seemed more stenotic by its thickened or dysplastic appearance on two-dimensional echocardiography. For coarctation of the aorta, the indications for angioplasty were similar to those for surgery, viz., heart failure or hypertension. Decision to dilate atrioventricular valves or pulmonary artery stenosis was made during cardiac catheterization after obtaining the appropriate angiograms and hemodynamic data. Coil embolization of aortopulmonary shunts were performed specifically for occluding the shunts in three patients with tetralogy of Fallot and in one patient with

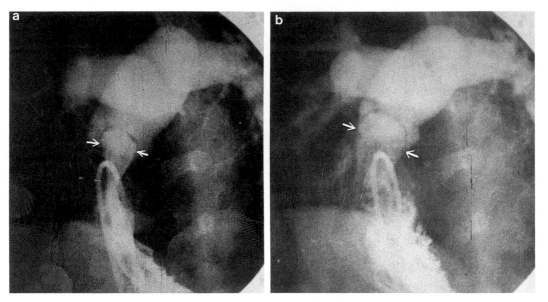

Fig. 1. Four-chamber view of right ventriculogram during midsystole (**a**) and early systole (**b**), demonstrating the differences in diameters (arrows) of the pulmonary annulus at the level of attachment of the valve leaflets.

pulmonary atresia and intact ventricular septum in whom the shunts were not divided during surgical correction.

General anesthesia was employed in all procedures except in eight older patients with pulmonary stenosis in whom local anesthesia was used, to be supplemented with intravenous ketamine when necessary just prior to the introduction of the balloon catheter. A peripheral arterial line and pulse oximeter were used to monitor patient blood pressure and oxygen saturations. We routinely gave the patient 100% oxygen for a few minutes before inflation of the balloon.[1]

Despite the availability of echocardiographic measurements, an angiogram was always obtained, and we measured the area of stenosis from developed cinefilms because we found it not only more reliable to choose the appropriate frame for measurement than from video playback but also more accurate in calculating

the diameter of the stenotic lesion, especially when the size of the catheter was used as a reference to correct for magnification. The waiting time for developing the cineangiogram was usually less than 15 minutes. Recently we tended to use a larger marker (a 10 cents coin, 17.5 mm in diameter) placed over the precordium as the reference.

For pulmonary valve stenosis, we found that the diameter of the pulmonary annulus at the attachment of the valve leaflets varies significantly during the cardiac cycle (Fig. 1). Most authors have suggested using balloon diameters 1.2–1.4 times the size of the pulmonary annulus or even larger [1,2]. None have mentioned any variations in the size of the pulmonary annulus during right ventricular contraction, nor have they indicated the phase of the cardiac cycle at which the measurement should be taken. Presumably the widest diameter was chosen, but Sullivan et al. [3] have indeed

---

[1]Editor's note: There is no theoretical reason for administering oxygen, and most authorities do not believe it is necessary

prior to balloon inflation. This may awaken an unanesthetized child.

stated that measurements were obtained "without specific regard to the phase of the cardiac cycle." During the course of our study we found that the pulmonary valve annulus was widest at end-diastole or early systole and narrowest at midsystole. The former was therefore used as the basis for the selection of balloon sizes, and we chose balloons with diameters equal to or one size (as available) larger then the maximal pulmonary annulus dimension. Such variations in annulus size was not encountered with aortic valve stenosis or with coarctation of the aorta.

The technique of balloon dilatation was basically similar to the standard procedures described in the literature. We have been using balloon catheters from either Schneider-Medintag AG or Cook Inc. For easy passage of the balloon catheter across the tricuspid valve and right ventricular outflow tract in pulmonary stenosis we found the use of the extra-stiff long exchange guidewire (Cook) or the back-up wire (Schneider-Medintag AG) very helpful. Hand injection of diluted contrast was used to inflate the balloon. The inflation pressures were not routinely measured except in about 20 patients in the beginning, and our experience showed that the inflation pressures would hardly exceed 5 atm. Usually a total of three inflations was performed for each dilatation. The duration of each inflation was timed by the assisting nurse and was less than 10 seconds. Measurement of pressure gradient by direct pullback across the stenotic lesion and repeat angiogram were done after the dilatation. Measurement of cardiac output by thermodilution was not routine.

RESULTS

Pulmonary Valve Stenosis

Sixty-eight dilatations were performed in 66 patients; they were divided into three subgroups. Group I consisted of 47 patients with typical pulmonary valve stenosis; mean age was 4.2 years (range, 7 weeks to 26 years), and seven were under 12 months. In one 5-month-old infant we were unable to advance an end-hole catheter across the pulmonary orifice after passage of a 0.021 inch guidewire. Group II included seven patients with dysplastic pulmonary valve, three of whom also had phenotypic features of Noonan's syndrome; mean age was 3.3 years (range, 4 months to 9 years). Group III included 12 patients with pulmonary atresia or critical pulmonary stenosis and intact ventricular septum who had previously received surgical valvotomy during the neonatal period. We have attempted but failed to pass a catheter through the pulmonary orifice in two neonates with critical pulmonary stenosis presenting with cyanosis after birth. Our current policy for these patients is to perform trans-ventricular close-heart surgical valvotomy as soon as possible and then elective patch repair of the right ventricular outflow tract or balloon dilatation for residual obstruction.

Table II shows the immediate and late results in these three groups of patients. We have restudied the first 20 patients in group I by cardiac catheterization at 6–27 (mean, 12) months after balloon dilatation. Subsequently we utilized Doppler ultrasound as the sole method for assessment of residual obstruction. Good reduction in transvalvular gradient was achieved in both group I and III patients but was unsatisfactory for group II patients with dysplastic valves. Only four patients (8.2%) in group I while four out of seven (57%) patients with dysplastic valves had a final gradient greater than 25 mmHg; two of the latter received surgery for relief of the stenosis.

As described above, we are inclined to use balloon sizes that are equal to or just slightly larger than the maximal pulmonary annulus diameters measured from the cineangiograms during late diastole or early systole. Table III compares the effect of various balloon sizes in 49 dilatations in patients with typical pulmonary valve stenosis. Statistical analysis showed no significant difference between those involving smaller balloons and the other groups involving large balloons. However, in the two patients who required a second dilatation the

TABLE II. Immediate and Late Results of Balloon Pulmonary Valvuloplasty[a]

Groups	Before	Follow-up		Percent drop
		Immediate	Late	
Right ventricular pressure				
I	86 (50–270)	51 (24–160)	40 (28–60)[b]	53[b]
II	67 (50–85)	55 (38–75)	NA	18
III	77 (40–120)	43 (14–80)	NA	43
RV–PA peak gradient				
I	69 (25–250	28 (0–135)	17 (0–40)[c]	76[c]
II	42 (25–65)	26 (15–50)	30 (15–55)	28
III	58 (24–105)	18 (10–50)	20 (10–40)	67

[a]NA not available; RV–PA, right ventricle-to-pulmonary artery.
[b]Based on 20 patients restudied by cardiac catheterization.
[c]Based on Doppler echocardiography.

balloon/annulus ratio was less than 1 (0.9 and 0.91, respectively) in the first attempt.[2] Although others have demonstrated the safety of using oversized balloons, most serious complications such as death [4], tricuspid valve damage [5], and conduction abnormalities [6] could be attributed to the use of large balloons.[3] Our experience suggested the importance of noting the variation in the size of the pulmonary annulus and that the use of balloons larger than its maximal dimension is probably not necessary.[2]

Twelve babies with pulmonary atresia (8) or critical pulmonary stenosis (4) and intact ventricular septum who survived a neonatal transventricular closed pulmonary valvotomy (group III) were catheterized at 5–18 (mean 10) months after surgery. Their diagnoses in the neonatal period were confirmed by two-dimensional echocardiography with both pulsed and continuous-wave Doppler flow studies. They all had echocardiographic evidence of a hypoplastic but tripartite right ventricle and possessed a good sized tricuspid valve annulus, right ventricular infundibulum, and main pul-

monary artery. At catheterization, balloon dilatation was attempted on all babies who had residual outflow tract obstruction with a right ventricular systolic pressure ≥40 mmHg. A small, 5 mm balloon was required in three babies for initial dilatation of an extremely narrowed opening of the pulmonary valve. However, the ultimate balloon size chosen for all babies was 1.0–1.3 times (8–13 mm) the maximal pulmonary annulus. In four infants, cardiac catheterization was repeated during the course of follow-up, and two of them underwent a second dilatation procedure. The ratio of right ventricular to left ventricular systolic pressures was used as a better hemodynamic index of the severity of right ventricular outflow obstruction. The ratio before valvuloplasty was compared with that immediately after or following the second interventional procedure.

Table IV shows the results of 12 dilatation procedures carried out in 10 babies. All except one achieved a significant drop in the peak systolic right-to-left ventricular pressure ratio ($P < 0.01$). Of these, in one baby the procedure

---

[2]Editor's note: The fact that both the patients requiring repeat dilatation had the procedure performed with balloons smaller than valve annulus suggests that balloons larger than annulus are should be used used for balloon pulmonary valvuloplasty.

[3]Editor's note: The complications reported, especially in references 5 and 6, are related to excessive length of the balloon rather than to excessive diameter of the balloon.

TABLE III. Comparison Between Balloon/Anulus Ratio and Gradient Reduction in Typical Pulmonary Stenosis[a]

Group	No.	BAR	RV–PA peak gradient (mean)		Percent drop
			Predilatation	Follow-up	
Ia	14	≤1.10	64	21	71
Ib	13	1.11–1.20	63	13	78
Ic	10	1.21–1.30	83	18	79
Id	7	1.31–1.40	82	17	78
Ie	5	≥1.41	52	16	68

[a]BAR, balloon/annulus ratio; RV-PA, right ventricle-to-pulmonary artery. $P > 0.3$ in all groups when compared with group Ia.

was complicated by embolization of a broken piece of guidewire after successful balloon valvuloplasty. The wire was removed by surgical exploration of the right pulmonary artery. In another baby, only a guidewire but not the balloon catheter could pass through the pinhole opening created by the previous valvotomy. He underwent successful right ventricular outflow reconstruction. One baby had a low right ventricular pressure (<40 mmHg), and no valvuloplasty was performed. The 10 babies were followed up for 1–24 (mean, 14.8) months. At the latest follow-up, all were well and showed no evidence of heart failure. Continuous-wave Doppler registered a residual gradient of ≤45 mmHg in all patients (8–45, mean 19 mmHg) except one, who had severe infundibular obstruction (55 mmHg).

TABLE IV. Balloon Dilatation for Pulmonary Atresia After Previous Valvotomy[a]

Case	Age at		Peak systolic pressures (mmHg)					
	Surgical valvotomy (days)	Cardiac catheterization and balloon dilatation (months)	Preangioplasty			Postangioplasty		
			RV	LV	RV/LV	RV	LV	RV/LV
1	3	9	70	75	0.93	35	75	0.47
2	4	16	50	90	0.56	37	90	0.41
3	3	15	75	60	1.25	14	60	0.23
4	2	18	40	75	0.53	34	75	0.47
5	2	14	75	75	1.00	40	75	0.53
6	5	5	120	75	1.60			
		17				40	80	0.50
7	25	7	90	70	1.28			
		18				65	75	0.87
8	2	12	90	90	1.00	80	80	1.00
9	3	6	65	80	0.81	38	80	0.45
10	1	5	90	90	1.00	50	75	0.67
11	2	11	80	60	1.33	—[b]		
12	10	15	24	100	0.24	Not attempted		

[a]LV, left ventricle; RV, right ventricle
[b]Only guidewire could pass through the stenotic pulmonary valve.

Pulmonary Valve Stenosis in Other Congenital Heart Diseases

Balloon dilatation of the pulmonary valve was attempted in two patients with pulmonary oligemia for palliation of cyanosis. The first patient had tetralogy of Fallot and was 11 months old at the time of cardiac catheterization. There was marked valvular as well as infundibular stenosis. The pulmonary annulus measured 10 mm, and a 10 mm diameter, 3 cm long balloon was used. Difficulty was encountered in advancing the balloon catheter across the right ventricular outflow tract. After one inflation–deflation cycle the patient developed persistent severe hypercyanotic spell with worsening hypoxemia and metabolic acidosis despite oxygen and other therapy under general anesthesia. An emergency modified Blalock-Taussig shunt was required to relieve the hypoxemia. The second patient was 3.5 years old and had double-inlet left ventricle with pulmonary stenosis and little subvalvular obstruction. The pulmonary annulus was 13 mm. A 10 mm balloon (balloon/annulus ratio-0.77) was chosen, with the aim of partially opening the stenotic pulmonary valve orifice and yet not to flood the lungs. The systemic oxygen saturation increased from 68% to 78% immediately after dilatation, although the pulmonary arterial pressure and transvalvular gradient remained unchanged. However, the oxygen saturation returned to predilatation levels within two days.[4] A modified Blalock-Taussig shunt was performed.

Aortic Stenosis

Ten patients (six boys and four girls) aged 3 months to 14 years with aortic stenosis were treated with balloon valvuloplasty (Table V). Five patients had valvular stenosis, 3 of which

were bicuspid. Three patients had discrete membranous subvalvular stenosis, and two patients had combined valvular and subvalvular obstructions. Other defects were present in three patients with aortic valve stenosis; two had a small ventricular septal defect, and one had previous operation for coarctation of the aorta and patent ductus arteriosus.

In patient 6 the gradient at rest was 20 mmHg but increased to 80 mmHg after isoprenaline infusion, and therefore balloon dilatation was conducted. In all cases retrograde left heart catheterization was performed via percutaneous puncture of the femoral artery. The left ventricle was entered with a pigtail catheter in the three cases with subvalvular stenosis, whereas for those patients with valvular stenosis a Gensini catheter together with a deflecting guidewire was utilized to traverse the aortic valve [7]. A single balloon was employed except in patient 3, in whom a trefoil balloon catheter was used. The balloon/aortic annulus ratio was limited to less than 1.1.

Mean gradient was reduced from 68 to 35 mmHg immediately after dilatation and was 36 mmHg at follow-up 3-25 (mean, 15) months later. Percentage decrease in gradient was 70% for isolated valvular stenosis but only 31% for those with subvalvular stenosis. In one patient (case 10) with combined stenosis, no gradient relief could be achieved. The residual gradient assessed by continuous wave Doppler at follow-up remained similar to that obtained by direct measurement immediately after dilatation. Aortic regurgitation was absent in all patients with valvular stenosis and was mild in three patients with subvalvular stenosis before dilatation. Aortic regurgitation developed in three patients with valvular stenosis after the procedure, being mild in two patients and moderate in the

[4]Editor's note: Use of balloons smaller than the valve annulus will only stretch and not tear valve raphae. Therefore, the O₂ saturation returned to normal. We (Rao and Brais, Am Heart J 115:1105-1110, 1988; Rao et al., Cathet Cardiovasc Diagn 25:16-24, 1992) advocate a balloon that is 1.2-1.4 times the size of the valve annulus. For further details, the reader is referred to Chapter 13 (this volume).

TABLE V. Balloon Dilatation for Aortic Stenosis

Patient No., sex, age	Stenosis	Balloon size (mm)	Balloon/ annulus ratio	Peak-to-peak gradient (mmHg)			Aortic regurgitation	
				Before	After	Follow-up[a]	Before	After
1. F/3 months	Valve	8	1.0	50	30	35	Nil	Nil
2. M/4 years	Bicuspid valve	15	1.0	50	6	10	Nil	Mild
3. M/5 years	Bicuspid valve	17[b]	1.1	100	40	35	Nil	Trace
4. M/4.8 years	Valve	15	1.1	60	20	20	Nil	Nil
5. F/4.5 years	Bicuspid valve	18	1.0	50	5	0	Nil	Moderate
6. M/9 years	Subvalvular membrane	17	1.1	70	34	30	Mild	Mild
7. M/4 years	Subvalvular membrane	13	1.1	90	40	60	Mild	Mild
8. F/14 years	Subvalvular membrane	13	1.0	20	20	20	Nil	Nil
9. F/14 years	Valve and subvalvular	15	1.1	90	55	45	Mild	Mild
10. F/13 years	Valve and subvalvular	15	1.0	100	100	100	Nil	Nil

[a]Doppler estimation.
[b]Trefoil balloon.

third. It remained the same in the three patients with subvalvular stenosis.

Mitral and Tricuspid Valve Stenosis

We have performed mitral valve dilatation in a 1.5-year-old boy with congenital mitral stenosis who had had congestive heart failure since age 9 months. Echocardiography showed thickened mitral leaflets with limited diastolic opening. The mitral annulus measured 15 mm, and the mitral valve area was estimated to be 0.9 cm² by Doppler half-time measurements. Right heart catheterization revealed systemic level pulmonary hypertension and raised pulmonary arterial wedge pressures. Retrograde left heart catheterization was normal, and left ventriculogram showed normal contractions and no mitral regurgitation. Left atrial catheterization was performed by transatrial septal puncture and, the mean left atrial pressure and transmitral gradient were 28 and 14 mmHg, respectively. The atrial septum was dilated with an 8 mm balloon, and then a 15 mm balloon was placed across the mitral valve and dilatation was achieved with obliteration of the "waist." The mean left atrial pressure

and transmitral gradient dropped to 14 and 4 mmHg, respectively, immediately after the procedure. Blood sampling in the right atrium showed no oxygen step-up, and a left atrial angiogram showed only a trace of left-to-right shunting. The pulmonary pressure fell to 15 mmHg below systemic pressure.

A repeat left ventriculogram showed mild mitral regurgitation. This was the youngest reported patient who underwent successful balloon valvuloplasty for congenital mitral stenosis. Despite a marked improvement in transvalvular gradient, the pulmonary artery pressure dropped only slightly. The patient has only been followed up for 4 months. Doppler assessment during the last visit showed a mean transmitral gradient of 9 mmHg and an estimated mitral valve area 1.5 cm². Although the long-term outcome awaits to be seen, the result demonstrated balloon dilatation for mitral stenosis is feasible even in the young child and permits omission or postponing mitral valve surgery to a later age.

Balloon dilatation for tricuspid stenosis was attempted in a 2-year-old girl with tricuspid stenosis complicating pulmonary atresia and intact ventricular septum. She had received closed pulmonary valvotomy and a modified Blalock-Taussig shunt on day 6 after birth followed by pericardial patch repair of the right ventricular outflow tract at 1.5 months of age. On follow-up she had persistent though mild cyanosis and hepatomegaly. Echocardiography showed a small tricuspid annulus (1.5 mm) and thickened tricuspid valve with restricted movements and a stretched foramen ovale. Although the small tricuspid annulus was considered the main reason for right ventricular inflow obstruction, an element of valve leaflet fusion appeared to be present and balloon dilatation was decided upon. At cardiac catheterization, the mean right atrial pressure was 16 mmHg and the right ventricular pressure was 40/12 mmHg. End-diastolic gradient across the tricuspid valve was 10 mmHg. Right ventriculogram demonstrated adequate right ventricular outlet dimensions and trace tricuspid regurgitation. Systemic oxygen saturation

was 90%. Dilatation of the tricuspid valve was done with an 18 mm balloon, but no definite waist was seen during balloon inflation. The right atrial and ventricular pressures and the systemic saturation remained unchanged after the procedure. The modified Blalock-Taussig shunt was occluded with a 3 mm coil embolus. Double balloons with combined diameters much greater than the tricuspid annulus were usually applied in successful dilatations for rheumatic tricuspid stenosis. In our experience the limiting tricuspid annulus rather than the size of the balloon was more likely the cause of failure to relieve the right ventricular inflow obstruction.

Coarctation of Aorta

Thirteen patients were treated with balloon angioplasty for coarctation of the aorta (Table VI). Nine were native coarctations, four of which were small infants presenting with heart failure; five were older asymptomatic children

TABLE VI. Balloon Dilatation for Coarctation of Aorta

Patient No., sex, age	Balloon size (mmHg)	Balloon coarctation ratio	Coarctation (mm) Before	Coarctation (mm) After	Gradient (mmHg) Before	Gradient (mmHg) After	Outcome
Native coarctation							
1. F/9 days	5	2.5	2	3.4	50	10	Aneurysm
2. M/33 days[a]	5	2.5	2	3.2	45	10	Restenosis, surgery at 3 months
3. M/37 days	4.2	2.3	1.8	3.0	55	5	Restenosis, repeat dilatation at 5 months
4. F/48 days[a]	5	2.8	1.8	3.7	45	5	Restenosis, surgery at 2 months
5. M/4.5 years	12	2.1	5.8	8.7	45	5	Aneurysm
6. F/11 years	12	2.1	5.6	10.2	40	0	Good
7. M/3 years	8	2.5	3.2	6.6	55	15	Good
8. M/12 years	18	2.3	8	12	40	0	Good
9. M/6 years	13	3.2	4.1	8.4	70	30	Good
Recoarctation							
10. M/7 months[a]	10	4	2.5	5.9	60	0	Good
11. M/7 years	10	1.8	5.5	7.7	40	10	Good
12. M/1 month	5	2.2	2.3	3.8	60	30	Good
13. M/2 months	6	3.2	1.9	3.5	40	20	Good

[a]Transvenous antegrade approach.

with incidental discovery of heart murmur and hypertension. Four patients were treated for recurrent coarctation after previous surgery by subclavian flap aortoplasty in three and end-to-end anastomosis in the other. Seven patients, including all five infants, had associated congenital heart lesions, patent ductus arteriosus in three, and ventricular septal defect in four. The transvenous antegrade approach [8] was possible in the three infants with ventricular septal defect, whereas retrograde catheterization via femoral artery puncture was used in the rest.

An aortogram was taken, and a balloon size not larger than the aortic arch above the coarctation segment was chosen. The mean balloon to coarctation ratio was 2.3 (range, 1.8–4.0). All experienced excellent gradient reduction, and the femoral arterial pulses that were absent or barely palpable initially became easily palpable immediately after dilatation. Repeat aortogram showed dramatic increase in width of the coarctation segment (mean, 75.2%; range, 40–106%). The good results, however, were not sustained in the young infants with native coarctation; three out of four developed severe restenosis clinically, which was confirmed by Doppler echocardiography within 3 months. Two of them underwent surgical correction, and a second dilatation was performed in the third, 4 months after the first procedure, with good results that have persisted up to 12 months of follow-up. The fourth infant with native coarctation did not develop restenosis, but at restudy 6 months later both showed presence of aneurysm formation at the site of the previous coarctation. Aneurysm occurred in one other older child after dilatation of native coarctation. On the other hand, the patients treated for recoarctation of aorta have good long-term results. The duration of follow-up has been 4–30 (mean, 14) months. We have failed to cross the coarctation antegradely in one other neonate with transposition of the great arteries and ventricular septal defect, and balloon angioplasty was abandoned.

Our experience with balloon angioplasty for coarctation of the aorta was similar to that in other reports in that failure rate and incidence of aneurysm formation were high with native coarctations.[5] We currently perform angioplasty for postoperative recoarctations and in older patients with native coarctation while surgery is the treatment of choice for the neonate or young infant.

Pulmonary Artery Stenosis

We have performed dilatation of stenotic pulmonary arteries in only two patients. Both had previous surgical correction for tetralogy of Fallot. The first patient was a 16-year-old girl with narrowing of the main pulmonary artery at the distal end of the pericardial patch repair of the right ventricular outflow tract. The obstruction was presumably due to inadequate extension of the repair to an originally hypoplastic main pulmonary artery. A single 19 mm balloon was used to dilate an 8 mm main pulmonary artery, which increased to 10.5 mm afterwards. Right ventricular systolic pressure dropped from 100 to 60 mmHg, and the systolic gradient dropped from 75 to 40 mmHg; the systemic blood pressure was unchanged. At restudy 9 months later, despite the fact that the width of the pulmonary artery remained enlarged, the right ventricular pressure and gradient across the narrow segment returned to preangioplasty values. No second attempt was tried, and the patient is awaiting surgery.

The second patient was a 15-year-old boy with discrete stenosis at the origin of the left pulmonary artery unnoticed during surgery. The stenotic site and the more distal artery measured 5 and 10 mm, respectively. Although at catheterization the gradient across the obstruction was only 15 mmHg, we decided to dilate it in view of the angiographic appearance of significant narrowing and also

---

[5]Editor's note: See Chapter 10 (this volume) for further discussion on these issues.

the reduction in perfusion to the left lung. A 13 mm balloon was used, which on repeated inflation still showed persistent presence of a waist. There was little change in the pressure gradient across the obstruction, but angiography showed an increase in width of the stenotic area from 5 to 7.5 mm. No further dilatation was attempted.

Our limited experience with angioplasty of pulmonary artery hypoplasia or branch stenosis appear unrewarding and might be the result of our rather small balloon to lesion diameter ratios (2.4 and 2.6). Balloons that are three to four (up to eight) times the size of the stenotic lesions had been used by those who reported greater successes.

Coil Embolization

Coil embolization to occlude polytetrafluoroethylene (PTFE) tubes used in modified Blalock-Taussig shunts was employed in three patients with tetralogy of Fallot and in one patient with pulmonary atresia and intact ventricular septum in whom the shunt was not divided during corrective surgery. The Gianturco occluding spring emboli (Cook Inc.) were used, and we chose a coil diameter one size bigger than the lumen of the shunt. Special coil positioning guidewires were used to position the coil in the shunt and to prevent the embolus from coiling up too early when being pushed out of the end of the catheter. Angiogram on the aortic side was performed before and after the procedure to verify shunt patency. Complete occlusion was achieved in two patients using two coils each, and a small residual shunt persisted in one patient despite the use of three coils. In one patient an 8 mm diameter coil was used on a 5 mm shunt, and the device failed to coil up inside the shunt and when released was dislodged and migrated to the right pulmonary artery. It was recovered at thoracotomy, and the shunt was divided at the same time. Our experience supports the effectiveness of coil embolization to occlude modified Blalock-Taussig shunts. Oversized coils, however, should not be used. Although small

coils are also at risk of being dislodged due to proximal vessel dilatation, PTFE tubes probably are less likely to develop this complication.

COMPLICATIONS

Complications have been few in our series, and there was no death related to the interventional procedures. Failure to negotiate the obstructive lesion was encountered in four patients with pulmonary stenosis and in one patient with coarctation (5/89 cases, 5.6%). Major complications during valvuloplasty or embolization procedures included precipitation of hypercyanotic spell (one case), breakage of guidewire (one), and dislodgement of coil embolus (one) requiring urgent surgical treatment.

Transient bradycardia, premature contractions, and hypotension during balloon inflation were commonplace in valve dilatations. These returned to normal rapidly upon deflation of the balloon without specific treatment. Persistent arrhythmias were found in three patients after pulmonary valvuloplasty. A 4-year-old girl developed complete heart block during balloon inflation that became permanent; the conduction abnormality was presumably due to the relatively long balloon that was used (4 cm; balloon/annulus ratio = 1.11). Two patients developed complete right bundle branch block; one lasted 4 months and the other persisted. Temporary loss of the femoral artery pulse after retrograde catheterization for aortic stenosis and coarctation of the aorta was evident immediately after the procedure in all 20 patients in whom the artery was punctured. Seventeen were given heparin infusion, and six required streptokinase thrombolysis. Permanent arterial occlusion with impalpable distal pulses and cold extremity was seen in one patient. The incidence of femoral vein occlusion was less clear. Of the 20 cases who were restudied after balloon pulmonary valvuloplasty, two (10%) were found to have blocked femoral veins.

SUMMARY AND CONCLUSIONS

Interventional catheterizations were performed in 101 patients. Apart from four coil embolizations of modified Blalock-Taussig shunts, all were done for dilatation of stenotic valves or great vessels. The procedure was abandoned in five cases due to inability to cross the obstructive site. The overall success rate in relieving the stenosis in 96 patients was 84.3%.

Although the scope of our work was limited, our experience corroborates that of others regarding the potential efficacy of transcatheter therapy for an increasing number of congenital or acquired cardiac anomalies. This is particularly true for pulmonary valve stenosis, and currently balloon valvuloplasty is our treatment of choice for this condition. Suboptimal results were obtained for other lesions, such as aortic stenosis and coarctation of the aorta. The double-umbrella occluding device for closure of the patent ductus arteriosus is just becoming available in Hong Kong, and it has not yet been used. The role of transcatheter treatment to replace surgery in these lesions remains to be established. Our policy on its indication is empirical and would likely change with accumulation of more experience in relation to outcome and complications.

REFERENCES

1. Radtke W, Keane JF, Fellows KE, Lang P, Lock JE (1986): Percutaneous balloon valvotomy of congenital pulmonary stenosis using oversized balloons. J Am Coll Cardiol 8:909-915.
2. Rao PS (1989): Balloon pulmonary valvuloplasty: A review. Clin Cardiol 12:55-74.
3. Sullivan ID, Robinson PJ, Macartney FJ, Taylor JFN, Rigby PG, Bull C, Deanfield JE (1985): Percutaneous balloon valvuloplasty for pulmonary valve stenosis in infants and children. Br Heart J 54:435-441.
4. Stanger P, Cassidy SC, Girod DA, Kan JS, Lababidi Z, Shapiro SR (1990): Balloon pulmonary valvuloplasty: Results of the valvuloplasty and angioplasty of congenital anomalies registry. Am J Cardiol 65:775-783.
5. Attia I, Weinhaus L, Walls JT, Lababidi Z (1987): Rupture of tricuspid valve papillary muscle during balloon pulmonary valvuloplasty. Am Heart J 114:1233-1234.
6. Lo RNS, Lau KC, Leung MP (1988): Complete heart block after balloon dilatation for congenital pulmonary stenosis. Br Heart J 59:384-386.
7. Lau KC, Leung MP, Lo RNS (1986): Retrograde transfemoral catheterisation of the left ventricle in children with aortic stenosis. Pediatr Cardiol 7:79-82.
8. Lo RNS, Leung MP, Lau KC (1989): Transvenous antegrade balloon angioplasty for recoarctation of the aorta in an infant. Am Heart J 117:1157-1159.

22d

Balloon Valvuloplasty/Angioplasty: The Indian Experience

Savitri Shrivastava, M.D., D.M., **and Vishva Dev**, M.D., D.M.

Department of Cardiology, Cardio-Thoracic Centre, All India
Institute of Medical Sciences, New Delhi 110 029, India

INTRODUCTION

Use of interventional catheterization with balloon dilatation catheters began in India in 1985. Since then it has been increasingly used, and presently at least six medical centers are actively involved in these procedures. We routinely perform balloon valvuloplasty in pulmonary, aortic, mitral, and tricuspid valvar stenosis and balloon angioplasty in coarctation of aorta and aortitis at our institution.

VALVAR PULMONIC STENOSIS

In the past 5 years we have attempted 96 valvuloplasty procedures in 93 patients with valvar pulmonic stenosis (PS). Three patients had redilatation. The pulmonary valve could not be crossed in two sick patients with critical PS with congestive failure and tricuspid regurgitation. Five patients were excluded from the study because they were found to have additional lesions requiring surgery: atrial septal defect in one, tight fibrous infundibular PS in three, and atrial septal defect with infundibular PS in one. Data from the remaining 89 procedures in 86 patients form the basis of this section. These patients included 58 males and 28 females aged 10 months to 53 years. Sixtynine of these were below 20 years of age, and 17 were above 20 years. Sixty percent of the patients were symptomatic; seven had right to left shunt at the atrial level with cyanosis and

three had gross right ventricular failure, tricuspid regurgitation, and congestive heart failure.

All of the patients were subjected to detailed two-dimensional and Doppler echocardiographic studies to measure pulmonary valve annulus, to study pulmonary valve morphology, to evaluate the infundibular area for any fixed obstruction, to exclude ventricular septal defect or any other associated cardiac anomalies, and to assess right ventricular function. The patients were then subjected to cardiac catheterization and balloon valvuloplasty as described in a previous publication [1]. At cardiac catheterization suprasystemic right ventricular peak systolic pressures were found in 50 patients and systemic or subsystemic in 39. The sizes of the pulmonary valve annulus ranged from 9.9 to 24 mm, and the effective sizes of the balloons used ranged from 12 to 34 mm. The balloon annulus ratio was 1.20 ± 0.19 (range, 0.68-1.9). Eighty one procedures were performed with a single balloon and eight with two balloons.

Immediate Results

Immediately after valvuloplasty the peak systolic gradient (PSG) fell from 115 ± 49 to 56 ± 45 mmHg; right ventricular systolic pressures (RVSP) fell from 137 ± 48 to 76 ± 43 mmHg; and the RVSP to aortic systolic pressure ratio (RVSP/ASP ratio) decreased from 110% ± 44% to 65% ± 39%.

The PSG fell below 50 mmHg in 53 pa-

Transcatheter Therapy in Pediatric Cardiology, pages 445–456
© 1993 Wiley-Liss, Inc.

tients. Twenty six patients had partial relief
(more than 50% decrease in gradient but a
residual gradient above 50 mmHg), and in 10
patients the PSG and RVSP had no change
immediately after valvuloplasty. The cardiac
output remained unchanged.

Follow-Up

The patients have been followed up for
periods varying from 2 months to 4 years
(mean follow-up, 19 months) On follow-up all
symptomatic patients became asymptomatic.
Congestive heart failure disappeared in all
three affected patients. Cyanosis disappeared
in six of the seven affected patients. A grade 2
to 3/6 pulmonary regurgitatioin (PR) murmur
was heard in 54% of patients. There were no
differences in the valvuloplasty results in patients with PR compared with those without.
The PR also did not seem to cause any significant adverse hemodynamic effects and did not
increase on follow-up.

During follow-up hemodynamic data on cardiac catheterization or on Doppler study (PSG)
were available for 59 patients at 3-6 months
and in 39 patients at 1-4 years. PSG in 39
patients at 1-4 years follow-up showed some
striking characteristics (Fig. 1). In this group
of patients there was a large decrease in gradient immediately after valvuloplasty (from 98 ±
42 mmHg to 47 ± 40 mmHg; $P < 0.001$). At
3-6 months there was a further decrease in
gradient to 35 ± 34 mmHg ($P < 0.02$), but
there was no further decrease at 1-4 years
follow-up (PSG, 32 ± 36 mmHg; P-NS). This
strongly suggests that 1) there is a gradual
reduction in infundibular obstruction over
time as hypertrophy and hypercontractility regress (this has been suggested by other workers
as well[1]) and 2) this regression in right ventricular outflow obstruction occurs over the initial
3-6 months. We did not observe any restenosis.

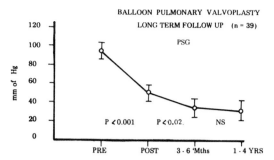

Fig. 1. Long-term follow-up after balloon pulmonary
valvuloplasty. There is a significant decrease in peak
systolic gradient (PSG) immediately after valvuloplasty.
A further decrease at 3-6 months was noted, but there
was no change in PSG thereafter.

There are two subgroups of patients who
require special mention. The first are those
with critical PS, gross congestive heart failure,
marked cardiomegaly, and tricuspid regurgitation. These are very high-risk candidates for
surgery, and their natural course is dismal.
There were three such cases in our study. All
three patients had a dramatic reduction in their
gradients and striking improvement in their
clinical conditions. Cardiomegaly regressed
over 3-6 months.

The other group of patients are those who
had no or an insignificant decreas in gradient
immediately after valvuloplasty despite adequate balloon size, satisfactory procedure, and
absence of any fixed subvalvular obstruction.
We had 36 such cases in our study. In most
of these the valvular gradient fell significantly,
but the infundibular gradient increased/ap-
peared possibly because of infundibular
spasm caused by the trauma of the large
balloon size. Of these 22 have been followed
up for 3 months to 4 years, and 12 of these
cases had a marked decrease and 5 had a
partial decrease in the gradients over the next
3-6 months, possibly due to regression of
infundibular obstruction. Five patients

[1]Editor's note: See Fontes VF et al. (1988): Am J Cardiol
62:977-979; and Thapar MK, Rao PS (1988); Am Heart J
118:99-103, for further details on regression of infundibular
hypertrophy following balloon pulmonary valvuloplasty.

showed no change over time. This regression occurred even without the use of β-blockers or verapamil. Whether giving these agents will alter the course of this regression can be answered only after a controlled trial, which we have recently begun. We did not observe any further reduction in gradients after 6 months.

Predictors of Response

Anatomy of the right ventricular outflow tract (RVOT) and pulmonary valve. Two-dimensional echocardiography clearly delineates the anatomy of the RVOT and the pulmonary valve. Dysplastic and thick pulmonary valves with no mobility of the cusps give poor results after valvuloplasty. All our patients had mildly thickened, clearly doming mobile pulmonary valve cusps. A narrow RVOT that does not dilate during diastole and produces a clear high velocity signal of obstruction below the pulmonary valve indicates organic infundibular PS, which rarely yields to valvuloplasty. A narrow annulus sometimes is the dominant site of obstruction and a cause of inadequate response to balloon valvuloplasty. Infundibular hypertrophy is common in valvar PS. In this situation the infundibular area dilates during diastole but may produce small dynamic late systolic gradient (a sickle-shaped Doppler velocity signal).

Balloon/annulus ratio. The optimal size of the balloon for pulmonary valvuloplasty is not clear, although it appears that it should be larger than the annulus of the pulmonary valve (PV). We measure PV annulus by echocardiography (except when echogenicity is poor). In a comparative study of 48 patients, we have found these measurements to have an excellent correlation with those obtained from angiogra-phy (r = 0.92) [2]. In our study the balloon/annulus ratio (BAR) ranged from 0.86 to 1.9. The BAR in 85% of the patients ranged from 1.0 to 1.5. The results of pulmonary valvuloplasty analyzed in relation to the BAR showed that there was no difference in the rate of immediate success in four subgroups (BAR <1.0, 1.0–1.25, >1.25–1.50, and >1.50). However, on follow-up more patients with BAR 1.25–1.50 had decreased gradients so that the total success rate at 3–6 months was significantly higher in this subgroup (BAR <1.0, 80%; 1–1.25, 84%; >1.25–1.50, 96%; >1.5, 83%). This may be explained by the occurrence of initial infundibular spasm by the larger sized balloons in this group, which regresses later. We conclude that a BAR of 1.25–1.50 may give the best results.[2] Larger-sized balloons will obviously also be required if the smaller balloon produces inadequate relief.

Preprocedure RVSP. In our experience, patients with suprasystemic RVSP behave differently from those with subsystemic RVSP. In the first group a higher proportion of patients have an inadequate initial decrease in gradient that regresses over 3–6 months. In the second group the gradient does not significantly change on follow-up. This may be related to a more severely hypertrophied infundibular area that is more prone to injury and spasm. All over success rate seems to be similar. Obviously patients with supra-systemic RVSP are much sicker, and the three deaths in our series were all in this subgroup.

Age. Analysis of our data shows that patients below 20 years of age tend to have marginally better response to valvuloplasty than do older patients. The reductions in their

---

[2]Editor's note: The recommendation for use of a balloon/annulus ration of 1.2–1.4 were initially made by Radtke et al. (J Am Coll Cardiol 8:909–915, 1986) and Rao (Texas Heart Inst J 14:57–61, 1987; Am Heart J 110:577–580, 1989; and Bri Heart J 60:507–511, 1988). The Radtke et al. recommen-dations are based on immediate results while those of Rao are based on immediate and follow-up results. For further discussion of these issues, the reader is referred to Chapter 6 (this volume).

RVSP, PSG, and RVSP/ASP ratio appear to be more than those in patients over 20 years of age. This is true for both immediate and follow-up (3–6 month) results.

Complications

We had three procedure-related deaths; all three had suprasystemic RVSP. Two of these patients had critical PS, gross tricuspid regurgitation, and congestive heart failure. The valve could not be crossed in either of them, and the procedure was abandoned. One of them developed hyperpyrexia and died, and the other died awaiting surgery. The third patient during redilatation with an oversized balloon (BAR > 1.4) developed infundibular spasm that was managed, but he also developed hyperpyrexia 12 hours after the procedure and died. There were no vascular problems or pulmonary embolization.

Other Studies

Arora et al. [3] reported their data from 66 patients (aged 2.5–33 years) with moderate to severe PS subjected to balloon valvuloplasty. The PSG fell from 102 ± 40 to 35 ± 27 mmHg immediately after the procedure. Follow-up at 3–40 months in 60 patients by Doppler echocardiography or cardiac catheterization revealed a further reduction in the PSG from 37 to 33 mmHg. On follow-up, PSG had decreased in 43%, remained the same in 50%, and increased in 7%. Pulmonary regurgitation was observed in 80% of patients. All of the patients were asymptomatic at follow-up. Shah et al. [4] reported 17 cases of valvuloplasty in pulmonic stenosis. The RVSP and PSG decreased from 132 ± 43 and 110 ± 47 mmHg to 50 ± 23 and 31 ± 20 mmHg, respectively. They did not observe PR in any of their patients after valvuloplasty.

Sharma et al. (personal communication) attempted balloon pulmonary valvuloplasty in 38 patients with success in 33 (aged 11 months to 12 years). The balloon size used was 120%–140% of the pulmonary annulus.

The PSG fell from 100 ± 40 to 30 ± 9 mmHg. Follow-ups after 6–30 months in 23 patients showed persistent benefit in all. Pulmonary regurgitation was detected in 55% of cases after valvuloplasty. None of these investigators have reported any fatal complications.

In summary, balloon pulmonary valvuloplasty is a safe and effective procedure and has emerged as the therapy of choice for valvular PS. Echocardiography helps in selecting appropriate patients and balloon sizes and in the follow-up of these patients.

JUVENILE RHEUMATIC MITRAL STENOSIS

In the past 5 years we have attempted balloon mitral valvuloplasty (BMV) in 40 patients with juvenile mitral stenosis (aged <20 years; range, 11–20 years; 17 males, 23 females.) Of these patients 31 had successful BMV [5]. The failures were related to failed atrial septal puncture in seven cases (inability to puncture in two, persistent hypotension without hemopericardium in two, and inability to dilate the atrial septum by the balloon in three) and inability to cross the mitral valve with a balloon dilatation catheter in two cases. We used the transseptal antegrade approach described by Lock et al. [6], except that we kept the guidewire in the left ventricular apex [7]. Pediatric transseptal needle was used for patients with body surface areas (BSA) less than 1 m². Our patients have small BSA (range, 0.9–1.65 M². The septal dilatation was performed using 8 mm balloons in 25 patients and 10 mm balloons in six. We choose the size of the balloon used for mitral valve dilatation on the basis of BSA; BSA 1.0 M² or less, 20 mm; >1.0–1.25 M², 23/25 mm; >1.25–1.50 M², double balloon 15 and 15 mm; >1.50–1.7 M², double balloon 15 and 18 mm. We used single-balloon technique in 21 patients (balloon size 20 mm in 6, 23 mm in 5, and 25 mm in 10) and double-balloon technique in 10 (two balloons of 15 and 15 mm in 5 and 15 and 18 mm in 5). If the results in any case was unsatisfactory the next larger sized balloon was used. The patients were followed up by clinical evaluation, two-dimensional and Doppler echocardiography, and hemodynamic evaluation.

Clinical Behavior

Of the 31 patients, 7 were in NYHA functional class II, 19 in class III, and 5 in class IV. Associated aortic regurgitation was present in 9 cases and tricuspid regurgitation in 11 cases. Moderate to severe pulmonary venous and arterial hypertension was present in all cases. After BMV all patient showed symptomatic improvement (to NYHA class I or II). The diastolic murmur became very short or disappeared, the opening snap moved away from the second sound, and tricuspid regurgitation and congestive failure improved. Five patients showed symptomatic worsening on follow-up

and were found to have restenosis on hemodynamic evaluation.

Hemodynamic Data

Hemodynamic data (Fig. 2) were obtained from all patients before and after BMV. The first 16 patients were catheterized at 1–2 weeks after BMV. This study was stopped after analysis showed no significant change over 1 week. Twelve patients were catheterized at 3–6 months, and 11 were studied 6 months to 4 years after the procedure. Immediately after BMV the pulmonary artery (PA) and pulmonary artery wedge (PAW) pressures fell from 46.2 ± 15.3 and 28.8 ± 5.6 mmHg to 33.7 ± 17.2 and 13.4 ± 4.4 mmHg, respectively. The end diastolic (EDG) and mean diastolic (MDG) gradients fell from 23.6 ± 6.1 and 21.6 ± 5.6 mmHg to 7.9 ± 5.3 and 7.6 ± 4.2 mmHg, respectively. The mitral valve area increased from 0.67 ± 0.23 to 1.77 ± 0.82 cm^2/M^2. The cardiac index increased. The pul-

BALLOON MITRAL VALVOPLASTY

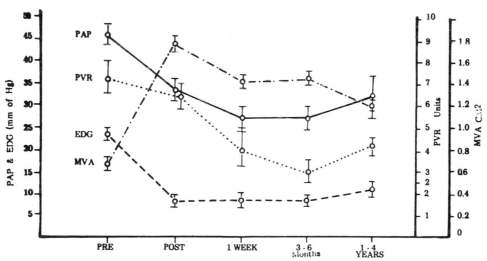

Fig. 2. Time courses of pulmonary artery pressure (PAP), pulmonary vascular resistance (PVR), end diastolic gradient (EDG) across the mitral valve, and mitral valve area (MVA) after balloon mitral valvuloplasty are shown. Note the improvement in all parameters listed.

monary vascular resistance fell from 7.2 ± 8.2 to 6.2 ± 5.2 units. At 1 week the PA and PAW pressures were 27.2. ± 10.3 and 14.1 ± 4.4 mmHg, respectively; the EDG and MDG were 8.3 ± 3.8 and 9.6 ± 3.8 mmHg, respectively; and the cardiac index and MVA were 3.2 ± 0.6 liters/min/M^2 and 1.4 ± 0.3 cm^2/M^2, respectively.

All of these findings were not significantly different from the respective observations in the same patient immediately after the procedure. The pulmonary vascular resistance 1 week after the procedure (4 ± 2.9 units) was significantly lower ($P < 0.01$) than that immediately after the procedure (6.3 ± 5.2 units). At 3–6 months follow-up there was a slight rise in the PA pressure (27.3 ± 8.0 mmHg) and PAW pressure (16.8 ± 4.7 mmHg). The EDG (8.1 ± 3.3 mmHg) and MDG (8.9 ± 4.1 mmHg) were not significantly different from the values immediately after the procedure. Similarly, the cardiac index (3.6 ± 0.9 liters/min/M^2) and MVA (1.45 ± 0.55 cm^2/M^2) remained unchanged. The pulmonary vascular resistance, however, showed a further decrease to 3 ± 1.6 units ($P < 0.05$). At long-term follow-up PAW (19.8 ± 7.0 mmHg) had increased and MVA (1.2 ± 0.5 cm^2/M^2) had decreased in the overall group. The other parameters showed no difference. Evidence of restenosis (MVA < 1.0 cm^2/M^2) was found in 2 of the 11 patients at 3–6 months and in 3 of 11 patients at 6 months to 4 years.

Mitral Regurgitation

Left ventricular angiography performed after BMV showed evidence of mitral regurgitation in 24 cases (trivial in 21, mild in 2, and severe in 1). Trivial and mild mitral regurgitation were associated with good relief of obstruction. The severe mitral regurgitation that developed in one case after BMV was caused by chordal rupture and was hemodynamically well tolerated.

Atrial Shunt

Pulmonary artery angiograms in hepatoclavicular view and oximetry were performed in all patients to detect the presence of an atrial shunt after the BMV. These were repeated on follow-up in all patients exhibiting the shunt initially. Angiographic atrial shunt was detected in 11 cases. Seven of these also had step-up in oximetry run. On follow-up after 6–18 months, three cases showed persistence of shunt (QP/QS ratios of 2:1, 2.4:1, and 2.2:1), respectively. Shunt disappeared in the others.

Valve Morphology and Response to Balloon Mitral Valvuloplasty

We have prospectively studied echocardiographic indices of the morphology of the mitral valve and subvalvular apparatus and correlated them with the results of BMV in 41 consecutive cases (both adults and children). The parameters analyzed include mitral valve annulus size; distances from the annulus to the tip of the domed mitral valve, to the tip of the papillary muscle, to the base of the papillary muscle, and to the apex of the left ventricle; chordal length; subvalvular ratio; and lengths and thicknesses of the anterior and posterior mitral leaflets (AML and PML). The patients were divided into "good responders" (group I, MVA after BMV > 2.0 cm^2) or "poor responders" (group II, MVA after BMV >2.0 cm^2). Multivariate discriminant analysis showed that the three parameters that best discriminated between the two groups are subvalvular ratio, distance between mitral valve annulus to the tip of the domed mitral valve, and PML mobility (over all discriminant value equal to 82.5%). Other parameters showed statistically insignificant independent discriminant power. There was no difference between adult or juvenile mitral stenosis in this analysis.

Complications

We encountered the following complications:

1. Cerebral embolism occurred in one patient, resulting in aphasia that receded over 3 months.

2. Pulmonary embolism occurred in two patients (symptomatic in one), confirmed by lung perfusion scan and successfully treated with intravenous heparin.

3. Pericardial effusion due to atrial injury occurred in two patients. One of them developed pericardial tamponade that required surgical drainage. There was no death in our series.

Overall, our experience shows a significant incidence of problems associated with BMV in juvenile mitral stenosis: failure to complete the procedure (9/40), severe mitral regurgitation (1/31), persistent atrial shunt (3/31), pericardial tamponade (1/31), pulmonary embolism (2/31), inadequate relief of mitral stenosis (2/31), and restenosis at 3-6 months (2/11) and at 6 months to 4 years (3/11). Some of these problems, especially failure to complete the procedure, were encountered in the initial period and reflect a learning curve of our experience and have significantly diminished by now. The higher incidence of atrial shunt detection in our series may be because 1) we do both angiography and oximetry for atrial septal defect detection and 2) we reuse balloon catheters whose deflated profiles are larger than the profiles of deflated new balloons.

The PVR followed a very interesting course. It steadily fell from immediately after the procedure to about 3-6 months. After this there was no further change.

BMV in juvenile mitral stenosis poses significant problems, but the procedure is feasible and effective. Its exact value vis à vis closed mitral valvotomy needs to be established. Also noteworthy is the fact that even single balloons give good results in juvenile mitral stenosis.

VALVAR AORTIC STENOSIS

Between September 1986 and December 1989, 37 patients with noncalcific valvar aortic stenosis were subjected to balloon valvuloplasty according a procedure described earlier [8]. The study included 27 males and 10 females be-tween 1 and 26 years of age (20 in the 1-10 year age group, 11 in the 11-20 year age group, and 6 above 20 years of age). All had isolated valvular aortic stenosis with gradients of more than 50 mmHg and a bicuspid pliable aortic valve. Single-balloon technique was used, the balloon diameter ranging from 71% to 100% of the size of the annulus measured at echocardiography/aortography. We have never used an effective balloon size larger than the size of the aortic annulus. In two patients the aortic valve could not be crossed. One of them developed hypotension. The procedure was successful in the other 35 cases. In these 35 patients the peak systolic gradient decreased from 107 ± 34 mmHg to 45 ± 32 mmHg. The aortic valve area increased from 0.34 ± 0.08 cm² to 0.69 ± 0.2 cm². The cardiac index did not change significantly (3.5 ± 0.9 liters/min² before the procedure and 3.6 ± 1.05 liters/min² after the procedure).

Aortic root angiography was performed in all patients before and after balloon dilatation. Before balloon aortic valvuloplasty 14 patients had trivial aortic regurgitation (1 +/4) and others had no aortic regurgitation. After valvuloplasty 17 had trivial aortic regurgitation, 8 had mild aortic regurgitation, 2 had moderate aortic regurgitation, and 8 had none. The aortic regurgitation was well tolerated in all cases. In one patient, aortic regurgitation increased from 1+ to 3+, and the gradient decreased from 50 to 25 mmHg. This possibly was related to progressive tear of the valve cusp with resultant increase in orifice and also regurgitation.

Complications

Transient weak femoral pulses occurred in five cases. Moderate aortic regurgitation occurred in two cases. There was one death during an attempt to cross the valve.

Follow-Up

The patients were followed up for a period of 1-42 months (mean, 18 ± 3.2 months). Follow-up evaluation included clinical assessment, echocardiography and Doppler studies, and cardiac catheterization (N = 15). Before balloon aortic valvuloplasty 3 patients were in NYHA class IV, 5 in class III, 13 in class II, and 13 in class I. On follow-up after valvuloplasty, 1 patient was in class IV, 2 in class II (both had moderate aortic regurgitation), and 30 in class I. Congestive heart failure was present in three cases before valvuloplasty and disappeared in two of them following valvuloplasty.

Doppler Echocardiography

In our experience comparative evaluation of gradients obtained at Doppler and at cardiac catheterization shows an excellent correlation between the two techniques. Doppler echocardiography was hence used for follow-up of these patients. Doppler studies were performed before valvuloplasty (N = 33), immediately after (N = 33); 3-12 months after (N = 25); and then 1-4 years after the procedure (N = 17). Immediately after the proce-

dure the peak instantaneous aortic valvar gradients decreased from 112 ± 18 to 48 ± 14 mmHg. At 3-12 months the gradients were 45 ± 13 mmHg, and in the 1-4 year follow-up group the gradient was 45 ± 15 mmHg (Fig. 3) Overall the group did not show a tendency for restenosis of the aortic valve. Analysis of the individual cases, however, showed evidence of restenosis in one patient at 3-12 months and in one patient at 1-4 years.

Doppler echocardiography was extremely useful in the detection and assessment of aortic regurgitation. Patients showed no change in the grade of aortic regurgitation on follow-up, except one patient in whom the regurgitation increased from 1+ to 3+. We had three patients with critical aortic stenosis and gross congestive heart failure with marked cardiomegaly. Two of these patients (aged 5 and 9 years) had a decreased gradient from 150 and 50 to 25 and 10 mmHg, respectively, immediately after the procedure. They showed progressive improvement

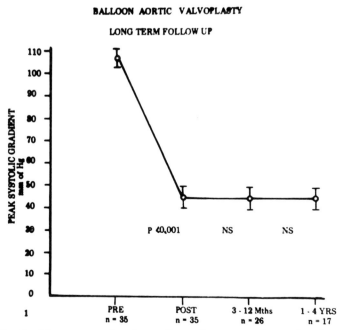

Fig. 3. Time course of peak systolic gradient across the aortic valve after balloon aortic valvuloplasty. There is a significant decrease in gradient after valvuloplasty, which remains unchanged on follow-up.

at 6 and 3 months follow-up, respectively, to normal sized heart and class I symptomatic status. In the third patient the gradient remained unchanged (108-100 mmHg) and was referred for surgery. His gradient after surgical valvotomy was still 70 mmHg. Balloon aortic valvuloplasty appears to be a very useful technique in this setting, because the risk of surgical valvotomy is high.

Predictors of Response in Balloon Aortic Valvuloplasty

Unicuspid valves respond poorly to balloon aortic valvuloplasty and may result in aortic regurgitation. All of our patients had bicuspid aortic valve on cross-sectional echocardiography. Valve thickness, valve mobility, and doming of the valve were assessed in all patients during echocardiography. All except five had mildly thickened valves, with good mobility and clear doming. Another five patients had thick valves with restricted mobility. Analysis of their hemodynamic responses did not suggest any difference either in the magnitude of the relief in obstruction with valvuloplasty or in the incidence of aortic regurgitation after valvuloplasty. Similarly, we analyzed various angiographic indices of valve morphology, but the results showed that angiographic indices had no predictive value for response to BAV.[3]

It appears that, in noncalcific aortic stenosis in the young, balloon aortic valvuloplasty is a safe and effective procedure that produces significant relief of obstruction and that there are no specific predictive factors to help select the suitable patients.[4]

DISCRETE SUBAORTIC STENOSIS

In the past 3 years 11 patients (seven females and four males, aged 4-24 years) were diagnosed to have discrete subaortic stenosis on clinical and echocardiographic evaluation. Symptomatically two patients were in NYHA class IV, four in class III, three in class II, and two in class I. Aortic regurgitation occurred in 10. It was trivial in seven and mild in three. One patient had severe pulmonary arterial hypertension and right to left shunt across a large ductus with congestive heart failure. They were subjected to cardiac catheterization and percutaneous transluminal balloon dilatation. The aortic annulus in these patients ranged from 15.2 to 20.2 mm.

Single balloons were used in nine cases; their sizes varied from 15 to 20 mm. In two patients a double-balloon technique was used (balloon sizes 10 and 10 mm and 10 and 12 mm; annulus sizes 15 and 16.8 mm). The effective BAR varied from 90% to 105%. A detailed echocardiographic evaluation was performed one day before the procedure, and the following data were especially looked for and recorded: 1) morphology of the obstructing segment—thickness and shape of the membrane, distance of its point of attachment from the aortic valve; 2) morphology of the aortic valve—number and thicknesses of cusps and fusion of commissures; 3) presence and grade of aortic regurgitation; 4) peak velocity of the jet across the obstruction to predict the gradient using a modified Bernoulli equation; 5) left ventricular function; and 6) other associated anomalies. Follow-up two-dimensional and Doppler echocardiographic studies were performed at 24 hours, 3 months, 6-12 months, and 18-24 months after the procedure. The outcome of the balloon dilatation immediately after the procedure and on follow-up was evaluated in relation to the morphologic features of the discrete subaortic stenosis observed at echocardiography.

---

[3]Editor's note: Rao et al. (Am J Cardiol 64:1356-11360, 1989) have found that an age less than 3 years and an immediate postvalvuloplasty residual gradient greater than 30 mmHg are predictors of poor result at follow-up. Valve morphology may also influence the results (Sholler et al.: Circulation 78:351-1360, 1988).

[4]See footnote 3.

Results

Echocardiographic data. On the basis of two-dimensional echocardiographic morphologic data of the membrane, the patients were divided into three groups (Fig. 4). Group I (seven patients) had uniform thin membrane (1-3 mm) obstructing the left ventricular outflow. One patient had slight nodular thickening (4 mm) at the tip, but the rest of the membrane was thin. Group II (two patients) had a thin membrane attached to a thick pyramidal ridge attached to the interventricular septum and projecting into the left ventricular outflow tract (intermediate type). Group III (two patients) had a thick ridge of tissue (6-8 mm) in the left ventricular outflow. The base of the obstructing segment was wider than the tip. The distance of the obstructing segment from the aortic root varied from 1 to 8 mm and was not different in the three groups. The aortic valve was thickened in two patients (one in group II and one in group III). In all patients the obstructing tissue was attached to the interventricular septum. The attachment to the anterior mitral leaflet was echocardiographically demonstrable in six patients. The other five (two in group III and three in group I) had noncircumferential attachment of the membrane. Four patients had hypokinesia of the left ventricle. All patients had aortic regurgitation before balloon dilatation (trivial in six, mild in four, and moderate in one). After balloon dilatation the membrane became frail in all of the patients in group I. The tip of the membrane became slightly frail in group II patients. Membrane morphology in group III patients remained unchanged. Aortic regurgitation increased from trivial to mild in two patients and remained unchanged in the rest. Left ventricular function improved in all four patients with poor function before the procedure.

Hemodynamic data. Hemodynamic response in the patients after balloon dilatation

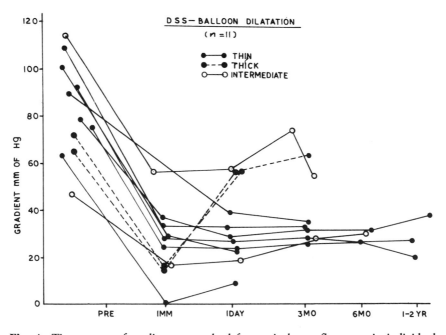

Fig. 4. Time course of gradient across the left ventricular outflow tract in individual patients after balloon dilatation of discrete subaortic stenosis (DSS) (see text for details).

varied between the three echocardiographic groups. In group I with thin membranes peak systolic gradient (PSG) decreased from 86 ± 17 to 24 ± 13 mmHg immediately after the procedure. On follow-up of 3–24 months by Doppler echocardiography or cardiac catheterization the PSG was 29 ± 16 mmHg. Only one patient had a significant increase in gradient (to 50 mmHg). In group II, with intermediate type membranes, the gradients fell from 40 and 116 mmHg to 18 and 58 mmHg, respectively. On follow-up at 3 months the gradients increased to 37 and 76 mmHg, respectively. In group III with thick membranes the gradients fell from 64 and 70 mmHg to 15 and 16 mmHg, respectively, immediately after balloon dilatation, but Doppler echocardiographic evaluation within 24 hours showed that the gradients had increased to 58 and 60 mmHg, respectively. On follow-up at 3 months the gradients were 64 and 60 mmHg, respectively.

Complications

Transient weak femoral and lower limb pulses on the side of balloon entry occurred in two cases. One patient with severe pulmonary artery hypertension and right to left shunt at the ductus level with gross left ventricular failure and cardiomegaly in addition to discrete subaortic stenosis gained partial relief of obstruction. She had vascular injury during an attempt at repeat dilatation and died after 12 hours.

Other Studies

Sharma (personal communication) reported four cases (aged 12–21 years) of discrete subaortic stenosis subjected to balloon dilatation using 12–18 mm balloons. The PSG across the membrane was reduced from 100 ± 20 (88–114) to 36 ± 15 (20–53) mmHg. The degree of aortic regurgitation remained unchanged in two and increased by one grade in two. Echocardiography before the procedure showed a thin membrane in all the patients. A tear in the membrane was identified on echocardiography after the procedure. Arora et al. [9] reported good results after balloon dilatation in three cases of discrete subaortic stenosis.

In summary, our results show that balloon dilatation efficacy in discrete subaortic stenosis is highly variable. The immediate response of the gradient to balloon dilatation cannot predict long-term behavior. Morphologic features of discrete subaortic stenosis detected on echocardiography, however, can predict response. Uniformly thin (1–3 mm) membranes responded well to dilatation. The relief was dramatic and long lasting. Thick fibromuscular shelves even if discrete do not respond well, and any decrease in gradient is transient. Patients with discrete subaortic stenosis of intermediate morphology have a partial response, and the benefit is likely to be lost over time.

COARCTATION OF AORTA

Our experience with balloon angioplasty of aortic coarctation over the last 2.5 years was limited to 18 patients. Associated lesions included right-side aortic arch in one, discrete subaortic stenosis in one, and mild valvar aortic stenosis in two. The study included 14 males and 4 females (aged 8 months to 22 years). One of these patients was a postoperative recoarctation. We used 6–15 mm diameter, 3 cm long balloons (Mansfield, Inc). The size of the balloon used was 90%–100% of the size of the aorta just above and just below the coarcted segment. The patients have been followed up for 3–24 months after balloon angioplasty. The follow-up included clinical evaluation, two-dimensional and Doppler echocardiography, and cardiac catheterization and angiography (in seven patients).

The peak systolic gradient across the coarctation of the aorta fell from 58 ± 18 to 23 ± 9 mmHg immediately after the angioplasty. Two patients had partial response (residual gradients of 30 and 50 mmHg), and one patient had no change in her gradient. Clinically all patients improved. The upper segment blood pressure normalized in 10 cases, with no requirement for antihypertensive therapy. In seven patients the blood pressure could be controlled with much smaller dosages of drugs. One patient had no change in her clinical status with angioplasty. In our experience (N = 18), contrary to the experience of some authors, there was a good correlation (r = 0.92) between Doppler-predicted gradients and those obtained at catheterization [10]. On follow-up at 3–24 months, the gradients across the coarctation in the overall group (N = 12) did not change significantly (26 ± 10 mmHg) compared with 22 ± 9 mmHg immediately after angioplasty). A review of the data from individual patients showed an increase in gradients in two patients.

Complications

Vascular complications. Transient weak femoral pulses on the side of balloon entry were identified in five patients. Persistent arterial insufficiency did not occur in any case. None required surgical repair. One patient developed minor dissection at the site of coarctation in an attempt to cross it. The procedure was abandoned and performed 4 weeks later.

Aneurysm formation. A small aneurysm at the site of coarctation dilatation was observed in one case on repeat angiography 3 months after angioplasty. No aneurysms were seen in the other six patients in whom follow-up angiography was performed.

Hypertensive response. We observed a hypertensive response in six cases immediately after angioplasty despite marked reduction in coarctation gradient and striking improvement in angiographic lumen. This was treated with sublingual nifedipine and intravenous propranolol. The hypertension was transient and settled down over the next 3–7 days. We did not observe any specific predictors for this response.

Restenosis. Two of 12 patients showed evidence of increased gradients to 41 and 50

mmHg on follow-up. Native coarctation of the aorta can be safely dilated by balloon angioplasty. However, in view of the inadequate response, restenosis, and aneurysm formation in some patients, this technique needs to be critically evaluated in comparison with surgery. The hypertensive response following angioplasty is similar to that seen after surgery and needs to be identified and treated promptly.

REFERENCES

1. Shrivastava S, Shyamsunder A, Mukhopathayay S, Rajani M (1987): Percutaneous transluminal balloon pulmonary valvoplasty for pulmonary valve stenosis. Int J Cardiol 17:303–314.
2. Dev V. Radhakrishnan S, Rajani M, Das G, Shyamsundar A, Sharma S, Shrivastava S (1990): Echocardiographic assessment of the size of aortic and pulmonary valve annulus before balloon valvoplasty. Indian Heart J 42:195–197.
3. Arora R, Kishore R, Kaul UA, Khalilullah M (1989): Follow up of results of balloon valvoplasty in pulmonic stenosis. Indian Heart J 41:373.
4. Shah LS, Khanolkar UB, Pinto RI (1989): Balloon dilatation of stenotic lesions and PTCA–A study of 41 cases. Indian Heart J 41:373.
5. Shrivastava S, Dev V, Vasan RS, Das GS, Rajani M (1991): Percutaneous balloon mitral valvuloplasty in juvenile rheumatic mitral stenosis. Am J Cardiol 67:892–894.
6. Lock JE, Khalilullah M, Shrivastava S, Bahl V, Keane JF (1985): Percutaneous catheter commissurotomy in rheumatic mitral stenosis. N Engl J Med 313:1515–1518.
7. Shrivastava S, Dev V, Das G, Sharma S, Rajani M (1991): Percutaneous balloon mitral valvuloplasty in rheumatic mitral stenosis: An experience of 50 patients in India. Clin Cardiol 14:237–241.
8. Shrivastava S, Das GS, Dev V, Sharma S, Rajani MI (1990): Follow up after percutaneous balloon valvoplasty for noncalcific aortic stenosis. Am J Cardiol 65:250–252.
9. Arora R, Goel PK, Lochan R, Mohan JC, Khalilullah M (1988): Percutaneous transluminal balloon dilatation in discrete subaortic stenosis. Am Heart J 116:1041–1042.
10. Vijaykumar M, Dev V, Saxena A, Shrivastava S (1989): Doppler evaluation of the pressure gradients in aortic coarctation. Indian Heart J 41:472.

22e

Balloon Valvuloplasty of Pulmonic Stenosis: The Saudi Arabian Experience[1]

M.A. Ali Khan M.D., F.R.C.P.(E.)

Division of Pediatric Cardiology, Riyadh Armed Forces Hospital, and Department of Pediatrics, King Saud University, Riyadh 11159, Saudi Arabia

INTRODUCTION

Balloon dilatation of valvular stenotic lesions by a pullback or dynamic technique was first described by Rubio and Limon-Lason [1] in 1954. Dotter and Judkins [2] in 1964 introduced the concept of dilating an atherosclerotic obstruction using a series of progressively larger catheters for the treatment of peripheral vascular disease. The first catheter intervention to be applied successfully to congenital heart disease, in 1966, was the Rashkind and Miller [3] balloon atrial septostomy for increasing interatrial mixing in transposition of the great arteries. In 1978, Gruntzig et al. modified the technique by placing a polyvinyl balloon on the tip of the catheter for renal artery stenosis. A smaller version of this dilatation catheter was then developed in 1979 for use within the coronary arterial tree [4]. In the same year, Semb et al. [5] reported the first successful pulmonary valvotomy by pulling a carbon dioxide–filled balloon from the pulmonary artery to the right ventricle. Since then interest in nonsurgical dilatation of stenotic pulmonary valves has rapidly increased, especially after the introduction of a new generation of dilating catheters made of polyethylene, which were first used for this purpose by Kan and Pepine and their associates in 1982 [6,7]. This spawned a new subspeciality in cardiology as well as a new industry in intravascular medical products.

The procedure of balloon dilatation of pulmonary stenosis was first introduced into the Riyadh Cardiac Centre, Armed Forces Hospital, in the Kingdom of Saudi Arabia, in August 1984 [8-12]. In this institution we also perform aortic and mitral valvuloplasty, balloon dilatation of native coarctation, balloon dilatation of venous cardiac chambers post-Mustard operation, umbrella closure of patent ductus arteriosus, endomyocardial biopsies, coil embolizations, and retrieval of foreign bodies from the cardiovascular system. In this chapter I will review only our experience of balloon dilatation of pulmonary stenosis in infants and children from August 1984 to October 1989. This will include our experience with a double balloon technique, graduated sequential balloon pulmonary valvuloplasty in infants with critical pulmonary stenosis, and palliative balloon pulmonary valve dilatation in complex cyanotic cardiac lesions. Recatheterization results postballoon dilatation will also be reviewed.

MATERIAL

Two hundred fifty-seven procedures were performed (Table 1). There were 11 technical failures because it was impossible to advance

---

[1]Despite the title, only experience at a single institution will be reviewed in this chapter.

Transcatheter Therapy in Pediatric Cardiology, pages 457–469

**TABLE I. PTBPV Riyadh Cardiac Centre
(August 1984 to October 1989)**[a]

Total procedures	257
Technical failures (including one complex lesion)	11
PS with complex lesions	14
Other lesions	
PFO	78
ASD	27
Hypoplastic RV	20
Tricuspid regurgitation (H-RV + TR = 9)	13
Dysplastic Pulmonary valve	19
Noonan's syndrome	4
Rubella syndrome	2
PAPVD	3
Small VSD	1

[a]Patients were ≤12 years old. ASD, atrial septal defect; H-RV, hypoplastic right ventricle; PAPVD, partial anomalous pulmonary venous drainage; PFO, patent foramen ovale; PTBPV, percutaneous transluminal balloon pulmonary valvuloplasty; RV, right ventricle; TR, tricuspid regurgitation; VSD, ventricular septal defect.

the catheter or the wire through the pulmonary valve. There were 14 patients with complex cyanotic cardiac lesions who required intentionally limited palliative balloon dilatation, as full annulus diameter would have been disadvantageous.

There were 232 procedures in patients with isolated pulmonary stenosis or with minor associated defects. These included 78 patent foramen ovale, 27 small atrial septal defects, and 20 hypoplastic right ventricles (RV), 13 tricuspid regurgitation that also included hypoplastic RV in nine patients. There were 19 dysplastic pulmonary valves, including 4 patients with Noonan's syndrome. In newborns and young infants there were 20 patients with a small patent ductus arteriosus.

The age range was from 1 day to 12 years, with a mean of 46 ± 44 months. There were 23 patients less than 1 month of age (10 being less than 1 week) and 61 patients between 1 and 12 months of age, giving a total of 84 patients under 12 months and 173 patients over 12 months of age. The weight range was between 2.4 to 46.8 kg, with a mean of 13.7

± 8.5 kg. There were 31 patients less than 5 kg, 80 patients between 6 and 10 kg, and 146 patients over 10 kg (Fig. 1).

METHOD

Most of the patients were admitted 1 day before the procedure, and electrocardiogram, chest x-ray, echocardiography, and blood work were performed before catheterization. Most patients received pethidine and promethazine intramuscularly 45 minutes prior to the commencement of the procedure. Patients also received additional ketamine hydrochloride intravenously during the procedure. Atropine was given when bradycardia was noted prior to or immediately after balloon dilatation.

The hemodynamic study was performed with a venous catheter in both the right and left femoral veins and an arterial monitoring line in a femoral artery. When the double-balloon technique was utilized, a third catheter was introduced percutaneously into the right brachial vein and advanced into the right ventricle. Cardiac output was measured by means of the Fick principle.

After the diagnosis of moderate to severe pulmonary valve stenosis was confirmed hemodynamically and defined angiographically, balloon valvuloplasty was begun. Anteroposterior and lateral markers were placed on the chest wall, to be used as reference points for pulmonary valve location.

Single Balloon

The method of valvuloplasty was the same for each patient regardless of age. In most cases, a 6 or 7 Goodale-Lubin (GL) catheter was advanced from a femoral vein to the right heart and then across the pulmonary valve into the left pulmonary artery, although sometimes in infants the catheter and wire were also placed in the right pulmonary artery. An angiographic catheter was advanced through the opposite femoral vein to the right ventricle and an arterial line inserted into a femoral artery usually in the left groin. The pressures in these

P T B P V
Aug 1984 to October 1989
n = 257

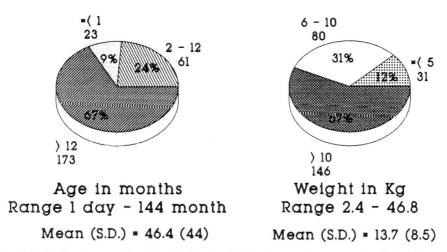

Age in months
Range 1 day - 144 month

Mean (S.D.) ▪ 46.4 (44)

Weight in Kg
Range 2.4 - 46.8

Mean (S.D.) ▪ 13.7 (8.5)

Fig. 1. Patient's age and weight distribution. PTBPV, percutaneous transluminal balloon pulmonary valvuloplasty.

locations were recorded simultaneously in a resting state.

Before the balloon dilatation, a 200 cm, 0.038 inch, flexible, curve-tipped exchange guidewire was advanced through the GL catheter into the distal left pulmonary artery. The GL catheter and venous sheath were removed, leaving the guidewire in place. The catheters utilized for the valvuloplasty were 5-9 Fr with a polyethylene balloon 5-20 mm in diameter. The size of the balloon was selected to be approximately 120%-130% larger than the pulmonary valve annulus as estimated by two-dimensional echocardiography and biplane angiocardiography. A grid factor was recorded on the angiogram or a marker catheter used to measure the actual diameter of the pulmonary valve annulus. The femoral vein was dilated with an appropriate size dilator passed over the guidewire. The valvuloplasty catheter was

advanced over the exchange wire and positioned across the stenotic pulmonary valve, leaving the guidewire in place in the left pulmonary artery.

Balloon rupture was common, though without any ill effect to the patient. Although mortality is extremely rare in pulmonary balloon valvuloplasty, two very sick infants with critical pulmonary stenosis died during the procedure.

Double Balloon Technique

In the double balloon technique, the angiocardiographic catheter is replaced with a second GL catheter, which is also maneuvered into the left pulmonary artery. A second 180-260 cm wire is passed through this catheter and left in place in the left pulmonary artery. In addition to these two wires, a 5 or 6 Fr sheath was introduced percutaneously into a right median basilic vein; an NIH catheter was introduced through this sheath and advanced into the heart and was positioned in the right ventricle. The balloons are carefully prepared to evacuate all air from the system. Appropriate balloon catheters were introduced from both groins (generally the combined diameter of the two balloons being 150% of the diameter of the pulmonary valve annulus, or the effective balloon diameter was measured as sum of two balloons multiplied by 0.8) into the femoral veins over the exchange wires and passed through the right heart to an area straddling the pulmonary valve. With the balloon catheters carefully positioned across the pulmonary valve, simultaneous inflations of the two balloons were performed inflating both balloons to approximately 5 atm pressure. In every procedure the balloon is inflated by hand through a 20 ml syringe filled with diluted (10%) contrast material. Inflation and deflation procedures were repeated approximately four to five times. In the last 200 procedures no gauge was utilized to check the pressures.[2] In every successful case the balloon was inflated until no "waisting" or "hourglass" deformity of the balloon was present. The inflation and deflation cycle was performed in a short duration of 10–15 seconds. During inflation and deflation cineangiograms at 30 frames per second and pressure monitoring were recorded. Balloon rupture[2] occurred frequently but with no detectable ill effects.

After valvuloplasty all of the patients had pulmonary valve pressure gradients recorded and repeat right ventricular angiograms performed in posteroanterior and lateral views to evaluate the right ventricular outflow tract. No patient was heparinized for the procedure except for the flush solution, which was mixed with a small amount of heparin. The patients usually were discharged on the day following the procedure.

Graduated Sequential Balloon Technique

Applications of balloon valvuloplasty in critical pulmonary stenosis has in the past been limited due to concerns about complete obstruction of the right ventricular outflow tract during the procedure if the ventricular septum is intact in infants who are already compromised by hypoxemia or acidemia. With this method, it was possible in these infants to introduce a smaller guidewire of only 0.014 inch and a coronary angioplasty balloon catheter as small as two millimeters in diameter for the initial dilatation. Subsequently these are replaced by 0.025–0.038 inch double-exchange guidewires and suitable sized balloons for definitive dilatation.

RESULTS AND OBSERVATIONS

Excluding the 12 technical failures and 14 complex lesions, in the remaining procedures preballoon valvuloplasty peak systolic gradients ranged from 30 to 310 mmHg with a mean of 97 ± 49 mmHg. Following balloon valvuloplasty the gradients ranged from 0 to 175 mmHg, with a mean of 22 ± 17, indicating a 77% reduction, and a P value of <0.001 (Fig. 2). There was 75%–100% reduction in gradient in 125 of 232 procedures (54%). There was 50%–75% reduction in gradient in 80 patients (35%), so that a total of 89% had a gradient reduced by 50% or more (Fig. 3).

The predilatation gradient of 310 mmHg is from a 9-year-old male who had reduction of the valve gradient to 2 mmHg but the infindibular gradient was 100 mmHg. This patient was recatheterized after 6 months, when the gradient at the pulmonary valve was 10 mmHg and the infundibular gradient was reduced to 25 mmHg.

A 12-year-old patient with Noonan's syndrome and dysplastic pulmonary valve had a

---

[2]Editor's note: Monitoring pressure of inflation (by placing a pressure gauge in series) and limiting pressure of inflation to avoid balloon ruptures is highly recommend by the editor and by many other interventional pediatric cardiologists.

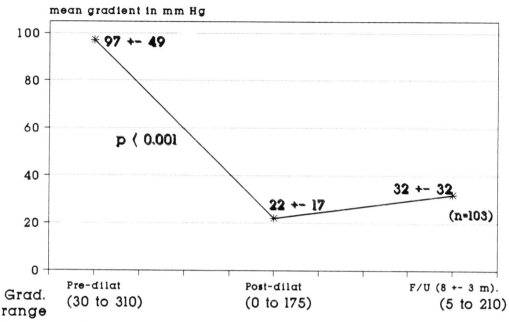

P T B P V (n = 232)
August 84 to October 89
Excludes 11 failures, 14 complex lesions

Fig. 2. Results of balloon dilatation showing pre- and postdilatation values and follow-up peak systolic pressure gradients. PTBV, percutaneous transluminal balloon pulmonary valvuloplasty; F/U, follow-up (months).

gradient of 240 mmHg. The postballoon gradient decreased to 175 mmHg. Six months later, on recatheterization the gradient had increased to 210 mmHg; redilatation was performed using the double-balloon technique. Eight months following reballoon the gradient returned to preballoon level, and surgery was performed.

A total of 103 children underwent recatheterization at an average period of 8 months after the initial procedures. The mean follow-up gradient was 32 ± 32 mmHg, slightly higher than that immediately after the dilatation. The maximum follow up has been 62 months (Fig. 4).

Note the reduction in gradient related to age distribution. The percentages of reduction are similar in all three age groups (Fig. 4).

A 6-year-old patient with a predilatation pulmonary valve gradient of 245 mmHg was found to have an immediate postdilatation gradient of 95 mmHg, but showed a severe infundibular reaction that did not respond to the usual doses of Inderal. On catheterization the following day the gradient had risen to over 200 mmHg. The patient underwent open pulmonary valvotomy on the third day. At surgery splitting was present at two commissures of the valve, and they appeared wide open. The patient underwent infundibular resection and an outflow patch, with full recovery.

Excluding technical failures and complex lesions, in the remaining 65 patients the preballoon gradient ranged between 30 and 220 mmHg, with a mean of 94 ± 41 mmHg; postballoon gradients ranged between 0 and

P T B P V
Percentage reduction in gradient
(n = 232)

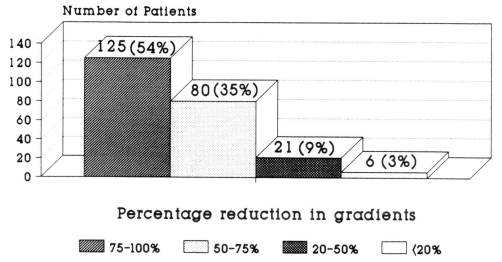

Fig. 3. Percentage reduction in peak systolic pressure gradients after initial balloon valvuloplasty. PTBPV, percutaneous transluminal balloon pulmonary valvuloplasty.

93, with a mean of 23 ± 17 mmHg ($P < 0.001$). In 33 patients, follow-up recatheterization (mean interval, 8 months), showed a mean gradient of 40 ± 31 mmHg. The arterial saturation also rose from a mean of 87% ± 12% to 91% ± 8% ($P < 0.01$).

In the double-balloon technique the age of the patients was between 3 days and 12 years. There were 24 patients with a mean pregradient of 87 ± 42 mmHg and a postballoon gradient mean of 25 ± 34 mmHg. Six patients had follow-up recatheterization, with a gradient mean of 65 ± 76 mmHg. Excluding the Noonan's syndrome mentioned previously, which was a failure due to the dysplastic valve, the mean recatheterization gradient was 36 ± 30 mmHg.

The technique of graduated sequential balloon dilatation was utilized in 19 patients under 1 year of age with critical pulmonary valve stenosis. These patients had the sequential use of one or more small balloons to open the valve prior to the full dilatation, with a final balloon diameter used between 80% and 130% of the measured pulmonary valve annulus [10]. There was one failure, in a 6-month-old patient who required surgery 1 month later. The ages ranged from 1 day to 12 months, with a mean of 5.1 ± 4.4 and a weight range of 2.9 to 9.8 kg, with a mean of 5.6 ± 2.2 kg.

Of the 19 patients, the preballoon gradient ranged between 55 and 220 mmHg, with a mean of 108 ± 43 mmHg. Immediately postballoon the gradient was 0 to 29 mmHg, with a mean of 18 ± 9 mmHg, ($P < 0.001$). The 8 month follow-up catheterization in nine of these patients showed a range of 17 to 110 mmHg (mean, 51 ± 36 mmHg). Four of these patients were reballooned with satisfactory re-

P T B P V
Recatheterization, 44%
(n = 103)

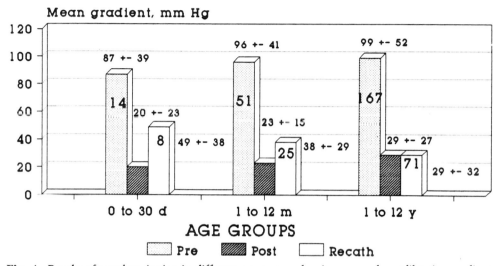

Fig. 4. Results of recatheterization in different age groups, showing pre- and postdilatation gradients and follow-up gradients on recatheterization. The numbers in the bars indicate the number of patients. PTBPV, percutaneous transluminal balloon pulmonary valvuloplasty; d, days; m, months; y, years.

sults. Two patients had surgery because of a dysplastic valve. The arterial O_2 saturation increased in these patients from a mean 80% ± 16% to 91% ± 5% ($P < 0.01$).

In the complex cyanotic cardiac lesions, 14 patients had an intentionally limited palliative balloon dilatation procedure. This group includes transposition of great arteries, tetralogy of Fallot, truncus arteriosus, double-inlet left ventricle, and Ebstein's anomaly. The balloons selected for these cases were purposefully the same size or smaller than the annulus.[3] The goal was to improve the pulmonary blood flow and avoid shunt operation or in postoperative cases to drop the pulmonary gradient further. There was an increase in the arterial saturation in the cyanotic group and a decrease in the pulmonary gradient in the postoperative patients.

A 1-day-old infant with transposition of the great arteries, ventricular septal defect, and pulmonary stenosis who had balloon dilata-

---

[3]Editor's note: Limiting the size of the balloon to the size of the pulmonary valve annulus will only stretch pulmonary valve leaflets without rupturing valve commissures or leaflets, and the favorable effect, if any, will be transient. I highly recommend a balloon size that is 1.2–1.4 times the size of the pulmonary valve annulus (Rao and Brais, Am Heart J 115:1105–1113, 1988; Rao et al. Cathet Cardiovasc Diagn 25:16–24, 1992). If one is concerned about overcirculation to the lungs, the presence of another obstruction in series should be required prior to attempting valvuloplasty. For further discussion of issues related to balloon dilatation in patients with cyanotic congenital heart disease, the reader is referred to Chapter 13 (this volume).

tion with a 5 mm balloon showed improvement in gradient as well as a 12% increase in arterial O_2 saturation. At the age of 12 months, because of a rise in hemoglobin to 20 g, he was reballooned and the arterial O_2 saturatuion again increased from 65% to 77%.

The second example is a 4-day-old infant with Ebstein's anomaly, valvular pulmonary stenosis, and large patent ductus arteriosus, with echo evidence of pulmonary stenosis, who had graduated balloon dilatation, starting with 2 up to 6.5 mm balloons. During the procedure the patient had ventricular tachycardia, supraventricular tachycardia, and 2:1 block, all of which improved with treatment. Arterial O_2 saturation rose from 69% to 73%. The heart size improved the next day. He is now being followed in another city.

There were three tetralogy of Fallot patients who had balloon dilatation and did not require a shunt operation. These patients subsequently had complete repair 6–9 months later.

A 9-month-old infant with double-inlet left ventricle, transposition of great arteries, and pulmonary stenosis had balloon dilatation. The arterial O_2 saturation rose from 44% to 81%. He had right Blalock-Taussig shunt 18 months later and is presently doing well.

The two postoperative patients, one with a 12 mm Hancock valve stenosis in a type I truncus arteriosus repair and another with tetralogy of Fallot repair, with residual supravalvular stenosis, both had successful balloon dilatation. The respective gradients were reduced from 75 to 22 mmHg and from 70 to 28 mmHg. The truncus case had a 20 mm conduit inserted 10 months later. The tetralogy of Fallot had no further surgery.

There are 21 patients who were reballooned who at the time of the initial balloon dilatation showed a significant drop in pulmonary gradient, from a mean of 107 $\pm$ 50 mmHg to a mean of 34 $\pm$ 20 mmHg. However, 6 months later the gradient increased again to a mean of 65 $\pm$ 20 mmHg. Reballoon dilatation was performed, and immediately the gradient fell to a mean of 24 $\pm$ 14 mmHg ($P < 0.001$).

Seven of these reballoon cases were further recatheterized 6 months later, and all are maintaining excellent results, with a mean gradient of 23 $\pm$ 24 mmHg (Fig. 5).

Restenosis, with an increase in gradient, occurred in four patients aged less than 1 month, in seven patients between 2 and 12 months, and in 10 patients aged over 1 year at the time of first balloon dilatation. These patients underwent reballooning with successful results. (The gradient reached maximum levels in the group below 1 month at the time of first balloon dilatation.)

COMPLICATIONS

The following complications occurred in 257 procedures. Balloon rupture (50 cases) during inflation was quite common and did not cause any known ill effects. Blood transfusion was given in 25 patients, some of whom were anemic prior to heart catheterization (Table II).

Intubation with ventilation was performed in 14 patients: 10 before catheterization and 4 requiring emergency intubation during catheterization. Infundibular reaction was also quite common and was seen in 71 patients. In some of these cases a gradient of over 100 mmHg was noted with little or no response to iv Inderal. Femoral vein thrombosis was a rare event; only 4 of 103 patients recatheterized showed occlusion of the vein. Dysrrhythmia was noted in 11 patients; two developed complete right bundle branch block, and nine patients developed bradycardia requiring intravenous atropine. Five patients developed serious arrhythmias, two supraventricular and two ventricular tachycardia requiring cardioversion. One of these patients had Ebstein's anomaly. One patient had a period of asystole requiring only cardiac massage, with full recovery. Sixteen patients required surgery, which included 12 technical failures and 4 inadequate relief of gradients postballoon dilatation, including dysplastic valves.

There were two deaths, one in a 5-month-old

P T B P V
Reballooning, (n = 21)

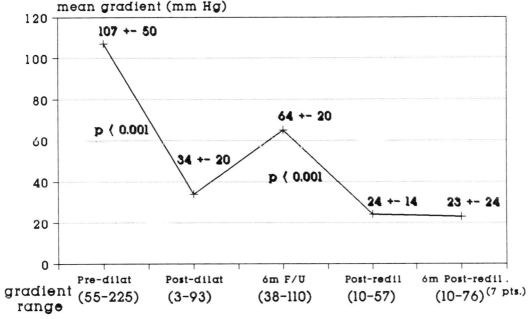

Fig. 5. Results of reballooning for restenosis after initial balloon valvuloplasty, showing pre- and postdilatation and follow-up gradients after initial dilatation and postredilatation and follow-up gradients. PTBV, percutaneous transluminal balloon pulmonary valvuloplasty.

TABLE II. PTBPV Complications (N = 257)[a]

Balloon rupture	50
Blood transfusion	25
Intubation, ventilation (emergency intub. = 4)	14
Infundibular reaction	71
Inderal after ballooning	13
Femoral vein thrombosis	4
Dysrhythmia	11
CRBBB	2
Bradycardia	9
SVT	2
VT	2
Asystole	1
Mortality	2

[a]CRBBB, complete right bundle branch block; PTBPV, percutaneous transluminal balloon pulmonary valvuloplasty; SVT, supraventricular tachycardia; VT, ventricular tachycardia.

infant weighing 5.5 kg with the gradient of 160 mmHg with critical pulmonary stenosis, hypoplastic right ventricle, and atrial septal defect arrested during the procedure with bradycardia and who could not be resuscitated; and the other in a 9-month-old, asymptomatic patient with a gradient of 50 mmHg. The annulus size was overestimated, with the result that the balloon size chosen was too large. The valve annulus was ruptured on inflation, leading to circulatory collapse and death.

DISCUSSION

Balloon pulmonary valvuloplasty has been well accepted and the technique has been very well described in the literature [6,9,13–25].

Although the indications for valvuloplasty are not clearly defined, it is generally agreed that the surgical indications for commissurotomy are accepted for balloon dilatation [17]. A peak systolic gradient of 50 mmHg or more even in an asymptomatic patient is an indication for balloon valvuloplasty. Occasionally we have not been adherent to this rule, and lower gradients have been accepted for this procedure. The mean gradient in our cases showed a drop from 97 ± 49 to 22 ± 17 mmHg, indicating 77% reduction with a P value of <0.001. Eighty-nine percent of our patients had a gradient reduced by 50% or more. In classic dysplastic pulmonary valves [26,27] our results have been at most mediocre. Long-term results in our patients show no beneficial effect. Our policy is to make an initial balloon dilatation attempt [11,15,23,28] since there may be different degrees of dysplasia [29]. Valves with partial dysplasia and commissural fusion do respond to dilatation. In general, we concur with several other groups who have reported excellent immediate and intermediate- to long-term results of this procedure [9,10,12,13,14,17,18,30]. Balloon size selection is an important feature of this procedure, since long-term results also depend on size of the balloon used in relation to the pulmonary valve annulus [30–33]. For better results, balloons larger than 120% of the pulmonary valve annulus but less than 140% should be used. If a double-balloon technique is utilized, generally the combined diameter of the two balloons is 140%–160% of the pulmonary valve annulus. We stopped using the pressure gauge after the first 60 procedures, as there was no added advantage. Balloons were inflated by the syringe until there was no waisting at the stenotic valve, and the total inflation/deflation procedure generally lasted for 5–10 seconds. We have noticed in our series that presence of foramen ovale or a small atrial septal defect has

been beneficial in maintaining the arterial pressure during inflation of the balloon. This is related to right to left shunting at the atrial level.

Infundibular reaction is not uncommon after surgical commissurotomy. A similar infundibular reaction is noted after balloon dilatation of pulmonary valve stenosis, more commonly in older patients and those with severe stenosis [9,34–36].[4] Twenty-five percent of the patients in our series had infundibular gradients soon after the dilatation. Some of these gradients reached over 100 mmHg. Most of the time the gradients regress within 6–12 months after adequate valvuloplasty. Propranolol had no consistent effect in improving the gradients.

The criteria for critical pulmonary valve stenosis include 1) angiographic and echocardiographic evidence of a very small stenotic pulmonary valve orifice (less than 2–3 mm diameter); 2) suprasystemic pressure in the right ventricle; and 3) right-to-left shunting across a patent foramen ovale, often associated with cardiomegaly and congestive heart failure in the neonate.

Potential technical difficulties in this group of patients include excessive radiation during the procedure, difficulty in guidewire positioning, perforation of the ventricular outflow tract or pulmonary valve sinuses, and inability to advance the necessary calibre of balloon across the small valve opening without causing bradycardia, hypoxemia, or acidemia.

In spite of all of the above potential problems, balloon valvuloplasty was successfully performed using a new technique of graduated sequential valve dilatation [10]. This was necessary in this subgroup of patients because of hemodynamic instability as a result of initial attempts to cross the valve.

The technique of graduated sequential dilatation allowed successful dilatation in the pres-

---

[4]Editor's note: This is well documented by Thapar and Rao (Am Heart J 118:99–103, 1989). For further discussion on issues related infundibular obstruction, the reader is referred to Chapter 6 (this volume).

ence of factors that in the past have limited interventional treatment. These include cyanosis, very small pulmonary valve orifice size, right ventricular hypoplasia, and inability to cross the valve with a size of catheter adequate for single balloon dilatation. We have found it necessary to support these patients aggressively during the procedure due to their tendency to develop bradycardia, hypotension, severe hypoxemia, and acidosis. Dilatation resulted in a prompt increase in O_2 saturation. Five of our newborns were kept on prostaglandin E_1 infusion during the procedure, and five patients were intubated and ventilated during the procedure.

The advantages of two balloons are [9] that smaller balloons are easier and smoother to introduce and remove and presumably cause less trauma to the femoral vessels; that smaller catheters are easier to manipulate and follow guidewires more easily and less likely to perforate or tear the structures; that double balloons extend the range of patients treatable with two balloons; that double balloons do not completely occlude the stenotic orifice during inflation; and that ventricles are vented and cardiac output is maintained. There is a significant pressure drop with the single-balloon technique compared with the use of double balloons. The main disadvantage is that more time is required for the procedure.

Limited palliative balloon dilatation in cyanotic heart disease and also in complex lesions is of benefit in improving arterial saturation and postponement of surgery or to avoid shunt operation [37–39]. It is especially beneficial when the valvular lesion is the dominant one. In over 14 patients there was definite improvement, and in some of our cases we have avoided shunt operation and have gone for total correction later on.

The complications of this procedure are few except in very sick infants with critical pulmonary stenosis. Many medical centers have reported transient bradycardia, premature beats, and systemic hypotension during inflation. We have noted complete right bundle branch block in two patients, bradycardia requiring atropine in nine patients, and supraventricular and ventricular tachycardia in two patients each; all of them recovered after cardiac massage or cardioversion. Femoral vein thrombosis was found in 4 of 103 patients recatheterized 6–12 months later. Balloon rupture was common, though without any ill effect to the patient. Although mortality is extremely rare in pulmonary balloon valvuloplasty, two very sick infants with critical pulmonary stenosis died during the procedure. Intubation and ventilation were performed in 10 patients (mostly newborns and infants) electively and in 4 as an emergency during the procedure.

Generally, balloon valvuloplasty of critical pulmonary stenosis in infants has a higher complication rate in comparison to older children. Although we had two deaths in our series, these are preventable if appropriate precautions are taken, preventing hypoxemia, acidosis correction, and judicial use of intubation and ventilation during the procedure. Of course, the experience of the operator plays a major role in preventing catastrophies.

SUMMARY AND CONCLUSIONS

The conclusions we have drawn from our experience with this procedure are that balloon dilatation of stenotic pulmonary valves in infants and children offers great promise in avoiding open heart surgery, besides being safe and effective and that a double-balloon technique is advantageous when the annulus is large or in infants in whom a large single balloon would be difficult to introduce. Valvuloplasty may be done in a very sick newborn with critical pulmonary valve stenosis and hypoplastic right ventricle. Graduated sequential balloon dilatation and controlled anesthesia with assisted ventilation may be required.

Poor long-term results are observed with dysplastic valves, even with good initial response to ballooning in some cases. Satisfactory long-term results can be achieved in patients without dysplastic valves or in patients with partial dysplasia regardless of age at the time of ballooning.

At the time of final revision of this manuscript, over 300 pulmonary balloon valvuloplasties had been performed in our institution with equally good results.

ACKNOWLEDGMENTS

The author acknowledges the contributions made by Dr. S. Al Yousef and the Locum staff in Paediatric Cardiology at the Armed Forces Hospital, Riyadh, Saudi Arabia. The author also appreciates the help of Dr. W. Sawyer in reviewing the manuscript and Mrs. Joan Nicholas for manuscript preparations.

REFERENCES

1. Rubio V, Limon-Lason R (1954): Treatment of pulmonary valvular stenosis and tricuspid stenosis using a modified catheter. Program Abstracts II, Second World Congress on Cardiology, Washington DC, p 205.
2. Dotter CT, Judkins MP (1964): Transluminal treatment of arteriosclerotic obstruction: Description of a new technique and a preliminary report of its application. Circulation 30:654-670.
3. Rashkind WJ, Miller WW (1966). Creation of an atrial septal defect without thoracotomy. JAMA 196:991-992.
4. Gruntzig AR, Senning A, Siegothaler WE (1979): Nonoperative dilation of coronary artery stenosis: Percutaneous transluminal coronary angioplasty. N Engl J Med 301:61-68.
5. Semb BKH, Tijonneland S, Stake G, et al. (1979): "Balloon valvulotomy" of congenital pulmonary valve stenosis with tricuspid valve insufficiency. Cardiovasc Radiol 2:239-241.
6. Kan JS, White RI Jr, Mitchell SE, et al. (1982): Percutaneous balloon valvuloplasty: A new method for treating congenital pulmonary valve stenosis. N Engl J Med 307:540-542.
7. Pepine CJ, Gessner IH, Feldman RL (1982): Percutaneous balloon valvuloplasty for pulmonic valve stenosis in the adult. Am J Cardiol 50:1442-1445.
8. Ali Khan MA, Al-Yousef S, Mullins CE (1986): Early experience with percutaneous transluminal balloon valvotomy of pulmonary valve stenosis. In Al-Fagih MR (ed): "Heart Disease in Neonates and Children. Cardiac Surgery Symposium Series." Oxford: Medical Education Services, pp 85-92.
9. Ali Khan MA, Al-Yousef S, Mullins CE (1986): Percutaneous transluminal balloon pulmonary valvuloplasty for the relief of pulmonary valve stenosis with special reference to double-balloon technique. Am Heart J 112:158-66.
10. Ali Khan MA, Al-Yousef S, Huhta JC, et al. (1989): Critical pulmonary valve stenosis in patients less than 1 year of age: Treatment with percutaneous gradational balloon pulmonary valvuloplasty. Am Heart J 117(5):1008-1014.
11. Ali Khan MA, Al Yousef S, Moore JW, Sawyer W (1990): Results of repeat percutaneous balloon valvuloplasty for pulmonary valvar restenosis. Am Heart J 120(4):878-881.
12. Ali Khan MA (1990): Balloon pulmonary valvuloplasty experience in infants and children. Bull Saudi Heart Assoc 2:59-61.
13. Rao PS (1986): Transcatheter treatment of pulmonic stenosis and coarctation of the aorta: The experience with percutaneous balloon dilatation. Br Heart J 56:250-258.
14. Rao PS, Fawzy ME, Solymar L, et al. (1988): Longterm results of balloon pulmonary valvuloplasty. Am Heart J 115:1105-113.
15. Rao PS (1988): Balloon dilatation in infants and children with dysplastic pulmonary valves: Short-term and intermediate-term results. Am Heart J 116:1168-1176.
16. Rao PS (1989): Balloon pulmonary valvuloplasty: A review. Clin Cardiol 12:55-74.
17. Tynan M, Baker EJ, Rohmer J, et al. (1985): Percutaneous balloon pulmonary valvuloplasty. Br Heart J 53:520-524.
18. Lababidi Z, Wu JR (1983): Percutaneous balloon pulmonary valvuloplasty. Am J Cardiol 52:560-562.
19. Kveselis DA, Rocchini AP, Snider AP, et al. (1985): Results of balloon valvuloplasty in the treatment of congenital valvar pulmonary stenosis in children. Am J Cardiol 56-527-532.
20. Miller GAH (1986): Balloon valvuloplasty and angioplasty in congenital heart disease. Br Heart J 54:285-289.
21. Sullivan ID, Robinson PJ, Macartney FJ, et al. (1986): Percutaneous balloon valvuloplasty for pulmonary stenosis in infants and children. Br Heart J 54:435-441.
22. Radtke W, Keane JL, Fellows KE, et al. (1986): Percutaneous balloon valvotomy of congenital pulmonary stenosis using oversized balloons. J Am Coll Cardiol 8:909-915.
23. Rey C, Marche P, Francart C, et al. (1988): Percutaneous transluminal balloon valvuloplasty of congen-

ital pulmonary valve stenosis, with a special report on infants and neonates. J Am Coll Cardiol 11:815–820.

24. Shrivastava S, Sundar AS, Mukhopadyaya S, *et al.* (1987): Percutaneous transluminal balloon pulmonary valvuloplasty: Long-term results. In J Cardiol 17:303–314.

25. Rocchini AP, Kveselis DA, Crowley D, *et al.* (1984): Percutaneous balloon valvuloplasty for treatment of congenital pulmonary valvar stenosis in children. J Am Coll Cardiol 3:1005–1012.

26. Jeffery RF, Moller JH, Amplatz K (1972): The dysplastic pulmonary valve: A new roentgenographic entity. Am J Roentgenol Radium Ther Nucl Med 114:322–39.

27. Koretzky ED, Moller JH, Korns ME, *et al.* (1969): Congenital pulmonary stenosis resulting from dysplasia of the valve. Circulation 60:42–53.

28. Marantz PM, Huhta JC, Mullins CE, *et al.* (1988): Results of balloon valvuloplasty in typical and dysplastic pulmonary valve stenosis: Doppler echocardiographic follow-up. J Am Coll Cardiol 12;476–479.

29. Musewe NN, Robertson MA, Benson LN, et al (1987): The dysplastic pulmonary valve: Echocardiographic features and results of balloon dilatation. Br Heart J 57:364–370.

30. Rao PS (1988): Further observations on the role of balloon size on the short-term and intermediate-term results of balloon pulmonary valvuloplasty. Br Heart J 60:507–511.

31. Rao PS (1987): Influence of balloon size on the short term and longterm results of pulmonary valvuloplasty. Texas Heart Inst J 14:57–61.

32. Ring JC, Kulik TJ, Burke RA, et al (1986): Morphologic changes induced by dilatation of pulmonary valve annulus with over-large balloons in normal newborn lamb. Am J Cardiol 55:210–214.

33. Yeager SB, Lock JE, Radtke W (1987): Balloon selection for double balloon valvotomy. J Am Coll Cardiol 9:467–468.

34. Fontes VF, Esteves CA, Eduardo J, *et al.* (1988): Regression of infundibular hypertrophy after pulmonary valvuloplasty for pulmonic stenosis. Am J Cardiol 62:977–979.

35. Griffith BP, Hardesty RL, Siewers RD, *et al.* (1982): Pulmonary valvotomy alone for pulmonic stenosis: Results in children with and without muscular infundibular hypertrophy. J Thorac Cardiovasc Surg 83:577–583.

36. Ben-Shachar G, Cohen MH, Sivakoff MC, *et al.* (1985): Development of infundibular obstruction after percutaneous pulmonary balloon valvuloplasty. J Am Coll Cardiol 5:754–756.

37. Boucek MM, Webster HE, Orsmond GS, *et al.* (1988): Balloon pulmonary valvuloplasty: Palliation for cyanotic heart disease. Am Heart J 115:318–322.

38. Qureshi SA, Kirk CR, Lamb R, *et al.* (1986): Balloon dilatation of the pulmonary valve in the first year of life in patients with tetralogy of Fallot: A preliminary study. Br Heart J 60:232–235.

39. Rao PS, Brais M (1988): Balloon pulmonary valvuloplasty for congenital cyanotic heart defects. Am Heart J 115:1105–1113.

22f

Balloon Valvuloplasty/Angioplasty: The Spanish Experience

José Suárez de Lezo, M.D., Alfonso Medina, M.D.,
Manuel Pan, M.D., Miguel Romero, M.D., Enrique Hernández, M.D.,
Djordje Pavlovic, M.D., and Francisco Melián, M.D.

Servicio de Cardiologia, Hospital Reina Sofía, University of
Córdoba, 14004 Córdoba (J.S.d.L., M.P., M.R., D.P.), and Unidad de
Cardiologia, Hospital del Pino, University of Las Palmas, Las Palmas
do Gran Canaria (A.M., E.H., F.M.), Spain

INTRODUCTION

The first Spanish report on angioplasty procedures in congenital heart disease was made by Pérez Martínez et al. [1] in 1983. For those who admired him, it was not a surprise that his last contribution before his premature death was the beginning of the "Spanish experience." Since then, several groups in our country have applied and reported different balloon techniques for the treatment of coarctation of the aorta [2–5], pulmonary valve stenosis [5–13], aortic valve stenosis [5,12,14,15], discrete subaortic stenosis [16], stenotic systemic to pulmonary shunts [17,18], ductus arteriosus [19], and stenotic pulmonary arteries [5].

The purpose of this chapter is to describe the results of cooperative experience from two Spanish groups (Córdoba and Las Palmas) with similar philosophies regarding interventional cardiology (The "Cor-Pal" experience). This experience relates to the following entities: 1) pulmonic stenosis, 2) valvular aortic stenosis, 3) discrete subaortic stenosis, and 4) coarctation of aorta.

PULMONIC STENOSIS

Following the initial experience of Kan et al. [20], several studies have shown excellent ini-tial results of pulmonary valvuloplasty in children and adults [21–26], with a low incidence of complications. Follow-up studies have shown a persistent pressure gradient relief in most patients [23,25,27–29]. The procedure is also effective in neonates with critical pulmonary stenosis and heart failure and may drastically change the clinical condition [24,29]; however, the incidence of complications in this group may be higher.

The Cor-Pal Experience

From 1983 to 1990 we have treated 70 patients with congenital pulmonary stenosis by percutaneous balloon valvuloplasty. The ages ranged between 2 days and 58 years (mean, 7.7 ± 10 years); eight were less than 1 year old, and all eight had critical pulmonary stenosis and presented with hypoxemia and heart failure. The remaining 62 patients older than 1 year were asymptomatic. The stenosis was valvular in 63 patients; in 2 of them the valve was dysplastic; the remaining 61 had a domed valve with commissural fusion. The stenosis was supravalvular in seven patients; all of them had hemodynamic and angiographic evidence of a localized and stenotic supravalvular ring without transvalvular gradient [30]. This particular group is discussed separately.

Immediate Results

The peak systolic pressure gradient (91 ± 38 vs. 35 ± 23 mmHg; P < 0.001) and the right ventricular peak systolic pressure (109 ± 40 vs. 61 ± 28 mmHg; P < 0.001) decreased significantly immediately after valvuloplasty. Angiographically, we observed a better valvular opening without a significant increase in pulmonary regurgitation. The systolic shortening of the infundibular diameter, as measured in lateral projection, increased significantly after dilatation; this created some mild and transient subvalvular gradients in seven patients. The right and left ventricular ejection fractions did not change significantly from when they were normal prior to valvuloplasty; however, in four patients with critical stenosis and depressed right ventricular function, significant improvements in ejection fraction occurred.

Complications

No major complications occurred in patients older than 1 year. One neonate who was successfully dilated died 4 hours after the procedure, following surgery for abdominal hemorrhage secondary to rupture of the right iliac artery.

Follow-Up

All our patients were followed for a period of 3 months to 6 years (mean, 3 ± 2 years). All of them remain asymptomatic. Serial non-invasive studies were performed in most patients. Hemodynamic re-evaluation was available in 38 patients at a mean follow-up of 12 ± 12 months. Figure 1 shows the progression of the mean Doppler and hemodynamic gradient; as can be seen, the gradient reduction persists on serial follow-up; no restenosis was detected. This persistent pressure relief led to a significant reduction in the degree of right ventricular hypertrophy, as detected by the electrocardiogram and vectorcardiogram [23,27].[1] Quantitative angiographic studies at follow-up in 37 patients showed a significant increase in the left ventricular end-diastolic

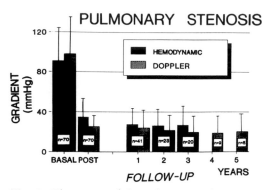

Fig. 1. The course of the pulmonary valve gradient following balloon valvuloplasty.

volume compared with basal values (43 ± 22 vs. 53 ± 18 cc/m²; P < 0.05). On the other hand, the systolic shortening of the infundibular diameter returned to baseline values, and no subvalvular gradients were detected. Finally, we did not observe significant changes in the angiographic degree of pulmonary regurgitation at follow-up.

Technical Details

A written informed consent was obtained prior to every interventional procedure. All patients were anticoagulated with heparin (1 mg/kg) when dilatations were initiated. All pediatric patients had mild anesthesia. We introduced three catheters (two venous, one arterial) percutaneously. The diagnostic phase always included right ventricular and pulmonary trunk angiograms in lateral projection, which was repeated after valvuloplasty. We always probed for the patency of the foramen ovale. After diagnostic procedures the balloon catheter was advanced over a long guidewire, positioned across the stenotic region, and inflated until complete disappearance of the stenotic notch. The diameter of the balloon used was, in most cases, slightly larger than the pulmonary valve annulus. The mean balloon/annu-

[1]Editor's note: For detailed electrocardiographic studies, the reader is referred to Rao and Solymar: J Interventional Cardiol 1:189-197, 1988 and to Chapter 6 (this volume).

lus ratio was 1.1 ± 0.1. A slight balloon oversize has been recommended in order to get an adequate gradient reduction [31], especially in dysplastic valves [29]. Sometimes this may require two balloon catheters introduced via both femoral veins [9,32]; in our work we used two balloon catheters in eight instances (11%); in two other patients we used a single multiballoon (bifoil or trefoil) catheter.

The antegrade passage of the balloon through the stenotic pulmonary valve is usually an easy procedure. Exceptions are in infants and neonates with critical stenosis, in whom repetitive attempts through a reactive infundibulum may increase the severity of hypoxemia. In such situation and after failing the antegrade approach, we have used the retrograde route through the ductus (Fig. 2). This alternative route through the patent ductus arteriosus was used in two patients; retrograde passage of the balloon catheter across the valve was surprisingly easy.

Physiopathology of Transient Right Ventricular Occlusion

Pulmonary valvuloplasty requires complete occlusion of the right ventricular outflow tract, temporarily stopping cardiac output during the period of inflation. Observations during transient balloon occlusions at the time of pulmonary valvuloplasty have shown that these procedures are well tolerated, although dramatic changes can occur [33]. The one-sided occluded heart can preserve a sinus rhythm. The ventricle seems to adapt suddenly by generating hypertensive and disynergic contractions with tricuspid regurgitation. The stagnant blood is partially emptied retrogradely. In the presence of a patent foramen ovale, right-to-left shunt through it becomes an important pathway of left ventricular filling.

Special Conditions

Discrete supravalvular pulmonary stenosis. Out of a total of 70 patients with congenital pulmonary stenosis who were treated by balloon dilatation, we identified a group of 7 (mean age = 4 ± 3 years) with hemodynamic and angiographic evidence of localized supravalvular stenosis. In all of them the stenotic ring was 1 cm above the pulmonary annulus, and no additional transvalvular gradient was detected. Following balloon dilatation in this particular group, the gradient decreased from 83 ± 42 to 24 ± 12 mmHg (P < 0.01). Angiographically, no significant increase in pulmonary regurgitation was observed. An improvement in the size of the lumen at the level of the stenotic area was also noted. The degree of right ventricular pressure relief was similar in these 7 patients to that observed in 63 patients with pulmonary valve stenosis. At follow-up studies (five hemodynamic, two Doppler) performed 19 ± 16 months later, the mean residual gradient was 20 ± 21 mmHg. Thus discrete supravalvular pulmonary stenosis can also be effectively treated by balloon dilatation, with results similar to those observed in patients with pulmonary valve stenosis.

Transluminal palliation for congenital heart defects with pulmonary oligemia and hypoxemia. Surgical treatment of several cyanotic heart defects includes initial palliative procedures in order to improve clinical conditions and prepare for an ultimate total surgical correction. In patients with severe pulmonary oligemia and hypoxemia, a cardiac catheterization study allows evaluation of patency of sources of pulmonary blood flow, namely, pulmonary valve, ductus arteriosus, and systemic-to-pulmonary shunts. In the course of these studies, it is also possible to perform transcatheter dilatation procedures that may palliate the clinical condition in a manner similar to that provided by palliative surgery [17]. Patients with severe pulmonic stenosis and ventricular septal defect may be palliated by a "controlled" valvuloplasty with undersized balloons [17,34–36].[2] Balloon an-

---

[2]Editor's note: See Chapter 13 (this volume) for further comments on the choice of balloon sizes in this subgroup of patients.

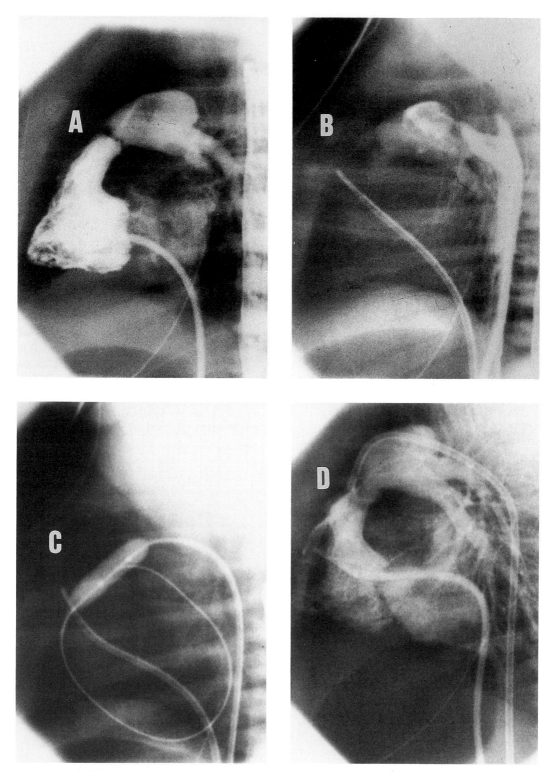

Fig. 2. Angiographic sequence (lateral projection) in a neonate with critical pulmonary stenosis in whom a retrograde approach was performed through a patent ductus arteriosus. **A:** Basal ventriculogram. **B:** Aortography showing ductus and pulmonary trunk anatomy. **C:** A retrogradely advanced balloon inflated across the right ventricular outflow tract. **D:** Ventriculogram after valvuloplasty.

gioplasty of a stenotic (or recently closed) ductus arteriosus [19] and stenotic Blalock-Taussig anastomosis [17,18,37] constitutes another transluminal alternative for palliation of severe hypoxemia.

Balloon valvotomy for pulmonary atresia. Pulmonary atresia with intact ventricular septum is a severe malformation with a high mortality rate within the first months of life. Besides medical treatment and atrial septostomy when required, different palliative surgical procedures depending on the anatomy and size of the right ventricle and pulmonary artery may be necessary. Systemic-to-pulmonary shunts may be necessary in addition to surgical opening of the atretic valve [38]. Surgical valvotomy could theoretically permit further development of the right ventricular cavity [39-41], which in turn may contribute to improved prognosis. We questioned whether it would be possible to perform transcatheter valvotomy in selected patients with pulmonary atresia [12,42,43]. In two patients, aged 1 month and 2.5 years, who had adequate annulus and ventricular sizes but without infundibular atresia, we performed puncture and perforation of the atretic valve tissue with a guidewire, through a catheter passed retrogradely through the ductus. The catheter tip was positioned at the level of the atretic membrane and orientated toward the right ventricular cavity. Then, the proximal hard tip of a coronary guidewire was advanced through the tip of the catheter to make the puncture. After perforating the atretic valve, a Mullins dilator was advanced, and the distal floppy end of the wire was passed and positioned in the right atrium or vena cava. This permitted retrograde passage of a balloon catheter. Inflation of the balloon produced rupture of the atretic tissue and opening of the natural pathway. This was demonstrated hemodynamically (Fig. 3) and angiographically in both patients. The older patient, who had a patent surgical shunt performed in the neonatal period, remained improved for 6 months after dilatation, with Doppler evidence of antegrade pulmonary flow. However, the procedure failed to prevent the need for surgery in the infant.

Other Spanish Contributions

Ubago et al. [6], from Santander, in 1984 published the first Spanish report of balloon pulmonary valvuloplasty. Seven patients aged 4-30 years were treated; the peak valvular gradient dropped from 72 ± 12 to 30 ± 6 mmHg; however, infundibular gradients were detected in two patients, which disappeared at short-term follow-up (10-31 days); no complications occurred. Macaya et al. [8], from Granada, reported similar findings in six patients with pulmonary stenosis; however, one neonate died. In a further analysis of 21 patients [11], the group from Granada found the balloon/annulus ratio greater than 1 and a thin pulmonary valve to be determinant factors of a good result. García Aguado et al. [5], from Madrid, in 1988 described their experience in 25 patients older than 1 year; the mean peak gradient was reduced from 71 ± 33 to 25 ± 11 mmHg. There were no complications in 24 patients; however, in one patient they observed a dissecting aneurysm of the pulmonary artery, which required elective surgery. This complication is unusual, even with large balloon/anulus ratios. More recently, Portis et al. [13], from Barcelona, reported the 4 year echo-Doppler follow-up results obtained in 10 patients treated by pulmonary valvuloplasty.

VALVULAR AORTIC STENOSIS

Percutaneous aortic valvuloplasty for the treatment of aortic stenosis was first introduced in 1984 by Lababidi et al. [44]. Since then, several studies have confirmed the efficacy of this technique in reducing the gradient [45-50], with a low incidence of significant worsening of aortic regurgitation. Initial results seem to be better in pliable and bicommissural

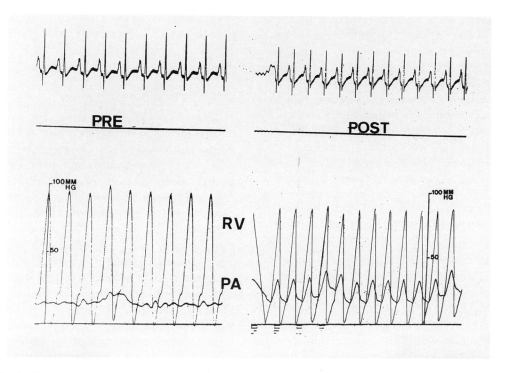

Fig. 3. Pressure tracings in a patient with pulmonary atresia with intact ventricular septum showing a phasic pulmonary artery pressure after perforation of the atretic valve and balloon valvuloplasty. PA, pulmonary artery; RV, right ventricle.

valves [47]. On the other hand, a balloon/annulus ratio greater than 1 is associated with a higher incidence of aortic insufficiency [47]. This method has also been successfully applied in children with restenosed aortic valves after previous surgery [49]. Similarly, the technique has been applied in neonates and infants with critical aortic stenosis [51–53].

The Cor-Pal Experience

Our experience with this treatment (1984–1990) was in 25 patients with congenital valvular aortic stenosis. Four of them were infants or neonates (mean age, 43 ± 83 days) with critical aortic stenosis and severe heart failure; two of them had an associated ventricular septal defect, and one had a combined aortic coarctation that was sequen-

tially dilated [54]. None of the infants survived.

The remaining 21 patients had better results. The ages ranged from 2 to 29 years (mean, 12 ± 6 years). Two of them (9.5%) had associated malformations (coarctation of aorta and mitral insufficiency). In one patient (5%) we performed a combined sequential dilatation of an associated coarctation of aorta. All patients were clinically and noninvasively studied prior to and following balloon valvuloplasty and at follow-up. Three patients (14%) had symptoms (effort dyspnea); the remaining 18 were asymptomatic.

Immediate Results

Following balloon valvuloplasty in children, the peak systolic pressure gradient across the aortic valve (93 ± 27 vs. 35 ± 23 mmHg; P < 0.0001) and the left ventricular peak systolic pressure (197 ± 36 vs. 141 ± 28 mmHg; P<0001) decreased significantly. The incidence of worsening of aortic regurgitation by more than one grade was 19% (4/21); however, one patient (5%) worsened to grade III. This incidence is similar to that observed by others [47–50].

Complications

Infants. One out of four infants died during the procedure following an irreversible cardiac arrest after balloon inflation; no causes of death, other than the severe cardiac abnormality itself, was found at necropsy. In the remaining three infants we obtained mild pressure reliefs that did not avoid the hospital mortality, irrespective of whether they had additional surgery (n = 2) or not (n = 1). This unfavorable experience in infants could be explained by two reasons: One is the severity of the condition itself, and the other is the lack of availability of large enough balloon diameters in low profile catheters to accomplish the procedure adequately. Nevertheless, other authors have reported good results in infants and neonates. In fact, in 38 infants in the American Registry [50] the initial survival rate was 87% compared with 43% observed in a recent surgical series [55]. Perhaps technical advances in catheter design may improve our results.

Children. No deaths occurred in children. A 19-year-old patient, without baseline aortic insufficiency, progressed to grade III after valvuloplasty; a retrospective analysis led us to suspect that this was a technical problem, induced by perforation of a cusp with a guidewire when trying to pass retrogradely into the left ventricle. Thus the inflation of the balloon was probably inadvertently made through this perforated leaflet. However, the patient tolerated the aortic insufficiency well and remains asymptomatic 24 months after valvuloplasty. Two other patients needed sur-

gery at the femoral artery puncture site because of thrombosis or pseudoaneurysm.

Follow-Up

Although initial results and clinical follow-up data are available from the literature [45,46], only a few studies have documented hemodynamic follow-ups [44,46,49,56]. The available information on the evolution of the aortic gradient (Doppler or hemodynamic) relates to a follow-up period that varied between 3 and 32 months in a total of 36 patients. In our series of 21 patients at clinical follow-ups of 3 months to 5 years (mean, 28 ± 17 months), all of them remained asymptomatic. Figure 4 shows the progression of the peak residual gradient (either Doppler or hemodynamic). As can be seen, no significant changes were observed in the degree of pressure gradient relief. Angiographic follow-up in nine patients also showed no significant changes in the degree of aortic regurgitation.

Technical Details

The technique has been described by Lababidi et al. [44]. In all pediatric patients the procedure was performed under mild anesthesia. After diagnostic procedures, heparin (100 IU/kg) was administered, and a single- or multiballoon catheter ranging in

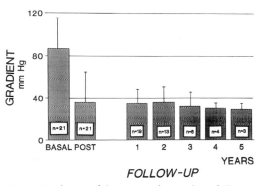

Fig. 4. Evolution of the aortic valve gradient following balloon valvuloplasty.

total diameter from 10 to 31 mm (mean, 22 ± 5 mm) was advanced over a guidewire across the aortic valve, where it was inflated until disappearance of the notch. We always tried to equate the balloon diameter to the angiographically measured aortic valve annulus size. The balloon/annulus ratio was 1 ± 0.3; however, this was not always possible to obtain in infants in whom the maximum balloon diameter available for use was 5 mm. The approach to the aortic valve was mostly retrograde, as described by Lababidi et al. [44], although in four patients we used the venoarterial circuit described by Babic et al. [57]. We also used an antegrade approach [58], through the venous route in one patient.

Physiopathology of Transient Systemic Occlusion

Transient left ventricular outflow occlusion is also well tolerated. During aortic valvuloplasty a dramatic decrease in systemic pressure coexists with significant increases in left ventricular and atrial pressures [33]. As with right ventricular occlusion, the left-sided occluded heart suddenly adapts by generating hypertensive and hypokinetic contractions, with mitral regurgitation. These acute situations may stimulate the homeostatic receptors involved in the immediate intravascular pressure and volume regulation. Abrupt releases of atrial natriuretic factor and vasopressin have been detected immediately after intracardiac occlusive periods in response to the acute and transient hemodynamic changes observed [59]. These extremely acute situations represent a potential model with which to investigate acute heart failure further.

Other Spanish Contributions

Macaya et al. [14] described their initial experience in three patients with severe aortic stenosis. The procedure was successful in two children and failed in one infant, probably secondary to undersized balloon. There were no complications. García-Aguado et al. [5],

from La Paz Hospital in Madrid, also reported their experience with six patients. Five of them were successfully relieved of their obstruction; one patient with an associated coarctation of the aorta was sequentially dilated. One procedure failed to decrease the gradient. Two patients had minor complications at the puncture site.

DISCRETE SUBAORTIC STENOSIS

Discrete subaortic stenosis has been considered a potentially progressive disease. Serial hemodynamic studies have shown that the left ventricular to aortic gradient usually increases over time in nonoperated patients. Besides, aortic regurgitation, infective endocarditis, and development of superimposed muscular obstruction can also complicate its natural course. Surgery is an effective and safe treatment. However, some operated patients may have residual gradients that require repeat outflow resection. Thus a method that could produce immediate and long-term relief of the subvalvular gradient at the time of cardiac catheterization could have substantial value.

Transluminal balloon dilatation for discrete subaortic stenosis was first described by our group in 1986 [16]. Since then, several studies have confirmed the initial good results in children and young adults [60–62]. Short-term follow-up studies have documented persistent gradient relief [16,60–62], and long-term results seem to be promising [63,64]. Better immediate results were observed in patients with smaller baseline gradients, a larger aortic annulus, and a larger valve-to-membrane distance [64].

The Cor-Pal Experience

From 1985 to 1990, we performed 33 dilatations in 27 patients. The ages ranged from 2 to 55 years (mean, 12 ± 9 years); 13 patients were younger than 12 years. Two patients had associated congenital mitral stenosis; both lesions were dilated in a sequential fashion [65]. Another patient who presented with an associated unoperated coarctation of the aorta was also sequentially dilated [54]. All patients underwent baseline noninvasive studies the day before cardiac catheterization. The mean Doppler gradient was 65 ± 28 mmHg. In most instances, a fixed subaortic membrane was clearly visualized by a two-dimensional echocardiogram. Quantitative left ventricular analysis was performed in every angiographic study; left ventricular volumes, mass, and ejection fraction were determined. The diastolic distance between the membrane and the aortic valve was measured. All values were corrected by body surface area.

Immediate Results

After balloon dilatation, the left ventricular to aortic peak-to-peak gradient decreased significantly, from 71 ± 32 to 21 ± 13 mmHg ($P < 0.001$); in one patient (3%) the gradient disappeared completely (Fig. 5), and in seven (26%) the immediate residual gradient was less than 10 mmHg. The mean percent gradient reduction was 67% + 21%. The left ventricular peak systolic pressure also decreased from 178 ± 33 to 143 ± 20 mmHg ($P < 0.01$). Angiographically, there were no significant changes in volumes and ejection fractions. No significant changes were observed in the degree of aortic regurgitation; in two patients it even disappeared after dilatation. In 23 patients a fluttering and widely mobile remaining membrane was clearly visualized after dilatation, suggesting membrane rupture (Fig. 6). The immediate residual gradient was lower in patients with a lesser baseline gradient ($P < 0.01$), larger annulus diameter ($P < 0.01$), and longer valve-to-membrane distance ($P < 0.01$). There were significant inverse correlations between the immediate residual gradient with the corrected annulus diameter ($r = -0.41$, $P < 0.05$) and with the valve-to-membrane distance ($r = -0.40$; $P < 0.05$).

Complications

One 8-year-old patient who had combined mitral valve and subaortic stenosis developed severe mitral regurgitation after mitral balloon valvuloplasty. He required surgery, which was performed 7 days later. Operative findings revealed a rupture of the anterior leaflet; the valve was replaced by a mechanical prosthesis, and the patient did well afterwards. The remaining 26 patients did not have major complications in 32 therapeutic procedures; three of them had a decreased femoral pulse at the puncture site without ischemic compromise. All patients without major complications (n = 32) were discharged within 2–6 days after a repeat noninvasive evaluation was performed.

Follow-Up

A close follow-up study was done on all patients. Serial echo-Doppler studies were available for 25 patients. We also performed 17 hemodynamic re-evaluations in 12 patients at a mean period of 26 ± 19 months after dilatation. A persistently dilated membrane was characterized by a fluttering and widely mobile structure in the outflow tract[16]. Restenosis was defined as the loss of 50% or more of the initial gain in the degree of pressure gradient relief. Six patients who demonstrated restenosis were redilated at a mean of 33 ± 19 months after the first attempt; in five of them redilation obtained similar benefits to those observed in the first attempt; 1 patient, in whom redilatation was unsuccessful, was operated on. Figure 7 shows the evolution of the mean residual gradient (either Doppler or hemodynamic) in nonrestenosed patients (upper panel). The evolution of the gradient in patients who restenosed is shown separately (lower panel). The only significant factor affecting the development of restenosis was the age [64]; 5 of 15 patients (33%) less than 12 years old restenosed, while only 1 of 18 patients (5%) older than 12 years did ($P < 0.05$). No

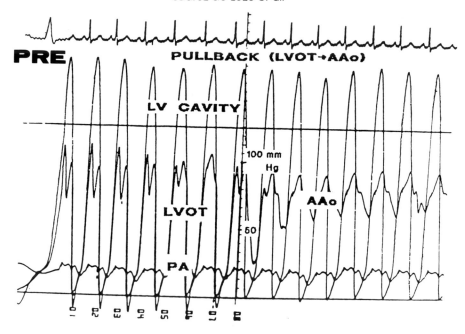

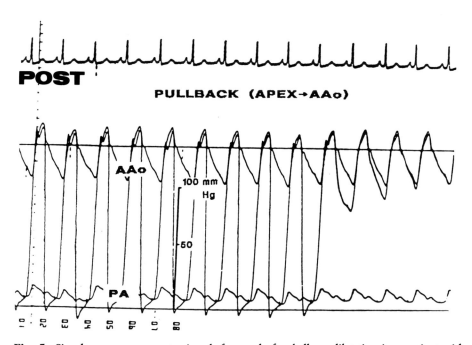

Fig. 5. Simultaneous pressure tracings before and after balloon dilatation in a patient with discrete subaortic stenosis. After the procedure, the gradient disappeared completely. AAo, ascending aorta; LV, left ventricle; OT, outflow tract; PA, pulmonary artery.

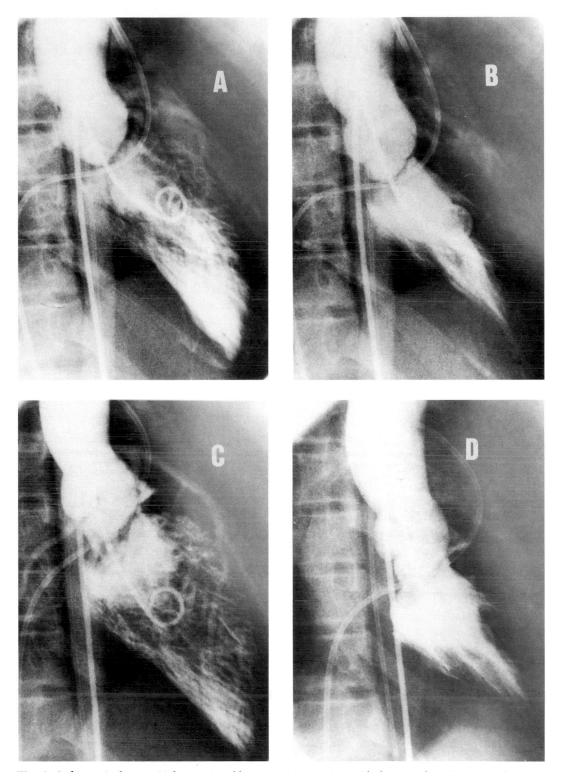

Fig. 6. Left ventriculogram (right anterior oblique view) in a patient with discrete subaortic stenosis showing a fixed membrane in diastole and systole (**A,B**), which became mobile and disrupted after dilatation (**C,D**)

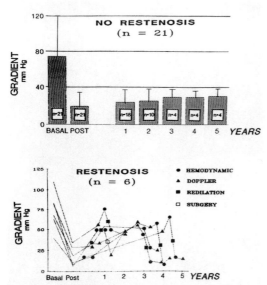

Fig. 7. Evolution of the mean gradient after dilatation in 27 patients with discrete subaortic stenosis. **Top:** No restenosis. **Bottom:** Restenosis.

who presented with aortic valve endocarditis complicating a severe discrete subaortic stenosis. At surgery, once the aortic valve was removed we performed an intraoperative balloon dilatation of the membrane which produced rupture, rather than stretching, of the fibrous structure (Fig. 8).

What subsequent anatomic changes in the torn and widely mobile membrane occur remains unknown. However, the pressure relief persists in most patients (78%) at a mean follow-up of 15 ± 15 months after dilatation. Restenosis can also occur (22%), as can happen in surgical patients. The persistent turbulence derived from residual stenosis could provoke recurrence of fixed subaortic obstruction. Interestingly, in our six restenosed patients the anatomic features of the membrane were similar to those observed at the first attempt. This suggests that restenosis may result from regrowth of fibrous tissue.

relevant changes were observed at late follow-up in the degree of aortic regurgitation, as assessed by either Doppler or angiography. The mass/volume ratio in re-evaluated patients was not significantly different from that observed in baseline conditions. The mean last documented residual gradient in 26 patients (either redilated or not) was 23 ± 9 mmHg after a mean period of 20 ± 18 months following the first dilatation.

Mechanism and Pathology

Two possible mechanisms may explain the pressure gradient relief obtained after balloon dilatation. First is stretching of the stenotic orifice [61], and the other is tearing of the fibrous tissue [60]. Our observations suggest that the latter mechanism seems to be applicable in most patients. After dilatation, the fixed subaortic structure becomes widely mobile and fluttering, in accordance with blood flow, thus relieving the subaortic obstruction. We could confirm this suspected mechanism in a surgical patient 22 years old

Technical Details

The technique has been previously described [16]. After diagnostic procedures, heparin (100 IU/kg) was administered, and a single or multiballoon catheter, ranging in total diameter from 15 to 38 mm, was retrogradely advanced into the left ventricular cavity over a long guidewire. Then the balloon was inflated until the notch disappeared. The guidewire was previously placed in the ventricle through a retrogradely advanced endhole catheter in 23 instances; in the remaining 10 instances the guidewire was passed through a venous catheter advanced transseptally to the left atrium, left ventricle, and aorta, where the guidewire was snared out of the body through the left femoral artery, as described by Babic et al. [57]. This venoarterial guidewire circuit allowed a much better stabilization of the balloon during inflation, and it also permitted a fast sequential dilatation of an associated mitral valve stenosis. Balloon size selection was based on the angiographically measured aortic annulus diameter. This required the balloon diameter to be almost identical to the aortic ring or even slightly greater when the pressure relief obtained was inadequate. The mean balloon/annulus ratio was 1.14 ± 0.1.

Clinical Implications

Our experience shows that balloon dilatation of discrete subaortic stenosis is a safe and effective procedure for reducing the left ventricular to aortic gradient, without substantial worsening of aortic valve competence. However, a close follow-up of these patients is needed, because some of them may require redilation or surgical resection. Since the clinical follow-up time (24 ± 19 months) of our series is shorter than the mean restenosis time, it is possible that some patients may develop restenosis with continued follow-up. Consequently, larger series studied over longer periods of time are needed to determine the long-term effectiveness of this treatment modality in the course of the disease.

COARCTATION OF AORTA

Following different experimental observations [66,67], Singer et al. [68] were the first to attempt balloon angioplasty in a newborn with severe coarctation of aorta. After this, several reports confirmed the efficacy of the procedure in reducing the gradient and the percentage angiographic stenosis, not only in native coarctation but also in restenosis after previous surgery [69]. In severely ill infants or neonates the pressure relief obtained is not usually maintained, but the procedure palliates hypertension and heart failure until better conditions for repair ensue [2]. In most children and adults balloon angioplasty can provide more prolonged relief than is documented for infants [70–75]. However, restenosis or a persistently high residual gradient at follow-up have also been detected [70,72,76]. Several factors may influence the residual gradient. The size of the isthmus may play a role [76]. Besides, the discrete type of coarctation and the induc-

tion of intimal tear are associated with lower residual gradient at follow-up [77]. On the other hand, there is generalized concern about the long-term anatomic changes in the aortic wall. Uncontrolled damage of the aorta may lead to aneurysm formation at the site of dilatation. The incidence of this long-term finding is not well known, and wide differences in frequency have been reported [71,74,77,78].

The Cor-Pal Experience

From 1982 to 1990, we have studied 75 patients with coarctation of aorta who were treated by balloon angioplasty. Thirty of them were infants (n = 10) or neonates (n = 20) in critical condition and with a high incidence of associated malformations (83%); the mean age at treatment for this group was 43 ± 57 days. The remaining 45 patients were children (n = 27) and adults (n = 18), with a mean age of 14 ± 8 years and a 20% incidence of associated lesions; all 45 presented with systemic hypertension, one with dyspnea and one with rupture of a cerebral aneurysm. Two patients had had previous surgery for coarctation; in the remaining 73 the coarctation had not been surgically treated. Three patients (4%) with combined stenotic lesions were sequentially dilated [54].

Immediate Results

Neonates and infants. Following angioplasty the mean transcoarctation gradient (52 ± 30 vs. 13 ± 20 mmHg; P < 0.001) and the left ventricular endiastolic pressure (17 ± 8 vs. 13 ± 5 mmHg; P < 0.05) decreased significantly. The angiographic percentage of stenosis was significantly reduced (67% ± 8% to 31% ± 14%; P < 0.001). In some patients, the stenosis disappeared completely (Fig. 9). This was associated with marked clinical improvements in 25 patients (83%); femoral pulses appeared in all of them. Five neonates died within a few days after angioplasty, two of them had had additional surgery.

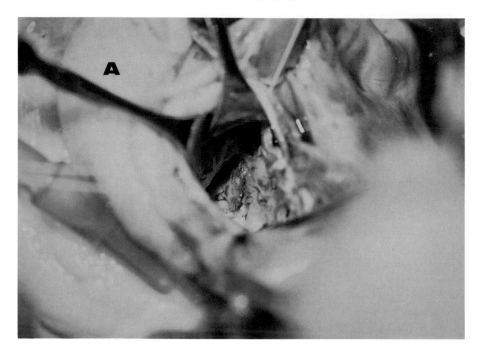

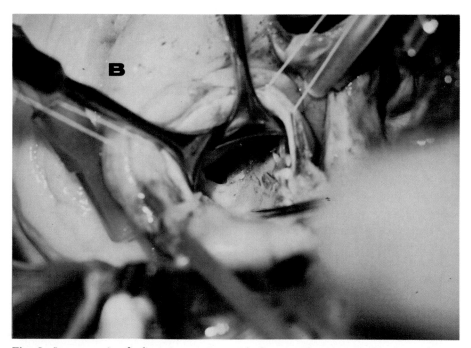

Fig. 8. Intraoperative findings in a patient with discrete subaortic stenosis who underwent balloon dilatation after resection of an infected aortic valve. Subaortic membrane before **(A)** and after **(B)** dilatation. Balloon inflated in the outflow tract **(C)**. After this, the membrane was also resected **(D)**.

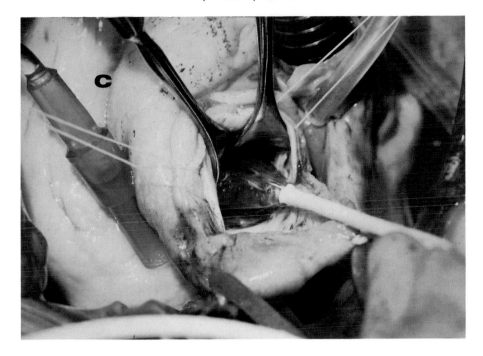

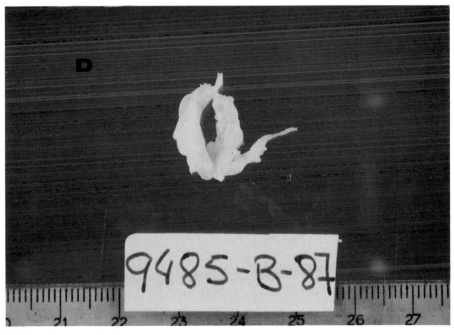

Fig. 8. *(Continued)*

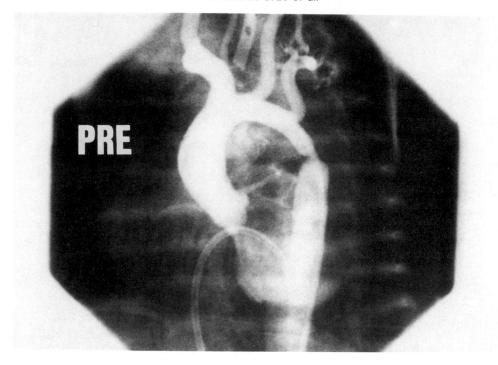

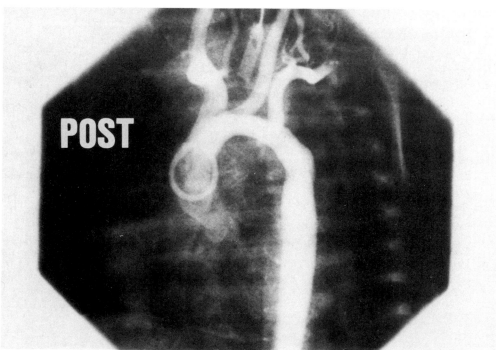

Fig. 9. Aortic angiograms before and after balloon angioplasty in a neonate with coarctation of the aorta.

Children and adults. Significant decreases in the peak-to-peak gradient (52 ± 18 vs. 9 ± 10 mmHg; P < 0.001) and the percent stenosis (69% ± 13% vs. 30% ± 15%; P < 0.0001) were also observed in this group. Angiographic intimal tears were identified in 15 patients (33%), although no further evidence of damaged aorta was detected at this time.

Complications

Neonates and infants. The mortality rate associated with the procedure was 5/30 (17%). Causes of death were ventricular fibrillation in one patient [2], refractory heart failure in two patients [54], and death after surgical intervention in two. Unexpected ventricular fibrillation in the hours following angioplasty was a frequent (10%) event in our experience. At the puncture site, the femoral pulse was poor in four patients, but no ischemic compromise appeared.

Children and adults. No patients died in this group. One (2%) had a brain embolism after angioplasty; three others (7%) had absent femoral pulses. Paradoxal hypertension appeared in nine (20%) patients within the first 24 hours after angioplasty. This was always immediately treated with antihypertensive agents to reduce the stretch on the dilated aortic wall and to prevent postcoarctectomy syndrome. Systemic blood pressures decreased and stabilized in all nine of them.

Follow-Up

All patients were closely followed. Figure 10 shows the observed actuarial event-free probabilities after angioplasty in both groups of patients.

Neonates and infants. Restenosis developed in all patients sooner or later, although the recurrence was not associated with heart failure. Fifteen patients were successfully operated on in stable conditions at a mean age of 8 ± 7 months; none of them died at operation or have restenosed since then. Two patients were effectively redilated 24 months later and

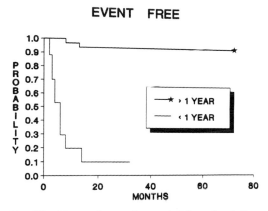

Fig. 10. Observed event-free probability after balloon angioplasty of coarctation of the aorta.

persist without further restenosis 51 and 22 months thereafter, respectively. Restenosis with normal weight curve was observed in the other eight patients, who remain asymptomatic under medical treatment 16 ± 13 months after angioplasty.

Children and adults. All patients remain asymptomatic and without hypertension 40 ± 20 months later; 27 patients (60%) were angiographically revaluated 11 ± 5 months after angioplasty. The residual gradient at that time varied between 0 and 40 mmHg (mean 9 ± 11 mmHg). One patient who had a persistently high residual gradient was operated on. No restenosis was detected in the remaining patients. Factors favorably influencing residual gradient were the discrete type of coarctation and angiographically identified intimal tear immediately after angioplasty. However, in our patients the size of the isthmus did not affect the residual gradient at follow-up. Small aneurysm formation at the site of dilatation was identified in four patients (9%). One of them was surgically repaired; at operation a complete rupture of the media progressing into a saccular aneurysm was observed [79]. The remaining three persist under close follow-up and have not been sent to surgery; two of them have been serially re-evaluated, and no angiographic evidence of progression was detected at 23 and

Suárez de Lezo *et al.*

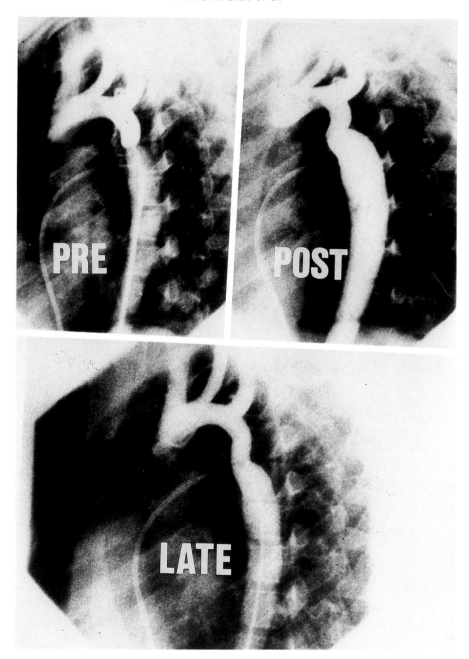

Fig. 11. Serial aortograms after balloon angioplasty in a patient with coarctation showing late realignment.

35 months, respectively, after angioplasty. On the other hand, changes in configuration of the aortic arch were clearly noted in 11 patients (42%). Our quantitative observations on serial aortograms [77,80] suggest that flow-dependent configuration changes may develop in the aorta after angioplasty, leading in some patients to realignment over time (Fig. 11).[3]

Technical Details

The coarctation was passed retrogradely. Diagnostic procedures always included hemodynamic and cardiac output measurements and left ventricular and aortic angiograms. After this, a single balloon catheter was retrogradely advanced over a guidewire previously positioned in the ascending aorta. The balloons ranged in diameter from 3 to 20 mm. Selection of balloon diameter was always based on angiographic measurements of the mean value between isthmic and distal aortic diameter (descending aorta distal to the poststenotic dilation). To avoid pain during angioplasty, mild anesthesia was applied at that point. To minimize the risk of hemorrhagic damage in the dilated aortic wall, we did not administer heparin. The balloon was placed across the stenotic area, and one or two balloon inflations were performed. Once the notch disappeared, the balloon catheter was rapidly exchanged over the guidewire with a diagnostic catheter. A repeat hemodynamic and angiographic evaluation was then performed.

Other Spanish Contributions

Following the initial description of Pérez Martínez et al. [1] on their experience in two infants, the group from Granada reported their acute results in 12 patients [4]; 11 were infants and one was 19 years old. No major complications occurred. The gradient decreased significantly. Three infants needed surgery later; in two additional patients restenosis was detected 2 months later. García-Aguado et al. [5] also reported 26 angioplasty procedures in 23 patients; 15 had native coarctation, and 11 were restenosis after previous surgery. In one patient with combined aortic stenosis a two-level sequential dilatation was performed. In native coarctation an adequate pressure relief was obtained in 11 patients, while in operated coarctation the procedure was effective in six. Minor complications at the puncture site were observed in two patients.

In conclusion, we think that the Spanish experience with balloon valvuloplasty/angioplasty procedures is extensive, began early, and has yielded results similar to those described in the literature.

REFERENCES

1. Pérez Martínez VM, García-Aguado A, Moreno Granados F, Castro Gusoni NC, Burgueros M (1983): Angioplastia transluminal con catéter de Gruntzig en la coartación de aorta. Rev Esp Cardiol 36:341–344.
2. Suárez de Lezo J, Fernández R, Sancho M, et al. (1984): Percutaneous transluminal angioplasty for aortic isthmic coarctation in infancy. Am J Cardiol 54:1147–1149.
3. Suárez de Lezo J, Herrera N, Sancho M, et al (1984): Angioplastia transluminal percutánea en la coartación aórtica del adulto. Rev Esp Cardiol 37:445–447.
4. Macaya C, Pérez de la Cruz JM, Prieto et al (1985): Tratamiento de la coartación aortica mediante angioplastia transluminal con catéter balón: Experiencia en 12 pacientes. Rev Esp Cardiol 38:415–420.
5. García-Aguado A, Benito Bartolomé F, Fernández-Ruiz A, et al. (1988): Angioplastia y valvuloplastia transluminal percutánea en diversas cardiopatías congénitas: Experiencia en 65 casos. Rev Esp Cardiol 41:223–232.
6. Ubago JLM, Figueroa A, Colman T, et al. (1984):

---

[3]Editor's note: For other types of remodelling of aorta after successful balloon angioplasty, the reader is referred to Rao and Carey (J Am Coll Cardiol 14:1312–1317, 1989) and to Chapter 10 (this volume).

Valvuloplastia pulmonar percutánea con catéter balón. Rev Esp Cardiol 37:354-358.

7. Suárez de Lezo J, Franco M, Concha M, et al (1985): Valvuloplastia transluminal en la estenosis pulmonar. Rev Esp Cardiol 38:213-217.

8. Macaya C, Pérez de la Cruz JM, Prieto J, et al. (1985): Valvuloplastia transluminal percutánea con catéter balón en la estenosis congénita de la válvula pulmonar. Rev Esp Cardiol 38:408-414.

9. Medina A, Bethencourt A, Coello I et al (1986): Valvuloplastia pulmonar con doble balón en la estenosis valvular pulmonar. Rev Esp Cardiol 39:199-202.

10. Medina A, Bethencourt A, Olalla E, et al. (1989): Intraoperative balloon valvuloplasty in pulmonary valve stenosis. Cardiovasc Intervent Radiol 12:199-201.

11. Melgares R, Prieto JA, Azpitarte J (1991): Success determining factors in percutaneous transluminal balloon valvuloplasty of pulmonary valve stenosis. Eur Heart J 12:15-23.

12. Suárez de Lezo J, Medina A, Pan M, et al. (1991): Papel de la valvuloplastia percutánea en enfermedades valvulares congénitas. Rev Esp Cardiol 44:35-50.

13. Portis MT, Esplugas E, García del Castillo H, Jara F (1990): Valvuloplastia pulmonar en el adolescente y el adulto: seguimiento a los dos años mediante Doppler continuo. Rev Esp Cardiol 43:619-623.

14. Macaya C, Santalla A, Pérez de la Cruz JM, et al. (1985): Valvuloplastia transluminal percutánea con catéter balón en la estenosis congénita de la válvula aórtica. Rev Esp Cardiol 38:396-399.

15. Suárez de Lezo J, Pan M, Herrera N, et al. (1985): Descompresión ventricular izquierda por vía transluminal en la estenosis aórtica congénita. Rev Esp Cardiol 38:400-407.

16. Suárez de Lezo J, Pan M, Sancho M, et al. (1986): Percutaneous transluminal balloon dilatation for discrete subaortic stenosis. Am J Cardiol 58:619-621.

17. Suárez de Lezo J, Concha M, Herrera N, et al. (1986): Paliación transluminal en cardiopatias con isquemia pulmonar e hipoxemia. Rev Esp Cardiol 39:296-302.

18. Descalzo A, Santos J (1991): Angioplastia con balón de fístulas de Blalock-Taussig estenosadas. Presentación de 4 casos. Rev Esp Cardiol 44:127-130.

19. Suárez de Lezo J, López Rubio F, Guzmán J, et al. (1985): Percutaneous transluminal angioplasty of stenotic ductus arteriosus. Cathet Cardiovasc Diagn 11:493-500.

20. Kan JS, White RI, Michell SE, Gardner TJ (1982): Percutaneous balloon valvuloplasty: A new method for treating congenital pulmonary valve stenosis. N Engl J Med 370:540-543.

21. Lababidi S, Wu JR (1983): Percutaneous balloon pulmonary valvuloplasty. Am J Cardiol 52:560-562.

22. Kan JS, White RI, Mitchell SE, et al. (1984): Percutaneous transluminal balloon valvuloplasty for pulmonary valve stenosis. Circulation 69:554-560.

23. Kveselis DA, Rocchini AP, Snider AP, et al. (1985): Results of balloon valvuloplasty in the treatment of congenital valvar pulmonary stenosis in children. Am J Cardiol 56:527-532.

24. Sullivan ID, Robinson PJ, Macartney FJ, et al. (1985): Percutaneous pulmonary valvuloplasty for pulmonary valve stenosis in infants and children. Br Heart J 54:435-441.

25. Schmaltz AA, Bein G, Grävinghoff L, et al. (1989): Balloon valvuloplasty for pulmonary stenosis in infants and children: Cooperative study of the German Society of Pediatric Cardiology. Eur Heart J 10:967-971.

26. Stanger P, Cassidy SC, Girod DA, et al. (1990): Balloon pulmonary valvuloplasty: Results of the valvuloplasty and angioplasty of congenital anomalies registry. Am J Cardiol 65:775-783.

27. Herrera N, Suárez de Lezo J, Sancho M, et al. (1985): Valvuloplastia pulmonar. Resultados a corto y medio plazo, abstracted. Rev Esp Cardiol 38(II):7.

28. Rao PS, Fawzy ME, Solymar L, Mardini MK (1988): Long-term results of balloon pulmonary valvuloplasty of valvar pulmonic stenosis. Am Heart J 115:1291-1296.

29. Rao PS (1988): Balloon dilatation in infants and children with dysplastic pulmonary valves: Short-term and intermediate-term results. Am Heart J 116:1168-1173.

30. Romero M, Jiménez F, Pan M, et al. (1990): Balloon angioplasty for discrete supravalvular pulmonary stenosis, abstracted. Eur Heart J 11:231.

31. Rao PS (1988): How big a balloon and how many balloons for pulmonary valvuloplasty? Am Heart J 116:577-580.

32. Al Kasab S, Ribeiro P, Al Zaibag M (1987): Use of a double balloon technique for percutaneous balloon pulmonary valvotomy in adults. Br Heart J 58:136-141.

33. Suárez de Lezo J, Pan M, Romero M, et al. (1988): Physiopathology of transient ventricular occlusion during balloon valvuloplasty for pulmonic or aortic stenosis. Am J Cardiol 61:436-440.

34. Boucek MM, Webster HE, Orsmond GS, Ruttenberg HD (1988): Balloon pulmonary valvuloplasty: Palliation for cyanotic heart disease. Am Heart J 115:318-322.

35. Rao PS, Brais M (1988): Balloon pulmonary valvuloplasty for congenital cyanotic heart defects. Am Heart J 115:1105-1113.

36. García Fernández E, Marañon R, Maroto C, et al.

(1991): Valvuloplastia pulmonar en niños con cardiopatías cianóticas. Rev Esp Cardiol 44:115-118.

37. Fisher DR, Park SC, Neches WH, et al. (1985): Successful dilatation of a stenotic Blalock-Taussig anastomosis by percutaneous transluminal balloon angioplasty. Am J Cardiol 55:861-862.

38. Kirklin JW, Pacifico AD (1978): Surgical treatment of congenital heart disease. In Hurst JW (ed): "The Heart, Arteries and Veins." New York: McGraw-Hill Book Company, pp 901-947.

39. Rowe RD, Freedom RM, Mehrizi A, Bloom KB (1981): Pulmonary atresia with intact interventricular septum. In Rowe RD, Freedom RM, Mehrizi A, Bloom KB (eds): "The Neonate With Congenital Heart Disease." Philadelphia: WB Saunders Company, pp 371-400.

40. Rudolf AM (1979): Pulmonary stenosis and atresia with intact ventricular septum. In Rudolf AM (ed): "Congenital Diseases of the Heart." Chicago: Year Book Medical Publishers Inc, pp 360-400.

41. Kirklin JW, Barrat-Boyes BG (1986): Pulmonary atresia with intact ventricular septum. In Kirklin JW, Barrat-Boyes BG (eds): "Cardiac Surgery." New York: John Wiley & Sons, pp 843-856.

42. Qureshi SA, Rosenthal E, Tynan M, et al. (1991): Transcatheter laser-assisted balloon pulmonary valve dilatation in pulmonic valve atresia. Am J Cardiol 67:428-431.

43. Latson LA (1991): Nonsurgical treatment of a neonate with pulmonary atresia and intact ventricular septum by transcatheter puncture and balloon dilation of the atretic valve membrane. Am J Cardiol 68:277-279.

44. Lababidi Z, Ku JR, Walls JT (1984): Percutaneous balloon aortic valvuloplasty: Results in 23 patients. Am J Cardiol 53:194-197.

45. Choy M, Beekman RH, Rocchini AP, et al. (1987): Percutaneous balloon valvuloplasty for valvar aortic stenosis in infants and children. Am J Cardiol 59:1010-1012.

46. Helgason H, Keane JF, Fellows KE, et al. (1987): Balloon dilatation of the aortic valve: Studies in normal lambs and in children with aortic stenosis. J Am Coll Cardiol 9:816-822.

47. Sholler GF, Keane JF, Perry SB, et al. (1988): Balloon dilation of congenital aortic valve stenosis: Results and influence of technical and morphological features on outcome. Circulation 78:351-360.

48. Beekman RH, Rocchini AP, Crowley DC, et al. (1988): Comparison of single and double balloon valvuloplasty in children with aortic stenosis. J Am Coll Cardiol 12:480-485.

49. Meliones JN, Beekman RH, Rocchini AP, Lacina SJ (1989): Balloon valvuloplasty for recurrent aortic stenosis after surgical valvotomy in childhood: Im-mediate and follow-up studies. J Am Coll Cardiol 13:1106-1110.

50. Rocchini AP, Beekman RH, Ben Schachar G, et al. (1990): Balloon aortic valvuloplasty: Results of the valvuloplasty and angioplasty of congenital anomalies registry. Am J Cardiol 65:784-789.

51. Rupprath G, Neuhaus KL (1985): Percutaneous balloon aortic valvuloplasty in infancy and childhood. Am J Cardiol 55:1855-1856.

52. Lababidi Z, Weinhaus L (1986): Successful balloon valvuloplasty for neonatal critical aortic stenosis. Am Heart J 112:913-916.

53. Wren C, Sullivan I, Ball C, Deanfield J (1987): Percutaneous balloon dilatation of aortic valve stenosis in neonates and infants. Br Heart J 58:608-612.

54. Pan M, Suárez de Lezo J, Herrera N, et al. (1987): Two-level left ventricular outflow balloon dilation: Sequential therapeutic approach. Am Heart J 114:162-165.

55. Pelech A, Dyck J, Freedom R, et al. (1984): Critical aortic stenosis in the neonate: Survival and management, abstracted. Circulation 70(Suppl II):II-132.

56. Rao PS (1989): Balloon dilatation in infants and children with cardiac defects. Cathet Cardiovasc Diagn 18:136-149.

57. Babic UU, Pejcic P, Djurisic Z, et al. (1986): Percutaneous transarterial balloon valvuloplasty for mitral valve stenosis. Am J Cardiol 57:1101-1104.

58. Medina A, Bethencourt A, Coello I, et al. (1989): Valvuloplastia aórtica utilizando la ruta transatrial en la estenosis valvular aórtica. Rev Esp Cardiol 42:274-277.

59. Suárez de Lezo J, Montilla P, Pan M, et al. (1989): Abrupt homeostatic responses to transient intracardiac occlusion during balloon valvuloplasty. Am J Cardiol 64:491-497.

60. Lababidi Z, Weinhaus I, Stoeckle H, Walls JT (1987): Transluminal balloon dilatation for discrete subaortic stenosis. Am J Cardiol 59:423-425.

61. Feldman T, Chiu C, Carroll, JD (1987): Catheter balloon dilatation for discrete subaortic stenosis in the adult. Am J Cardiol 60:403-405.

62. Arora R, Goel PK, Lochan R, et al. (1988): Percutaneous transluminal balloon dilatation in discrete subaortic stenosis. Am Heart J 116:1091-1092.

63. Suárez de Lezo J, Medina A, Pan M, et al. (1990): Long-term results after balloon dilation for discrete subaortic stenosis, abstracted. Circulation 82:583.

64. Suárez de Lezo J, Pan M, Medina A, et al. (1991): Immediate and follow-up results after transluminal balloon dilatation for discrete subaortic stenosis. J Am Coll Cardiol 18:1309-1315.

65. Medina A, Bethencourt A, Coello I, et al. (1989): Combined percutaneous mitral and aortic balloon valvuloplasty. Am J Cardiol 64:620-624.

66. Sos T, Sniderman KW, Rettek-Sos B, *et al.* (1979): Percutaneous transluminal dilatation of coarctation of thoracic aorta post-mortem. Lancet 2:970–971.

67. Lock JE, Niemi T, Burke B, *et al.* (1982): Transcutaneous angioplasty of experimental aortic coarctation. Circulation 66:1280–1286.

68. Singer MI, Rowen M, Dorsey TJ (1982): Transluminal aortic balloon angioplasty for coarctation of the aorta in the newborn. Am Heart J 103:131–132.

69. Kan JS, White RI, Mitchell SE, *et al.* (1983): Treatment of restenosis of coarctation by percutaneous transluminal angioplasty. Circulation 68:1087–1094.

70. Lababidi Z, Daskalopoulos D, Stoeckle H (1984): Balloon coarctation angioplasty: Experience with 27 patients. Am J Cardiol 54:1288–1291.

71. Allen HD, Marx GR, Ovitt TW, Goldberg SJ (1986): Balloon dilation angioplasty for coarctation of aorta. Am J Cardiol 57:828–832.

72. Cooper RS, Ritter SB, Rothe WB, *et al.* (1987): Angioplasty for coarctation of the aorta: Long-term results. Circulation 75:600–604.

73. Kan JS, White RI, Mitchell SE, *et al.* (1983): Treatment of restenosis of coarctation by percutaneous transluminal angioplasty. Circulation 68:1087–1094.

74. Saul JP, Keane JF, Fellows KE, Lock JE (1987): Balloon dilation angioplasty of postoperative aortic obstructions. Am J Cardiol 59:943–948.

75. Morrow WR, Vick GW III, Nihill MR, *et al.* (1988): Balloon dilatation of unoperated coarctation of the aorta: Short- and intermediate-term results. J Am Coll Cardiol 11:133–138.

76. Rao PS, Thapar MK, Kutayli F, Carey P (1989): Causes of recoarctation after balloon angioplasty of unoperated aortic coarctation. J Am Coll Cardiol 13:109–115.

77. Suárez de Lezo J, Sancho M, Pan M, *et al.* (1989): Angiographic follow-up after balloon angioplasty for coarctation of aorta. J Am Coll Cardiol 13:689–695.

78. Wren C, Peart I, Bain H, Hunter S (1987): Balloon dilatation of unoperated aortic coarctation: Immediate results and one year follow-up. Br Heart J 58:369–373.

79. Medina A, Bethencourt A, Coello I, *et al.* (1987): Cirugía tras dilatación transluminal en la coartación aórtica por la formación de un aneurisma. Rev Esp Cardiol 40:216–219.

80. Pavlovic DJ, Suárez de Lezo J, Medina A, *et al.* (1992): Sequential transcatheter treatment of combined coarctation of aorta and persistent ductus arteriosus. Am Heart J 123:249–250.

23

Conclusions and Future Directions

P. Syamasundar Rao, M.D.

Department of Pediatrics, Division of Pediatric Cardiology,
University of Wisconsin Medical School, University of Wisconsin
Children's Hospital, Madison, Wisconsin 53792-4108

The conventional treatment option for congenital or acquired lesions of the heart is surgical correction. Since the early 1950s, concurrent with the development of surgical techniques, investigators have attempted to replace the more invasive surgical techniques with less invasive transcatheter treatment modes. In 1953 and 1954, Rubio-Alvarez and his colleagues described a technique by which pulmonary and tricuspid valve stenoses could be relieved via a catheter; they used a ureteral catheter with a wire. A decade later, Dotter and Judkins introduced a gradual dilatation technique to open up stenotic atherosclerotic lesions of the peripheral arteries. In the next decade, Grüntzig and his coworkers extended these principles and developed a double-lumen catheter with a nonelastic balloon and used it to dilate stenotic lesions of the iliac, popliteal, femoral, renal, and coronary arteries. Shortly thereafter, in 1982, Kan and her associates extended these dilatation techniques to children with pulmonary valve stenosis. This appears to have produced a rapid increase in the use of balloon dilatation techniques in the pediatric patient. Concurrent with the development of these techniques, other investigators attempted either to open or to close cardiac septal defects. In 1966, Rashkind and Miller described a dynamic balloon dilatation technique to enlarge the patent foramen ovale. This life-saving technique was extensively used in neonates with transposition of the great arteries. For patients in whom this balloon

septostomy technique is not adequate, Park et al. developed a blade septostomy technique. This is useful in older infants and children and in patients with thick interatrial septae. Porstmann (1967), King (1976), Rashkind (1979, 1983), and their associates, on the other hand, developed devices that could be deployed via catheters and occlude atrial and ventricular septal defects and patent ductus arteriosus. These initial historic attempts have been followed by clinical trials and refinement of techniques by many investigators around the world.

Rashkind's balloon atrial septostomy has been used extensively in the palliation of the neonate with complete transposition of the great arteries. The improved mixing at the atrial level allowed the transposition patients to grow up to an age and size at which a venous switch procedure (Mustard or Senning) could safely be performed. Since the advent and extensive use of the arterial switch procedure (Jatene) in the early neonatal period, balloon septostomy has not been used as extensively as in the past. But, this procedure is still useful in temporizing a sick, hypoxemic, and acidotic neonate. It is also used for palliation if the arterial switch procedure cannot be performed on an urgent basis. The septostomy technique is also useful in the management of other conditions such as tricuspid or mitral atresia, hypoplastic right or left heart syndrome, and total anomalous pulmonary venous connection, all with interatrial obstruction. Balloon

Transcatheter Therapy in Pediatric Cardiology, pages 493–501
© 1993 Wiley-Liss, Inc.

atrial septostomy is the initial procedure of choice in all situations in which an adequate interatrial communication is deemed necessary.

While the balloon atrial septostomy is generally successful, it does fail to create an adequate interatrial opening in some patients. By and large, this appears to be related to a thick interatrial septum, especially in older infants and children. To circumvent this problem, Park developed a blade septostomy catheter that can be utilized to cut (literally) the interatrial septum, which is then followed up by balloon atrial septostomy to enlarge the atrial defect further. The majority of time the procedure is carried out through an open, but restrictive, atrial defect. However, the procedure can also be performed in patients with an intact atrial septum following transseptal puncture. Park's initial clinical trials, collaborative studies, and experience reported by multiple other workers around the world have demonstrated that the method is feasible, effective, and safe. Attention to details of the technique and biplane fluoroscopy are essential to the safety and success of the procedure.

The technique of balloon angioplasty/valvuloplasty used in relieving obstructive lesions is reasonably well standardized. The indications for employing these procedures are similar to those used for surgical intervention. Obtaining informed consent from the parents and/or patient is essential. An intravenous line and type and cross-match for blood are generally required. Surgical stand-by is generally not recommended. We perform the procedure with sedation of the patient with a mixture of meperidine, promethazine, and chlorpromazine (supplemented with intermittent doses of midazolam), while a limited number of interventional pediatric cardiologists use ketamine or general anesthesia. The procedure involves positioning a balloon dilatation catheter across the site of obstruction and inflating it. Sequential balloon inflation with 3, 4, and 5 atm of pressure of 5 second duration, 5 minutes apart is recommended. Higher inflation pressures

may be used if the balloon catheter manufacturer states that higher pressures are tolerated by the balloon. Appropriate choice of balloon size remains critical to achieving good results and preventing complications. Further miniaturization of balloon/catheter systems and meticulous attention to the details of the technique are necessary for successful relief of obstruction and the reduction of complication rates. Limited applications of newer transcatheter technologies, such as double-blade valvotomy, laser, and atherectomy catheter device, have been reported in the treatment of children with heart disease.

While the interventional cardiologist does not need to become a physicist, some understanding of the catheter and balloon material, dilating forces of the balloon, and implications of use of different sizes, types, and numbers of balloons is necessary to optimize the effects of balloon dilatation procedures. The effects of complete but transient obstruction to blood flow during balloon inflation are minimal and are well tolerated by most patients. Minimizing adverse effects of such obstruction while maximizing the benefits of radial forces of balloon dilatation is the key to the success of the balloon dilatation procedures. The response of the stenotic site depends not only on the radial forces of balloon dilatation but also on the morphology and pathologic process of the lesion being dilated. Commissural splitting is the most frequently observed response following balloon valvuloplasty. However, valve tears and dehiscence of valve leaflets have also been reported. These latter effects are likely to be problematic when aortic or mitral valves are the sites of damage. Such adverse effects may be secondary to unicommissural valve or related to the technique of valvuloplasty. Disruption of intimal and medial layers of the aortic wall appears to be the mechanism of action of controlled injury by balloon dilation of aortic coarctation.

Pulmonary valve stenosis is one of the first congenital stenotic lesions to be balloon dilated and is one of the first for which balloon valvuloplasty is generally accepted as a therapeutic procedure of choice. There is some difference of opinion as to the indications for balloon therapy. I believe that indications for balloon intervention should be similar to those for surgery. A moderate degree of pulmonary valve obstruction with a gradient ≥ 50 mmHg and a normal cardiac index are what I would require for considering balloon intervention. Previous surgery, mild pulmonary valve dysplasia, and Noonan syndrome are not contraindications for balloon valvuloplasty. Excellent relief of obstruction of valve stenosis by pulmonary balloon valvuloplasty has been documented in neonates, infants, children, and adults. Immediate and intermediate-term results are available, but there are limited long-term follow-up data. Electrocardiographic and echo-Doppler evaluations at follow-up are reflective of the results; recatheterization may not be necessary to evaluate results. The results of balloon valvuloplasty are either comparable with or better than those reported with surgical valvotomy. Complications of the procedure are minimal. The causes of restenosis have been identified, and appropriate modification of the technique, particularly use of a balloon/annulus ratio of 1.2–1.5, may produce better results than previously documented. Infundibular reaction may be present in older patients and in patients with severe obstruction and can most often be treated with adequate valvuloplasty and β-blocking drugs, with rare need for surgery. Further miniaturization of the balloon/catheter systems, further refinements of the procedure, and meticulous attention to details of the technique may further increase the success rate and decrease the complication rate. Documentation of favorable results for 5–10 years following balloon dilatation is necessary. Balloon pulmonary valvuloplasty is an excellent alternative to open or closed heart surgery in most, if not all, patients with pulmonary stenosis.

Balloon valvuloplasty was initially utilized for aortic stenosis by Lababidi, but has not been used as frequently as balloon pulmonary valvuloplasty. Several workers have utilized it for relief of aortic valve obstruction in neonates, infants, children, and adults. Immediate and intermediate-term results have produced reduction of aortic valve gradients by 60% of prevalvuloplasty valves. Previous surgical valvotomy does not adversely affect the result. Complications are minimal, although the potential for complications, such as arterial occlusion, especially in young children, and aortic insufficiency should be recognized. Significant restenosis rates at intermediate-term follow up have been reported and could be minimized by reducing risk factors associated with recurrence. Echo-Doppler studies are helpful in follow-up evaluation of balloon dilatation of aortic valve. The balloon therapy compares favorably with surgical valvotomy. The indications for balloon valvuloplasty are essentially the same as those used for surgical intervention, namely, peak-to-peak gradients ≥ 70 mmHg, irrespective of symptoms, and gradients ≥ 50 mmHg with associated symptoms and/or ST–T wave abnormalities suggestive of myocardial ischemia. The procedure is particularly useful in neonates and young infants in view of the high mortality rate associated with surgery in these sick infants. Thus far, only short-term follow-up results are available. Five to 10 year follow-up results to document longer term effectiveness of balloon aortic valvuloplasty are needed. Some reduction in the size of the balloon catheter systems has taken place. Further decrease in the size of the catheter and greater rapidity of inflation/deflation of balloons are necessary for increasing the safety and effectiveness of the balloon dilatation procedures, particularly in younger children.

Inoue introduced balloon mitral valvotomy to relieve mitral valve obstruction in 1984, shortly after the introduction of balloon valvuloplasty to treat congenital valvar obstructions. The majority of the reported experience is in adult patients with rheumatic mitral stenosis. In general, the indications for balloon intervention are symptoms in patients with moderate to severe stenosis (mitral valve area

≤ 1.5 cm^2) without evidence for left atrial thrombus or moderate to severe mitral regurgitation. Balloon dilatation with conventional single and double balloons and with Inoue balloons has been reported. The balloons are most commonly inserted antegrade by transseptal technique. Decrease in pressure gradient across the mitral valve, increase in mitral valve area, and improvement in symptoms have been documented after balloon mitral valvuloplasty. Complication rate is low and includes minimal mortality (<2%), cardiac tamponade (1%–3%), thromboembolism (0%–4%), and severe mitral insufficiency requiring surgery (1%–4%). Residual atrial septal defects with left-to-right shunting have been noted, but these are small, with negligible hemodynamic consequence. Short-term follow-up results are encouraging; long-term results are not available. Based on the available data, percutaneous balloon mitral valvuloplasty appears to be a valid alternative to surgical commissurotomy in the relief of stenotic mitral valve. Balloon valvuloplasty has also been applied to rheumatic tricuspid valve stenosis. The reported experience is small but favorable. An increase in cardiac output and improvement in symptoms were noted in most cases. Complications are minimal. Percutaneous tricuspid valvuloplasty appears to be a reasonable alternative to surgery for the relief of tricuspid valve stenosis unless there is associated severe tricuspid regurgitation.

Suarez de Lezo *et al.* in 1986 applied balloon dilatation techniques to relieve discrete subaortic stenosis. Several other workers have since used this technique with success. Because of the potential for development of aortic insufficiency, indication for intervention is set at a slightly lower level of obstruction (peak-to-peak gradients ≥ 40 mmHg) than for valvar stenosis. The immediate results appear excellent, as are the intermediate-term follow-up results when the subaortic membrane is discrete and thin (type I). When the subaortic obstruction is a fibromuscular (type II) or tunnel (type III) type, both the immediate and follow-up results are poor. With the discrete, thin subaortic membrane, balloons larger than the aortic valve annulus may be safely used, provided there is no associated valvar aortic stenosis. The mechanism of action is tearing of the subaortic membrane. Balloon angioplasty may be a preferable initial procedure in the treatment of membranous subaortic obstruction.

Because of the initially reported poor result and concern for the development of aneurysms, there is considerable controversy with regard to use of balloon angioplasty for treatment of native aortic coarctation. This initial concern seems to be abating, and at present, more medical centers are performing this procedure than in the past. Immediate and intermediate-term follow-up results of balloon angioplasty are generally good, with a small chance for recoarctation and aneurysmal formation at the site of coarctation. Echo-Doppler and nuclear magnetic resonance imaging techniques are useful adjuncts to cardiac catheterization and selective cineangiography in the evaluation of follow-up results. The causes of recoarctation have been identified and include age <1 year, hypoplasia of the aortic isthmus, and a very small coarcted segment prior to and immediately after balloon angioplasty. The aorta appears to remodel itself to approach a near-normal aortic shape following successful balloon dilatation. Complications of the procedure are modest in degree, although arterial complications in the neonate and young infant may be significant. A substantial miniaturization of balloon catheter systems has taken place. Further miniaturization may be necessary to decrease the arterial complications. Meticulous attention to the technique, including appropriate balloon choices and avoidance of manipulation of the tips of catheters and guidewires in the region of freshly dilated coarctation, are likely to reduce the complication rate further. Despite some of these problems, I consider balloon angioplasty to be an effective and safe alternative to surgical intervention for native coarctation, particularly in the neonate and young infant. Periodic assessment of this recommendation is in order as more data are accumulated. Five to 10 year follow-up data, assessment of the causes and the natural history of aneurysms occurring after balloon angioplasty, and actuarial evaluation of surgical versus balloon angioplasty are needed to achieve this objective.

Balloon dilatation of aortic recoarctation following previous surgery is next only to valvar pulmonic stenosis with regard to the acceptability by cardiologists as a therapeutic alternative to surgery. Immediate results seem excellent with an acceptable complication rate. The results and risks appear comparable with those seen with repeat surgical intervention. Follow-up results are available in only a limited number of patients, with recurrence and aneurysmal formation rates of 25% and 9%, respectively. The high recurrence rates appear to be related to the use of small balloons in the early experience of some of the investigators. These and arterial complication rates are likely to diminish because of progressive improvement of the balloon catheter technology and a greater understanding by cardiologists of the angioplasty technique. Most cardiologists agree that balloon angioplasty is the treatment of choice for management of aortic recoarctations. A peak-to-peak systolic pressure gradient across the operative site in excess of 20 mmHg with angiographic demonstration of discrete narrowing is an indication for balloon dilatation. Use of heparin, appropriate choice of balloon diameter, and avoidance of manipulation of the tips of guidewire and catheter in the vicinity of freshly dilated recoarctation are important technical features of balloon angioplasty. Periodic evaluation for evidence of renarrowing and for development of aneurysms is necessary; these may be performed by clinical, echo-Doppler, nuclear magnetic resonance, and angiographic studies. The mechanism of effectiveness of angioplasty appears to be intimal and medial disruption produced by controlled injury through radial forces of balloon inflation. Further miniaturization of bal-

loon/catheter systems, a better understanding of the technique of balloon angioplasty, longer duration of follow-up in a larger number of patients than is currently available, and cause and natural history of aneurysm formation following angioplasty are important in further advancing balloon angioplasty as a successful therapeutic option for the management of postoperative aortic recoarctation.

Peripheral pulmonary artery stenosis is one of the few lesions in which balloon dilatation has not produced excellent results. This is related to the elastic nature of branch pulmonary artery stenotic lesions in the congenital obstructions and fibrosis around the pulmonary artery in the postsurgical obstructions. It is generally more difficult to position a balloon dilatation catheter across branch pulmonary artery stenotic lesions than across other lesions. With the availability of extra-stiff guidewires and low-profile balloon angioplasty catheters, this technical difficulty has decreased. Even with adequate technique, balloon angioplasty success can be expected in approximately 50% of the patients. However, the follow-up studies are few, and therefore long-term results are unknown. Recently, balloon-expandable stents have been used with success in relieving branch pulmonary artery stenoses. Although there is limited experience with stents, they are likely to be useful in patients in whom balloon angioplasty is not successful.

Transcatheter treatment methodology appears useful in the management of several types of cyanotic congenital heart defects. The role of Rashkind's balloon atrial septostomy and Park's blade atrial septostomy in promoting interatrial mixing and relieving atrial obstruction has already been alluded to. Cyanotic children with interatrial right-to-left shunting secondary to severe valvar pulmonary stenosis respond to balloon pulmonary valvuloplasty in a manner similar to that observed with isolated pulmonary valve stenosis. In these patients, balloon valvuloplasty is the treatment of choice and may be corrective in the majority of patients. In a substantial proportion of patients with interventricular right-to-left shunting secondary to pulmonary outflow tract obstruction, balloon pulmonary valvuloplasty may be an effective palliative procedure, obviating the need for palliative shunt. Balloon dilatation of narrowed classic or modified Blalock-Taussig shunts is also feasible and augments pulmonary blood flow and improves systemic arterial oxygen saturation. I would recommend either balloon valvuloplasty of the stenotic pulmonary valve or narrowed Blalock-Taussig shunt if the patient's size or cardiac anatomy make a cyanotic heart defect unsuitable for safe total surgical correction. In patients with pulmonary atresia, opening of the atretic pulmonary valve by either laser or initial surgery and follow-up with balloon dilatation are potentially beneficial in reducing the total number of surgical procedures that these children are likely to require. The preliminary data seem to indicate potential for these methods; further clinical trials are required prior to adopting them for general use.

Calcific degeneration and obstruction of bioprosthetic valves have been documented; this appears to occur more frequently and more rapidly in younger children than in older children and adults. Conventional treatment of choice is repeat valve replacement. Recently, balloon valvuloplasty techniques have been utilized to relieve the obstruction of the biological valves in an attempt to avoid or postpone surgery for repeat valve replacement. All varieties of heterografts and homografts can be balloon dilated. The largest experience is with bioprosthetic valve conduits in the pulmonary position. Although the results are not uniformly successful, repeat valve replacement was avoided or at least postponed for several years in some patients. The indication for intervention is a peak-to-peak systolic pressure gradient ≥ 50 mmHg across the pulmonary bioprosthetic valve. A balloon size equal to the size of the bioprosthesis should be used. Relief of valvar obstruction may unmask additional obstructive lesions at the proximal or distal anastomoses. These should be sought and, if feasible, balloon dilated concurrently. The high incidence of balloon rupture associated with pulmonary heterograft dilatation is of concern; appropriate precautions should be taken to prevent or reduce balloon ruptures. Follow-up results are few and are needed. There are also reports of balloon dilatation of stenotic heterografts in the tricuspid position. Acute improvement in valve stenosis was observed in most, but nearly one-half of them required additional intervention within months after balloon valvuloplasty. Because of limited experience with this lesion, definitive recommendations with regard to the role of balloon dilatation of tricuspid heterograft stenosis cannot be made. Balloon dilatation of mitral and aortic heterograft valve stenosis has also been performed. The results are unpredictable. This and the potential for dislodgement of calcific debris and fractured valve cusps and the consequent systemic embolization warrant a limited role of balloon valvuloplasty procedures in the management of left heart bioprosthetic valve obstruction. However, development of an embolic-protecting device may resolve the latter issue. Mechanisms of relief of obstruction following balloon dilatation have been studied and include commissural splitting and valve leaflet fracture. Because of limited experience with balloon dilatation of prosthetic biologic valve stenoses, it is imperative that careful documentation of both immediate and follow-up results is made. Additional clinical trials are necessary prior to adoption of the balloon valvuloplasty technique as a procedure of choice in the management of bioprosthetic valve stenosis.

As discussed above, balloon angioplasty/valvuloplasty techniques have been applied with reasonable success in relieving several congenital and acquired stenotic lesions of the heart and great vessels. There are other lesions that are either uncommon or for which balloon dilatation has not frequently been utilized. These lesions, namely, congenital tricuspid and mitral valve stenosis, truncal valve stenosis, stenotic ductus arteriosus, restrictive patent foramen ovale, subvalvar pulmonic stenosis, supravalvar pulmonic stenosis (congenital or postoperative), stenosis of the aorta (Takayasu's arteritis), baffle obstructions following a Mustard or Senning procedure (both systemic venous and pulmonary venous), superior and inferior venal caval obstructive lesions, pulmonary vein stenosis, pulmonary veno-occlusive disease, pulmonary venous obstruction following repair of total anomalous pulmonary venous obstruction, cor triatriatum dexter, and coronary artery stenotic lesions post-Kawasaki disease, can also be balloon dilated. The indications are generally those used for surgical intervention. The reported experience with each of the above lesions is limited. In most, there is effective relief of obstruction after balloon dilatation. Follow-up results are scanty. Further clinical trials are necessary to advocate the use of balloon dilatation technique as a preferred alternative to surgical intervention. There have also been attempts to devise pulmonary bands that could initially be placed surgically to produce effective relief of pulmonary overcirculation and later opened up (dilated) by balloon angioplasty if the offending lesion (e.g., ventricular septal defect) resolves spontaneously.

While the balloon dilatation techniques have rapidly been adopted in effecting enlargement of stenotic lesions of the heart, transcatheter methods of closure of septal defects have not gained quick acceptance. This is related in part to the cumbersome nature of the techniques and in part to leaving a foreign body in the heart. Since King's initial description of paired umbrellas to close the atrial septal defects, a variety of devices have been developed and tested in animal models and in clinical trials. Until recently, Clamshell Septal Umbrella and "buttoned" devices are the only two atrial septal defect closing devices approved by the FDA for investigational use. Approximately 400 Clamshell devices have been implanted in a multicenter trial. At the time of this writing, the FDA suspended clinical trials with this device because of breakage of wire hinges at follow-up. Therefore, the buttoned device is the only atrial septal defect closure prosthesis currently under approval for clinical trials. To date, approximately 100 buttoned devices have been implanted, with success in 90% of the patients. With further clinical trial and further refinement of the device, it is likely to be clinically useful in the treatment of atrial septal defects. There are also multiple types of patent ductus arteriosus closing devices, many were tried in animal models, and a few of these have been applied to human subjects. Porstmann's Ivalon plug and Rashkind's double-disc device are available for use. In the United States, Rashkind's device is available for investigational use; it is likely to be released soon by the FDA for general use. A "buttoned" device, similar to that used for atrial septal defect closure, has also been utilized for closure of patent ductus arteriosus as a custom-made device; approval by the FDA for clinical trials of this device is awaited. Closure of the ventricular septal defects, though more cumbersome than atrial septal defect and patent ductus arteriosus closure, can be accomplished by use of several of the above-described devices. Much larger clinical experience than is currently available is needed for adopting the method for general use. In summary, attempts to replace surgical treatment of cardiac septal defects with transcatheter methods began more than 25 years ago. Several types of devices and device delivery systems have been developed and refined to some degree. Safety and efficacy have been reasonably good, but most of the available devices and delivery systems are bulky and cumbersome. Some miniaturization of the devices has taken place, and some are more suitable for clinical use today than in the past. Further clinical trials to examine the safety and effectiveness and further miniaturization of the devices are required prior to routine application of these techniques in the treatment of certain cardiac septal defects.

Transcatheter embolization techniques were initially developed for treatment of neurovascular conditions. These have since been extended to a variety of vascular abnormalities seen in pediatric patients. Multiple types of embolic materials have been utilized; however, Gianturco coils and detachable balloons are most commonly used. Systemic collateral vessels to the lungs in patients with tetralogy of Fallot, pulmonary atresia, pulmonary arteriovenous malformations, Blalock-Taussig shunt that is no longer needed, systemic arteriovenous fistulae, vein of Galen malformation, coronary arteriovenous fistula, and systemic vessels supplying the sequestered lung in Scimitar syndrome are but some of the lesions that have been successfully treated by transcatheter embolization techniques. There is a limited number of reports on a limited number of patients, but the acute results are generally good. Complications are rare, but include embolization to an undesirable site, transient infarction, and infection. There are extremely few reports on long-term effects. These embolization techniques do have advantage over surgery, but no systematic study comparing the two modes has been made. However, based on the available data, the embolization techniques are considered as the initial choice for treatment of these conditions.

Since the initial introduction by Myers in 1945 of indwelling intravascular catheters, polyethylene catheters have become a source of inadvertent embolization. The incidence of embolization has increased with the widespread use of these catheters in critically ill patients for the purpose of monitoring and fluid administration. Recognition of this problem resulted in the modification of the catheter systems, with improvement. But new sources of emboli have emerged with widespread use of catheterization and, more recently, with interventional procedures. Retained intravascular/intracardiac foreign bodies cause serious complications, including death. The consensus at this time is that all foreign bodies should be retrieved. Initially, a surgical approach was

necessary to extract the foreign bodies. Since the first description by Thomas and colleagues in the mid 1960s of percutaneous, nonsurgical removal of the foreign body, several other types of retrieval sets have been described. Guidewire loop snare (or a modification of it), helical baskets, and endoscopic forceps are the most commonly utilized retrieval devices. Approximately 90% of the foreign bodies can be retrieved through transcatheter methods. Complications associated with foreign body retrieval are minimal. The prevention of embolization through meticulous attention to the details of the technique of placing, securing, and removal of intravenous lines is important. Use of radiopaque catheters is a must so that they can be easily visualized and removed through transcatheter techniques in the event of inadvertent embolization. Initially, the retrieval devices were bulky, but their sizes have been reduced for safe usage in the pediatric patient.

Refractory dysrhythmias are now amenable through transcatheter treatment. Multiple forms of energy, including direct current, laser, microwave, cryothermia, and radiofrequency, have been used in catheter ablation. Currently, radiofrequency ablation appears to be the most commonly utilized. Ablation techniques have been used in the treatment of both automatic focus and re-entry tachycardias in childhood. Accurate diagnosis through careful mapping studies is needed prior to transcatheter ablation. Although there is limited experience with these techniques, the experience is encouraging and compares favorably to that with surgical ablation.

In the last section of this book, several international experts describe their experiences with balloon dilatation of stenotic lesions of the heart. The results are generally similar to those reported by the U.S. workers. These international experiences enrich the discussions presented in the preceding chapters.

In this book, I have included most, if not all, transcatheter techniques available for treatment of congenital and acquired cardiac anomalies seen in infancy and childhood. Many of these techniques are equally applicable to adult patients. There has not been an extensive experience with the transcatheter techniques, mostly because of the relatively recent availability of the techniques to the the practicing cardiologist. There is also a need for better understanding by the practicing cardiologist of the balloon technology, with particular reference to the types and sizes of balloon catheters, the balloon sizes available, and the choice of balloon size that is most appropriate in a given case. Acute results have been generally good. There is a limited number of reports, on a limited number of patients, describing intermediate-term follow-up results. There are practically none describing long-term results. The long-term results are needed to assess the efficacy of the techniques.

For the most part, the catheter systems are bulky and have a high potential for vascular injury. Recently, a significant miniaturization of the catheter systems has taken place, and, I believe, with further research and development, additional reduction in the size of the catheters, balloons, and devices is feasible. This would increase the safety and effectiveness of the transcatheter treatment modes.

Many of the catheter modes of treatment are replacing "standard" surgical procedures. However, there has not been a careful, prospective comparison between surgical and transcatheter therapeutic modalities. It is doubtful if such a comparative study is feasible at this stage of technology development.

While it may not be feasible to have a double-blind, controlled comparison of surgical versus transcatheter therapy, it is certainly possible to collect data prospectively to evaluate the immediate and follow-up results. Because the number of patients treated at each institution is small, registries have been established in the United States and Europe. While such registries increase the numbers, vagaries of variations in the technique and difficulties in data acquisition have been stumbling blocks to the rapid acquisition of results. Further miniaturization of catheter systems and careful, long-term (at least 5 and 10 year) follow-up studies are, I believe, feasible and should be attempted.

For lesions that are not currently amenable to presently available transcatheter methods, other methods should be sought. Some attempts in this direction are being made, and include stents and laser application. Such efforts should continue.

Index

Page numbers followed by a "t" designate tables.

Ablation therapy in childhood dysrhythmias, 393–398;
    see also Dysrhythmias
Age
    for balloon atrial septostomy, 12
    for pulmonary valvuloplasty, 67–70, 69t, 71t
Alagille's syndrome, 217, 227
Anesthesia and sedation: general, 30
Aneurysm: post balloon coarctation angioplasty, 183,
    187, 428, 456
Aortic aneurysm. See Aneurysm
Aortic angioplasty
    in discrete subaortic stenosis, 453–455, 478–483,
        496
    Spanish studies, 478–483
    see also Aortic coarctation angioplasty
Aortic atresia, 8–9
Aortic coarctation angioplasty
    acute results
        children +1 year, 160–164
        neonates and infants -1 year, 158–160
    applicability to adults, 168–169
    balloon technique vs. surgery, 169–171
        in children +1 year, 171
        complication rates, 171–172
    Brazilian studies, 414–417
    British studies, 423–426
    complications
        acute, 172–174
        follow-up, 174–175
    conclusions and future directions, 496–497
    follow-up results
        children +1 year, 166–168
        neonates and infants -1 year, 164–166
    history, 153–155
    Hong Kong studies, 440t, 440–441
    Indian studies, 455–456
    indications for balloon angioplasty, 155–156
    influence of technical factors, 176–177
    mechanism, 172
    noninvasive follow-up evaluation

        aneurysm formation, 183, 187
        aortic remodeling, 181, 184t
        Doppler studies, 177–181, 182t
        intravascular ultrasound, 188–189
        NMR imaging, 181
    restenosis
        acute results, 199t, 199–200, 205–205t
        aneurysm formation, 209
        balloon angioplasty vs. surgery, 201
        causes, 175t, 175–176, 207
        complications, 206–207
        follow-up results, 201.206t
        indications for treatment, 198–199
        intravascular ultrasound, 209
        mechanism of angioplasty, 206
        noninvasive follow-up evaluation, 208–209
        pathogenesis of recurrence, 197–198
        technical influences, 207–208
        technique, 199
    in restenosis, 427–428
    results, 199t
    Spanish studies, 483–489
    summary and conclusions, 188
    technique of balloon angioplasty, 156–158
    tissue properties in, 54–55
Aortic stenosis
    in prosthetic valves, 270
    tissue properties and, 53–54
Aortic valvuloplasty, 292–293
    age applicability
        adults, 115
        infants, 116
        in utero techniques, 116
        neonates, 113–115, 114t
        premature infants, 116
    Brazilian studies, 410–414
    complications
        acute, 118–119
        follow-up, 119
    conclusions and future directions, 495

history, 105–106
Hong Kong studies, 438–439, 439t
Indian studies, 451–453
indications for, 60
instrumentation and outcome, 119–120, 120t
mechanism of, 117–118
noninvasive follow-up evaluation, 120–122
restenosis in, 116, 120
results
    acute, 107t, 109–110
    follow-up, 110–113, 112t
Spanish studies, 475–478
subaortic stenosis, 122, 147–151; *see also* Discrete
    subaortic stenosis
summary and conclusions, 123
technique, 106–109
transesophageal echocardiography in, 122–123
vs. surgical treatment, 117
Aortopulmonary shunts. *See* Shunt narrowing
Arrhythmias, cardiac. *See* Dysrhythmias
Arterial transposition, 285–287
atrial septostomy in, 7–8
post Mustard/Senning baffle obstruction, 293–301;
    see also Mustard/Senning baffle obstruction
Arteriovenous fistulae, 372, 375
Atherectomy catheter technique, 40, 238
Atherosclerotic aortic lesions, 169
Atrial septal defects
anatomy and natural history, 7–8
atrial septostomy with
    balloon, 7–13
    blade, 17–26
conclusions and future directions, 499
historical aspects, 2, 3–4
occlusion techniques
    Bard clamshell septal umbrella, 337–348
    "buttoned" devices, 349–356, 499
    devices compared, 349–356
    King and Mills umbrella, 335
    Rashkind ASD Occluder, 336–337
post balloon mitral valvotomy, 135–136
pulmonary valvuloplasty in, 238–242, 242t; *see
    also* Pulmonary valvuloplasty
see also Atrial septostomy
Atrial septostomy
balloon, 2–3, 7–13, 285–287
    applicability and age, 12
    complications, 11–12
    conclusions and future directions, 494
    immediate and follow-up results, 10–11
    indications for, 8–9
    mechanism, 12
    noninvasive follow-up evaluation, 12–13
    summary and conclusions, 13
    technique, 9–10
    vs. surgical therapy, 13
blade, 3–4

age applicability and limitations, 23–24
complications, 23
immediate results, 23
indications for, 17–18
mechanism, 23
noninvasive follow-up results, 25–26
restenosis in, 25
technique and instrumentation, 18–23
vs. surgical therapy, 26
see also Atrial septal defects
Atrioventricular valve stenosis, 54

Baffle obstruction, 293–301, 428–429, 498–499; *see
    also* Mustard/Senning baffle obstruction
Balloon atrial septostomy. *See* Atrial septostomy:
    balloon
Balloon selection
for aortic coarctation angioplasty, 176t, 176–177,
    177t
for aortic valvuloplasty, 411
for atrial septal defect closure, 363
conclusions and future directions, 494
diameter, 35–35
double balloons, 36, 459–460, 467
for embolization procedures, 371–372
general principles of inflation and manipulation,
    48–50, 49t
graduated sequential balloon technique, 460
inflation material, 38
inflation pressure, number, and duration, 38–39
length, 35–36
material
    distention characteristics, 46
    heat characteristics, 46–47
    profile, 46
    strength, 46
    yield strength, 45–46
for mitral valvotomy, 130–131
for peripheral pulmonary angioplasty, 214
for pulmonary valvuloplasty, 80–84, 402, 447
Saudi Arabian studies, 458–460
single balloons, 458–459
trefoil and bifoil balloons, 36–37
Balloon valvuloplasty/angioplasty
alternative methods
    atheterectomy catheter method, 40–41
    laser techniques, 40
    Yang double-blade technique, 40
conclusions and future directions, 493–501
indications, 29–30
international experience
    Brazil, 402–417
    Hong Kong, 433–443
    India, 445–456
    overview, 401–402
    Saudi Arabia, 457–468
    Spain, 471–489

United Kingdom, 421–430
  see also International studies
  mechanical aspects
    balloon material, 45–47
    dilating forces, 47–48
    instrumentation principles, 46–50, 49t
    physiology of intracardiac occlusion, 50–52
    tissue properties, 52–54
  predilatation preparation, 30
  procedure
    balloon selection, 33–37
    catheter insertion site, 31–32
    catheter positioning, 32
    general description, 30–31
    heparinization, 32–33
    inflation substance, 38
    monitoring, 37–38
    in multiple obstructions, 39–40
    pressure, number, and duration of inflations,
      38–39
  see also specific disorders and techniques
Bard clamshell septal umbrella ASD closure device
  comparative studies, 349–356
  design and rationale, 337–338
  indications for use, 347–348
  long-term results, 346–347
  problems, 344–346
  technique, 338–344
Bifoil balloons, 36–37, 50
Bioprosthetic stenoses
  aortic position, 270
  British studies, 430
  conclusions and future directions, 498
  history and pathophysiology, 255–256
  mitral position, 265, 268–269t, 270
  pulmonary position, 260–261t, 263t
    acute results, 258–262
    comments, 264
    complications, 263–264
    follow-up results, 262–263, 263t
    indications for dilatation, 256
    technique, 256–258
  tricuspid position, 264–265, 266–267t
Bioprosthetic valve obstruction
Blalock-Taussig shunt occlusion, 244–251, 372–375,
  429–430, 442
Brazilian studies, 403–417; see also International
  studies
British studies, 421–430; see also International studies
Budd-Chiari syndrome (inferior vena caval
  obstruction), 303–304
"Button" ASD-closure devices, 348–356, 499; see also
  Atrial septal defects

Cardiac arrhythmias. See Dysrhythmias
Catheter ablation in childhood dysrhythmias, 393–398;
  see also Dysrhythmias

Catheters for blade atrial septostomy, 18, 18t, 19
Clamshell ASD occlusion device, 337–356, 499; see
  also Bard clamshell septal umbrella ASD
  closure device
Coil embolization, 442
Complications
  of aortic angioplasty, 479
  of aortic coarctation angioplasty, 455–456
    acute, 172–174
    follow-up, 174–175
  of aortic valvuloplasty, 477
  of atrial septostomy
    balloon, 11–12
    blade, 23
  of balloon mitral valvuloplasty, 450–451
  of pulmonary bioprosthetic stenosis dilatation,
    263–264
  of embolization therapy, 375
  of foreign body embolization, 386
  in Hong Kong studies, 442
  of mitral balloon valvotomy, 134t, 134–135
  of mitral balloon valvuloplasty, 279–280
  of peripheral pulmonary angioplasty, 219–220,
    223t
  of pulmonary shunt–opening procedures, 248–250
  of pulmonary valvuloplasty, 73–75, 236–237, 405,
    472
  in Saudi Arabian studies, 464–465, 465t
  of transcatheter cardiac defect closure, 362
  of tricuspid balloon valvotomy, 139
  of tricuspid balloon valvuloplasty, 276–277
Conduit restenoses. See Bioprosthetic stenoses
Cordoba/Los Palmas studies, 471–489; see also
  International studies: Spanish
Coronary artery fistulae, 375
Coronary artery stenosis, 310
Cor-Pal studies, 471–489; see also International
  studies: Spanish
Cor triatriatum dexter, 310
Cyanotic congenital defects, 429–430, 473–474, 499
  narrowed systemic-to-pulmonary shunts, 243–251
  pulmonary atresia, 242–243
  pulmonary stenosis with atrial right-to-left shunt
    (intact ventricular septum), 238–242
  pulmonary stenosis with right-to-left shunt
    (ventricular septal defect), 229–238
  summary and conclusions, 251
  see also Pulmonary stenosis; Pulmonary
    valvuloplasty

Dilating force mechanics, 47–48
Discrete subaortic stenosis, 147–151, 150t, 453–455,
  478–483, 496
Doppler studies
  in aortic coarctation restenosis, 208–209
  in aortic stenosis, 120–122, 452–453
  intravascular ultrasound, 187–188, 209

for mitral valvotomy, 131–132
post pulmonary valvuloplasty, 88–91
in pulmonary valvuloplasty, 88–91, 239–241
tranesophageal echocardiography, 364–365
Double-balloon techniques, 36, 50
Ductus arteriosus
  catheter occlusion
    anatomic considerations, 322–324
    historical considerations, 321–322
    Rashkind technique, 324–330
    transfemoral plug closure (Portsmann), 330–332
  patent
    balloon dilatation procedures, 2–3, 280–285, 281t
    transcatheter closure and "button" devices, 356–361
Dysrhythmias
  catheter ablation therapy
    conclusions, 398
    energy sources, 396–397
    history and mechanism, 393
    indications for, 395–396
    technique, 394–395
  as complication of balloon atrial septostomy, 10
  conclusions and future directions, 500
  post embolization therapy, 386

Ebstein's anomaly, 2, 239
Echocardiography. See Doppler studies;
    Transesophageal echocardiography
Electrocardiography post pulmonary valvuloplasty,
    84–88
Embolization therapy
  complications, 375
  conclusions and future directions, 500
  foreign body retrieval
    complications, 386
    history and pathogenesis, 377–380
    prevention of embolization, 386–388
    results, 385–386, 387t
    summary and conclusions, 388
    techniques, 380–385
  instrumentation, 371–372
  malformations treated
    Blalock-Taussig shunts, 243–251, 372–375
    coronary artery fistulae, 375
    pulmonary arteriovenous lesions, 372
    pulmonary collateral vessels, 372
    systemic arteriovenous fistulae, 375
    vein of Galen lesions, 375

Fistulae
  coronary artery, 375
  mammary artery/portal vein, 375
  pulmonary arteriovenous, 372
  systemic arteriovenous, 375

Fixed discrete subaortic stenosis, 147–151, 150t
Foreign body embolization, 377–388, 387t, 500; see
    also Embolization therapy
Future directions of balloon techniques, 493–501

Grafts. See Bioprosthetic stenoses
Grüntzig PTCA-technique, 4

Heparinization, 32–33, 472
Heterografts. See Bioprosthetic stenoses
Historical aspects, 1–5
Homografts. See Bioprosthetic stenoses
Hong Kong studies, 433–444; see also International
    studies
Hypoplasia
  left heart syndromes: balloon atrial septostomy in,
    8–9
  right heart syndromes: balloon atrial septostomy in,
    7

Indian (All India Institute of Medical Sciences) studies,
    445–456; see also International studies
Inferior vena caval obstruction, 303–304
Informed consent, 30
Infundibular obstruction, 95–98, 96t, 466
International studies
  Brazil
    aortic coarctation, 414–417
    aortic stenosis, 410–414
    pulmonic stenosis, 403–410
  conclusions and future directions, 500–501
  Hong Kong
    aortic stenosis, 438–439, 439t
    coarctation of the aorta, 440t, 440–441
    coil embolization, 442
    complications, 442
    mitral and tricuspid stenosis, 439–440
    pulmonary artery stenosis, 441–442
    pulmonary valve stenosis, 435–438, 436t, 437t
    summary and conclusions, 443
    technique, 433–444
  India
    aortic coarctation angioplasty, 455–456
    aortic valvuloplasty, 451–453
    discrete subaortic stenosis, 453–455
    juvenile rheumatic mitral stenosis, 448–451
    pulmonary valvuloplasty, 445–448
  Saudi Arabia
    complications, 464–465, 465t
    discussion, 465–467
    instrumentation, 457–458
    results and observations, 460–464
    technique, 458–460
  Spanish (Cor-Pal)
    aortic angioplasty, 478–483
    aortic coarctation angioplasty, 483–489
    aortic valvuloplasty, 475–478

pulmonary valvotomy, 475
pulmonary valvuloplasty, 471–475
United Kingdom
aortic valve stenosis, 423–426
aortopulmonary shunt obstruction, 429–430
atrial baffle/Mustard procedure restenosis,
428–429
balloon procedures as alternative to surgery,
421–427
balloon procedures in restenosis, 427–430
bioprosthetic valve obstruction, 430
coarctation of the aorta, 426–428
pulmonary atresia, 423
pulmonary valve stenosis, 421–422
supravalvar pulmonary restenosis, 430
tetralogy of Fallot, 422–423
Intravascular/intracardiac foreign bodies, 377–388; see
also Embolization therapy

Jatene procedure, 410
Junctional automatic ectopic tachycardia, 394–395; see
also Dysrhythmias
Juvenile rheumatic mitral valve stenosis, 448–451; see
also Mitral balloon valvuloplasty

Kan pulmonary valvuloplasty, 4–5
Kawasaki disease, 310
King and Mills umbrella ASD-closure device, 335

Laser techniques, 40

Magnetic resonance imaging. See NMR imaging
Mammary artery/portal vein fistulae, 375
Mechanical aspects of valvuloplasty/angioplasty, 45–
54; see also Balloon valvuloplasty/angioplasty
Mitral atresia, 8–9
Mitral regurgitation
in mitral valve stenosis, 130–131
post procedure, 131–132, 134–135, 450
Mitral stenosis
balloon valvotomy in
complications, 134t, 134–135
Doppler/echocardiographic evaluation, 131–133
future of, 137
mechanism, 129–130
patient selection/indications, 129, 133t
procedure and balloon selection, 130–131
results, 133t, 133–135
vs. surgical valvotomy, 136–137
balloon valvuloplasty in
comments, 279–280
history and pathogenesis, 277–278
Hong Kong studies, 439–440
Indian studies, 448–450
indications for, 278
mechanism, 279
results and complications, 278–279

technique, 278
bioprosthetic restenosis, 265, 268–269t, 270
conclusions and future directions, 495–496
Monitoring: general, 37–38
MRI imaging. See NMR imaging
Mustard/Senning baffle obstruction
British studies, 428–429
conclusions and future directions, 498–499
pulmonary venous obstruction
comments, 301
indications and technique of dilatation, 300
results and complications, 300–301
systemic venous obstruction
comments, 298
indications and technique of dilatation, 293–294
results, 294–298, 296t

NMR imaging in aortic coarctation, 181, 209

Paradoxical embolism, 366
Park atrial septostomy technique, 3–4
Patent ductus arteriosus
balloon dilatation in, 281–284
historical aspects, 2–3
history and pathogenesis, 280–281, 281t
stent procedures in, 284–285
see also Ductus arteriosus
Patent foramen ovale, 238–242, 242t, 285–287, 366;
see also Pulmonary valvuloplasty
Peripheral arteritis, 1–2
Portsmann transfemoral plug closure technique,
330–332
Preparation: general technique, 30
Pulmonary arteriovenous fistulae, 372, 375
Pulmonary artery angioplasty
complications, 219–220, 223t
in peripheral lesions
pathology, 213
recommendations, 226–227
results
acute, 214–217
follow-up, 220–222
stainless steel stenting, 223–226
technique, 213–214
Pulmonary artery band dilatation, 308–310
Pulmonary artery stenosis: Hong Kong studies,
441–442
Pulmonary atresia, 242–243, 475
British studies, 423
Pulmonary bioprosthesis restenosis, 260–261t,
260–264, 263t
Pulmonary dysplasia, 91–94, 94t
Pulmonary stenosis
with atrial shunt/intact ventricular septum, 238–242
discrete supravalvar, 473
peripheral, 497
supravalvular, 430

with ventricular septal defect, 229–238
Pulmonary valvotomy
    balloon valvuloplasty following, 243
    history, 1, 4
    restenosis in, 70
    Spanish studies, 475, 478
Pulmonary valvuloplasty
    in atrial defect or patent foramen ovale
        acute results, 239–241, 242t
        comments, 241
        conclusions, 241–242
        indications for, 238
        technique, 238–239
    Brazilian studies, 403–410
    British studies, 421–422
    conclusions and future directions, 494–495
    history, 4–5, 59–60
    Hong Kong studies, 435–437, 436t, 437t
    Indian studies, 445–448
    in isolated lesions
        acute results, 64
        age group applicability, 67–70, 69t, 71t
        complications, 73–75
        with dysplastic valve, 91–94, 94t
        follow-up results, 64–67, 66t, 69t, 71t
        indications for, 60–61
        with infundibular obstruction, 95–98, 96t
        instrumentation, 77–84
        mechanism, 72–73
        in postsurgical restenosis, 70
        restenosis mechanisms, 75–77, 76t, 78t
        summary and conclusions, 96
        technique, 61–64
        vs. surgical treatment, 70–72
    noninvasive follow-up
        Doppler echocardiography, 88–91
        ECG, 84–88
    in pulmonary atresia, 242–243
    in shunt narrowing
        Blalock-Taussig, 244–251, 372–375
        Waterston, 243–244
    Spanish studies, 471–475
    in subvalvar lesions, 287–288
    in supravalvar lesions
        comments, 290–292
        history and pathogenesis, 288
        indications and technique, 289
        results, 289–290
    in ventricular septal defect
        acute results, 230–233, 233t
        comments, 237–238
        complications, 236–237
        conclusions, 238
        follow-up results, 233–236
        indications for, 230
        new developments, 238
        technique, 230

Pulmonary vein stenosis
    congenital, 304–305
    obstructed total anomalous pulmonary/systemic
        connection, 306–307
        post-reconstruction stenosis, 307–308
    pulmonary veno-occlusive disease, 305–306
Pulmonary venous anomaly
    atrial septostomy in, 9
    balloon atrial septostomy in, 9
    post Mustard/Senning baffle procedure, 301, 428–
        429
Pulmonic stenosis
    subvalvar, 287–288
    supravalvar, 288–292

Rashkind ASD Occluder and modifications, 336–337,
    353–357
Rashkind Double-Disk device, 357–358
Rashkind ductus arteriosus closure technique, 324–330
Restenosis
    in aortic coarctation
        British studies, 427–428
        causes, 207
        treatment; see also Aortic coarctation
            angioplasty
    in aortic coarctation angioplasty, 456
        causes, 175t, 175–176
        treatment, 197–210
    in atrial blade septostomy, 25
    in bioprostheses
        aortic, 270
        mechanism of balloon dilatation, 270–271
        mitral, 265, 268–269t, 270
        pulmonary, 260–261t, 260–264, 263t
        tricuspid, 264–265, 266–267t
    British studies, 427–430
    post pulmonary valvuloplasty, 75–77, 76t
    post surgical pulmonary valvotomy, 70

Saudi Arabian studies, 457–467; see also International
    studies
Sedation and anesthesia: general, 30
Semb pulmonary valvotomy, 4
Shunt narrowing, 244–251, 372–375, 429–430
Spanish studies, 471–489; see also International
    studies
Stenting techniques
    in ductal disorders, 284–285
    in peripheral pulmonary stenosis, 223–226
Subaortic stenosis, 122, 147–151, 150t, 453–455,
    478–483, 496
    balloon dilatation, 147–151, 150t
    clinical features, 145–146
    pathogenesis, 143–144
    pathology: type I through IV, 144–145
    surgical treatment, 146–147
    see also Discrete subaortic stenosis

Subvalvar pulmonic stenosis, 287–288
Superior vena caval obstruction, 301–303
Supravalvar pulmonic stenosis, 288–292, 430; *see also*
     Pulmonary valvuloplasty

Takayasu's disease, 169
Technique: general description, 29–41; *see also*
     Balloon valvuloplasty/angioplasty
Tetralogy of Fallot: British studies, 422–423
Transarterial embolization, 371–375
Transesophageal echocardiography
     in aortic stenosis, 122–123
     in atrial septal defects closure, 364–365
Transposition of great arteries. *See* Arterial
     transposition
Trefoil balloons, 36–37, 50
Tricuspid atresia, 9
Tricuspid stenosis
     balloon valvotomy in
          complications, 139
          mechanism, 137–138
          patient selection/indications, 137
          procedure, 138
          results, 138–139
     balloon valvuloplasty in
          comments, 277
          history and pathogenesis, 275–276
          indications for, 276
          mechanism, 277
          results and complications, 277
          technique, 276
     bioprosthetic restenosis, 264–265, 266–267t
     history, 1
Tricuspid valvuloplasty: Hong Kong studies, 439–440

Truncal valve stenosis, 280

Ultrasound studies. *See* Doppler studies
United Kingdom studies, 421–430; *see also*
     International studies

Valvotomy
     atrioventricular
          balloon mitral, 129–137
          balloon tricuspid, 137–139
          balloon vs. surgical, 136–137
     in atrioventricular stenoses, 129–139
     pulmonary, 1, 4
          restenosis following, 70
     Semb, 4
     Yang double-blade, 40
     see also individual procedures
Vena caval obstruction
     inferior, 303–304
     post Mustard/Senning baffle obstruction, 293–298,
          428–429
     superior, 301–303
Venous thrombosis, 11
Ventricular septal defect
     closure devices, 361–362
     pulmonary valvuloplasty in, 229–238, 233t

Waterston shunt narrowing, 243–244
William's syndrome, 217, 227; *see also* Pulmonary
     peripheral angioplasty
Wolff-Parkinson-White disease, 393–398; *see also*
     Dysrhythmias

Yang double-blade valvotomy, 40